Medical Coding Fundamentals

Medical Coding Fundamentals

Susan Goldsmith, CPC, CPC-H, CPC-P, CPC-I, CCP, CCS-P, CPEHR

Marc Leib, MD, JD

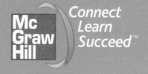
McGraw Hill

Connect
Learn
Succeed™

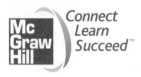

The McGraw·Hill Companies

Connect
Learn
Succeed™

MEDICAL CODING FUNDAMENTALS

Published by McGraw-Hill, a business unit of The McGraw-Hill Companies, Inc., 1221 Avenue of the Americas, New York, NY, 10020.

Some ancillaries, including electronic and print components, may not be available to customers outside the United States.

This book is printed on acid-free paper.

1 2 3 4 5 6 7 8 9 0 QDB/QDB 1 0 9 8 7 6 5 4 3 2

ISBN   978-0-07-337498-7
MHID   0-07-337498-9

Vice president/Director of marketing: *Alice Harra*
Editorial director: *Michael S. Ledbetter*
Senior sponsoring editor: *Natalie J. Ruffatto*
Director, digital products: *Crystal Szewczyk*
Managing development editor: *Michelle L. Flomenhoft*
Development editor: *Raisa Priebe Kreek*
Executive marketing manager: *Roxan Kinsey*
Digital development editor: *Katherine Ward*
Director, Editing/Design/Production: *Jess Ann Kosic*
Project manager: *Kathryn D. Wright*
Buyer II: *Sherry L. Kane*

Senior designer: *Srdjan Savanovic*
Senior photo research coordinator: *John C. Leland*
Photo researcher: *LouAnn Wilson*
Manager, digital production: *Janean A. Utley*
Media project manager: *Brent dela Cruz*
Media project manager: *Cathy L. Tepper*
Cover design: *Ellen Pettengell*
Typeface: *10.5/12 ITC Berkeley*
Compositor: *Aptara®, Inc.*
Printer: *Quad/Graphics*
Cover credit:© Steve McAlister, Getty Images

Credits: The credits section for this book begins on page C1 and is considered an extension of the copyright page.

Library of Congress Cataloging-in-Publication Data

Goldsmith, Susan.
    Medical coding fundamentals / Susan Goldsmith, Marc Leib.
       p. ; cm.
    Includes index.
    ISBN-13: 978-0-07-337498-7 (alk. paper)
    ISBN-10: 0-07-337498-9 (alk. paper)
    I. Leib, Marc. II. Title.
    [DNLM: 1. International classification of diseases. 9th revision. Clinical modification.
 2. International statistical classification of diseases and related health problems. 10th revision.
 Clinical modification. 3. International statistical classification of diseases and related health
 problems. 10th revision. Procedure coding system. 4. Clinical Coding—Problems and Exercises.
 5. International Classification of Diseases—Problems and Exercises. W 18.2]
    616.001'2—dc23

                                                                            2011043844

All brand or product names are trademarks or registered trademarks of their respective companies.

CPT five-digit codes, nomenclature, and other data are © 2011 American Medical Association. All rights reserved. No fee schedules, basic unit, relative values, or related listings are included in the CPT. The AMA assumes no liability for the data contained herein. CPT codes are based on CPT 2012.

ICD-9-CM codes are based on ICD-9-CM 2012. ICD-10-CM codes are based on ICD-10-CM 2012. ICD-10-PCS codes are based on ICD-10-PCS 2012.

All names, situations, and anecdotes are fictitious. They do not represent any person, event, or medical record.

The Internet addresses listed in the text were accurate at the time of publication. The inclusion of a website does not indicate an endorsement by the authors or McGraw-Hill, and McGraw-Hill does not guarantee the accuracy of the information presented at these sites.

www.mhhe.com

Dedication

To our families and friends, whose love and understanding were constantly with us, even as we spent hundreds of hours hunched over computers surrounded by coding manuals. Their sacrifices made this project possible and without them we could never have brought this book to life. Thank you.

—Susan Goldsmith and Marc Leib

About the Authors

Susan Goldsmith, CPC, CPC-H, CPC-P, CPC-I, CCS-P, CCP, CPEHR

Susan Goldsmith is a leading national expert in healthcare coding, education, and system implementation. With over 25 years of experience in healthcare, Susan provides consulting, education, and analysis of healthcare claims processing systems for private insurance companies and State Medicaid agencies. She is certified in both physician and facility coding through the American Academy of Professional Coders (AAPC) and AHIMA and obtained certification at UCLA in Electronic Medical Record implementation. Susan co-authored the CPC-P test guidance material available from AAPC.

Marc Leib, MD, JD

Dr. Marc Leib practiced anesthesiology for nearly 20 years before graduating law school and working on healthcare policy issues in Washington, D.C. He later returned to Arizona as the Chief Medical Officer for the state's Medicaid program. In that position he is responsible for coding and coverage policy decisions, the oversight of contracted health plans, quality improvement and medical management activities, and has undertaken major revisions of the claims system. Over the last 10 years, Dr. Leib has drafted diagnosis and procedure codes that have been adopted for inclusion in the coding manuals. He approaches coding issues as a provider and a payer, giving him a balanced perspective of these issues.

BRIEF CONTENTS

Preface xvi

1 Medical Terminology, Anatomy, and Physiology 1

PART I: ICD-9-CM AND ICD-10-CM 35

2 Introduction to ICD-9-CM 36

3 ICD-9-CM Chapter-Specific Guidelines, Part I: Chapters 1–10 54

4 ICD-9-CM Chapter-Specific Guidelines, Part II: Chapters 11–19 82

5 Introduction to ICD-10-CM and ICD-10-PCS 111

PART II: CPT AND HCPCS 129

6 Introduction to CPT 130

7 Modifiers 151

8 Evaluation and Management Services, Part I: Guidance and Theory 188

9 Evaluation And Management Services, Part II: Code Selection 210

10 Anesthesia Services 254

11 Radiology Services 284

12 Surgery Codes: Coding for Surgical Procedures on Specific Organ Systems 305

Module 12.1 General and Integumentary System 308

Module 12.2 Musculoskeletal System 326

Module 12.3 Respiratory, Cardiovascular, Hemic, and Lymphatic Systems; Mediastinum and Diaphragm 343

Module 12.4 Digestive System 366

Module 12.5 Urinary System, Male and Female Genital Systems, and Maternity Care and Delivery 383

Module 12.6 Endocrine, Nervous, Ocular, and Auditory Systems 400

13 Pathology and Laboratory Services 422

14 Medicine Services 440

15 Introduction to the Healthcare Common Procedure Coding System (HCPCS) 470

PART III: PRACTICUM 495

16 Putting It All Together 496

Appendix: Common Medical Abbreviations A-1

Glossary G-1

Credits C-1

Index I-1

CONTENTS

About the Authors v
Preface xvi
Guided Tour xxii
Acknowledgments xxiv

1 MEDICAL TERMINOLOGY, ANATOMY, AND PHYSIOLOGY 1

Introduction 2

1.1 Word Elements 2
Root Words 2
Combining Vowels and Combining
    Forms 2
Prefixes 5
Suffixes 6

1.2 Eponyms, Abbreviations, and Acronyms 7
Eponyms 7
Abbreviations and Acronyms 8

1.3 Anatomy and Physiology 9
Integumentary System 11
Musculoskeletal System 12
Cardiovascular System 13
Lymphatic System 16
Respiratory System 17
Digestive System 18
Urinary System 19
Reproductive System 20
Nervous System 21
Endocrine System 23
Hemic System 24

1.4 ICD-10-CM and Medical Terminology 25
Chapter Review 27

PART I ICD-9-CM and ICD-10-CM 35

2 INTRODUCTION TO ICD-9-CM 36

Introduction 37

2.1 The Structure of the ICD-9-CM Manual 37

2.2 Using Volumes 1 and 2 to Determine Diagnosis Codes 38
Volume 2: Alphabetic Index of
    Diseases 38
Volume 1: Tabular List of Diseases 40
Volume 3: Tabular List and
    Alphabetic List for Procedure
    Codes 41

2.3 ICD-9-CM Conventions 42
Abbreviations 43
Punctuation 43
Instructional Notations 43
"Use Additional Code"
    Instruction 43
"Code First Underlying Disease"
    Instruction 43
Update Notations 44
Additional Digit Specificity
    Indicator 44
Diagnosis Code–Specific Color
    Highlights 44
Age Conflict Edits 44
Sex Conflict Edits 44
Hospital-Acquired Condition (HAC)
    Indicator 44
"Other" and "Unspecified"
    Codes 45
"See" and "See Also" Instructions 45
Signs and Symptoms 45
Combination Codes 45

2.4 Outpatient Coding Principles 46
Specific Guidelines for Coding
    Outpatient Encounters 47
Chapter Review 48

3 ICD-9-CM CHAPTER-SPECIFIC GUIDELINES, PART I: CHAPTERS 1–10 54

Introduction 55

3.1 Coding Diseases and Disorders, Chapters 1–3 (000–279) 55

    Chapter 1: Infectious and Parasitic Diseases 55

    Chapter 2: Neoplasms 57

    Chapter 3: Endocrine, Nutritional, and Metabolic Diseases and Immunity Disorders 60

3.2 Coding Diseases and Disorders, Chapters 4–6 (280–389) 63

    Chapter 4: Diseases of the Blood and Blood-Forming Organs 63

    Chapter 5: Mental Disorders 64

    Chapter 6: Diseases of the Nervous System and Sense Organs 65

3.3 Coding Diseases, Chapters 7–8 (390–519) 67

    Chapter 7: Diseases of the Circulatory System 67

    Chapter 8: Diseases of the Respiratory System 70

3.4 Coding Diseases, Chapters 9–10 (520–629) 72

    Chapter 9: Diseases of the Digestive System 72

    Chapter 10: Diseases of the Genitourinary System 73

Chapter Review 76

4 ICD-9-CM CHAPTER-SPECIFIC GUIDELINES, PART II: CHAPTERS 11-19 82

Introduction 83

4.1 Coding Conditions and Complications of Pregnancy, Chapter 11 (630–679) 83

    Chapter 11: Pregnancy, Childbirth, and the Puerperium 83

4.2 Coding Diseases, Chapters 12–13 (680–739) 88

    Chapter 12: Diseases of the Skin and Subcutaneous Tissue 88

    Chapter 13: Diseases of the Musculoskeletal System and Connective Tissue 89

4.3 Coding Abnormalities and Unusual Conditions, Chapters 14–17 (740–999) 91

    Chapter 14: Congenital Anomalies 91

    Chapter 15: Certain Conditions Originating in the Perinatal Period 92

    Chapter 16: Symptoms, Signs, and Ill-Defined Conditions 93

    Chapter 17: Injury and Poisoning 94

4.4 V-Codes and E-Codes, Chapters 18–19 (V01–E999) 98

    Chapter 18: Supplemental Classification of Factors Influencing Health Status and Contact with Health Services 98

    Chapter 19: Supplemental Classification of External Causes of Injury and Poisoning 100

Chapter Review 104

5 INTRODUCTION TO ICD-10-CM AND ICD-10-PCS 111

Introduction 112

5.1 Transitioning to the ICD-10-CM Coding System 112

    General Equivalence Mapping 112

5.2 Diagnosis Code Structure 114

    Laterality 114

    Trimesters 115

    Initial Treatment, Subsequent Encounter and Sequelae 115

5.3 Structure of the ICD-10-CM Manual 116

5.4 ICD-10-CM Conventions and General Guidelines 118

    Conventions 118

    General Guidelines 119

5.5 Introduction to ICD-10-PCS 120

    Breakdown of Sections 120

Chapter Review 122

PART II: CPT and HCPCS 129

6 INTRODUCTION TO CPT 130

Introduction 131

6.1 Structure of the CPT Manual 131
Code Sections 132

6.2 Code Format and Additional Information 133
Indented Code Structure 133
Symbols 134
Parenthetical Notes 134
Modifiers 135
Separate Procedure 135

6.3 Other Information Included in the CPT Manual 136
Index 136
Appendices 137
Introductory Pages 140
Information Listed on the Inside Front and Back Covers 140

6.4 Reporting Category II Codes and Using Category II Modifiers 140
Format of Category II Codes 141
Types of Category II Performance Measurement Codes 142

6.5 Reporting Category III Codes 143
Chapter Review 144

7 MODIFIERS 151

Introduction 152

7.1 The Function and Use of Modifiers 152

7.2 Services Provided during the Global Period 154
Modifier 24 155
Modifier 25 156
Modifier 57 157
Modifier 58 158
Modifiers 76 and 77 158
Modifier 78 159
Modifier 79 160

7.3 Reporting Portions of a Procedure or Service 161
Professional and Technical Components 162
Surgical Procedure Components 163

7.4 Reporting Multiple Services on the Same Date 164
Modifier 50 164
Modifier 51 165
Modifier 59 166
Modifier 91 168

7.5 Identifying Additional Providers Involved in Procedures 169
Modifiers 80, 81, and 82 169
Modifier 62 170
Modifier 66 170

7.6 Reporting Procedures Involving Significantly More or Less Work than Is Typical 171
Reporting Procedures Involving More Work than Is Typical 171
Reporting Procedures Involving Less Work than Is Typical 173

7.7 Reporting Mandatory Services, Physical Status, and Genetic Tests 174
Mandatory Services 174
Physical Status Modifiers P1 through P6 175
Genetic Modifiers 175

7.8 HCPCS Modifiers 176
Anatomical Modifiers 176
Ambulance Modifiers 177
Equipment Modifiers 178
Chapter Review 179

8 EVALUATION AND MANAGEMENT SERVICES, PART I: GUIDANCE AND THEORY 188

Introduction 189

8.1 Categories and Subcategories of E/M Services 189
Categories of E/M Services 189
Subcategories of E/M Services 190

8.2 Defining Key Terms in E/M Coding 191
New vs. Established Patient 191
Chief Complaint 191
Concurrent Care and Transfer of Care 191
Counseling 191

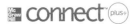

Family History 192
History of Present Illness (HPI) 192
Nature of the Presenting Problem 192
Past History 192
Review of Systems 193
Physical Examination 193
Medical Decision Making 193
Social History 193
Time 193
Unlisted Services 194
Special Report 194

8.3 Selecting the Level of E/M Service 195
8.4 Working with Histories 196
Elements of History 196
8.5 The Physical Examination 197
8.6 The Complexity of Medical Decision Making 198
8.7 Selecting the Correct Level of E/M Services 200
Determining Coding Requirements 200
Special Situations 201
Chapter Review 202

9 EVALUATION AND MANAGEMENT SERVICES, PART II: CODE SELECTION 210

9.1 Outpatient Services Coding for New or Established Patients (99201–99215) 211
New Patient 211
Established Patient 212
9.2 Categories and Subcategories of Hospital Services (99217–99239) 213
Hospital Observation Services 213
Hospital Inpatient Services 215
Observation or Inpatient Care Services (Including Admission and Discharge) 217
Hospital Discharge Services 218
9.3 Consultation Services (99241–99255) 219
Office or Other Outpatient Consultations 219
Inpatient Consultations 220

9.4 Emergency Department Services (99281–99288) 222
E/M Services for New or Established Patients 222
Other Emergency Services 222
9.5 Reporting Critical Care Services (99291–99292) 223
Services Included in Critical Care 224
9.6 Reporting E/M Codes in Other Settings (99304–99350) 225
Nursing Facility Services 225
Domiciliary, Rest Home (e.g., Boarding Home), or Custodial Care Services 227
Home Services 228
9.7 Prolonged Services and the Time Factor (99354–99360) 229
Prolonged Physician Service with Direct Patient Contact 229
Prolonged Physician Service without Direct Patient Contact 230
Physician Standby Services 231
9.8 Case Management and Care Plan Oversight Services (99363–99380) 231
Case Management Services 231
Care Plan Oversight Services 232
9.9 Preventive Medicine Services (99381–99429) 233
New Patient 234
Established Patient 234
Counseling Risk Factor Reduction and Behavior Change Intervention 235
9.10 Special E/M Services (99441–99456) 236
Telephone Services 236
Online Medical Evaluation 237
Other Special E/M Services 237
9.11 Coding E/M Services for Pediatric Patients (99460–99479) 238
Newborn Services 238
Inpatient Neonatal Intensive Care and Pediatric/Neonatal Critical Care 239
Chapter Review 241

10 ANESTHESIA SERVICES 254

Introduction 255

10.1 Selecting Anesthesia CPT Codes Based on the Surgical Procedure 255

10.2 Anesthesia Time Units 258

10.3 Secondary Aspects of Anesthesia Coding 259

    Physical Status Modifiers 259

    Modifiers Identifying Professional Credentials of Anesthesia Providers 260

    Modifiers Describing Reasons for Monitored Anesthesia Care (MAC) 260

    Qualifying Circumstances Add-on Codes 261

10.4 Calculating Total Anesthesia Units 262

10.5 Selecting Anatomy-Based Anesthesia CPT Codes (00100–01860) 263

    Head 263

    Neck 264

    Thorax (Chest Wall and Shoulder Girdle) 264

    Intrathoracic Region 265

    Spine and Spinal Cord 266

    Upper Abdomen 266

    Lower Abdomen 267

    Perineum 267

    Pelvis (Except Hip) 268

    Upper Leg (Except Knee) 269

    Knee and Popliteal Area 269

    Lower Leg (Below Knee, Includes Ankle and Foot) 270

    Shoulder and Axilla 270

    Upper Arm and Elbow 271

    Forearm, Wrist and Hand 272

10.6 Coding for Specific Procedures (01960–01999) 273

    Radiological Procedures 273

    Burn Excisions or Debridement 273

    Obstetrical Anesthesia 274

    Other Procedures 275

Chapter Review 276

11 RADIOLOGY SERVICES 284

Introduction 285

11.1 Positions, Projections, and Planes 285

11.2 Reporting Radiology Services 286

    Unlisted Codes 287

11.3 Modifiers 287

11.4 Radiology CPT Coding (70010–79999) 288

    Diagnostic Radiology (Diagnostic Imaging) 289

    Diagnostic Ultrasound 290

    Radiologic Guidance 291

    Breast, Mammography 292

    Bone/Joint Studies 292

    Radiation Oncology 292

    Nuclear Medicine 293

Chapter Review 295

12 SURGERY CODES: CODING FOR SURGICAL PROCEDURES ON SPECIFIC ORGAN SYSTEMS 305

Introduction 306

    Follow-up Care 306

    Multiple Procedures and "Separate Procedures" 306

    Structure of the Surgical Section of the CPT 307

Module 12.1 General and Integumentary System 308

    Introduction 309

    12.1.1 Reporting Procedures of the Skin and Subcutaneous Tissues (10021–11983) 309

    12.1.2 Wound Repair (Closure) (12001–13160) 313

    12.1.3 Skin Repair Procedures (14000–16036) 315

    12.1.4 Destruction of Lesions (17000–17999) 317

    12.1.5 Procedures on the Breast (19000–19499) 319

    12.1.6 Anesthesia Associated with Procedures on the Integumentary System 321

Module Review 322

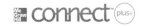

Module 12.2 Musculoskeletal System 326

Introduction 327

12.2.1 Musculoskeletal System Treatments 327

12.2.2 General Codes and Codes Describing Procedures on the Head, Neck, and Thorax (20005–21899) 329

12.2.3 Codes Describing Procedures on the Back and Flank, Spinal Column, and Abdomen (21920–22299) 331

12.2.4 Codes Describing Procedures on the Extremities and Joints (23000–28899) 333

12.2.5 Casting, Strapping, Endoscopy, and Arthroscopy (29000–29999) 336

12.2.6 Anesthesia Associated with Procedures on the Musculoskeletal System 337

Module Review 339

Module 12.3 Respiratory, Cardiovascular, Hemic, and Lymphatic Systems; Mediastinum and Diaphragm 343

Introduction 344

12.3.1 Procedures on the Respiratory System (30000–32999) 344

12.3.2 Procedures on the Heart and Pericardium (33010–33999) 347

12.3.3 Procedures on the Arteries and Veins (34001–37799) 352

12.3.4 Procedures on the Hemic and Lymphatic Systems, Mediastinum, and Diaphragm (38100–39599) 358

12.3.5 Anesthesia for Procedures in the 30000 Code Series 359

Module Review 362

Module 12.4 Digestive System 366

Introduction 367

12.4.1 Procedures on the Mouth and Throat (40490–42999) 367

12.4.2 Procedures on the Gastrointestinal Tract from the Esophagus to the Anus (43020–46999) 369

12.4.3 Procedures on Organs Connected to the Digestive Tract (47000–49999) 374

12.4.4 Anesthesia for Procedures Included in the 40000 Series of CPT Codes 377

Module Review 379

Module 12.5 Urinary System, Male and Female Genital Systems, and Maternity Care and Delivery 383

Introduction 384

12.5.1 Procedures on the Urinary System (50010–53899) 384

12.5.2 Procedures on the Male Genital System (54000–55899) 387

12.5.3 Procedures on the Female Genital System (56405–58999) 390

12.5.4 Maternal Care and Delivery (59000–59899) 392

12.5.5 Anesthesia for Procedures Described by Codes in the 50000 Series 395

Module Review 396

Module 12.6 Endocrine, Nervous, Ocular, and Auditory Systems 400

Introduction 401

12.6.1 Endocrine System (60000–60699) 401

12.6.2 Procedures on the Skull, Meninges, and Brain (61000–62258) 402

12.6.3 Procedures on the Spine and Spinal Cord (62263–63746) 405

12.6.4 Procedures on Extracranial Nerves, Peripheral Nerves, and the Autonomic Nervous System (64400–64999) 409

12.6.5 Procedures on Ocular Structures (65091–68899) 411

12.6.6 Procedures on the Auditory System; Operating Microscope (69000–69990) 413

12.6.7 Coding for Anesthesia for Procedures in the 60000 Series 416

Module Review 418

13 PATHOLOGY AND LABORATORY SERVICES 422

Introduction 423

13.1 Organ or Disease-Oriented Panels (80047–80076) 423

13.2 Lab Tests Involving Drugs or Medicines (80100–80440) 426

Drug Testing 426

Therapeutic Drug Assay 427

Evocative/Suppression Testing 427

13.3 Reporting Other Lab Tests (80500–87999) 428

Consultations (Clinical Pathology) 428

Urinalysis 428

Chemistry 429

Molecular Pathology 429

Hematology and Coagulation 429

Immunology 430

Transfusion Medicine 430

Microbiology 430

13.4 Coding for Pathology Services (88000–89398) 431

Anatomic Pathology 431

Cytopathology and Cytogenetic Studies 432

Surgical Pathology 432

In Vivo Laboratory Procedures 433

Reproductive Medicine Procedures 433

Chapter Review 434

14 MEDICINE SERVICES 440

Introduction 441

14.1 Medicine Chapter Structure and General Guidelines 441

Multiple Procedures 442

Add-on Codes 442

Separate Procedures 442

Unlisted Services or Procedures 443

Materials Supplied by Physician 443

14.2 Immune Globulins; Immunization Administration for Vaccines/ Toxoids; Vaccines, Toxoids (90281– 90749) 444

Immune Globulins 444

Immunization Administration for Vaccines/Toxoids 444

Vaccines, Toxoids 445

14.3 Psychiatry; Biofeedback; Dialysis; Gastroenterology; Ophthalmology, and Otorhinolaryngological Services (90801–92700) 446

Psychiatry 446

Biofeedback 447

Dialysis 447

Gastroenterology 448

Ophthalmology 448

Special Otorhinolaryngologic Services 449

14.4 Cardiovascular, Immunological, and Neurological Services (92950– 96155) 450

Cardiovascular 450

Noninvasive Vascular Diagnostic Studies 454

Pulmonary 454

Allergy and Clinical Immunology 454

Endocrinology 455

Neurology and Neuromuscular Procedures 455

Medical Genetics and Genetic Counseling Services 456

Central Nervous System Assessments/Tests 456

Health and Behavior Assessment/ Intervention 456

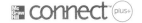

14.5 Injections and Infusions;
Therapeutic Services; Rehabilitation;
Moderate Sedation; Home Health and
Medication Therapy Management
Services (96360–99607) 457

Hydration, Therapeutic Injections
and Infusions, and
Chemotherapy 457
Photodynamic Therapy 458
Special Dermatological
Procedures 459
Physical Medicine and
Rehabilitation 459
Medical Nutrition Management 459
Acupuncture 459
Osteopathic Manipulative
Treatment 460
Chiropractic Manipulative
Treatment 460
Education and Training for Patient
Self-Management 460
Non-Face-to-Face NonPhysician
Services 460
Special Services, Procedures, and
Reports 460
Qualifying Circumstances for
Anesthesia 460
Moderate (Conscious)
Sedation 460
Home Health Procedures/
Services 461
Medication Therapy Management
Services 461
Chapter Review 463

15 INTRODUCTION TO THE HEALTHCARE
COMMON PROCEDURE CODING SYSTEM
(HCPCS) 470

Introduction 471
15.1 HCPCS Codes 471
Functions of HCPCS Codes 471
Uses of HCPCS Codes 472
Index and Tabular List of
Services 472

Calculating Multiple Units of
Service 472
Identifying Services Described by
Each Category of HCPCS
Codes 473
15.2 HCPCS A-, B-, C-, and
E-Codes 474
A-Codes: Transportation Services
Including Ambulance; Medical
and Surgical Supplies;
Administrative, Miscellaneous
and Investigational 474
B-Codes: Enteral and Parenteral
Therapy 476
C-Codes: Outpatient Prospective
Payment System (OPPS)
Codes 477
D-Codes: Dental Procedures 477
E-Codes: Durable Medical
Equipment 477
15.3 HCPCS G-, H-, J-, K-, L-, and
M-Codes 478
G-Codes: Procedures/Professional
Services (Temporary); Physician
Voluntary Reporting Program
Codes; Last-Minute Additions 478
H-Codes: Alcohol and Drug Abuse
Treatment Services 479
J-Codes: Drug Administered Other
Than Oral Method 480
K-Codes: Temporary Codes 480
L-Codes: Orthotic and Prosthetic
Procedures 481
M-Codes: Other Medical Services 482
15.4 HCPCS P-, Q-, R-, S-, T-, and
V-Codes 482
P-Codes: Pathology and Laboratory
Services 482
Q-Codes: Miscellaneous Services
(Temporary) 483
R-Codes: Diagnostic Radiology
Services 483
S-Codes: Temporary National Codes
(Non-Medicare) 483
T-Codes: National T-Codes
Established for State Medicaid
Agencies 484

V-Codes: Vision Services, Hearing Services, and Speech-Language Pathology Services 485

15.5 HCPCS Modifiers and HCPCS Manual Appendixes 485

Anatomical Modifiers 485

DME and Other Equipment Modifiers 486

Radiology Modifiers 486

Place of Service Modifier 486

Appendixes 486

Chapter Review 488

PART III: PRACTICUM 495

16 PUTTING IT ALL TOGETHER 496

Introduction 497

Coding Scenarios 497

Chapter Review 507

Appendix: Common Medical Abbreviations A-1

Glossary G-1

Credits C-1

Index I-1

PREFACE

No matter where you work, every day you have the potential for an encounter with the healthcare system. This may be as simple as a routine annual exam in your doctor's office or as critical as an accident requiring emergency treatment. But healthcare doesn't stop when your doctor's visit is over or you leave the emergency department. From the careful management of patient information and protection of patient privacy to the payment of insurance claims, healthcare involves ongoing communications between numerous entities that make up the healthcare system. The medical coder plays a vital role in this process, helping to translate complex clinical information into the language of medical codes to communicate with medical offices and payers. Coders enable reimbursement for services and, by generating trackable data about healthcare encounters, contribute to improving patient care on national and global levels. As a result, medical coding is a healthcare field that continues to be in high demand.

In order to become a skilled coder, it is crucial to be able to navigate the tools of the trade—the ICD, CPT, and HCPCS code manuals. Knowing what to look for in these manuals, including the terminology to search for, is just as important. Beginning with a review of anatomy, physiology, and medical terminology, *Medical Coding Fundamentals* walks you through the structure of each manual. It shows you hands-on examples of how to use each manual to find codes for diagnoses or procedures. The final chapter provides a series of scenarios for you to practice what you have learned—a key step toward becoming a proficient medical coder.

Here's What Instructors and Students Can Expect from *Medical Coding Fundamentals*

- A book by Susan Goldsmith, an experienced coder and instructor, and Marc Leib, a physician with years of clinical and coding expertise.
- Comprehensive coverage of both diagnosis coding and procedure coding in one book.
- Clear, readable language that takes the mystery out of the coding process.
- Step-by-step walkthroughs of how to code scenarios.
- Frequent opportunities to practice coding with exercises that build in complexity.
- Opportunities to go "beyond the code" by thinking critically about code selection and the implications of choosing those codes.
- A review of anatomy, physiology, and medical terminology—essential tools in translating documentation into codes.
- Dedicated chapters about ICD-10-CM/ICD-10-PCS and HCPCS.

Here's How Instructors Have Described *Medical Coding Fundamentals*

"An innovative approach to coding that utilizes up-to-date information and has excellent coverage of coding topics in today's world. It is written from the perspective of somebody who has witnessed first-hand what the students are looking for and the specific material that is important to cover."
Amy Ensign, CMA (AAMA), RMA (AMT), Baker College of Clinton Township

"This is an excellent textbook for use in teaching students how to code in an out-patient setting, especially geared towards physician offices, clinic settings, and other ambulatory facilities. The material is written in easy to understand language, has lots of coding examples, and follows a logical format in each chapter. It is perfectly suited for the current coding environment which requires coders to know and understand ICD-9-CM coding while preparing for ICD-10 and still needing to know CPT."
Georgina Sampson, RHIA, Anoka Technical College

"User-friendly and easy to follow. It gives great depth and explanation into the guidelines for the specific body systems."
Kathleen Coraspe, RHIT, Upper Valley Career Center

"I really like this approach. It takes it a step at a time, explains a lot, and gives details for better understanding. I'm very excited about this text."
Karen McAbee, CMA (AAMA), CPC, Miami-Jacobs Career College

"A very thorough textbook that could be used as a refresher course or a solid introductory course in medical coding. It offers plenty of explanation and examples that allow the student to develop a good understanding of both diagnostic and procedural coding. Additionally, the text provides perspectives from fellow coders that enable the student to gain insight into real-life coding. The text provides a good amount of practice to serve as reinforcement."
Monica Jarabeck Johnson, BA, M.Ed., Westmoreland County Community College

Organization of Medical Coding Fundamentals

Medical Coding Fundamentals consists of a review chapter followed by three parts, as shown in the following table.

Part	Coverage
Medical Terminology, Anatomy, and Physiology	Chapter 1 provides an overview of anatomical systems, basic physiology, and medical terminology, including common prefixes and suffixes.
I: ICD-9-CM and ICD-10-CM	Part I covers the format and guidelines of the ICD-9-CM code set. It walks through the use of ICD-9-CM to assign diagnosis codes. It also introduces the transition to ICD-10-CM and ICD-10-PCS, along with basic information about code assignment in the new code set.
II: CPT and HCPCS	Part II describes the format and guidelines of the CPT and HCPCS code sets. It explains the process for selecting modifiers and E/M codes. It includes comprehensive, modular coverage of surgical procedures as they relate to body systems.
III: Practicum	Part III offers additional, concentrated coding practice in the form of 25 clinical scenarios.

Content Highlights of *Medical Coding Fundamentals* by Chapter

(Information about the book's pedagogical elements appears in the Guided Tour, starting on page xxii.)

- **Chapter 1** provides an overview of anatomical systems, basic physiology, and medical terminology, all of which are key factors in code selection.
- **Chapter 2** introduces the format of the ICD-9-CM code set. It describes the process of finding and selecting codes from this code set, including general guidelines about sequencing and grouping codes.

- **Chapter 3** describes how to select codes for conditions classified in the first half of the ICD-9-CM manual, including infectious diseases, neoplasms, blood disorders, and conditions of various anatomical systems.

- **Chapter 4** walks through the code selection process for situations involving pregnancy and childbirth, skin and muscle disorders, congenital disorders, signs and symptoms, and injuries and poisonings. It also explains the use of E-codes and V-codes.

- **Chapter 5** describes the transition to ICD-10-CM and ICD-10-PCS with a walk-through of the code format in each set.

- **Chapter 6** introduces the organization of the CPT manual, including the codes themselves, the index, and appendixes. It differentiates between Category I, Category II, and Category III codes.

- **Chapter 7** thoroughly explains how to select modifiers to describe services in additional detail or to report unusual characteristics of services. It includes a section about HCPCS modifiers.

- **Chapter 8** begins the discussion of evaluation and management (E/M) codes by describing the guidelines for choosing these codes and factors affecting those choices—history, examination, and decision making.

- **Chapter 9** dives deeper into the process of evaluating factors in order to select E/M codes. It provides details about each type of E/M service, including office and other outpatient services, inpatient services, emergency services, care management, preventive medicine, telephone and online consultations, and services for newborns.

- **Chapter 10** describes how to select anesthesia codes. It walks through the calculation of base and time anesthesia units, the selection of modifiers and add-on codes, and the coding for specific sites and procedures.

- **Chapter 11** discusses codes for radiology services, including the code selection process, modifiers to radiology codes, and parameters around coding for radiology services.

- **Chapter 12** provides an in-depth look at coding for surgical procedures on various anatomical systems. Each of six modules walks through the factors to be considered in each body system. Each module ends with a section about coding for anesthesia related to the procedures covered in that module.

- **Chapter 13** shows how to differentiate between organ-oriented and disease-oriented panels, in addition to explaining the coding process for laboratory tests and pathology services.

- **Chapter 14** describes how to code for the administration of various types of medicine services, including dialysis, vaccinations, specific medicine procedures, and the management of medications.

- **Chapter 15** explains the use and format of HCPCS codes, including how to identify and report scenarios in which modifiers are appropriate.

- **Chapter 16** provides an opportunity to apply what has been learned throughout the book in preparation for the certification exam. Twenty-five real-life clinical scenarios, ranging from simple to complex, prompt critical thinking in order to select the right codes for each case.

To the Instructor

McGraw-Hill knows how much effort it takes to prepare for a new course. Through focus groups, symposia, reviews, and conversations with instructors like you, we have gathered information about what materials you need in order to facilitate successful courses. We are committed to providing you with high-quality, accurate instructor support.

Instructor Resources

You can rely on the following materials to help you and your students work through the exercises in the book:

- Instructor Edition of the Online Learning Center at **www.mhhe.com/goldsmithleib**. Your McGraw-Hill sales representative can provide you with access and show you how to "go green" with our online instructor support. The OLC contains a number of resources to assist you in teaching your course:

Resource	Description
Instructor's Manual	Course overview; lesson plans; sample syllabi; answer keys for end-of-section and end-of-chapter questions; and correlations to competencies from several organizations, such as ABHES, CAAHEP, and CAHIIM.
PowerPoint slides	Slide presentation for each chapter. Teaching notes correlated to Learning Outcomes. Each presentation seeks to reinforce key concepts and provide a visual for students. The slides are excellent for in-class lectures.
Test bank	A variety of question types, with each question linked directly to its Learning Outcome, Bloom's Taxonomy, and difficulty level. Both a Word version and a computerized version (EZ Test) of the test bank are provided.
Asset map	These online chapter tables are organized by Learning Outcome and allow you to find instructor notes, PowerPoint slides, and even test bank suggestions with ease! Asset maps label and organize course material for use in a multitude of learning applications.

- *Connect Plus:* McGraw-Hill *Connect Plus* is a revolutionary online assignment and assessment solution, providing instructors and students with tools and resources to maximize their success. Through *Connect Plus*, instructors enjoy simplified course setup and assignment creation. Robust, media-rich tools and activities, all tied to the textbook Learning Outcomes, ensure you'll create classes geared toward achievement. You'll have more time with your students and spend less time agonizing over course planning.

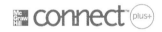

CodeitRightOnline™: Your Online Coding Tool

So that your students can gain experience with the use of an online coding tool, they will have access for a 29-day period to CodeitRightOnline, produced by Contexo Media, a division of Access Intelligence. CodeItRightOnline is available online at **www.codeitrightonline.com**.

Features

These are the general features that are offered with a subscription:

- CodeitRightOnline Search—The ability to find a CPT, HCPCS Level II, and ICD-9-CM code either using the Index or Tabular search sections, by code terminology, description, keyword, or code number to locate the correct code. Plus, the Single Search Feature allows you to locate all codes related to a particular term.
- Fully customizable—Provides note capability, LCD customization, personalized searches and fee schedules, and specialty-specific code sets.

- Coding Crosswalks—Essential coding links from CPT codes to ICD-9-CM to HCPCS Level II codes and to Anesthesia codes.

- Articles—We have compiled articles from CMS, OIG, carriers, intermediaries, payers, and other government websites along with newsletter articles from AMA, AHA, Decision Health, Coding Institute, and others.

- Medicare LCD/NCD policies and codes, Medicare's payment policy indicators, and, of course, CPT®, HCPCS Level II, and ICD-9-CM codes with full descriptions and our Plain English Definitions.

- ICD-10-CM/PCS Code Sets—Help you prepare for 2013 mandatory implementation with ICD-10-CM/PCS full code sets and descriptions.

- NCCI Edits Validator™—Validates codes to help you remain in compliance with the correct coding guidelines established by the Centers for Medicare & Medicaid Services (CMS).

- Automatic Updates—Ensure that CodeitRightOnline contains the most up-to-date, real-time information.

- Build-A-Code™—Allows students to build codes from the ground up, helping them understand how ICD-10 codes are constructed.

- Click-A-Dex™—Helps index searches for easy future reference.

- Comprehensive Medicare Resource—Contains local coverage determination (LCD) and national coverage determination (NCD) information, contact information for comprehensive list of Medicare providers, and information on how to bill for procedures allowed by Medicare's Physician Quality Reporting Initiative (PQRI) program.

- ABC Codes and Descriptions—Provide access to the alternative medicine codes you need to describe services, remedies, and/or supplies required during patient visits.

- Educational Games and Learning Tools—Games and interactive tools that help to reinforce the student's knowledge of anatomy.

Using the Online Coding Tool

Go to **www.codeitrightonline.com** to complete the steps needed to begin. The following screen will appear:

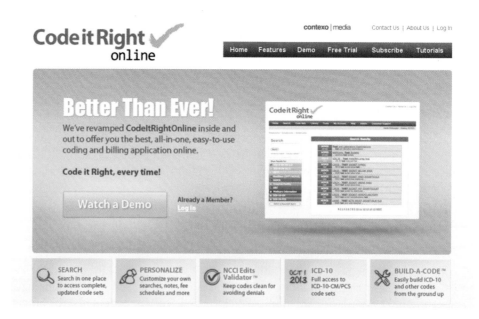

Click on the Free Trial tab at the top right-hand corner of the screen. On the page that appears, enter your name, e-mail address, school, phone, and address. Next, click on "Use account contact information" for your account administrator information, a one-time process that optimizes CodeitRightOnline for your particular location. Choose a username and password you will remember. Next, read the Terms and Conditions, including the AMA Agreement. After accepting these Terms and Conditions, click Continue. You will then receive an e-mail containing an activation link. Clicking on the link will activate your account. From that page, follow the "Click here" link to sign in with the account information you selected. This will take you to the CodeitRightOnline home page—you're in!

These actions set up your trial subscription. Now, to use the online coding tool to locate codes, click Search and select the appropriate code set. Next, choose the start point for your code search. For example, select ICD-9-CM Vol 1, 2 and Vol 3 in the Show Results For box, enter the term Fracture, and click Search. CodeitRightOnline will return a list of the various fracture entries for your selection. To see how it works, choose Fracture of Ribs, Closed and click the code number to review the Tabular List entry.

Do More Now

McGraw-Hill Higher Education and Blackboard have teamed up. What does this mean for you?

1. **Your life, simplified.** Now you and your students can access McGraw-Hill's *Connect Plus* and Create right from within your Blackboard course—all with one single sign-on. Say goodbye to the days of logging in to multiple applications.

2. **Deep integration of content and tools.** Not only do you get a single sign-on with *Connect Plus* and Create, but you also get deep integration of McGraw-Hill content and content engines right in Blackboard. Whether you're choosing a book for your course or building *Connect Plus* assignments, all the tools you need are right where you want them—inside Blackboard.

3. **Seamless gradebooks.** Are you tired of keeping multiple gradebooks and manually synchronizing grades into Blackboard? We thought so. When a student completes an integrated *Connect Plus* assignment, the grade for that assignment automatically (and instantly) feeds your Blackboard grade center.

4. **A solution for everyone.** Whether your institution is already using Blackboard or you just want to try Blackboard on your own, we have a solution for you. McGraw-Hill and Blackboard can now offer you easy access to industry-leading technology and content, whether your campus hosts it, or we do. Be sure to ask your local McGraw-Hill representative for details.

Do More

Need Help? Contact McGraw-Hill Higher Education's Customer Experience Team

Visit our Customer Experience Team Support website at www.mhhe.com/support. Browse our FAQs (Frequently Asked Questions) and product documentation, and/or contact a Customer Experience Team representative. The Customer Experience Team is available Sunday through Friday.

GUIDED TOUR

Chapter Opener ·

The **chapter opener** sets the stage for what will be learned in the chapter.

Learning Outcomes are written to reflect the revised version of Bloom's Taxonomy and to establish the key points the student should focus on in the chapter. In addition, major chapter heads are structured to reflect the Learning Outcomes and are numbered accordingly.

Key Terms are first introduced in the chapter opener so the student can see them all in one place.

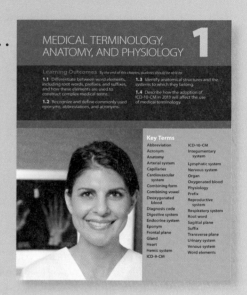

MEDICAL TERMINOLOGY, ANATOMY, AND PHYSIOLOGY **1**

Learning Outcomes *By the end of this chapter, students should be able to:*

1.1 Differentiate between word elements, including root words, prefixes, and suffixes, and how these elements are used to construct complex medical terms.

1.2 Recognize and define commonly used eponyms, abbreviations, and acronyms.

1.3 Identify anatomical structures and the systems to which they belong.

1.4 Describe how the adoption of ICD-10-CM in 2013 will affect the use of medical terminology.

Key Terms

Abbreviation
Acronym
Anatomy
Arterial system
Capillaries
Cardiovascular system
Combining form
Combining vowel
Deoxygenated blood
Diagnosis code
Digestive system
Endocrine system
Eponym
Frontal plane
Gland
Heart
Hemic system
ICD-9-CM

ICD-10-CM
Integumentary system
Lymphatic system
Nervous system
Organ
Oxygenated blood
Physiology
Prefix
Reproductive system
Respiratory system
Root word
Sagittal plane
Suffix
Transverse plane
Urinary system
Venous system
Word elements

Learning Aids ·

anatomy
The physical structure of the body.

physiology
How anatomical structures function in a living person.

Although coders are not physicians, the language of medicine is used extensively throughout the healthcare profession, so it is important for coders to understand this language, too. Coders encounter anatomical, conditional, and procedural terms, in addition to many acronyms, symbols, and abbreviations, during the course of their professional duties. Therefore, mastery of this language is vital to coding. Coders also must understand **anatomy** (the physical structure of the body) and **physiology** (how the anatomical structures function in a living person) to properly interpret medical records and report procedures and services provided to patients by healthcare professionals.

Key Terms are bolded and defined in the margin so that students will become familiar with the language of coding. These are reinforced in the **Glossary** at the end of the book.

Tips ·

Coder's Tips highlight helpful information for students.

CODER'S TIP

When studying medical terminology, be alert to repetition of certain prefixes, suffixes, root words, and/or combining elements throughout this text and coding books. Most of the medical terms available are a combination of two or more of word elements. The interpretation of a medical term involves examining each separate word part. The sum of the parts gives meaning to the entire word when each part is translated separately and recombined.

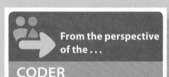

From the perspective of the . . .

CODER

While anatomy is difficult to learn, once the structures and relationships are understood, they almost never change. The coding system changes every year, but anatomy remains constant.

From the perspective of . . . provides insight from coders, physicians, specialized providers, and payers. This feature gives students practical coding advice and shows how coding fits into the overall healthcare process.

Coding Examples walk students through how to code a clinical scenario, from identifying the main terms to selecting the right code, sequencing codes correctly, and adding appropriate modifiers.

CODING EXAMPLE

A patient is diagnosed with COPD and asthma. At first it might appear that two codes are necessary to report these diseases. Turn to the Alphabetic Index and look under "asthma" to identify the codes that identify this disease. The first code listed is 493.9 (asthma, unspecified). However, looking farther down the list, you will see code 493.2 (chronic obstructive asthma), which is followed by a notation that it describes asthma with COPD. Since this describes the patient's condition, this would be the correct code.

It is not correct to report 493.2 with 496 (chronic airway obstruction, not elsewhere classified) to report these two diagnoses, because the code descriptor for 493.2 includes COPD. Therefore, a separate code designation is not necessary. A notation under code 496 identifies codes that are excluded, including asthma (493.2).

Exercises

Exercises within the chapter provide students with hands-on practice in coding diagnoses and procedures.

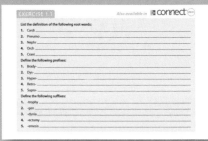

End-of-Chapter Resources

The **Chapter Summary** is in a tabular, step-by-step format with page references to help with review of the materials.

The **Chapter Review** contains the following types of questions, all tagged by Learning Outcome: terminology, multiple-choice, short answer (code manual navigation and code selection), and Thinking It Through exercises to test students' critical-thinking skills.

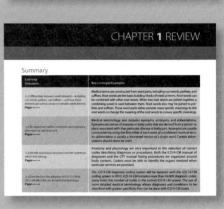

Using Terminology

Match the key terms with their definitions.

_____ 1. L01.1 Word element
_____ 2. L01.1 Root word
_____ 3. L01.1 Prefix
_____ 4. L01.1 Suffix
_____ 5. L01.1 Combining form
_____ 6. L01.1 Combining vowel
_____ 7. L01.2 Eponym
_____ 8. L01.2 Acronym
_____ 9. L01.2 Abbreviation
_____ 10. L01.3 Anatomical system
_____ 11. L01.3 Organs

A. Adding a combining vowel to a root word
B. Describes anatomical disorders or physiological malfunction
C. Parts of words that ma
D. International Classifica Modification
E. Attached to the beginn
F. Usually indicates a pro comes at the end of a v
G. Networks of organs th
H. An *o* or *i* added to a ro
I. Structures that have sp

Checking Your Understanding

Select the answer that best completes the statement or answers the question.

1. L01.1 Which of the following enable(s) the coder to define medical terms?
   a. Building up components
   b. Root words
   c. Anatomical structures
   d. Complex vocabulary

2. L01.1 Which of the following is true regarding a combining vowel?
   a. It joins a prefix, root word, and suffix.
   b. It is attached to the beginning of a word to modify or alter its meaning.
   c. It is always used to join the root word to the suffix.
   d. It is always used when two or more root words are joined.

3. L01.1 Which of the following is true regarding the suffix of a word?
   a. It indicates time or number.
   b. It often indicates a condition or disease.
   c. It is the base from which a definition grows.
   d. It always contains a combining vowel.

Applying Your Skills

Fill in the blank with the word(s) to complete each sentence.

1. L01.1 The basic building block of medical terms that can be combined to form other words is referred to as a(n) _____.

2. L01.1 _____ is the root word for the bladder.

3. L01.1 Words that are constructed from word parts, including root words, prefixes, and suffixes, are called

4. L01.2 A disease, anatomical structure, and/or surgical procedure scientist who discovered it is referred to as a(n) _____

5. L01.2 Beginning letters of multiword terms that are commonly f

6. L01.2 A short form of a commonly used word is called a(n) ____

7. L01.2 _____ is the acronym for the administration of

8. L01.2 _____ is the abbreviation for calcium.

9. L01.2 _____ is an abbreviation for a fracture.

10. L01.1, L01.2 A recording of the electrical conductivity of the hear

11. L01.3 A 56-year-old man with atherosclerotic heart disease has a

Thinking It Through

Use your critical-thinking skills to answer the questions below.

1. L01.4 Identify several elements you must comprehensively understand in order to effectively code using the ICD-10-CM manual.
   _____

2. L01.4 Which factors do you need to consider when coding for diabetes?
   _____

3. L01.4 Identify relevant elements that coders should look for within the medical record.
   _____

4. L01.4 Identify a diagnosis for which the procedure is being performed. Using your knowledge of medical terminology, explain the relationship between the diagnosis and the procedure.
   _____

ACKNOWLEDGMENTS

Suggestions have been received from faculty and students throughout the country. We rely on this vital feedback with all of our books. Each person who has offered comments and suggestions has our thanks. Special thanks are due to Edward O'Beirne, Eva Oltman, Angela Suarez, and Cynthia Ward for their work on the end-of-chapter exercises.

The efforts of many people are needed to develop and improve a product. Among these people are the reviewers and consultants who point out areas of concern, cite areas of strength, and make recommendations for change. In this regard, the following instructors provided feedback that was enormously helpful in preparing the first edition of *Medical Coding Fundamentals*.

Symposia

An enthusiastic group of trusted faculty members active in this course area attended a symposium to provide crucial feedback.

Paz Liduvina M. Beech, CPC, NRCCS
Sanford Brown Institute

Becky Buegel, RHIA, CHP, CHC
Brookline College

Nikita Carr, CPC
Centura College

Chetan Deshmukh, MBA, OTR/L, CPC, CCA, CHDA, CIPP
Vastaccess, Inc

Regina L. Hall, RMA, NCICS
MedVance Institute

Yolanda Levy, BS, RHIT
Sanford Brown College

Charlotte Gale Sheppeard, AA, BS, M.Ed.
Holmes Community College

Angela R. Suarez, BA, CPC, RMA, DHCE
National College

Workshops

In 2010 and 2011, McGraw-Hill conducted 13 health professions workshops, providing an opportunity for more than 700 faculty members to gain continuing education credits as well as to provide feedback on our products.

Book Reviews

Many instructors participated in manuscript reviews throughout the development of the book.

Dodie Anderson, CPC, CMRS
Career Learning Center of the Black Hills

Stacey M. Ashford, AAS, CPC, CCA
Remington College

Katherine E. Baus, RHIA, CCS-P
Southwest Florida College

Gerry A. Brasin, AS, CMA (AAMA), CPC
Premier Education Group

Sue Butler, CPC, CIMC
Lansing Community College

Mary M. Cantwell, RHIT, CPC, CPC-I, CPC-H, CPC-P, HIMS Coordinator
Metro Community College

Karen Collins Gibson, RHIA, MSA
Delaware County Community College

Kathleen Coraspe, RHIT
Upper Valley Career Center

Jennifer de Zayas Carmean, MBA, CPC, CPC-H, CCS-P
American Intercontinental University Online

Barbara Donnally, CPC
University of Rio Grande

Amy Ensign, CMA (AAMA), RMA (AMT)
Baker College of Clinton Township

Patti A. Fayash, CCS
St. Mary Medical Center and Luzerne County Community College

Terri Gilbert, BSBA, CMAA, CEHRS
ECPI University, Medical Careers Institute

Jacquelyn Harris, ME.d, CMA (AAMA), ACA, AHI
Bryan College

Traci Hotard, RHIA
South Central Louisiana Technical College

Rhonda Johns, CMA (AAMA), MS
Baker College

Debi Kenney, NCMA, NCBCS
Premier Education Group, Harris School of Business

Fannie Sue Martin, CPC
YTI Career Institute

Rebecca C. Martinez, PharmD, MS, RPh
Kaplan University

Karen M. McAbee, CMA (AAMA), CPC
Miami Jacobs Career College

Wilsetta McClain, RMA, NCPT, Ph.D
Baker College of Auburn Hills

Eva Oltman, CPC, EMT, CMA
Jefferson Community and Technical College

Barbara Parker, CMA (AAMA), CPC, CCS-P
Olympic College

Andrea Robins, MS
Keiser University eCampus

Diane Roche Benson, CMA (AAMA), BSHCA, MSA, CFP, NSC-SCFAT, ASE, CMRS, CPC, CDE, AHA BCLS/First Aid-Instructor, PALS, ACLS, CCT, NCI-I
Johnston County Community College, University of Phoenix, Wake Technical Community College

Georgina Sampson, RHIA
Anoka Technical College

Leslie S. Schwanfelder, BS, CPC
Ridley-Lowell Business and Technical School

Gene Simon, RHIA, RMD
Florida Career College

Mary Jo Slater
Community College of Beaver County

Patricia A. Stich, MA, CCS-P
Waubonsee Community College

Mary B. Valencia, CPC, CMC, CMOM
University of Texas at Brownsville/Texas Southmost College

Lori Warren Woodard, MA, RN, CPC, CPC-I, CCP, CLNC
Spencerian College

Accuracy Panel

A panel of instructors completed a technical edit and review of all content in the book page proofs to verify its accuracy.

Gerry A. Brasin, AS, CMA (AAMA), CPC
Premier Education Group

Carol Hendrickson, MS Ed., CCS-P
Pasco Hernando Community College

Karen McAbee, CMA, CPC
Miami-Jacobs Career College

Andrea Robins, MS
Keiser University eCampus

Lori Warren Woodard, MA, RN, CPC, CPC-I, CCP, CLNC
Spencerian College

Workbook

Special thanks are due to Mary Cantwell, Deborah Kenney, Edward O'Beirne, Eva Oltman, Selinda McCumbers, and Angela Suarez for their help in developing the exercises in the *Workbook for use with Medical Coding Fundamentals*.

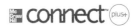

A panel of instructors reviewed the contents of the workbook page proofs and answer keys for accuracy.

Terri Franklin, CPC
Everest College

Jane M. O'Grady, MSEd, RN, CMA, CPC
Northwestern Connecticut Community College

Deena Pebley, CCS, CPC-A, CBCS, CMAA
New Horizons

Acknowledgments from the Authors

Thanks to all the individuals at McGraw-Hill whose tireless efforts have moved this project forward from the first blank pages to final publication. We especially want to thank the McGraw-Hill editorial team—Michael S. Ledbetter, Natalie J. Ruffatto, Michelle L. Flomenhoft, and Raisa Priebe Kreek—for their encouragement and support throughout this process.

We also want to thank other McGraw Hill staff who provided invaluable assistance, including project manager Kathryn Wright, executive marketing manager Roxan Kinsey, digital development editor Katherine Ward, buyer Sherry Kane, senior designer Srdjan Savanovic, senior photo research coordinator John Leland, digital production manager Janean Utley, and media production managers Brent dela Cruz and Cathy Tepper. Without them, this book would not have been possible.

To the students and instructors using this first edition, thank you in advance for your feedback and suggestions to make the next edition better.

To all of our friends and families, we could not have done this without your support. Thank you.

Susan Goldsmith and Marc Leib

A COMMITMENT TO ACCURACY

You have a right to expect an accurate textbook, and McGraw-Hill invests considerable time and effort to make sure that we deliver one. Listed below are the many steps we take to make sure this happens.

OUR ACCURACY VERIFICATION PROCESS

First Round—Development Reviews

STEP 1: Numerous **health professions instructors** review the draft manuscript and report on any errors that they may find. The authors make these corrections in their final manuscript.

Second Round—Page Proofs

STEP 2: Once the manuscript has been typeset, the **authors** check their manuscript against the page proofs to ensure that all illustrations, graphs, examples, and exercises have been correctly laid out on the pages, and that all codes have been updated correctly.

STEP 3: An outside panel of **peer instructors** completes a review of content in the page proofs to verify its accuracy. The authors add these corrections to their review of the page proofs.

STEP 4: A **proofreader** adds a triple layer of accuracy assurance in pages by looking for errors; then a confirming, corrected round of page proofs is produced.

Third Round—Confirming Page Proofs

STEP 5: The **author team** reviews the confirming round of page proofs to make certain that any previous corrections were properly made and to look for any errors they might have missed on the first round.

STEP 6: The **project manager,** who has overseen the book from the beginning, performs **another proofread** to make sure that no new errors have been introduced during the production process.

Final Round—Printer's Proofs

STEP 7: The **project manager** performs a **final proofread** of the book during the printing process, providing a final accuracy review. In concert with the main text, all supplements undergo a proofreading and technical editing stage to ensure their accuracy.

RESULTS

What results is a textbook that is as accurate and error-free as is humanly possible. Our authors and publishing staff are confident that the many layers of quality assurance have produced books that are leaders in the industry for their integrity and correctness. *Please view the Acknowledgments section for more details on the many people involved in this process.*

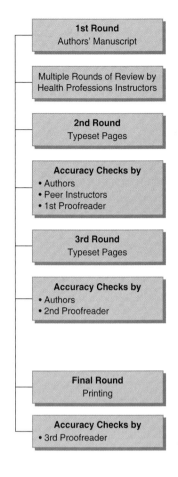

MEDICAL TERMINOLOGY, ANATOMY, AND PHYSIOLOGY

1

Learning Outcomes   *After completing this chapter, students should be able to:*

1.1 Differentiate between word elements, including root words, prefixes, and suffixes, and understand how these elements are used to construct complex medical terms.

1.2 Recognize and define commonly used eponyms, abbreviations, and acronyms.

1.3 Identify anatomical structures and the systems to which they belong.

1.4 Describe how the adoption of ICD-10-CM in 2013 will affect the use of medical terminology.

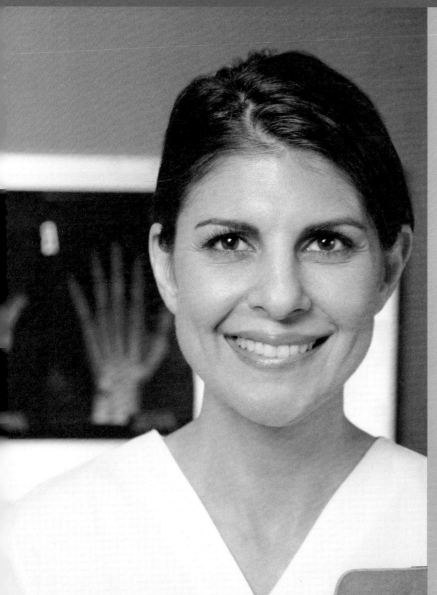

Key Terms

Abbreviation	ICD-10-CM
Acronym	Integumentary system
Anatomy	
Arterial system	Lymphatic system
Capillaries	Nervous system
Cardiovascular system	Organ
	Oxygenated blood
Combining form	Physiology
Combining vowel	Prefix
Deoxygenated blood	Reproductive system
Diagnosis code	Respiratory system
Digestive system	Root word
Endocrine system	Sagittal plane
Eponym	Suffix
Frontal plane	Transverse plane
Gland	Urinary system
Heart	Venous system
Hemic system	Word elements
ICD-9-CM	

Introduction

Medical coding is essential to the healthcare delivery process. Based on medical documentation, professional coders select the appropriate diagnosis and procedure codes to report a patient's diagnoses and any procedures that were performed. One use for these codes is to ensure accurate reimbursement for services rendered, even a basic doctor's visit, by making sure that medical necessity (the diagnosis) justifies those services. Codes are also used to track data related to public health and healthcare: diagnosis codes help show the occurrence and spread of diseases, and procedure codes track how often particular services are provided. Tracking these aspects of healthcare is a way to improve the healthcare delivery process for everyone, from stopping the spread of epidemics to streamlining the way that procedures are provided and paid for.

The language of medicine is used extensively throughout the healthcare profession, so it is important for coders to understand this language, too. Coders encounter anatomical, conditional, and procedural terms, in addition to many acronyms, symbols, and abbreviations, during the course of their professional duties. Therefore, mastery of this language is vital to coding. Coders also must understand **anatomy** (the physical structure of the body) and **physiology** (how the anatomical structures function in a living person) to properly interpret medical records and report procedures and services provided to patients by healthcare professionals.

anatomy
The physical structure of the body.

physiology
How anatomical structures function in a living person.

1.1 Word Elements

Learning medical terminology begins by understanding **word elements,** or parts of words, that make up the medical language. This chapter reviews the basic elements of medical terminology, including root words, combining vowels, combining forms, prefixes, and suffixes.

Words used to describe anatomical structures and medical procedures often are complex and as difficult to spell as they are to pronounce. These words may be formulated by joining two or more word elements to create a complex vocabulary. Although these words are often complex, coders should be able to break them into their common components to identify their meanings.

Tables throughout this section list examples of common word elements for review. Table 1.1 lists root words with their meanings and examples of use. Tables 1.2 and 1.3 provide similar lists for commonly used prefixes and suffixes. These lists are not exhaustive, but provide a review of these word elements.

word elements
The words and word parts that combine to form medical terms.

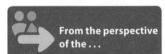

CODER

A minor change, even a single letter in a word, prefix, or suffix, can completely change the meaning of a word. For example, the prefixes *intra-* and *inter-* are similar but have opposite meanings, as do the prefixes *ecto-* and *endo-*. Everyone using medical terminology must choose the correct words and write them clearly enough to avoid mistakes in how the words are read.

Root Words

A **root word** is the base from which a term's definition grows. The root contains the basic meaning of the word. It usually, but not always, indicates the involved body part. More than one root word may be combined together to create new words. Adding a prefix at the beginning and suffix at the end of the root word provides greater specificity. Table 1.1 lists common root words.

root word
The base from which a term's definition grows.

combining vowel
A vowel added to a root or base word to facilitate pronunciation.

combining form
A word element consisting of a root word and a combining vowel.

Combining Vowels and Combining Forms

A **combining vowel,** such as an *o* or *i*, is often added to a root or base word to facilitate pronunciation. Adding a combining vowel to a root word creates a **combining form.** A combining vowel may be used to connect or join a root word and a suffix. When the suffix begins with a consonant, it is appropriate to use a combining vowel. For example, joining the root word *neur* (nerve) with the suffix *-plasty* (surgical repair) requires the combining vowel *o* to form the term *neuroplasty* (surgical repair of the nerve).

TABLE 1.1 Root Words

Root	Meaning	Example	Root	Meaning	Example
abdomin	abdomen	abdominal	cheil	lip	cheilitis
acou	hearing	acoustic	chole	gallbladder	cholecystectomy
acr	extremities or height	acral	cholangi	bile duct	cholangiography
actin	ray or radius	actinic	chondr	cartilage	chondroplasty
aden	gland	adenocarcinoma	chrom	color	chromatogenous
adren	adrenal gland	adrenaline	colp	vagina	colposcopy
aer	air or gas	aerosol	core	pupil or eye	corectopia
algesi	pain	analgesic	cost	rib	costicervical
ambly	dull or dim	amblyopia	crani	head or skull	craniotomy
andr	male	androgen	cutane	skin	subcutaneous
angi	vessel	angina	cysto, cysti, cyst	bladder	cystogram
aniso	unequal or dissimilar	anisochromatic	dacry	tear or tear duct	dacryoadenitis
ankyl	crooked, bent, or fused	ankylosed	dactyl	fingers or toes	dactylolysis
antr	cavity or chamber	antronasal	dent	tooth	dentition
arche, archi	first or beginning	archicerebellum	derm	skin	dermis
arthr	joint	arthritis	dextro	right	dextrocardia
articul	joint	articulate	diaphor	sweat	diaphoresis
atel	imperfect or incomplete	atelectasis	diplo	two or double	diploid
ather	yellowish or fatty plaque	atheroma	dips	thirst	dipsosis
aur	ear	auricular, aural rehab	ectop	located away from usual place	ectopia
aut	self	autism	encephal	brain	encephalitis
axill	armpit	axilla	enter	intestine	enterogenous
blephar	eyelid	blepharoplasty	erythr	red	erythrocyte
brachi	arm	brachialgia	gastro	stomach	gastritis
bucc	cheek	buccal	gingiv	gum	gingivitis
carcin	cancer	carcinoma	gloss	tongue	glossitis
cardi	heart	cardiac	gnath	jaw	gnathocephalus
caud	toward the lower part of the body, tail	caudal	gyn	woman	gynecology
cephal	head	encephalitis	hem	blood	hemocyte
			hepat	liver	hepatitis
			hyster	uterus, womb	hysterectomy

(Continued)

TABLE 1.1 *(Concluded)*

Root	Meaning	Example
irid	iris	iridectomy
isch	deficiency or blockage	ischemia
kal	potassium	hypokalemia
kerat	cornea or horny tissue; hard	keratotomy, keratosis
kyph	hump	kyphosis
laparo	loins or abdomen	laparoscopy
laryng	larynx	laryngitis
lei	smooth	leiomyoma
leuk	white	leukocyte
lith	stone or calculus	lithotripsy
macr	abnormal largeness	macromelia
mamm	breast	mammography
mast	breast	mastitis
meat	opening	meatus
melan	black	melanoma
myel	bone marrow or spinal cord	myeloma
myo	muscle	myoma
narc	stupor	narcotic
nas	nose	nasal
necr	death	necrotic
nephr	kidney	nephrectomy
neur	nerve	neuropathy
ocul	eye	ocular
olig	scanty or few	oligemia
onych	nail	onychogenic
orch	testis or testicle	orchiectomy
orth	straight	orthocephalic
oste	bone	ostealgia
ot	ear	otitis
pachy	thick	pachycephalic
pector	chest	pectoralgia
phac	lens of eye	phacolysis

Root	Meaning	Example
phag	eat or swallow	dysphagia
phas	speech	aphasia
pneumo	lung or air	pneumonia
pod	foot	podagra
proct	anus or rectum	proctalgia
pseud	fake or false	pseudopolyp
pulmo	lung	pulmonary
pyel	renal pelvis	pyelogram
pyr	fever or heat	pyrogenic
radic	nerve root	radiculopathy
ren	kidney	renal
rhabd	rod shaped or striated	rhabditis
rhino	nose	rhinitis
salping	tube (usually uterine)	salpingocele
sarco	flesh or connective tissue	sarcoma
scoli	crooked or curved	scoliosis
somn	sleep	insomnia
spir	breathe or breathing	spirometry
spondylo	vertebra or spinal or vertebral column	spondylosis
stomato	mouth	stomatoplasty
tomo	cut or section	tomography
thorac	chest	thoracotomy
thrombo	clot	thrombus
trich	hair	trichoid
tympan	eardrum or middle ear	tympanoplasty
ungu	nail	ungual
vaso	vessel or duct	vasospasm
vesico	bladder or sac	vesical
viscer	internal organs	viscera
xanth	yellow	xanthoma
xero	dry	xerosis

A combining vowel is not used when the suffix begins with a vowel. For example, the root word *neur* joined with the suffix *-itis* (inflammation) forms the term *neuritis* (inflammation of a nerve).

A combining vowel is always used when two or more root words are joined. For example, joining the root words *gastr* (stomach) and *enter* (small intestine) with the combining vowel *o* and adding the suffix *-itis* (inflammation) creates the term *gastroenteritis* (inflammation of the stomach and small intestine).

Prefixes

A **prefix** is attached to the beginning of a word to modify its meaning. Not all medical terms contain a prefix. Prefixes often (but not always) indicate location, position, time, or number. For example, joining the prefix *epi-* (above) to the root *dermis* (skin) creates the term *epidermis* (the topmost layer of skin). Table 1.2 provides a list of commonly used prefixes.

prefix
A word part attached to the beginning of another word to modify its meaning.

TABLE 1.2 Prefixes Commonly Used in Medical Terminology

Prefix	Meaning	Example	Prefix	Meaning	Example
a-	without or absence of	anemia	hex-	six	hexon
ab-	away from	abneural	homo-	same	homozygous
ad-	toward	adaxial	hyper-	excessive, above	hyperactive, hypertension
ambi-	both	ambilateral	hypo-	deficient, below	hypotension, hypoxia
an-	without or absence of	anaerobic	infra-	below, under	inframamillary
ana-	up, again, or backward	anaphoresis	intra-	within	intravenous
aniso-	unequal	anisogamy	ipsi-	same	ipsilateral
ante-	before	antepartum	iso-	equal	isoteric
apo-	upon	aponeurotic	mal-	bad, poor	malformation
bi-	two	bilateral	megalo-	large	megaloblast
brady-	slow	bradycardia	meso-	middle	mesocord
cata-	down	catatonic	meta-	after, beyond, transformation	metastatic
con-	together	concurrent	mono-	one	mononucleosis
contra-	against	contraceptive	pan-	all or total	pancytopenia
diplo-	double	diplogenesis	per-	through	percutaneous
dys-	bad, painful, difficult	dysphagia	peri-	surrounding	perivascular, perineuropathy
ecto-, exo-	outside	ectopic, exogenous	quadr-	four	quadrant
endo-	within	endoscopy	retro-	behind, back	retrograde, retroperitoneal
epi-	upon	epidemic, epidermis	supra-	above	supraclavicular
eso-	inward	esotropia	uni-	one	unilateral
eu-	good, normal	euplasia			
hetero-	different	heterozygous			

Suffixes

suffix
A word part attached to the end of another word to modify its meaning.

A **suffix** comes at the end of a word. Usually a suffix indicates a procedure, condition, disorder, or disease. A suffix also can be used to change the word's use in sentence structure. By adding *-ing* to a noun (name of a thing), you create a verb that describes an action with that thing. For example, adding *-ing* to the noun *suture* (the name of a material used to place surgical stitches) creates *suturing* (the act of placing surgical stitches). Table 1.3 contains a list of commonly used suffixes.

TABLE 1.3 Suffixes Commonly Used in Medical Terminology

Suffix	Meaning	Example	Suffix	Meaning	Example
-algia	pain	fibromyalgia	-oma	tumor	lymphoma
-apheresis	removal	leukapheresis	-osis	abnormal condition of	diverticulosis
-asthenia	weakness	neurasthenia, myoasthenia	-ostomy	new permanent opening	colostomy
-cele	hernia or protrusion	enterocele	-otomy	to open temporarily, then close	arthrotomy
-centesis	puncture a cavity to remove fluid	arthrocentesis	-paresis	weakness	hemiparesis
-desis	surgical fixation or fusion	arthrodesis	-pathy	disease	myopathy
-dynia	pain	arthrodynia	-pepsia	digestion	dyspepsia
-ectasis	stretching out, dilation, or expansion	bronchiectasis	-phagia	eating or swallowing	dysphagia
-ectomy	surgical removal or excision	tonsillectomy	-physis	growth	hypophysis
-emesis	vomiting	hematemesis	-plasia	growth	dysplasia
-emia	blood	anemia	-plasty	surgical repair	rhinoplasty, angioplasty
-gen	agent that produces or causes	pathogen	-plegia	paralysis	quadriplegia
-genesis	origin or cause	iatrogenesis	-pnea	breathing	apnea
-ial	pertaining to	arterial	-poiesis	formation	hematopoiesis
-iasis	condition of	amebiasis	-prandial	meal	postprandial
-ictal	seizure or attack	postictal	-ptosis	dropping, sagging, or prolapse	splanchnoptosis
-itis	inflammation	rhinitis, appendicitis	-rrhea	flow or discharge	amenorrhea, rhinorrhea
-lysis	destruction or breakdown	adhesiolysis	-rrhexis	rupture	capsulorrhexis
-lytic	destroy or break down	osteolytic	-sclerosis	hardening	atherosclerosis
			-stalsis	contraction	peristalsis
-malacia	softening	chondromalacia	-stasis	control or stop	hemostasis
-megaly	enlargement	hepatosplenomegaly	-tripsy	surgical crushing	lithotripsy
			-trophy	nourishment	atrophy
-oid	like, similar to	carcinoid	-uria	urine or urination	proteinuria

EXERCISE 1.1

Also available in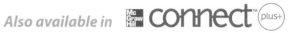

List the definition of the following root words:

1. Cardi _____

2. Pneumo _____

3. Nephr _____

4. Orch _____

5. Crani _____

Define the following prefixes:

1. Brady- _____

2. Dys- _____

3. Hyper- _____

4. Retro- _____

5. Supra- _____

Define the following suffixes:

1. -trophy _____

2. -gen _____

3. -dynia _____

4. -ectomy _____

5. -emesis _____

1.2 Eponyms, Abbreviations, and Acronyms

Eponyms

An **eponym** is a word derived from the name of a person, real or fictional, that is used to identify something associated with that person. Some eponyms are based on the name of a place. In medicine, an eponym may be associated with a:

- Disease (e.g., Alzheimer's disease, first described by German psychiatrist Alois Alzheimer in 1901).
- Anatomical structure (e.g., Achilles tendon, named for the character Achilles from Greek mythology [Figure 1.1]).
- Surgical procedure (e.g., the Monti procedure, named for Brazilian urologist, Paulo Ricardo Monti).

eponym
A name derived from the existing name of a person or location.

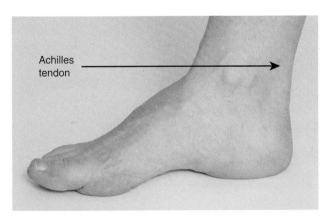

FIGURE 1.1 Many medical terms come from names of people or places. The Achilles tendon is named after Achilles, a character in Greek mythology.

Eponyms are commonly used in medical terminology. Other examples include but are not limited to:

- Lou Gehrig's disease (named for a famous baseball player diagnosed with the disease).
- Lyme disease (named after Lyme, Connecticut).
- Colles' fracture (first described by Abraham Colles in 1814).
- Baker's cyst (named after William Baker, the surgeon who first described this condition).
- Blalock-Hanlon procedure (a procedure developed by Alfred Blalock and C. Rollins Hanlon).
- Parkinson's disease (named after the English physician who first described the disorder in 1817).
- Down or Down's syndrome (described by English physician John Down in 1866).

Abbreviations and Acronyms

abbreviation
A shortened form of a commonly used word.

acronym
An abbreviation consisting of the beginning letters of a multiword term.

Coders must be familiar with the numerous medical abbreviations and acronyms they use in their day-to-day work. An **abbreviation** is a shortened form of a commonly used word. An **acronym** usually is made up of the beginning letters of a multiword term. Healthcare professionals use abbreviations and acronyms frequently in both oral and written communication. See Appendix A at the end of this book for a list of commonly used abbreviations and acronyms.

According to The Joint Commission (TJC), one of the major organizations that accredit healthcare entities, some abbreviations and acronyms should not be used because they can be misinterpreted and cause errors in the delivery of healthcare services. The Joint Commission established a list of these dangerous abbreviations, acronyms, and symbols that should not be used (see Table 1.4). Coders should be aware of these abbreviations and avoid using them even if others have used them in the medical record.

TABLE 1.4 Abbreviations, Acronyms, and Symbols to Avoid in Medical Documentation

Abbreviation	Potential Problem	Preferred Term
U (for unit)	Mistaken as zero, four, or cc	Write "unit"
IU (for international unit)	Mistaken as IV (intravenous) or 10 (ten)	Write "international unit"
Latin abbreviations: Q.D. (once daily) Q.I.D. (four times a day) Q.O.D. (every other day)	Mistaken for each other. The period after the "Q" can be mistaken for an "I" and the "O" can be mistaken for "I."	Write "daily", "four times a day", or "every other day."
Trailing zero (X.0 mg) [Note: Prohibited only for medication-related notations]; Lack of leading zero (.X mg)	Decimal point is missed.	Never write a zero by itself after a decimal point (X mg), and always use a zero before a decimal point (0.X mg).
MS (morphine sulfate) MSO_4 (morphine sulfate) $MgSO_4$ (magnesium sulfate)	Confused for one another.	Write "morphine sulfate" or "magnesium sulfate."

© The Joint Commission, 2011. Reprinted with permission.

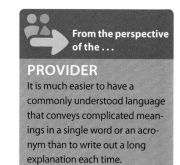

From the perspective of the . . .

PROVIDER

It is much easier to have a commonly understood language that conveys complicated meanings in a single word or an acronym than to write out a long explanation each time.

EXERCISE 1.2

Also available in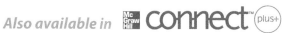

Define the following abbreviations.

1. COPD _____
2. CABG _____
3. CA _____
4. BP _____
5. IM _____
6. EBV _____
7. vWD _____
8. ASD _____
9. ALS _____
10. OSD _____

1.3 Anatomy and Physiology

Successful coding requires a thorough knowledge of human anatomy and basic physiology. Anatomy is the study of body parts, including structures that make up the musculoskeletal system, **organs** that perform specific functions, and **glands** that secrete substances that act elsewhere in the body. Physiology is the study of how those body parts perform their functions in the body and how those functions affect other anatomical systems.

organ
Anatomical structure or tissue that serves a specific function within the body.

gland
Tissue that secretes hormones.

Medical terminology is used to describe locations of anatomical parts in relation to each other. It is important for coders to know the names of the anatomical structures as well as their relationships to one another. These relationships often describe where one structure lies in relation to other structures. Some terms to review are listed in Table 1.5.

Anatomical drawings or actual images (e.g., x-rays, CT scans, or MRIs) may be made from a number of different angles or perspectives. Various planes divide the body into sections, including the frontal (or coronal) plane, sagittal plane, and transverse plane. The **frontal plane** runs through the body vertically from side to side, dividing the body into front and back portions. The **sagittal plane** runs through the

frontal plane
A plane dividing the body into anterior and posterior portions.

sagittal plane
A plane dividing the body into right and left portions.

TABLE 1.5 Common Directional Terms

Directional Term	Definition
Anterior (Ventral)	At or near the front surface of the body
Posterior (Dorsal)	At or near the back surface of the body
Superior or cephalic	Above, toward the head of the body
Inferior or caudal	Below, away from the head or toward the lower part of the body
Medial	Nearer to the midline
Lateral	Side of the body or away from the midline
Proximal	Nearer to the center of the body, closer to the hips or shoulders
Distal	Further from the center of the body, further from the hips or shoulders
Superficial	Toward the surface of the body
Deep	Away from the surface
Supine	Face up or palm up
Prone	Face down or palm down
Contralateral	On the opposite side of the body
Coronal or frontal plane	A plane dividing the body into anterior and posterior portions
Transverse plane	A plane dividing the body into upper and lower portions
Sagittal plane	A plane dividing the body into right and left portions

transverse plane
A plane dividing the body into upper and lower portions.

body vertically from front to back, dividing the body into right and left sides. The **transverse plane** runs through the body horizontally, dividing the body into top and bottom portions. Figure 1.2 illustrates these positions and planes.

Systems are groups of organs that work together to perform complex functions. The study of anatomy usually is divided into the study of specific systems.

FIGURE 1.2 (a) Anatomical Positions with Directional Terms (b) Anatomical Planes

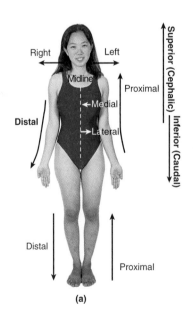

(a)

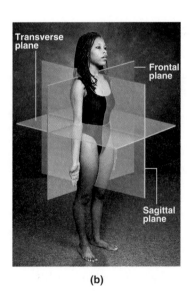

(b)

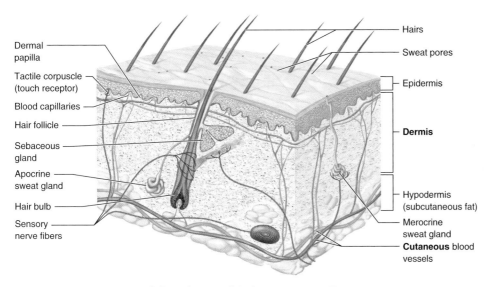

Dermal papilla

Tactile corpuscle (touch receptor)

Blood capillaries

Hair follicle

Sebaceous gland

Apocrine sweat gland

Hair bulb

Sensory nerve fibers

Hairs

Sweat pores

Epidermis

Dermis

Hypodermis (subcutaneous fat)

Merocrine sweat gland

Cutaneous blood vessels

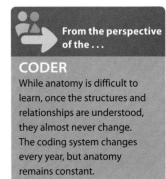

FIGURE 1.3 Structure of the Skin and Subcutaneous Tissue

Integumentary System

The **integumentary system** includes the skin (*Figure 1.3*) and the accessory organs of hair, nails, and glands. This is the largest organ system in the body, providing the following functions:

- Protection from injury, fluid loss, and microorganisms.
- Temperature regulation.
- Fluid balance.
- Sensation. Table 1.6 provides a list of common medical terms related to the integumentary system.

integumentary system
Network of organs, including the skin, that provide protection, sensation, and temperature regulation.

TABLE 1.6 Medical Terms Related to the Integumentary System

Term	Definition
Alopecia	Loss of hair
Cutaneous	Pertaining to the skin
Dermatology	Study of skin
Decubitus	Pressure ulcer (known as bedsore)
Ecchymosis	A condition in which blood seeps into the skin causing discoloration
Epidermis	Most superficial layer of the skin
Hypodermic	Under the skin
Intradermal	Within the skin
Jaundice	Yellowness of skin
Melanin	Pigment that gives color to the skin
Mole	Benign area of melanin-producing cells
Pruritis	Itching
Subcutaneous	Below the skin
Transdermal	Going across or through the skin

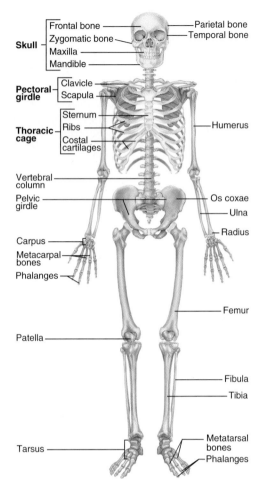

FIGURE 1.4 The Skeletal System

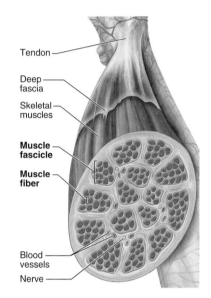

FIGURE 1.5 Structure of Skeletal Muscle

Musculoskeletal System

The skeletal system (*Figure 1.4*) provides structure to the body and protection to vital structures within the body. For example, the skull protects the brain, and the rib cage protects the heart and lungs. The muscles (*Figure 1.5*) provide the means to move the bones and joints in relationship to each other. Together the musculoskeletal system provides support, form, strength, protection, and movement. Table 1.7 provides a list of common medical terms related to the musculoskeletal system.

CODER'S TIP

The skeletal system also provides references for other anatomical structures. Many of these are named for skeletal structures in their vicinity. For example, the radial artery, posterior tibial artery, femoral vein, and parietal lobe of the brain are named for nearby skeletal structures. Coders should pay particular attention to the relationship of anatomical structures to each other.

TABLE 1.7 Medical Terms Related to the Musculoskeletal System

Term	Definition
Abduction	Movement away from the midline
Adduction	Movement toward the midline
Ankylosis	Condition of stiffening of a joint
Arthralgia	Pain in a joint
Arthrodesis	Surgical fixation of a joint
Arthroscope	Endoscope used to visualize the interior of a joint
Arthroscopy	Visual examination of a joint, usually with an arthroscope
Bursitis	Inflammation of a bursa
Cartilage	Connective tissue usually found in joints
Chondral	Pertaining to cartilage
Coccygeal	Pertaining to the coccyx
Cortex	Outer portion of a bone
Epiphyseal plate	Area of bone where growth occurs, usually near ends of bones
Extension	Straightening a joint, increasing the joint angle
Flexion	Bending a joint, decreasing the joint angle
Kyphosis	Humpback
Ligament	Tissue connecting two bones together
Lordosis	Abnormal anterior curvature of the spine
Marrow	Tissue in the cavities of bones in which blood is formed
Metacarpal	Bones of the hand
Metatarsal	Bones of the foot
Osteochondritis	Inflammation of bone and cartilage
Osteoporosis	Condition resulting in reduction of bone mass
Osteopenia	Decreased calcification of bones
Osteorrhaphy	Suture of bone
Pathologic fracture	Fracture occurring in area weakened by disease, such as cancer
Tendon	Tissue connecting muscle to bone

Cardiovascular System

The **cardiovascular system** includes the **heart** (Figures 1.6 and 1.7), **arterial system**, **capillaries**, and **venous system**. The cardiovascular system is also known as the circulatory system. Table 1.8 provides a list of common medical terms related to the cardiovascular system.

cardiovascular system
Network that includes the heart, blood vessels, and blood.

heart
Organ that pumps deoxygenated blood into the pulmonary system to be oxygenated and pumps oxygenated blood into tissues in the body.

arterial system
Network of arteries that carry blood from the heart to the organs.

capillaries
Tiny blood vessels between the arterial and venous systems.

venous system
Network of veins that carry blood from the body back to the heart.

FIGURE 1.6 External Anatomy of the Heart, Frontal View

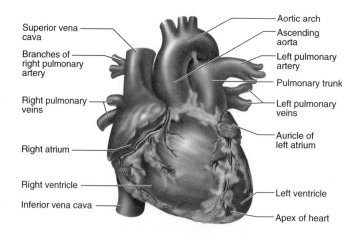

- Superior vena cava
- Branches of right pulmonary artery
- Right pulmonary veins
- Right atrium
- Right ventricle
- Inferior vena cava
- Aortic arch
- Ascending aorta
- Left pulmonary artery
- Pulmonary trunk
- Left pulmonary veins
- Auricle of left atrium
- Left ventricle
- Apex of heart

FIGURE 1.7 Internal Anatomy of the Heart, Frontal View

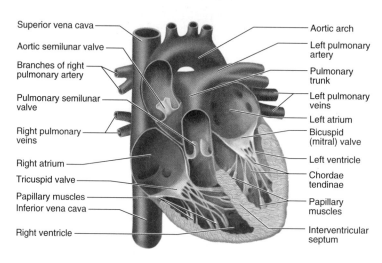

- Superior vena cava
- Aortic semilunar valve
- Branches of right pulmonary artery
- Pulmonary semilunar valve
- Right pulmonary veins
- Right atrium
- Tricuspid valve
- Papillary muscles
- Inferior vena cava
- Right ventricle
- Aortic arch
- Left pulmonary artery
- Pulmonary trunk
- Left pulmonary veins
- Left atrium
- Bicuspid (mitral) valve
- Left ventricle
- Chordae tendinae
- Papillary muscles
- Interventricular septum

TABLE 1.8 Medical Terms Related to the Cardiovascular System

Term	Definition
Angina	Severe pain around the heart
Aneurysm	Abnormal dilation of a blood vessel
Angioplasty	Mechanical widening of a narrowed blood vessel
Aorta	Major blood vessel from the heart to the body
Arteriosclerosis	Thickening and hardening of the walls of an artery
Atrium	Chambers where blood enters the right and left sides of the heart
Bradycardia	Slow heartbeat
Cardiogenic	Pertaining to the heart
Cardiomegaly	Enlargement of the heart
Cardiomyopathy	Disease of the heart muscle
Carditis	Inflammation of the heart

Term	Definition
Cyanosis	Bluing of the skin, lips, and mucous membranes caused by lack of oxygen
Edema	Abnormal swelling due to excessive fluid in the body tissue
Electrocardiogram (ECG or EKG)	Recording of the electrical signals of the heart
Hematoma	Mass of blood outside a vessel caused by a break in a blood vessel
Myocardium	Heart muscle
Pericardium	Saclike structure around the heart
Pulmonary circulation	Pertaining to the blood supply through the lungs
Vena cava	One of the two large veins bringing blood from the body to the heart
Ventricles	Chambers of the heart that pump blood out to the body or lungs

The primary purpose of the cardiovascular system is the circulation of blood and delivery of oxygen and other nutrients to the body. The heart pumps **deoxygenated blood** into the pulmonary system, where it becomes oxygenated and then returns to the heart. The heart then pumps the **oxygenated blood** away from the heart through the arteries, beginning with the aorta, to provide oxygen to the rest of the tissues in the body. Deoxygenated blood moves back toward the heart through the venous system and eventually into the right atrium, where the cycle begins again.

Coders should understand the flow of blood through the heart. Deoxygenated blood returns from the body through the superior and inferior vena cava, entering the right atrium. The atrium forces this blood into the right ventricle. The right ventricle pushes the blood into the pulmonary artery and then through the lungs, where the blood is oxygenated and returns to the left atrium of the heart. After moving from the left atrium to the left ventricle, blood is forced from the heart and circulates through the arterial system (Figure 1.8), beginning with the aorta. When the blood gets to the smallest arteries, it travels through capillaries and the oxygen is transferred to body tissues and organs. The blood then moves into the venous system (Figure 1.9), returning to the right side of the heart.

deoxygenated blood
Blood that has released its oxygen and is returning to the pulmonary system to be oxygenated.

oxygenated blood
Blood that has received oxygen from the pulmonary system and is pumped back into the body.

CODER'S TIP

Most editions of the Current Procedural Terminology (CPT) manual and ICD-9-CM manual include illustrations of the flow of blood through the heart. Coders should locate this information in their own manuals for future use.

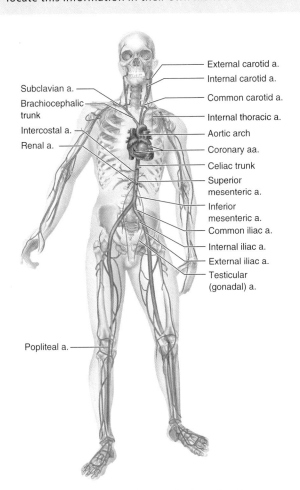

FIGURE 1.8 The Major Systemic Arteries (a. = artery; aa. = arteries)

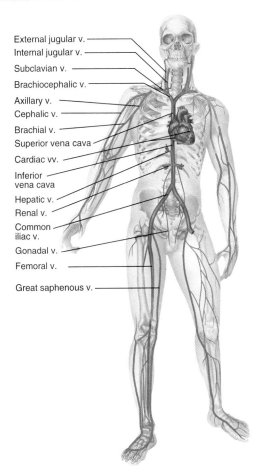

FIGURE 1.9 The Major Systemic Veins (v. = vein; vv. = veins)

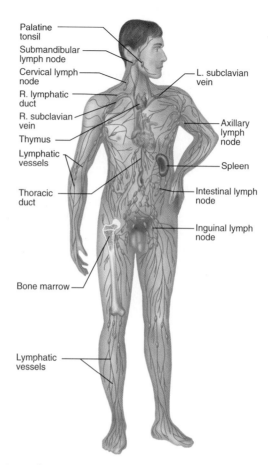

Palatine tonsil
Submandibular lymph node
Cervical lymph node
R. lymphatic duct
R. subclavian vein
Thymus
Lymphatic vessels
Thoracic duct
Bone marrow
Lymphatic vessels

L. subclavian vein
Axillary lymph node
Spleen
Intestinal lymph node
Inguinal lymph node

FIGURE 1.10 The Lymphatic System (R. = right; L. = left)

Lymphatic System

lymphatic system
Network of vessels and nodes that aid in fighting infection.

The **lymphatic system** (Figure 1.10) is made up of lymphatic vessels and nodes. The lymphatic system collects excess interstitial fluid and returns it to the heart. It also aids in fighting infections. This system operates without a pump by using a series of valves to ensure that the fluid travels in one direction back to the heart. Table 1.9 provides a list of common medical terms related to the lymphatic system.

TABLE 1.9 Medical Terms Related to the Lymphatic System

Term	Definition
Adenoid	Mass of lymphatic tissue in the midline at the back of the throat
Interstitial fluid	Fluid that is outside the vascular system between the cells of the body
Lymph	Clear fluid collected by the lymphatic system and returned to the heart
Lymphedema	Swelling of tissues due to obstruction of the lymphatic circulation

Term	Definition
Lymphoma	Neoplasm of lymphatic tissue
Node	A mass of tissue
Spleen	Lymphatic organ in the left upper quadrant of the abdomen
Splenectomy	Excision of the spleen
Tonsil	Mass of lymphatic tissue on either side of the throat

Respiratory System

The primary function of the **respiratory system** (Figures 1.11 and 1.12) is to exchange carbon dioxide and waste products for oxygen. During this exchange, oxygen is supplied to the body and carbon dioxide is expelled.

Structures of the respiratory system include the nose, pharynx, larynx, trachea, bronchi, bronchioles, and lungs. The right lung has three lobes (superior, middle, and inferior), whereas the left lung is divided into two lobes (superior and inferior). Table 1.10 provides a list of common medical terms related to the respiratory system.

respiratory system
Network of organs that take in oxygen and release carbon dioxide.

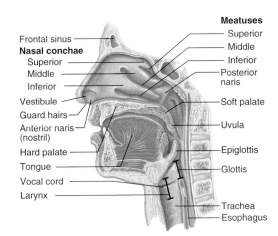

FIGURE 1.11 The Upper Respiratory Tract

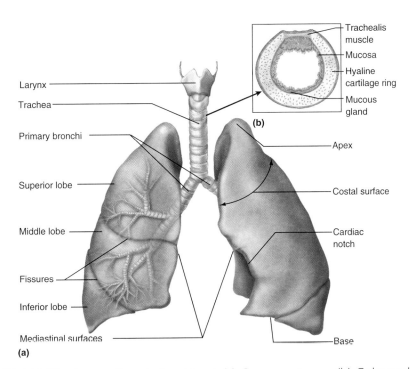

FIGURE 1.12 The Lower Respiratory Tract. (a) Gross anatomy; (b) C-shaped tracheal cartilage

TABLE 1.10 Medical Terms Related to the Respiratory System

Term	Definition
Apnea	Cessation of breathing
Asthma	Difficulty breathing due to constricted airways
Auscultation	Listening to sounds within the body
Cyanosis	Blue discoloration of skin and lips due to low oxygen (hypoxia)
Dyspnea	Difficulty breathing
Hemoptysis	Blood in the sputum
Hyperpnea	Rapid or excessive breathing
Hypoxia	Below normal levels of oxygen in the tissues or blood
Inspiration/Expiration	Breathing in and out
Larynx	Organ that produces vocal sounds and speech
Lobectomy	Surgical excision of a lobe of the lung
Orthopnea	Difficulty breathing unless sitting upright
Pharynx	Back of the throat
Pulmonary edema	Collection of fluid in the lungs
Rhinorrhea	Discharge from the nose
Tachypnea	Fast breathing
Thoracentesis	Removal of fluid from the lung via surgical puncture
Thoracotomy	Incision into the chest

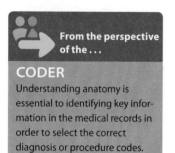

From the perspective of the . . .

CODER

Understanding anatomy is essential to identifying key information in the medical records in order to select the correct diagnosis or procedure codes.

digestive system
Network of organs that break down nutrients and remove food waste.

Digestive System

The **digestive system,** also known as the gastrointestinal system (Figure 1.13), includes a tubelike structure that starts at the mouth and ends at the anus. The back of the mouth is the pharynx, which empties into the esophagus. The esophagus runs through the thorax and joins the stomach. The pyloric sphincter separates the stomach from the small intestine. The small intestine is divided into thirds—the first portion is the duodenum, the second is the jejunum, and the third is the ileum. The cecum connects the ileum to the colon. The colon is comprised of several segments, including the ascending, transverse, descending, and sigmoid colon. The sigmoid colon connects to the rectum, and the digestive tract terminates at the anus. The digestive system also includes the accessory organs (mainly glands) that secrete fluids and enzymes into the digestive tract.

The major functions of the digestive system are to break down foods into basic elements, absorb nutrients to provide fuel, and eliminate waste from the body. Table 1.11 provides a list of common medical terms related to the digestive system.

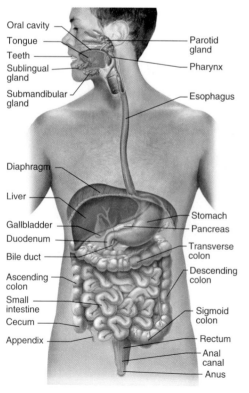

Oral cavity
Tongue
Teeth
Sublingual gland
Submandibular gland
Parotid gland
Pharynx
Esophagus
Diaphragm
Liver
Gallbladder
Duodenum
Bile duct
Ascending colon
Small intestine
Cecum
Appendix
Stomach
Pancreas
Transverse colon
Descending colon
Sigmoid colon
Rectum
Anal canal
Anus

FIGURE 1.13 The Digestive System

TABLE 1.11 Medical Terms Related to the Digestive System

Term	Definition	Term	Definition
Amylase	A digestive enzyme that aids in breaking down starch	Hepatitis	Inflammation of the liver
Ascites	Collection of fluid in the abdominal cavity	Ileum	Third part of the small intestine
Buccal	Pertaining to the cheek	Jaundice	Yellow appearance due to increased bilirubin and other elements
Cholecystectomy	Surgical excision of the gallbladder	Jejunum	Second part of the small intestine
Cholecystitis	Inflammation of the gallbladder	Lipase	A digestive enzyme that breaks down fats
Colectomy	Excision of part of the colon	Pancreatitis	Inflammation of the pancreas
Duodenum	First portion of the small intestine	Portal vein	Blood vessel from the intestines to the liver
Dysphagia	Difficulty in swallowing	Pyloris	The exit from the stomach to the duodenum
Emesis	Vomit	Rectocele	Hernia of part of the rectum into the vagina
Epigastric	Region around the stomach, upper part of the abdomen	Reflux	Backward flow (e.g., from the stomach back into the esophagus)
Gastralgia	Pain in the stomach	Splenomegaly	Enlarged spleen
Gastritis	Inflammation of the lining of the stomach	Stomatitis	Inflammation of the mouth
Hematemesis	Vomiting blood		

Urinary System

The **urinary system** (Figure 1.14) removes metabolic waste and maintains fluid and electrolyte balance within the body. The primary structures of the urinary system include the kidneys, ureters, urinary bladder, and urethra. Blood flows through the kidneys, which filter out waste and adjust fluid and electrolytes. Waste materials are discharged from the kidneys in urine that flows through the ureter to the bladder. Urine exits the body through the urethra. Table 1.12 provides a list of common medical terms related to the urinary system.

urinary system
Network of organs that remove waste from the body.

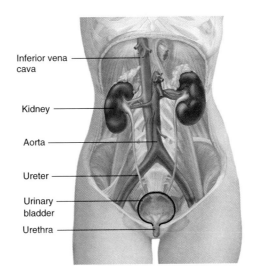

Inferior vena cava
Kidney
Aorta
Ureter
Urinary bladder
Urethra

FIGURE 1.14 The Urinary System

TABLE 1.12 | Medical Terms Related to the Urinary System

Term	Definition
Bacteriuria	Bacteria in the urine
Bladder	Hollow organ that holds urine
Cystectomy	Excision of the bladder or part of the bladder
Cystitis	Inflammation of the bladder
Cystocele	Hernia of the bladder
Dialysis	Artificially separating waste materials from the blood
Dysuria	Difficult or painful urination
Hematuria	Blood in the urine
Hydronephrosis	Dilation of the kidney pelvis and calyces
Incontinence	Inability to retain urine

Term	Definition
Kidney	Organ that removes waste from the blood system
Nephritis	Inflammation of the kidney
Polyuria	Excessive urination
Pyuria	Pus in the urine
Ureter	Tube connecting the kidney to the bladder
Ureteroplasty	Surgical repair of the ureter
Urethra	Tube that allows urine to leave the bladder and exit the body
Urethritis	Inflammation of the urethra
Wilms' tumor	Malignant tumor of the kidney that usually appears in childhood

Reproductive System

reproductive system
Network of organs that control reproduction.

The organs related to reproduction, or the **reproductive system,** differ by gender. Male external genitalia include the following structures: testes, epididymis, vas deferens, scrotum, and penis. Internal organs include the prostate gland, seminal vesicle, and Cowper's glands. Figure 1.15 shows the anatomy of the male reproductive system.

External genitalia for the female include the vulva, labia majora and minora, clitoris, external opening of the vagina, opening of the urethra, Skene's glands, and Bartholin's glands. Internal organs for the female genital system include the vagina, uterus, fallopian tubes, and ovaries. Figure 1.16 depicts the organs of the female reproductive system.

Table 1.13 provides a list of common medical terms related to the male and female reproductive systems.

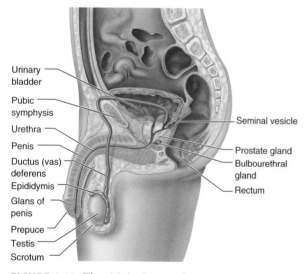

FIGURE 1.15 The Male Reproductive System

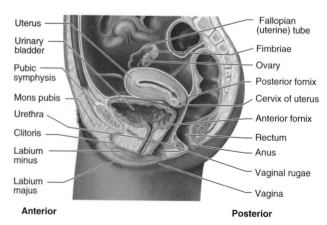

FIGURE 1.16 The Female Reproductive System

TABLE 1.13 Medical Terms Related to the Male and Female Reproductive Systems

Term	Definition
Amenorrhea	Absence of menstruation
Cervix	Lower portion of the uterus
Clitoris	Erectile organ of the vulva
Colporrhaphy	Suture of the vagina
Dysmenorrhea	Painful or difficult menstruation
Epididymis	Coiled tube attached to the testis
Fibroma	Fibrous tumor
Hypospadias	Urethral opening on the proximal ventral surface of the penis
Menorrhagia	Excessive blood flow during menstruation
Orchiectomy	Surgical excision of a testicle
Prostatitis	Inflammation of the prostate
Salpingectomy	Surgical excision of the fallopian tubes
Scrotum	External sac containing the testes
Torsion	Result of twisting
Vaginitis	Inflammation of the vagina
Varicocele	Varicose veins of the spermatic cord
Vas deferens	Tube through which sperm travel from epididymis to the urethra
Vasectomy	Removal of a segment of the vas deferens resulting in male sterility
Vulva	External female genitalia

Nervous System

The **nervous system** is composed of the central and peripheral nervous systems. The brain (Figure 1.17) and spinal cord (Figure 1.18) make up the central nervous system (CNS). The peripheral nervous system (PNS) includes the cranial and spinal nerves. In many cases, parts of several spinal nerves combine to form the peripheral nerves.

nervous system
Network that functions as the regulator and central intelligence of the body.

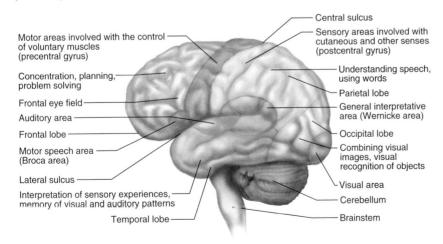

FIGURE 1.17 The Cerebral Cortex, Functional Regions

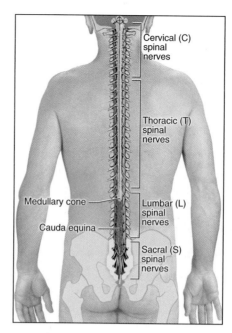

FIGURE 1.18 The Regions of the Spinal Cord

The nervous system functions as the regulator and central intelligence of the body. It regulates bodily functions, and it provides for an internal method of communication between the brain and other organs, as well as between the organism and the environment. Peripheral nerves connect the central nervous system to muscles to initiate and control movement. The nervous system also regulates involuntary body functions such as heart rate, respiration, body temperature, and peristalsis of the intestines. Table 1.14 provides a list of common medical terms related to the nervous system.

TABLE 1.14 Medical Terms Related to the Nervous System

Term	Definition	Term	Definition
Autonomic	Involuntary self-governing peripheral nervous system	Occipital lobe	Posterior portion of the cerebral hemispheres
Craniectomy	Removal of a part of the skull	Paraplegia	Paralysis of both lower extremities
Craniotomy	Surgical incision into the skull	Parasympathetic	Part of the autonomic nervous system
Dysphasia	Speech impairment	Parietal lobe	Area of the brain under the parietal bone
Epilepsy	Seizure disorder	Psychosis	Abnormal condition of the mind
Frontal lobe	Area of the brain behind the frontal bone, forehead	Quadriplegia	Paralysis of all four extremities
Hemiparesis	Weakness on one side of the body	Radiculitis	Inflammation of the spinal nerve roots
Meningitis	Infection of the brain	Sensory nerves	Nerves that carry sensory information from the body to the brain
Motor nerves	Nerves that send information from the brain to the muscles and glands	Sympathetic	Part of the autonomic nervous system
Myelitis	Inflammation of the spinal cord	Temporal lobe	Portion of the brain behind the temporal bone
Neuralgia	Pain in the nerve		

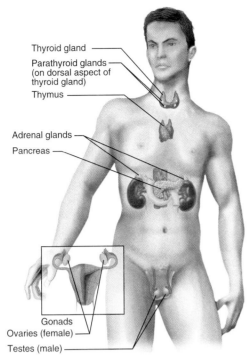

FIGURE 1.19 Major Endocrine Glands

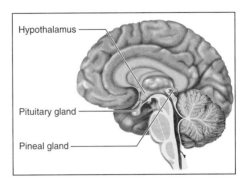

FIGURE 1.20 Hypothalamus, Pituitary Gland, and Pineal Gland

Endocrine System

The **endocrine system** is comprised of glands (Figure 1.19) that secrete or excrete chemicals called hormones. These hormones elicit an effect on tissues other than the glands that secrete them. Each gland and its associated hormone have a cause and effect that is unique. The major endocrine glands include the hypothalamus, pituitary, pineal (Figure 1.20), thyroid, parathyroids, thymus, adrenals, pancreas, ovaries, and testes. Table 1.15 provides a list of common medical terms related to the endocrine system.

endocrine system
Network of glands that secrete or excrete chemicals called hormones.

TABLE 1.15 Medical Terms Related to the Endocrine System

Term	Definition
Adrenal gland	Gland attached to the upper part of the kidneys
Antidiuretic	A substance that decreases urine production
Diabetes	Disease that causes poor control of blood sugar levels
Euthyroid	Normal thyroid gland activity
Hyperkalemia	Excessive potassium in the blood
Hyperthyroidism	Excessive secretion of the thyroid gland
Hypoglycemia	Abnormally low blood sugar level
Hypopituitarism	Deficiency of one or more pituitary hormones

Term	Definition
Hypothyroidism	Deficient secretion of the thyroid gland
Insulin	Hormone that regulates blood sugar levels
Ketoacidosis	Excessive ketone production, making the blood acidic
Pancreatic islet cells	Cells that secrete insulin and glucagon
Parathyroid	Gland located behind the thyroid gland
Pheochromocytoma	Adrenal gland abnormality that causes excessive catecholamine secretion
Thymitis	Inflammation of the thyroid gland
Thyroxine	One of the thyroid hormones

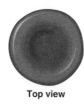
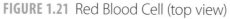

FIGURE 1.21 Red Blood Cell (top view)

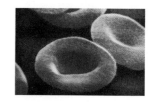

FIGURE 1.22 Red Blood Cells

Hemic System

hemic system
Network of blood vessels and blood cells.

The **hemic system** involves blood and blood cells, including:

- Red cells (Figures 1.21 and 1.22), which contain hemoglobin, a protein that delivers oxygen throughout the body.
- White cells, which provide defense against infection.
- Platelets, which assist in the clotting process.

Blood also includes plasma fluid and various proteins. Table 1.16 provides a list of common medical terms related to the hemic system.

TABLE 1.16 Medical Terms Related to the Hemic System

Term	Definition
Albumin	One of the proteins in the blood
Anemia	A reduction in the number of circulating red blood cells
Erythrocyte	Red blood cell
Hematocrit	Blood test that measures the volume of blood made up of red blood cells when they are separated from the plasma using a centrifuge
Hematopoietic	Pertaining to the making of red blood cells
Hemoglobin	The component of red blood cells that carries oxygen to the tissues
Hemolysis	Destruction of red blood cells
Hemostasis	Control of bleeding
Hyperglycemia	Excessive amount of sugar in the blood
Hypoxia	Lower than normal oxygen levels in the blood and tissues
Leukemia	Overproduction of leukocytes that results in a malignant state
Leukocyte	White blood cell
Oxyhemoglobin	Hemoglobin combined with oxygen
Plasma	Main fluid component of blood
Polycythemia	Too many red blood cells
Splenectomy	Surgical removal of the spleen
Septicemia	Pathogenic bacteria in the blood
Thrombosis	Blood clot

Also available in McGraw Hill **connect** plus+

Identify the body system to which each of the following anatomical structures belongs.

1. Aorta _____
2. Large intestine _____
3. Adrenal gland _____
4. Axillary lymph nodes _____
5. Bladder _____
6. Trachea _____
7. Ureters _____
8. Pharynx _____
9. Right ventricle _____
10. Fallopian tube _____
11. Ovary _____
12. Occipital lobe _____
13. Blood _____
14. Hormones _____
15. Spinous process _____
16. Seminal vesicles _____
17. Kidneys _____
18. Cerebral cortex _____
19. Hair _____
20. Pineal gland _____

1.4 ICD-10-CM and Medical Terminology

In 2013, the U.S. healthcare system will undergo major changes as it converts from the use of the International Classification of Diseases, 9th Revision, Clinical Modification (**ICD-9-CM**) to the significantly more robust system of **ICD-10-CM**. The current ICD-9-CM system includes approximately 14,000 **diagnosis codes**. This will expand to more than 69,000 diagnosis codes under ICD-10-CM. Although ICD-10-CM is thought to have many advantages over the 30-year-old ICD-9-CM system, these changes will require significant effort on the part of everyone who uses diagnosis codes. All coders, from those just beginning their careers to those with decades of experience, will need to become familiar with an entirely new coding system.

Although the differences between these two coding systems will be discussed in more detail in Chapter 5 of this text, for the purposes of this chapter, it is necessary to understand how this change will impact the use of medical terminology. Coders will be expected to understand a more extensive set of medical terms for ICD-10-CM than is required for ICD-9-CM.

ICD-9-CM
Abbreviated title of *International Classification of Diseases, Ninth Revision, Clinical Modification.*

ICD-10-CM
Abbreviated title of *International Classification of Diseases, Tenth Revision, Clinical Modification.*

diagnosis code
Code that identifies a patient's diagnosed condition or other underlying factor in a healthcare encounter.

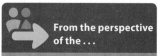

CODER'S TIP

There are 32 separate ICD-9-CM codes that describe femoral fractures. These codes contain approximately 10 specific medical terms that describe anatomical structures of the femur. Each of these terms is used in several of the femoral fracture codes. In contrast, ICD-10-CM describes femoral fractures in much more detail, including separate codes to describe each different fracture type and increased differentiation of fracture location. There are over 2,400 separate ICD-10-CM codes describing femoral fractures, in which 40 to 50 medical terms provide anatomical detail with greater specificity than the codes in ICD-9-CM.

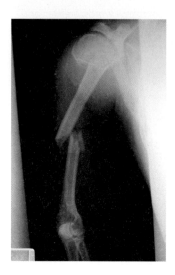

Using ICD-10-CM, coders will need to report greater specificity in diagnoses. For example, fractures will need to be classified by level of injury.

During the transition to ICD-10-CM, coders will have to learn a completely new coding system while also becoming familiar with many more medical terms. Under ICD-9-CM, it is only necessary to use medical terms to the specificity that the codes themselves require. In the femoral fracture example discussed in this section's Coder's Tip, under ICD-9-CM it is only necessary to ascertain that the injury is an open fracture. Under ICD-10-CM, however, open fractures are classified according to a system that divides those fractures into five separate levels, depending on the degree of injury. Coders will need to be able to evaluate those injuries based on the medical terminology included in the medical records.

EXERCISE 1.4   *Also available in*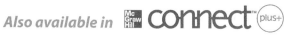

Insert the word or words that best complete(s) the following sentences.

1. ICD-9-CM will be used until _____.

2. ICD-10-CM will include over _____
diagnosis codes.

3. The use of more detailed medical terminology will allow diagnosis codes to describe conditions in much greater _____.

Summary

Learning Outcome	Key Concepts/Examples
1.1 Differentiate between word elements—including root words, prefixes, and suffixes—and how these elements are used to construct complex medical terms. **Pages 2–7**	Medical terms are constructed from word parts, including root words, prefixes, and suffixes. Root words are the basic building blocks of medical terms. Root words can be combined with other root words. When two root words are joined together, a combining vowel is used between them. Root words also may be joined to prefixes and suffixes. These word parts either provide more specific meanings to the root words or change the meaning of the root words to convey specific meanings.
1.2 Recognize and define commonly used eponyms, abbreviations, and acronyms. **Pages 7–9**	Medical terminology also includes eponyms, acronyms, and abbreviations. Eponyms are names of diseases or body parts that are derived from a person or place associated with that particular disease or body part. Acronyms are usually constructed by using the first initial of each word of a multiword medical term. An abbreviation is usually a shortened version of a single word. Certain abbreviations should never be used.
1.3 Identify anatomical structures and the systems to which they belong. **Pages 9–25**	Anatomy and physiology are very important to the selection of correct codes describing diagnoses or procedures. Both the ICD-9-CM manual of diagnoses and the CPT manual listing procedures are organized around body systems. Coders must be able to identify the organs involved when particular services are provided.
1.4 Describe how the adoption of ICD-10-CM in 2013 will affect the use of medical terminology. **Pages 25–26**	The ICD-9-CM diagnosis coding system will be replaced with the ICD-10-CM coding system in 2013. ICD-10-CM includes more than 69,000 diagnosis codes, many times the number of codes in the current ICD-9-CM system. The use of more detailed medical terminology allows diagnoses and conditions to be described with greater specificity than can be done with ICD-9-CM codes.

Using Terminology

Match the key terms with their definitions.

_____ **1.** L01.1 Word element

_____ **2.** L01.1 Root word

_____ **3.** L01.1 Prefix

_____ **4.** L01.1 Suffix

_____ **5.** L01.1 Combining form

_____ **6.** L01.1 Combining vowel

_____ **7.** L01.2 Eponym

_____ **8.** L01.2 Acronym

_____ **9.** L01.2 Abbreviation

_____ **10.** L01.3 Anatomical system

_____ **11.** L01.3 Organs

A. Adding a combining vowel to a root word

B. Describes anatomical disorders or physiological malfunction

C. Parts of words that make up medical language

D. International Classification of Diseases, Tenth Revision, Clinical Modification

E. Attached to the beginning of a word to modify or alter its meaning

F. Usually indicates a procedure, condition, disorder, or disease and comes at the end of a word

G. Networks of organs that interact with one another

H. An *o* or *i* added to a root or base word to facilitate pronunciation

I. Structures that have specific functions within the body

_____ **12.** L01.3 Glands

_____ **13.** L01.4 ICD-10-CM

_____ **14.** L01.4 Diagnosis codes

J. Identifies the person responsible for discovering the disease, structure, or procedure

K. Consists of the beginning letters of a multiword term

L. Shortened form of a commonly used word

M. Secrete substances that act elsewhere in the body

N. Contains the basic meaning of the word

Checking Your Understanding

Select the answer that best completes the statement or answers the question.

1. L01.1 Which of the following enable(s) the coder to define medical terms?

   a. Building up components
   b. Root words
   c. Anatomical structures
   d. Complex vocabulary

2. L01.1 Which of the following is true regarding a combining vowel?

   a. It joins a prefix, root word, and suffix.
   b. It is attached to the beginning of a word to modify or alter its meaning.
   c. It is always used to join the root word to the suffix.
   d. It is always used when two or more root words are joined.

3. L01.1 Which of the following is true regarding the suffix of a word?

   a. It indicates time or number.
   b. It often indicates a condition or disease.
   c. It is the base from which a definition grows.
   d. It always contains a combining vowel.

4. L01.1 Which of the following is true with regard to interpretation of a medical term?

   a. One should interpret each separate word part.
   b. The suffix defines the word.
   c. Prefixes are always interpreted.
   d. Repetition of certain words should be avoided.

5. L01.1 A coder need not be aware of which of the following when defining medical terms?

   a. Minor changes in a word's meaning
   b. Spelling and defining component parts
   c. Anatomical structures and functions
   d. Cellular biochemical reactions

6. L01.2 Which of the following is true of an eponym?

   a. Eponyms are made up of the beginning letters of a multiword term.
   b. Eponyms are a type of abbreviation.
   c. Eponyms are usually based on or derived from a person's name.
   d. Eponyms are not commonly used in medical terminology.

7. L01.2 Which of the following is true of acronyms and abbreviations?

    a. They are used in both written and oral communication.
    b. They are never misinterpreted.
    c. You can make up your own short version.
    d. They are not used very often in healthcare.

8. L01.2 Which of the following is an eponym?

    a. Q.I.D.
    b. MS
    c. Lou Gehrig
    d. I.U.

9. L01.2 Which of the following is a medical abbreviation?

    a. NAFTA
    b. WHO
    c. CABG
    d. TANF

10. L01.3 Which of the following topics is absolutely necessary for coders to understand?

    a. Basic physiological functions of organ systems
    b. Eponyms and abbreviations
    c. The relationships between anatomical structures
    d. All of the above

11. L01.3 Which of the following is true regarding organ systems?

    a. They are groups of organs that work together to perform complex functions.
    b. The study of anatomy is divided into the study of specific systems.
    c. The relationships between anatomical structures almost never change.
    d. All of the above are true.

12. L01.3 The musculoskeletal system:

    a. Provides support and protection.
    b. Contains vital organs.
    c. Provides references for other anatomical structures.
    d. Generates hormones that affect organs.

13. L01.3 Coders should understand which of the following with regard to the flow of blood through the heart?

    a. Oxygenated blood returns from the body through the superior and inferior vena cava.
    b. The left ventricle pushes the blood into the pulmonary artery, then through the lungs.
    c. The heart pumps deoxygenated blood into the pulmonary system, where it becomes oxygenated.
    d. The left ventricle pushes the blood into the pulmonary artery and then through the lungs.

14. L01.3 Which of the following is not true about the lymphatic system?

    a. It collects excess fluid from the interstitial space and returns it to the heart.
    b. Lymph contains white blood cells that fight infection.
    c. The lymphatic system is made up of lymph vessels and nodes.
    d. It aids in fighting infection.

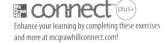

15. L01.3 The respiratory system's primary function is to:

    a. Fight infection.
    b. Warm the air.
    c. Exchange gases.
    d. Clean the air.

16. L01.3 Which of the following anatomical structures does the digestive system contain?

    a. Ancillary organs
    b. Waste
    c. Fluid and enzymes
    d. Gastric juices

17. L01.3 Which of the following structures is not a primary structure of the urinary system?

    a. Urethra
    b. Bladder
    c. Gallbladder
    d. Kidneys

18. L01.3 Which of the following statements describes how the urinary system functions?

    a. Urine is filtered by the kidneys.
    b. Blood is filtered by the kidneys.
    c. Electrolytes are eliminated by the kidneys.
    d. Urine flows from the bladder to the ureter.

19. L01.3 The male genitalia include which of the following?

    a. Ovaries
    b. Prostate gland
    c. Urinary bladder
    d. Skene's glands

20. L01.3 The female genitalia include which of the following?

    a. Thymus
    b. Vulva
    c. Abscess
    d. Bladder

21. L01.3 Which of the following is not true regarding the nervous system?

    a. The nervous system is comprised of the CNS and PNS.
    b. It regulates movement, but does not influence involuntary actions like heart rate or body temperature.
    c. It provides an internal method of communication.
    d. It regulates involuntary and voluntary body functions.

22. L01.3 Which of the following mechanisms of action is voluntary?

    a. Musculoskeletal
    b. Heart rate
    c. Blood pressure
    d. Respiration

23. L01.3 Which of the following is/are not part of the endocrine system?

a. Hormones
b. Hypothalamus
c. Pituitary gland
d. Kidney

24. L01.3 The hemic system contains which of the following structures and substances?

a. Red blood cells
b. Lymph
c. Bile
d. HCl

25. L01.3 Which of the following is the difference between anatomy and physiology?

a. Anatomy is the function and physiology is the structure of organ systems.
b. Anatomy includes visceral organs and physiology includes organ systems.
c. Anatomy is the structure and physiology is the function of organ systems.
d. Anatomy is the function of the body and physiology is electrochemical physics.

26. L01.4 A change from the ICD-9-CM to the ICD-10-CM coding system will impact medical terminology in which of the following ways?

a. The coding system will stay essentially the same with minor revisions.
b. Coders will be expected to understand a more extensive set of medical terms.
c. Reporting of codes will not require coding to the maximum degree of specificity.
d. Coders will not be required to read medical records as thoroughly as before.

27. L01.4 What main advantage will ICD-10-CM have over the existing ICD-9-CM coding system?

a. ICD-10-CM will be more specific and less vague or unclear.
b. ICD-10-CM will require more specific documentation by providers.
c. ICD-10-CM will require coders to understand anatomy and physiology.
d. ICD-10-CM will require coders to have a greater degree of clinical knowledge.

28. L01.4 What can be said about femoral fractures under the ICD-10-CM code system?

a. There are only 10 fracture codes.
b. There are about 2,400 fracture codes.
c. There are about 50 fracture codes.
d. There are 32 fracture codes.

29. L01.4 One benefit of ICD-10-CM's use of more detailed medical terminology is:

a. A more documentable diagnosis.
b. Less work for coders.
c. Greater specificity to describe conditions.
d. More work for physicians.

30. L01.4 How will diagnostic coding change in the near future?

a. The number of medical terms will be much greater.
b. There will be a heavier reliance upon anatomy and physiology.
c. There will be increased specificity.
d. All of these statements are true.

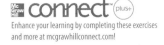
Enhance your learning by completing these exercises
and more at mcgrawhillconnect.com!

CHAPTER 1 | MEDICAL TERMINOLOGY, ANATOMY, AND PHYSIOLOGY   31

Applying Your Skills

Fill in the blank with the word(s) to complete each sentence.

1. L01.1 The basic building block of medical terms that can be combined to form other words is referred to as a(n) _____.

2. L01.1 _____ is the root word for the bladder.

3. L01.1 Words that are constructed from word parts, including root words, prefixes, and suffixes, are called _____.

4. L01.2 A disease, anatomical structure, and/or surgical procedure that is usually derived from the name of the scientist who discovered it is referred to as a(n) _____.

5. L01.2 Beginning letters of multiword terms that are commonly found within medical record documentation are _____.

6. L01.2 A short form of a commonly used word is called a(n) _____.

7. L01.2 _____ is the acronym for the administration of a medication twice per day.

8. L01.2 _____ is the abbreviation for calcium.

9. L01.2 _____ is an abbreviation for a fracture.

10. L01.1, L01.2 A recording of the electrical conductivity of the heart is called a(n) _____.

11. L01.3 A 56-year-old man with atherosclerotic heart disease has an enlarged heart known as _____.

12. L01.3 A child has infected and swollen tonsils needing to be removed by _____.

13. L01.3 A burn patient receives a foreign graft from another species known as a(n) _____.

14. L01.3 A cholecystectomy is removal of the _____.

15. L01.3 A patient with inflammation of the gallbladder is said to have _____.

16. L01.3 A menopausal woman with absence of menstrual flow is said to have _____.

17. L01.3 A cytotechnologist studies _____.

18. L01.3 A surgical operation to reduce the size of the nose is called _____.

19. L01.3 A slow heart rate is called _____.

20. L01.3 Inflammation of brain cells is called _____.

21. L01.3 An inflamed heart muscle is called _____.

22. L01.3 A 36-year-old female needs outpatient surgery of the abdomen called _____.

23. L01.3 A diabetic patient experiences low blood sugar, which is known as _____.

24. L01.3 A patient who has difficulty breathing is said to have _____,

25. L01.3 Inflammation of the stomach and intestines is referred to as _____.

26. L01.3 A patient undergoes eye surgery whereby an incision is made into the cornea called _____.

27. L01.3 The septum between the right and left ventricles of the heart is called the _____.

28. L01.3 Worn-out red blood cells turn into _____.

29. L01.3 A patient with traumatic brain injury and grand mal episodes is said to have _____.

30. L01.2, L01.4 A(n) _____ _____ of medical terminology will be more important after the U.S healthcare system converts from the ICD-9-CM to the ICD-10-CM and ICD-10-PCS coding systems in 2013.

Thinking It Through

Use your critical-thinking skills to answer the questions below.

1. L01.4 Identify several elements you must comprehensively understand in order to effectively code using the ICD-10-CM manual.

_____

_____

2. L01.4 Which factors do you need to consider when coding for diabetes?

_____

_____

3. L01.4 Identify relevant elements that coders should look for within the medical record.

_____

_____

4. L01.4 Identify a diagnosis for which the procedure is being performed. Using your knowledge of medical terminology, explain the relationship between the diagnosis and the procedure.

_____

_____

5. L01.4 What might be the complications of the following diseases?
   a. Diabetes mellitus (DM) _____
   b. Cerebrovascular accident (CVA) _____
   c. Atherosclerotic heart disease (ASHD) _____

6. L01.4 What might be the effects of the following diseases?
   a. Diabetes mellitus (DM) _____
   b. Cerebrovascular accident (CVA) _____
   c. Atherosclerotic heart disease (ASHD) _____

7. L01.4 What common question(s) do you need to ask yourself when coding for fractures using the ICD-10-CM coding manual?

_____

_____

8. L01.4 How would you educate a physician with regard to medical record documentation for ICD-10-CM?

_____

_____

Mc Graw Hill connect™ (plus+)

Enhance your learning by completing these exercises and more at mcgrawhillconnect.com!

CHAPTER 1 | MEDICAL TERMINOLOGY, ANATOMY, AND PHYSIOLOGY   33

ICD-9-CM AND ICD-10-CM

2 Introduction to ICD-9-CM

3 ICD-9-CM Chapter-Specific
Guidelines, Part I:
Chapters 1–10

4 ICD-9-CM Chapter-Specific
Guidelines, Part II:
Chapters 11–19

5 Introduction to
ICD-10-CM and
ICD-10-PCS

2 INTRODUCTION TO ICD-9-CM

Learning Outcomes *After completing this chapter, students should be able to:*

2.1 Explain the structure of the ICD-9-CM manual.

2.2 Describe how to use Volumes 1 and 2 to determine diagnosis codes.

2.3 Define the conventions in Volumes 1 and 2 that help coders identify correct diagnosis codes.

2.4 Discuss general outpatient coding principles to select appropriate diagnosis codes.

Key Terms

Alphabetic Index of Diseases (Volume 2)

Encounter

First-listed diagnosis

Hypertension Table

NEC (not elsewhere classifiable)

Neoplasm Table

NOS (not otherwise specified)

Principal diagnosis

Secondary diagnosis

Sign

Supplemental classification

Symptom

Table of Drugs and Chemicals

Tabular List of Diseases (Volume 1)

Visit

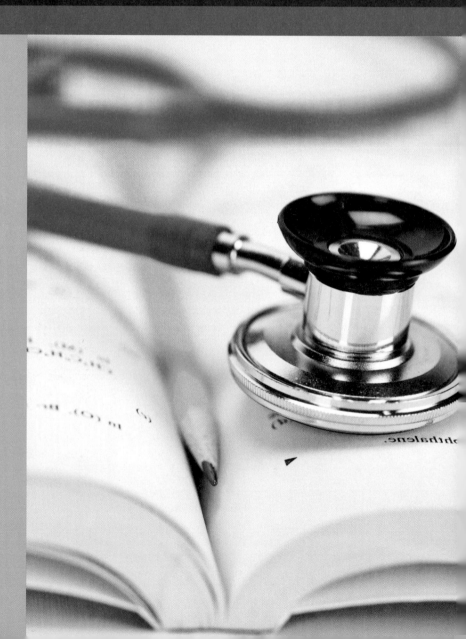

Introduction

Describing medical services completely requires the use of at least two out of three separate coding systems. Two coding systems—Current Procedural Terminology (CPT) and Healthcare Common Procedural Coding System (HCPCS)—describe the actual services provided and are discussed in later chapters of this book. A third system, the International Classification of Diseases, 9th Revision, Clinical Modification (ICD-9-CM or ICD-9), describes the reasons those services were provided. These three coding systems can be thought of as the "what" and the "why" regarding the services provided.

The ICD-9-CM coding system is based on the official version of the World Health Organization's (WHO) ninth revision of the International Classification of Diseases (ICD-9). The World Health Organization no longer maintains ICD-9, publishing instead the ICD-10. Two federal agencies—the National Center for Health Statistics and the Centers for Medicare and Medicaid Services—maintain ICD-9-CM through the ICD-9-CM Coordination and Maintenance Committee, which publishes annual updates of the ICD-9-CM manual in October of each year. These two entities are responsible for converting the ICD-9-CM coding system to two new systems, ICD-10-CM (Diagnoses) and ICD-10-PCS (Procedures), scheduled to begin on October 1, 2013.

Correct diagnosis coding facilitates payment for services, tracks disease and associated healthcare usage, advances research, and aids patient care. Diagnosis codes should be reported to the highest level of specificity known and accurately represent information in the medical record. It is important to review the medical record sufficiently to ascertain all the conditions treated. The ICD-9-CM diagnosis codes support the medical necessity of the treatments provided to the patient.

Reporting diagnosis codes will change significantly in 2013 when the ICD-10-CM code set replaces the ICD-9-CM codes. ICD-10-CM will be discussed in detail in Chapter 5. Some instructors may choose to teach ICD-9-CM and ICD-10-CM together, whereas others may separate the two. To accommodate multiple approaches to learning the current coding system as well as the future codes, exercises in Chapters 3 and 4 will include answers for both.

CODER'S TIP

Many payers have claim edits in their adjudication (claims processing) systems that establish "diagnosis to procedure code" relationships to justify payments for the claimed procedure. Coders should be familiar with the specific requirements for each payer. When preparing a claim, review all diagnosis codes associated with the patient and visit to make sure that important information for reporting the particular service is not overlooked.

2.1 The Structure of the ICD-9-CM Manual

The ICD-9-CM code manual consists of three volumes. Volume 1 (Tabular List of Diseases) and Volume 2 (Alphabetic Index of Diseases) are used together to determine appropriate diagnosis codes. These codes are used to report diagnoses in all settings. Volume 3, which contains both a tabular and alphabetical list of procedure codes, is used by hospitals to identify procedures performed on patients in their facilities. Physicians and other professionals do not use Volume 3 to report procedures.

Each volume is divided into chapters, tables, or appendices. The chapters in Volume 1 cover codes describing specific diseases and conditions. Volume 2 includes several tables with information necessary to identify codes describing particular conditions. Chapters in Volume 3 describe procedures on specific body systems. Each of these is discussed in more detail below.

EXERCISE 2.1

Also available in McGraw Hill **connect** plus+

Use the ICD-9-CM manual to answer the following questions.

1. How many volumes are included in the ICD-9-CM manual? _____

2. Identify the volumes by name and number. _____

3. Which healthcare entities use the codes in Volume 3? _____

2.2 Using Volumes 1 and 2 to Determine Diagnosis Codes

Tabular List of Diseases (Volume 1)
Volume 1 of the ICD-9-CM manual, which covers codes describing specific diseases and conditions.

Alphabetic Index of Diseases (Volume 2)
Volume 2 of the ICD-9-CM manual, which includes several tables with information necessary to identify codes describing particular conditions.

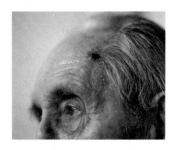

When assigning codes for neoplasms, begin with the Neoplasm Table that appears in Volume 2 of the ICD-9-CM manual.

Volume 1 is the **Tabular List of Diseases**. Volume 2 is the **Alphabetic Index of Diseases**. Coders use both volumes in tandem to determine correct diagnosis codes. When selecting a code to describe a diagnosis, coders actually use the Alphabetic Index in Volume 2 first to identify possible diagnosis codes, and then use the list of individual codes and their descriptors in Volume 1 to select the most appropriate code from among them. Because coders should always use the volumes in this order, Volume 2 is presented first, then Volume 1.

Volume 2: Alphabetic Index of Diseases

The Alphabetic Index of Diseases lists diseases, conditions, and injuries along with their accompanying codes. It is used as a guide in finding the correct codes. In most manuals, Volume 2 actually precedes Volume 1, and the two volumes are always used together to validate or refine the code selection. Volume 2 has three discrete sections:

• Section 1: Alphabetic Index to diseases, conditions and injuries. This section includes the **Hypertension Table** and **Neoplasm Table,** which coders use to select the correct codes to describe related conditions. Figure 2.1 shows an example of entries in the Alphabetic Index.

• Section 2: **Table of Drugs and Chemicals,** which includes an extensive list of drugs, industrial solvents, corrosive gases, noxious plants, pesticides, and other toxic agents. Coders use this table to identify poisonings and external causes of adverse affects.

• Section 3: Alphabetic Index to External Causes of Injury and Poisoning (E-codes), a list of codes and terms that describe environmental circumstances, such as accidents or acts of violence, and other conditions that may be the cause of injury or other adverse effects.

FIGURE 2.1 Example of Alphabetic Index Entries

C
Cacergasia 300.9
Cachexia 799.4
  cancerous - *see also* Neoplasm, by site,
     malignant 799.4
  cardiac - *see* Disease, heart
    dehydration 276.51
     with
       hypernatremia 276.0
       hyponatremia 276.1
  due to malnutrition 799.4
  exophthalmic 242.0 5th
  heart - *see* Disease, heart
  hypophyseal 253.2
  hypopituitary 253.2
  lead 984.9
    specified type of lead - *see* Table of
      Drugs and Chemicals
  malaria 084.9
  malignant *see also* Neoplasm, by site,
    malignant 799.4
  marsh 084.9
  nervous 300.5
  old age 797
  pachydermic - *see* Hypothyroidism
  paludal 084.9
  pituitary (postpartum) 253.2
  renal (*see also* Disease, renal) 593.9
  saturnine 984.9
    specified type of lead - *see* Table of
      Drugs and Chemicals
  senile 797
  Simmonds' (pituitary cachexia) 253.2
  splenica 289.59
  strumipriva (*see also* Hypothyroidism) 244.9
  tuberculous NEC (*see also* Tuberculosis)
    011.9 5th
Café au lait spots 709.09
Caffey's disease or syndrome (infantile
  cortical hyperostosis) 756.59
Caisson disease 993.3
Caked breast (puerperal, postpartum)
  676.2 5th
Cake kidney 753.3
Calabar swelling 125.2
Calcaneal spur 726.73
Calcaneoapophysitis 732.5
Calcaneonavicular bar 755.67
Calcareous - *see* condition
Calcicosis (occupational) 502
Calciferol (vitamin D) deficiency 268.9
  with
    osteomalacia 268.2
    rickets (*see also* Rickets) 268.0

Diagnosis codes that identify the main reason for the encounter should be listed first. When coding for professional services provided in the outpatient setting, the major diagnosis is usually referred to as the **first-listed diagnosis**. For hospital coding, the major diagnosis is often referred to as the **principal diagnosis**. Because this text primarily addresses outpatient coding, the main diagnosis will be referred to as the first-listed diagnosis. Additional or **secondary diagnosis** codes may be listed to identify other conditions that are present.

CODER'S TIP

It is imperative to use both Volumes 1 and 2 to determine the correct ICD-9-CM code. Always start with Volume 2. After finding codes in Volume 2 that may describe the condition, refer to those code sections in Volume 1 for critical guidance regarding the use of additional digits, alternative codes, or additional codes.

CODING EXAMPLE

A patient presents with a migraine headache. Turning to Volume 2, coders can look under "migraine" to find a list of four-digit codes ranging from 346.0 to 346.9 that describe different conditions associated with migraines. Each of these codes includes a symbol indicating that a fifth digit is necessary.

Volume 1 includes additional information regarding codes 346.0–346.9, including lists of conditions included under each code and specific excluded conditions. It is not possible to determine the correct code without reviewing these inclusions and exclusions, as well as the fifth digits necessary to completely describe the patient's condition.

Hypertension Table
A table containing a complete list of all conditions that are either due to or associated with hypertension.

Neoplasm Table
A table used to select correct codes for neoplasms.

Table of Drugs and Chemicals
A table that includes an extensive list of drugs, industrial solvents, corrosive gases, noxious plants, pesticides, and other toxic agents to identify poisonings and external causes of adverse effects.

first-listed diagnosis
The major diagnosis used to identify the main reason for outpatient or professional services.

principal diagnosis
The major diagnosis used to identify the main reason for the service when coding for the hospital.

secondary diagnosis
Additional diagnoses used to identify conditions that are present in addition to the major diagnosis.

Volume 1: Tabular List of Diseases

The Tabular List of Diseases (Volume 1) consists of three parts:

- Disease classification by **etiology** (cause) or anatomical (body) site
- Supplementary classification (V- and E-codes)
- Appendices

etiology
The origins and causes for the development of a disease.

Diseases are primarily classified by their causes or the anatomical sites affected by those diseases. This section of Volume 1 is divided into 17 individual chapters containing categories and subcategories of codes that describe diseases (see Table 2.1).

Each category is designated by three-digit codes. In most cases, this is not sufficient to accurately report the diagnosis or condition. Subcategories include codes with either a fourth character or fourth and fifth characters to identify the diagnosis in sufficient detail for reporting purposes. Figure 2.2 provides an example of entries in the Tabular List.

The second part of Volume 1 is comprised of Chapters 18 and 19. Codes in these chapters describe **supplemental classifications**, which provide additional information beyond the diagnosis codes, including:

supplemental classification
Additional information beyond the diagnosis codes used to fully describe the reason a patient encountered the healthcare system.

18. Supplementary Classification of Factors Influencing Health Status and Contact with Health Services (V01–V91)
19. Supplementary Classification of External Causes of Injury and Poisoning (E800–E999)

The use of V- and E-codes will be discussed in greater detail below.

TABLE 2.1 Tabular List Organization

Chapter Descriptive Title	Categories
1. Infectious and Parasitic Diseases	001–139
2. Neoplasms	140–239
3. Endocrine, Nutritional, and Metabolic Diseases and Immunity Disorders	240–279
4. Diseases of the Blood and Blood-Forming Organs	280–289
5. Mental Disorders	290–319
6. Diseases of the Nervous System and Sense Organs	320–389
7. Diseases of the Circulatory System	390–459
8. Diseases of the Respiratory System	460–519
9. Diseases of the Digestive System	520–579
10. Diseases of the Genitourinary System	580–629
11. Complications of Pregnancy, Childbirth, and the Puerperium	630–679
12. Diseases of the Skin and Subcutaneous Tissue	680–709
13. Diseases of the Musculoskeletal System and Connective Tissue	710–739
14. Congenital Anomalies	740–759
15. Certain Conditions Originating in the Perinatal Period	760–779
16. Symptoms, Signs, and Ill-Defined Conditions	780–799
17. Injury and Poisoning	800–999

FIGURE 2.2 Example of Tabular List Entries

4th 585 Chronic kidney disease (CKD)
  Includes Chronic uremia
  Code first *hypertensive chronic kidney disease, if applicable,*
    (403.00-403.91, 404.00-404.93)
  Use additional code to identify:
    kidney transplant status, if applicable (V42.0)
    manifestation as:
    uremic:
      neuropathy (357.4)
      pericarditis (420.0)
  585.1 Chronic kidney disease, Stage I
  585.2 Chronic kidney disease, Stage II (mild)
  585.3 Chronic kidney disease, Stage III (moderate)
  585.4 Chronic kidney disease, Stage IV (severe)
  585.5 Chronic kidney disease, Stage V%
    Excludes *chronic kidney disease, stage V requiring*
      chronic dialysis (585.6)
  585.6 End stage renal disease,
    Chronic kidney disease, stage V requiring chronic dialysis
  585.9 Chronic kidney disease, unspecified
    Chronic renal disease
    Chronic renal failure NOS
    Chronic renal insufficiency

The third part of Volume 1 includes four separate appendices:

- Appendix A: Morphology of Neoplasms
- Appendix C: Classification of Drugs by American Hospital Formulary Services List Number and Their ICD-9-CM Equivalents
- Appendix D: Classification of Industrial Accidents According to Agency
- Appendix E: List of Three-Digit Categories

Note that there is no Appendix B.

CODER'S TIP

Appendix B (The Glossary of Mental Disorders) was officially deleted on October 1, 2004, and is no longer included in the ICD-9-CM manual.

Volume 3: Tabular List and Alphabetic List for Procedure Codes

As mentioned earlier in this chapter, Volume 3 of the ICD-9-CM manual is used only in hospital settings. CPT codes are used to describe procedures reported by professionals. These will be discussed in great detail later in this book.

The approximately 4,000 codes in Volume 3 are divided into 17 chapters designated as 0 through 16. Each chapter contains one or more two-digit sections describing particular types of procedures. Specific procedure codes include either a third digit or third and fourth digits for specificity. In each Volume 3 code, there is a decimal after the second digit, and coders must code to the greatest level of specificity if more detailed information is available. The 17 chapters of Volume 3 include broad categories of procedures designated by one or more two-digit sections:

- 00 Procedures and Interventions, Not Elsewhere Classified
- 01–05 Operations on the Nervous System
- 06–07 Operations on the Endocrine System
- 08–16 Operations on the Eye
- 18–20 Operations on the Ear
- 21–29 Operations on the Nose, Mouth, and Pharynx
- 30–34 Operations on the Respiratory System
- 35–39 Operations on the Cardiovascular System
- 40–41 Operations on the Hemic and Lymphatic System
- 42–54 Operations on the Digestive System
- 55–59 Operations on the Urinary System
- 60–64 Operations on the Male Genital Organs
- 65–71 Operations on the Female Genital Organs
- 72–75 Obstetrical Procedures
- 76–84 Operations on the Musculoskeletal System
- 85–86 Operations on the Integumentary System
- 87–99 Miscellaneous Diagnostic and Therapeutic Procedures

Exercise 2.2

Also available in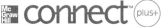

1. List the contents of Volume 2 of the ICD-9-CM manual. _____
2. Describe the structure of Volume 1 of the ICD-9-CM manual. _____
3. In general terms, describe the process that coders use to select the correct diagnosis code to describe the condition for which the patient encountered the healthcare system. _____

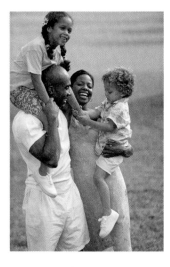

Some diagnosis or procedure codes are only appropriate for patients of a particular age or gender. When looking up the code for a condition, pay attention to the instructions listed for that code.

2.3 ICD-9-CM Conventions

The ICD-9-CM manual is constructed with conventions intended to guide coders when identifying diagnosis or procedure codes. Most editions of the manual include a guide to these conventions at the beginning of the manual. The most common conventions span a wide range:

- Abbreviations
- Punctuation
- Instructional notations
- "Use additional code" instruction
- "Code first underlying disease" instruction
- Update notations
- Additional digit specificity indicator
- Diagnosis code-specific color highlights
- Age conflict edits
- Sex conflict edits
- Hospital-acquired condition (HAC) indicators

These and other commonly encountered conventions are discussed on the following pages, including when coders are likely to encounter the use of these conventions in the ICD-9-CM manual.

Abbreviations

NEC (not elsewhere classifiable) identifies codes that are used when the available information indicates a specific diagnosis but the listed codes do not identify the specific condition present in that patient.

NOS (not otherwise specified) indicates codes that are used when there is not enough information to allow a specific diagnosis.

Punctuation

[ ] Brackets enclose synonyms, alternative wording, or explanatory phrases that may be useful in identifying the correct diagnosis codes associated with a condition. *Note:* Red brackets [ ] appear in some codes in the Tabular List of Diseases. As explained below, these have a different use than black brackets, and the two should not be confused.

[ ] Italic brackets indicate that a separate code included within the italicized brackets must be listed as an additional diagnosis code to indicate an associated manifestation.

( ) Parentheses indicate that the enclosed words may be either present or absent in the description of a condition without affecting the code used to designate that diagnosis.

: Colons are used after an incomplete term in the Tabular List of Diseases to indicate that one or more of the modifiers following the colon is necessary to assign that code.

Instructional Notations

Includes Conditions following this notation are included in that category.

Excludes Conditions following this notation are NOT described by that code, and other codes must be used to designate those conditions.

"Use Additional Code" Instruction

This instruction is included in the Tabular List when the code is insufficient on its own to describe the diagnosis and additional code(s) must be listed. When this instruction appears, the choices of the required additional codes appear in parentheses following the instruction.

"Code First Underlying Disease" Instruction

This instruction indicates that the code describes a manifestation that cannot be used as the first-listed diagnosis. A manifestation is a condition that results from the underlying disease. The code describing a manifestation cannot be sequenced before the underlying disease. This instruction only appears in the Tabular List and requires that the etiology or underlying disease must be listed first and the manifestation to which the instruction is attached listed secondarily.

CODER'S TIP

It is important that coders understand the difference between the "use additional code" and the "code first underlying disease" instructions. The "use additional code" instruction indicates that the selected code is not sufficient on its own to describe the first-listed diagnosis and other codes must be listed. Choices of additional codes are listed in parentheses following the instruction. However, the "code first underlying disease" instruction indicates that the code does not indicate a diagnosis. These codes cannot be the first-listed diagnosis. Instead these codes are listed as secondary diagnoses after the first-listed diagnosis.

NEC (not elsewhere classifiable)
Identifies codes that are used when the available information indicates a specific diagnosis, but the listed codes do not identify the specific condition present in that patient.

NOS (not otherwise specified)
Indicates codes that are used when there is not enough information to allow a specific diagnosis.

Update Notations

- • A bullet in the Tabular List indicates a new category, subcategory, or code.
- ▲ A triangle symbol in the Tabular List indicates that the category, subcategory, or code has been revised.

<u>Text</u> Newly added text is indicated with underlining.

~~Text~~ Newly deleted text is indicated with strikethrough.

Additional Digit Specificity Indicator

When a 4th or 5th symbol appears with three-digit or four-digit codes, an additional digit is necessary to designate a more specific code. In most cases, the specific codes with the additional necessary digits follow the code with the indicator.

In general, three-digit numbers identify categories of codes. In most cases, the three-digit number is not a specific diagnosis code. Most category numbers have an associated symbol indicating that a fourth digit is required to code correctly (see below for a complete discussion of required digits indicators). A few three-digit codes are sufficient to identify a specific disease and no "4th digit required" symbol is present. Four-digit numbers may identify a specific disease code or identify a subcategory of codes, each of which is identified with a five-digit code number. When a fifth digit is required, a "5th digit required" symbol is added to the four-digit subcategory number.

In some cases, multiple codes have common fourth or fifth digits to indicate the specificity required for correct code selection. In these instances, the common code designations are listed once in red at the beginning of the code section. Not all of the common code designations necessarily apply to every code in that section. When only some of the common code designations listed at the beginning of the code section are applicable, those that apply are listed in red parentheses (#) as a range or list of designations following the code.

Diagnosis Code–Specific Color Highlights

In some editions of the ICD-9-CM manual, certain diagnosis codes may include a color designation to indicate that the code cannot be used as the first-listed diagnosis. A code with a blue background describes a manifestation of an underlying disease, not the disease itself. A code with a red background describes circumstances that influence an individual's health but are not a current illness or injury. Codes with these backgrounds are not acceptable as the first-listed diagnosis.

Age Conflict Edits

Some diagnosis codes are only indicated for certain age ranges. In these cases, an age indicator is included with the code to specify the appropriate ages for that diagnosis. The age indicators include:

- • N (Newborn): 0 years of age, newborns and neonates only
- • P (Pediatric): 0–17 years of age
- • M (Maternity): 12–55 years of age
- • A (Adult): 15 years of age and older

Sex Conflict Edits

Some diagnosis or procedure codes are only indicated for one gender, either male or female. When this is the case, a gender symbol (male: ♂, female: ♀) is included with the code descriptor to indicate the appropriate gender.

Hospital-Acquired Condition (HAC) Indicator

Medicare and Medicaid are prohibited from paying for care provided to treat or correct some conditions that were not "present on admission" to the hospital. Diagnoses with the

HAC indicator (an "H" printed on a light-blue background in most ICD-9-CM manuals) are not considered secondary diagnoses for purposes of hospital payments unless that condition is coded as having been present when the patient was admitted to the hospital.

"Other" and "Unspecified" Codes

"Other" or "other specified" diagnosis codes are often indicated with an 8 as the fourth digit or 9 as the fifth digit. These are used when the information in the record provides enough information to indicate what the specific diagnosis is, but a separate code describing that diagnosis does not exist. The use of NEC in the index indicates that the condition should be designated with an "other" code.

"Unspecified" diagnosis codes are usually indicated with a 9 as the fourth digit or 0 as the fifth digit. These codes are used when the information available is insufficient to determine the exact diagnosis.

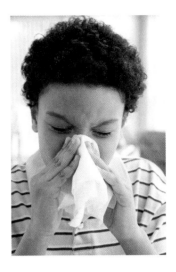

"See" and "See Also" Instructions

The "see" instruction indicates that another term should be utilized to identify the correct diagnosis code. Coders should refer to the term identified in the "see" instruction before choosing a diagnosis code to describe the condition.

The "see also" instruction indicates that another term may be referenced for additional information, but it is not necessary to do so. This means that the term that includes the "see also" instruction may be used as the correct diagnosis.

If clinical documentation indicates a specific diagnosis, do not report codes for associated signs or symptoms. However, signs or symptoms can be assigned codes if there is no specific diagnosis, or if they are not associated with the diagnosis.

Signs and Symptoms

ICD-9-CM diagnosis codes that describe **signs** and **symptoms**, rather than specific diseases, may be used as the first-listed diagnosis when a specific diagnosis has not been established for the patient. Many of the codes in Chapter 16 of ICD-9-CM Volume 1 (780.0–799.9) describe symptoms.

Signs and symptoms commonly associated with a specific reported diagnosis should not be listed as additional diagnosis codes. However, signs and symptoms not usually associated with a specific diagnosis may be listed if present.

sign
Objective evidence of disease.

symptom
Subjective manifestation of disease.

Combination Codes

A combination code is a single code that designates two diagnoses, a single diagnosis combined with one or more manifestations, or a single diagnosis with an associated complication. Individual codes should not be used when a combination code exists that accurately describes the patient's condition. Combination codes can be identified by the entries in the Alphabetic Index, or by referring to the inclusion and exclusion notes in the Tabular List.

Each of the 17 etiology and anatomical disease-specific chapters and the two supplemental classification chapters have specific guidance or instructions associated with them. These specific instructions will be covered in subsequent chapters of this book.

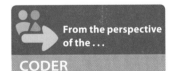

From the perspective of the . . .

CODER

To code accurately, it is important to understand the symbols and instructional notes located in the Tabular List found in Volume 1.

EXERCISE 2.3   *Also available in*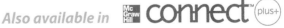

1. Define the meaning or use of the following common ICD-9-CM conventions:
   a. **Includes** _____
   b. **Excludes** _____
   c. [ ] _____
   d. ( ) _____

(Continued)

2. Distinguish between the "see" instruction and the "see also" instruction.
_____

3. Distinguish between the code definition of "other" and the meaning of "unspecified."
_____

4. When is it appropriate to assign a code that describes signs and symptoms?
_____

5. What does it mean when the instructional notes state, *"Code first underlying disease"*? Where in the ICD-9-CM manual is this instruction found?
_____

6. Describe the meaning of a combination code. _____

7. What do the symbols 4ᵗʰ and 5ᵗʰ indicate? _____

2.4 Outpatient Coding Principles

Outpatient coding includes reporting *professional* services provided in offices, outpatient hospital settings, and inpatient hospital settings. Hospitals also use outpatient codes to report hospital services provided in the outpatient setting. Hospitals do not use outpatient codes to report hospital services provided in the inpatient setting.

The major reason for a health system encounter or visit is reported as the first-listed condition. The terms "**encounter**" and "**visit**" generally mean the same thing and will be used interchangeably in this text. The first-listed condition is selected to the greatest degree of specificity that can be ascertained from the medical record.

A specific diagnosis may not be available after the first visit, but may be determined at a later date. When no specific diagnosis is documented in the medical record, codes describing signs and/or symptoms may be the first-listed condition. Many ICD-9-CM codes describing signs/symptoms are listed in Chapter 16 (Symptoms, Signs, and Ill-Defined Conditions). These will be discussed in greater detail in subsequent chapters.

For example, a patient may present with nonspecific signs or symptoms that do not allow a definitive diagnosis, even after a physical exam. In those cases, the manifestations of the disease (signs/symptoms) may be reported as the first-listed condition for that visit. If a more definitive diagnosis can be made after the results of lab tests are obtained, the more definitive diagnosis is reported as the first-listed condition on subsequent visits.

encounter
A patient's interaction with the healthcare system for a service or procedure.

visit
Term often used interchangeably with "encounter" to describe an interaction with the healthcare system for a service or procedure.

CODER'S TIP

At times it is not possible to determine a specific diagnosis from the medical records. For example, a patient may present with ecchymoses on his arms and legs. No specific cause could be determined and none is documented in the medical record. The first-listed condition is identified by the presenting signs/symptoms and is reported as 782.7 (spontaneous ecchymoses, petechiae). Lab work is ordered and the results come back several days later revealing a low platelet count.

When the patient returns for a follow-up visit, the first-listed condition is reported as 287.5 (thrombocytopenia, unspecified).

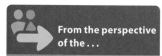

From the perspective of the . . .

CODER

To correctly report surgical procedures, it is necessary to know the reason (diagnosis) the surgeon performed the procedure.

If a patient undergoes outpatient surgery, the reason for the surgery is reported as the first-listed condition. This code is reported even if the surgery is subsequently canceled because of another condition or contraindication. The other condition may be reported as an additional diagnosis.

If a patient is admitted for observation of a medical condition, the medical condition for which the observation is occurring should be coded as the first-listed condition. When a patient undergoing outpatient surgery develops a complication that requires observation, the reason for the surgery should be reported as the first-listed condition, followed by codes for the complication necessitating the observation.

Diagnosis codes may have three, four, or five digits. Diagnosis codes must be reported to the greatest level of specificity that may be determined from the medical records. When fourth or fifth digits are necessary to accurately report a diagnosis, indicators are included to alert coders to this. Three-digit diagnosis codes cannot be reported as definitive diagnosis codes unless the three-digit code is not further subdivided. If fourth- and fifth-digit codes are available, they must be reported.

Some encounters occur for circumstances other than for the diagnosis and treatment of diseases or injuries. Those encounters are usually reported with codes from the Supplementary Classification of Factors Influencing Health Status and Contact with Health Services (V01–V91). These codes will be discussed in detail in Chapter 4.

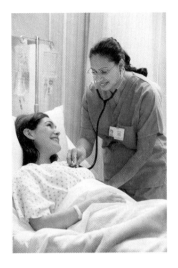

Codes listed in Volumes 1 and 2 of the ICD-9-CM manual are used to report the diagnoses associated with professional services provided in offices, outpatient hospital settings, inpatient hospital settings, and other healthcare settings.

Specific Guidelines for Coding Outpatient Encounters

If a patient receives only diagnostic services during an encounter or visit, the first-listed condition should be the medical diagnosis or condition for which the diagnostic services are performed. Other conditions may be reported with additional codes. V-codes may be used to report lab tests and/or radiological studies in the absence of specific diagnoses, signs, or symptoms. If the results of lab tests or radiological studies are known at the time of the encounter and the report of those results is available, codes identifying confirmed diagnoses should be reported. Codes describing signs and symptoms are not reported in addition to the definitive diagnosis codes.

If a patient receives only therapeutic services during an encounter, the code describing the diagnosis or condition for which the treatment is provided should be the first-listed condition. Codes identifying other conditions may be listed as additional diagnoses. The only exception to this instruction is when the primary reason for the visit is chemotherapy, radiation therapy, or rehabilitation, in which case the appropriate V-code is the first-listed diagnosis followed by the code identifying the underlying reasons for those treatments.

EXERCISE 2.4

Also available in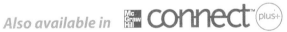

1. What is the major factor that determines which code should be identified as the first-listed condition? _____

2. What criteria are used to determine the first-listed condition if the medical record does not include a diagnosis for the visit? _____

3. If the patient currently has a condition that is not the reason for the visit or that is not causing the patient any difficulties at the time of the visit, are those conditions reported? If so, what codes are generally used to report those conditions? _____

4. If a patient is admitted for observation of a medical condition, what would be the first-listed diagnosis? _____

5. What would be the first-listed diagnosis code if a patient receives only diagnostic services during an encounter or visit? _____

6. Diagnosis codes must be reported to the _____ that can be determined from the medical records

7. The major reason for a health system encounter or visit is reported as the _____.

CHAPTER **2** REVIEW

Summary

Learning Outcome	Key Concepts/Examples
2.1 Explain the structure of the ICD-9-CM manual. **Pages 37–38**	The ICD-9-CM manual is divided into three volumes. Volume 1 is the Tabular List of Diseases. Volume 2 is the Alphabetic Index of Diseases. Volume 3 lists procedures reported by hospitals. The codes in Volume 3 are not used to report procedures on physician or outpatient claims.
2.2 Describe how to use Volumes 1 and 2 to determine diagnosis codes. **Pages 38–42**	Volumes 1 and 2 are used together to determine the correct diagnosis code(s) to describe any medical condition. Coders begin with Volume 2 to locate possible diagnosis codes in the Alphabetic Index. Volume 1 is then used to determine which of these codes is most appropriate to report the diagnosis. These codes are used to report the diagnoses of patients in any healthcare setting.
2.3 Define the conventions utilized in Volumes 1 and 2 that help coders identify correct diagnosis codes. **Pages 42–46**	Several conventions and notations are used in Volumes 1 and 2 to help coders determine the correct diagnosis codes, including abbreviations, punctuation, notations, and specific instructions regarding how a particular code may be used. Specific instructions list conditions that are included or excluded under a particular code. Indicators specify age limits, sex limits, and whether a third, fourth, or fifth digit is necessary to accurately report that condition.
2.4 Discuss general outpatient coding principles to select appropriate diagnosis codes. **Pages 46–47**	General guidelines are outlined to select diagnosis codes for reporting conditions in the outpatient setting, including professional services. The first-listed condition should identify the main reason the patient was seen. In most cases, this will identify a specific diagnosis. In some cases, a specific diagnosis is not known at the time the patient is seen, particularly on a first visit. In that case, codes identifying signs and/or symptoms may be reported as the first-listed condition. When the actual diagnosis is known, that is reported instead of codes describing signs or symptoms. When a patient undergoes outpatient surgery, the reason for the surgery is the first-listed condition, not the surgery itself. Sometimes patients encounter the healthcare system for reasons other than to diagnose or treat an underlying condition. These encounters are reported using codes in categories V01–V91.

Using Terminology

Match the key terms with their definitions:

_____ 1. L02.1 Tabular List of Diseases (Volume 1)
_____ 2. L02.1 Alphabetic Index of Diseases (Volume 2)
_____ 3. L02.1 Hypertension Table
_____ 4. L02.1 Neoplasm Table
_____ 5. L02.1 Table of Drugs and Chemicals
_____ 6. L02.1 First-listed diagnosis

A. Codes that provide additional information beyond diagnosis codes (e.g., V- and E-codes)
B. Not elsewhere classifiable
C. ICD-9 volume used to validate selection of diagnosis codes
D. List used to identify poisoning and external causes of adverse effects
E. Not otherwise specified
F. Outpatient/professional coding, major or primary diagnosis
G. Codes used to identify other conditions present

_____ **7.** L02.1 Principal diagnosis

_____ **8.** L02.1 Additional diagnosis

_____ **9.** L02.1 Supplemental classification

_____ **10.** L02.2 NEC

_____ **11.** L02.2 NOS

_____ **12.** L02.3 Sign

_____ **13.** L02.3 Symptom

_____ **14.** L02.3 Encounter

H. ICD-9 volume that lists diseases, conditions, etc., and acts as a guide to identifying a diagnosis code

I. Hospital coding, major or primary diagnosis

J. Term used to describe an outpatient service

K. Objective evidence of disease

L. Subjective manifestation of disease

M. Table used to identify diagnosis for a tumor

N. Table used to identify diagnosis for hypertensive chronic renal disease

Checking Your Understanding

Select the answer that best completes the statement or answers the question.

1. L02.1 Which volume of ICD-9 would be used first to identify the code for a patient with congestive heart failure?

a. Volume 1

b. Volume 2

c. Volume 3

d. CPT

2. L02.2 Which instruction indicates that another term should be utilized to identify the correct diagnosis?

a. See

b. See also

c. NEC

d. Includes

3. L02.1 Where is the Neoplasm Table located within the ICD-9 manual?

a. Appendices

b. Volume 3

c. Volume 1

d. Volume 2

4. L02.3 Which of the following should a coder use to assign a code when the outpatient medical record does not state a definitive diagnosis?

a. Signs and symptoms

b. "Probable" diagnosis

c. "Rule out" diagnosis

d. "Suspected" liver failure

5. L02.3 In which of the following settings would you use outpatient coding principles?

a. Physician office

b. Inpatient services

c. Hospital services

d. Skilled nursing facility

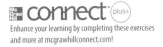

6. L02.3 A patient presented to the outpatient clinic with cough, chest congestion, and a fever. A chest x-ray was performed and a diagnosis of bronchitis was made. The first-listed diagnosis in this scenario would be which of the following?

   a. Cough

   b. Chest congestion

   c. Bronchitis

   d. Fever

7. L02.2 When looking up a code for abdominal pain in the Alphabetic Index of the ICD-9 manual, the 5th symbol appears next to the code for 789.0. What does this symbol indicate?

   a. The code has been deleted.

   b. The code is new.

   c. The code requires additional digit(s).

   d. The patient required moderate conscious sedation.

8. L02.2 Which convention means that the physician's documentation was not specific enough to give the diagnosis a more detailed code?

   a. NEC

   b. NOS

   c. Includes

   d. Excludes

9. L02.2 Which convention provides additional descriptions, terms, or phrases that are included in the description of the code?

   a. Brackets

   b. Parentheses

   c. Braces

   d. Colons

10. L02.1 ICD-9-CM codes identify:

   a. The "why" of a healthcare encounter.

   b. The "who" of a healthcare encounter.

   c. The "where" of a healthcare encounter.

   d. The "when" of a healthcare encounter.

11. L02.1 Which of the following qualifies as "medical necessity"?

   a. The procedure does not meet insurance payer criteria for coverage based upon the correct diagnostic code linkage.

   b. A preexisting condition was treated under HIPAA Administrative Simplification I.

   c. The provider was qualified to provide the service or treatment.

   d. The medical service can be substantiated based upon correct code linkage between procedure and diagnosis.

12. L02.3 Which of the following information is used to code from a physician's report?

   a. A definitive diagnosis

   b. Subjective reasons for the visit (symptoms)

   c. Objective reasons for the visit (signs)

   d. All of these

13. L02.1 Which of the following is another way to describe V-codes?

   a. Poisoning codes
   b. Adverse effect codes
   c. Supplemental classification codes
   d. Morphology codes

14. L02.2 Coding to the highest level of specificity for a disease means coding to which digit?

   a. Third digit
   b. Fourth digit
   c. Third, fourth, or fifth digit
   d. Always the fifth digit

15. L02.2 Where would the code describing a benign skin lesion on the back be found?

   a. Neoplasm Table
   b. Volume 1 (Tabular List)
   c. Volume 3
   d. HCPCS manual

16. L02.2 Which of the following statements is true?

   a. A coder may use the Alphabetic Index to assign a code.
   b. A coder should use the Tabular List first when searching for code assignment.
   c. A coder may only use the Alphabetic Index to Disease and Injuries when assigning a code.
   d. A coder must reference the Alphabetic Index and then assign a code from the Tabular List.

17. L02.2 Which fifth-digit subclassification is for use with code 550.1, bilateral inguinal hernia with obstruction, without mention of gangrene or recurrence?

   a. 0
   b. 1
   c. 2
   d. 3

18. L02.3 Which of the following would be the main term to look for in the Alphabetic Index (Volume 2) of the ICD-9-CM manual when the diagnosis is "congestive heart failure"?

   a. Congestive
   b. Heart
   c. Failure
   d. Disease

19. L02.1 Where in the ICD-9-CM manual can you find an extensive list of drugs, gases, pesticides, and other toxic agents used to identify poisonings and external causes of adverse effects?

   a. Alphabetic Index to External Causes of Injury and Poisoning
   b. Table of Drugs and Chemicals
   c. Volume 3
   d. Appendices

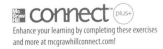

20. L02.1 Where in the ICD-9-CM manual would codes be found to describe environmental circumstances and conditions contributing to injury or other adverse effects?

    a. Index to External Causes of Injury and Poisoning (E-codes)
    b. Table of Drugs and Chemicals
    c. Volume 3
    d. Appendices

Applying Your Skills

Fill in the blank with the word(s) to complete each sentence.

1. L02.1 ICD-9-CM Volume 1 is also known as the _____.

2. L02.1 ICD-9-CM Volume 2 is also known as the _____.

3. L02.1 ICD-9-CM Volume 3 is also identified as the _____.

4. L02.1 Third-party payers look for diagnostic codes that are appropriately linked with their corresponding procedures in order to meet _____ _____ criteria for reimbursement.

5. L02.1 Agencies that make up the ICD-9-CM Coordination and Maintenance Committee are the _____ and _____.

6. L02.2 A coder would look up _____ as the main term in Volume 2 (Alphabetic Index) when a patient is seen in the office for migraine headaches.

7. L02.1 The three sections of Volume 2 are _____, _____, and _____.

8. L02.1 The three sections of Volume 1 are _____, _____, and _____.

9. L02.1 The code range used for diseases of the digestive system is _____.

10. L02.1 To report a congenital anomaly, the coder would use code range _____.

11. L02.2 In Volume 3, the decimal occurs after the _____ digit.

12. L02.2 A bullet next to a code in the Tabular Index indicates _____.

13. L02.2 An italic bracket next to a code indicates that a _____ must also be coded.

14. L02.2 The abbreviation for a hospital-acquired condition is _____.

15. L02.2 The age range included in the age indicator for maternity (M) is _____.

16. L02.2 The age range included in the age indicator for a newborn (N) is _____.

17. L02.3 If a patient undergoes outpatient surgery, the _____ is reported as the first-listed diagnosis.

18. L02.3 The _____ _____ instruction indicates that another term may be referenced for additional information.

19. L02.3 A patient's appointment for a service or procedure is referred to as an _____ or visit.

20. L02.3 When a patient's medical record states that the patient has a diagnosis of rapid heart rate, the main term the coder would look for in Volume 2 (Alphabetic Index to Diseases) is _____.

21. L02.3 If you do not know the definitive diagnosis at the time of the encounter or visit, it is permissible to code _____.

22. L02.3 When a surgery is canceled because of another condition or complication, the first-listed diagnosis is the
_____.

23. L02.3 If a patient undergoes surgery and develops a complication that requires observation, the first-listed diagnosis would be the _____ and the second code would be for the _____.

24. L02.3 During an encounter, a patient receives diagnostic services only. The first-listed diagnosis should be for the
_____.

25. L02.3 When reporting lab tests and radiological studies in the absence of a specific diagnosis or signs and symptoms, the coder may report a _____.

26. L02.3 When a patient receives only therapeutic services during an encounter, the code describing the diagnosis or condition for which the treatment is provided is the _____.

27. L02.1 The _____ diagnosis is defined as the reason the encounter occurred.

28. L02.2 The symbol that indicates that one or more modifiers of a diagnosis code follow is a _____.

29. L02.2 Conditions following the _____ notation are among the specific conditions described by that diagnosis code.

30. L02.2 Conditions following the _____ notation are among the specific conditions that are not described by that diagnosis code.

Thinking It Through

Use your critical-thinking skills to answer the questions below.

1. L02.1 How does a coder know that a code from Volume 1 or 2 requires a fourth or fifth digit?

_____

_____

2. L02.1, L02.2 Why are codes carried out to specific digits in certain cases?

_____

_____

3. L02.2 Explain the necessity for the designation of a hospital-acquired condition (HAC).

_____

_____

4. L02.2 Using Volume 2 of your ICD-9 manual, find and list an example of each of the following conventions: NEC, NOS, and Excludes.

_____

_____

5. L02.2 Using your ICD-9 manual, identify symbols for the following—revised code, new code, and deleted code.

_____

_____

connect plus+

Enhance your learning by completing these exercises
and more at mcgrawhillconnect.com!

CHAPTER 2 | INTRODUCTION TO ICD-9-CM   53

3 ICD-9-CM CHAPTER-SPECIFIC GUIDELINES, PART I: CHAPTERS 1–10

Learning Outcomes
After completing this chapter, students should be able to:

3.1 Identify the most appropriate diagnosis codes to report infectious and parasitic diseases; neoplasms; endocrine, nutritional, and metabolic diseases; and immune system disorders.

3.2 Recognize diagnosis codes for diseases of the blood and blood-forming organs,

mental disorders, and disorders of the nervous system and sense organs.

3.3 Name the correct diagnosis codes to describe diseases of the circulatory and respiratory systems.

3.4 List diagnosis codes for diseases of the digestive and genitourinary systems.

Key Terms
Asymptomatic HIV
Carcinoma in situ
Chronic kidney disease
End-stage renal disease (ESRD)
HIV-positive patient
HIV-related condition
Methicillin-resistant *Staphylococcus aureus* (MRSA)
Primary malignant tumor
Secondary diabetes
Secondary malignant tumor
Sepsis
Septic shock
Septicemia
Severe sepsis
Systemic inflammatory response syndrome (SIRS)
Type I diabetes
Type II diabetes

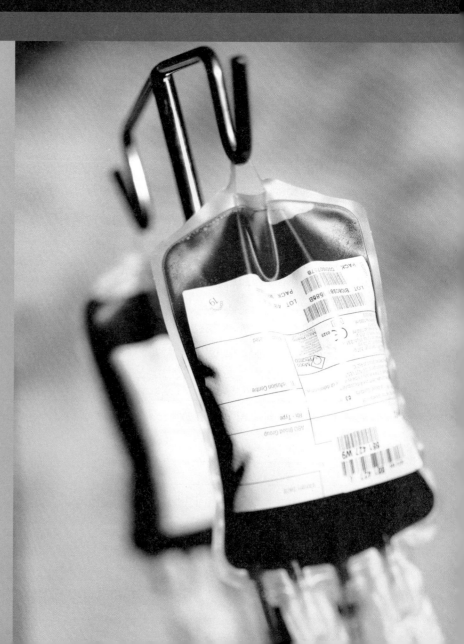

Introduction

Almost every chapter in the ICD-9-CM manual has associated chapter-specific guidelines with information applicable to that chapter. These guidelines indicate when a particular code requires additional consideration, specification, or replacement with a combination code.

This chapter includes the following ICD-9-CM chapters and categories:

- Infectious and Parasitic Diseases (001–139)
- Neoplasms (140–239)
- Endocrine, Nutritional, and Metabolic Diseases and Immunity Disorders (240–279)
- Diseases of the Blood and Blood-Forming Organs (280–289)
- Mental Disorders (290–319)
- Diseases of the Nervous System and Sense Organs (320–389)
- Diseases of the Circulatory System (390–459)
- Diseases of the Respiratory System (460–519)
- Diseases of the Digestive System (520–579)
- Diseases of the Genitourinary System (580–629)

Note that reporting diagnosis codes will change significantly in 2013, when the ICD-10-CM code set will replace the ICD-9-CM codes. ICD-10-CM is discussed in detail in Chapter 5 of this book.

3.1 Coding Diseases and Disorders, Chapters 1–3

Chapter 1: Infectious and Parasitic Diseases (001–139)

Chapter 1 of ICD-9-CM includes instructions on selecting and reporting diagnosis codes for several specific infections, examples of which are shown in Figures 3.1–3.3.

Human Immunodeficiency Virus (HIV) Infections HIV should only be listed as a diagnosis code in confirmed cases of HIV infection. If the patient is admitted for an **HIV-related condition,** the first-listed diagnosis should be reported as 042, followed by the codes for any related conditions.

HIV-related condition
A condition related to the presence of human immunodeficiency virus (HIV).

> **CODER'S TIP**
>
> Confirmation of HIV does not require documentation of positive serology. A statement from the provider that the patient is HIV positive or has an HIV-related illness is sufficient to report code 042 as the first-listed diagnosis or secondary diagnosis.

If an **HIV-positive patient** is admitted for reasons other than an HIV-related condition, that diagnosis code should be listed as the first-listed diagnosis, with diagnosis code 042 reported as a secondary diagnosis, along with codes for existing HIV-related conditions.

A patient with **asymptomatic HIV** infection is identified using the supplemental classification code V08. This code may be used for patients identified as "HIV positive," "known HIV," or similar statements as long as no HIV-related conditions are present. This code cannot be used to identify a patient with a diagnosis of AIDS, because that is not an asymptomatic condition.

HIV-positive patient
A patient diagnosed with human immunodeficiency virus (HIV).

asymptomatic HIV
An infection within HIV-positive patients with no HIV-related conditions present.

Septicemia, Systemic Inflammatory Response Syndrome, Sepsis, Severe Sepsis, and Septic Shock

septicemia
A systemic disease caused by the presence of bacteria in the bloodstream.

systemic inflammatory response syndrome (SIRS)
The systemic response to infection, burns, trauma, or other severe insult. Symptoms may include fever, tachycardia, tachypnea, and leukocytosis (elevated white blood cells).

sepsis
Systemic inflammatory response syndrome secondary to infection.

severe sepsis
Sepsis associated with acute organ dysfunction.

septic shock
Circulatory failure associated with severe sepsis.

methicillin-resistant *Staphylococcus aureus* **(MRSA)**
A strain of bacteria that is resistant to all penicillins.

Septicemia is a systemic disease caused by the presence of bacteria in the bloodstream.

Systemic inflammatory response syndrome (SIRS) is a systemic response to infection, burns, trauma, or other severe insult. Symptoms may include fever, tachycardia, tachypnea, and leukocytosis (elevated white blood cells). **Sepsis** refers to SIRS secondary to infection. **Severe sepsis** is associated with acute organ dysfunction. **Septic shock** refers to circulatory failure associated with severe sepsis.

Reporting SIRS requires the use of two codes, one to describe the underlying cause, such as infection or trauma, and the other a code from subcategory 995.9. The code describing the underlying etiology is always listed before subcategory 995.9.

Methicillin-Resistant *Staphylococcus aureus*

Infections due to **methicillin-resistant** *Staphylococcus aureus* **(MRSA)** are usually identified with ICD-9-CM code 041.12 (methicillin-resistant *Staphylococcus aureus*). Some MRSA infections are identified with specific combination codes that identify the type of infection and indicate that it is caused by MRSA. For example, septicemia due to MRSA is designated with code 038.12 (methicillin-resistant *Staphylococcus aureus* septicemia). Similarly, pneumonia due to MRSA is reported with code 482.42 (methicillin-resistant pneumonia due to *Staphylococcus aureus*). When the diagnosis code identifies MRSA as part of the code descriptor, code 041.12 is not reported as an additional code. If the underlying condition cannot be described with a combination code that identifies the presence of MRSA, the most specific code is listed as the first-listed diagnosis, with code 041.12 listed as an additional code.

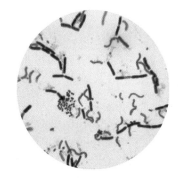

FIGURE 3.1 Bacteria Displayed by a Gram Stain

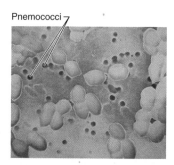

FIGURE 3.2 Spherical Bacteria of Pneumococcus

From the perspective of the . . .

CODER
It is important to understand both the causes and different manifestations of infectious diseases.

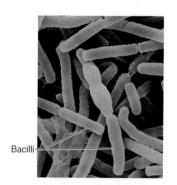

FIGURE 3.3 *Bacillus anthracis*

Using your ICD-9-CM manual, assign the correct code(s) for each diagnosis.

1. Amebic infection of the appendix _____

   (ICD-10-CM: _____)

2. Primary progressive tuberculosis with tuberculous pleurisy

   _____

   (ICD-10-CM: _____)

3. Listeriosis, septicemia due to meningitis

   _____

   (ICD-10-CM: _____)

4. Methicillin-resistant *Staphylococcus aureus* _____

   (ICD-10-CM: _____)

5. Whipple's disease _____

   (ICD-10-CM: _____)

6. Acute poliomyelitis _____

   (ICD-10-CM: _____)

7. *H. pylori* _____

   (ICD-10-CM: _____)

8. Human immunodeficiency virus (HIV) infection _____

   (ICD-10-CM: _____)

9. Coxsackie carditis, unspecified _____

   (ICD-10-CM: _____)

10. Trench fever _____

    (ICD-10-CM: _____)

Chapter 2: Neoplasms (140–239)

Chapter 2 contains ICD-9-CM diagnosis codes for all malignant and most benign tumors. Some benign tumors are included in chapters containing diagnosis codes based on the anatomical site of the disease. The code ranges included in this chapter contain diagnosis codes based on the type of tumor:

- 140–195   Primary malignant tumors except lymphatic and hemopoietic tumors
- 196–198   Secondary malignant tumors of specified sites
- 199   Malignant tumors without specific sites
- 200–208   Malignant tumors of lymphatic and hemopoietic tissues
- 209   Neuroendocrine tumors
- 210–229   Benign neoplasms
- 230–234   Carcinoma in situ
- 235–238   Neoplasms of uncertain behavior
- 239   Neoplasms of unspecified nature

The starting point for locating the correct code to describe neoplasms is the Neoplasm Table in Volume 2 (see Table 3.1). This table identifies tumors by anatomical site. Six diagnosis codes are listed for each anatomical site, corresponding to three types of malignant tumors (**primary malignant tumors, secondary malignant tumors,** and

primary malignant tumor
The original site of a tumor and the original tissue type.

secondary malignant tumor
A metastatic tumor or spread of a tumor from its original site to another location.

carcinoma in situ); benign tumors; tumors with uncertain behavior; and unspecified tumors. These codes are then located in the Tabular List of Diseases to verify the code selection and to ascertain whether there are codes describing the specific tumor. If the actual type of tumor is identified in the medical record, coders may look up the specific tumor in the Alphabetic Index for guidance to the correct code selection. Figures 3.4–3.6 provide visual examples of carcinomas.

TABLE 3.1 Excerpt from the Neoplasm Table

	Malignant					
	Primary	**Secondary**	**Carcinoma in situ**	**Benign**	**Uncertain Behavior**	**Unspecified**
Neoplasm						
breast (connective tissue) (female) (glandular tissue) (soft parts)	174.9	198.81	233.0	217	238.3	239.3
areola	174	198.81	233.0	217	238.3	239.3
male	175	198.81	233.0	217	238.3	239.3
axillary tail	174.6	198.81	233.0	217	238.3	239.3
central portion	174.1	198.81	233.0	217	238.3	239.3
contiguous sites	174.8			-		-
ectopic sites	174.8	198.81	233.0	217	238.3	239.3
inner	174.8	198.81	233.0	217	238.3	239.3
lower	174.8	198.81	233.0	217	238.3	239.3
lower-inner quadrant	174.3	198.81	233.0	217	238.3	239.3
lower-outer quadrant	174.5	198.81	233.0	217	238.3	239.3
male	175.9	198.81	233.0	217	238.3	239.3
areola	175.0	198.81	233.0	217	238.3	239.3
ectopic tissue	175.9	198.81	233.0	217	238.3	239.3
nipple	175	198.81	233	217	238.3	239.3
mastectomy site (skin)	173.5	198.2		-		
specified as breast tissue	174.8	198.81		-		-
midline	174.8	198.81	233.0	217	238.3	239.3
nipple	174	198.81	233.0	217	238.3	239.3
male	175	198.81	233.0	217	238.3	239.3
outer	174.8	198.81	233.0	217	238.3	239.3
skin	173.5	198.2	232.5	216.5	238.2	239.2
tail (axillary)	174.6	198.81	233.0	217	238.3	239.3
upper	174.8	198.81	233.0	217	238.3	239.3
upper-inner quadrant	174.2	198.81	233.0	217	238.3	239.3
upper-outer quadrant	174.4	198.81	233.0	217	238.3	239.3

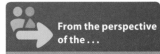

From the perspective of the . . .

If the treatment provided is directed at the tumor, the malignancy generally should be reported as the first-listed diagnosis. If the treatment is radiation therapy, chemotherapy, or immunotherapy, the first-listed diagnosis is reported as V58.0 (encounter for radiation therapy), V58.11 (encounter for antineoplastic chemotherapy), or V58.12 (encounter for antineoplastic immunotherapy), with the particular tumor as the secondary diagnosis. If complications occur during any of these therapies, diagnosis codes describing the complications are listed as additional secondary diagnoses.

If a patient's treatment involves surgical resection of a primary or secondary tumor followed by radiation, chemotherapy, or immunotherapy, the tumor should be identified with diagnosis codes from the 140–198 or 200–203 code series.

If the patient has a primary malignancy that has metastasized and the treatment is directed at the metastasis (secondary) site only, the secondary tumor should be listed as the first-listed diagnosis code, even if the primary tumor is still present.

If a primary tumor has been previously excised and is no longer present, diagnosis codes from the V10.0–V10.9 series (personal history of malignant neoplasm) should be used to identify the primary site of the tumor. Extensions or metastatic disease may be listed as secondary diagnoses. Alternatively, the secondary tumor may be listed as the first-listed diagnosis and the V10 code listed as a secondary diagnosis.

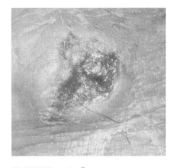

FIGURE 3.4 Squamous Cell Carcinoma

CODING EXAMPLE

A patient is diagnosed with a neoplasm of uncertain behavior of the central portion of the breast.

Using the Neoplasm Table, 238.3 is identified as the ICD-9 code. Before assigning this code, it is necessary to consult the Tabular Index to ensure there are no additional guidelines to follow.

	| Malignant |					
	Primary	Secondary	Carcinoma in situ	Benign	Uncertain Behavior	Unspecified
Neoplasm (_Continued_)						
breast (connective tissue) (female) (glandular tissue) (soft parts)	174.9	198.81	233.0	217	238.3	239.3
areola	174.0	198.81	233.0	217	238.3	239.3
axillary tail	174.6	198.81	233.0	217	238.3	239.3
central portion	174.1	198.81	233.0	217	238.3	239.3
contiguous sites	174.8			–		–
ectopic sites	174.8	198.81	233.0	217	238.3	239.3
inner	174.8	198.81	233.0	217	238.3	239.3
lower	174.8	198.81	233.0	217	238.3	239.3
lower-inner quadrant	174.3	198.81	233.0	217	238.3	239.3

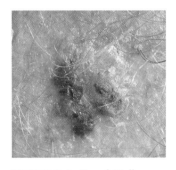

FIGURE 3.5 Basal Cell Carcinoma

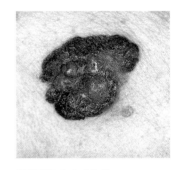

FIGURE 3.6 Malignant Melanoma

Using your ICD-9-CM manual, assign the correct code(s) for each diagnosis.

1. Malignant neoplasm, base of the tongue _____
   (ICD-10-CM: _____)
2. Breast cancer, site unspecified, estrogen receptor–negative _____
   (ICD-10-CM: _____)
3. Prostate cancer _____
   (ICD-10-CM: _____)
4. Cancer of the temporal lobe of the brain _____
   (ICD-10-CM: _____)
5. Benign carcinoid tumor of the ascending colon _____
   (ICD-10-CM: _____)
6. Benign neoplasm of the lip _____
   (ICD-10-CM: _____)
7. Hemangioma of the skin of the newborn's right arm _____
   (ICD-10-CM: _____)
8. Neoplasm of uncertain behavior of the trachea and lung _____
   (ICD-10-CM: _____)
9. Carcinoma in situ of the areola _____
   (ICD-10-CM: _____)
10. Neoplasm of uncertain behavior of the bone _____
    (ICD-10-CM: _____)

Chapter 3: Endocrine, Nutritional, and Metabolic Diseases and Immunity Disorders (240–279)

Although multiple endocrine, metabolic, and immunity disorders are included in this chapter, most of the instructions involve proper coding of diabetes. However, coders should be aware that many codes contain notations that the code **Excludes** certain diagnoses. Where this occurs, the description and code number of the excluded diagnosis is included to direct coders to the proper code.

Diabetes Mellitus Diabetes is identified with codes from the range of 250.0–250.9. Each of these codes requires a fifth digit to indicate whether the diagnosis is **type I diabetes** or **type II diabetes** and whether the diabetes is controlled, uncontrolled, or not specified as either. The fifth digits used with diagnosis codes designating diabetes are:

0—Type II or unspecified type, controlled or not identified as uncontrolled
1—Type I (juvenile type), controlled or not identified as uncontrolled
2—Type II or unspecified type, uncontrolled
3—Type I (juvenile type), uncontrolled

The 10 diagnosis codes included in the 250.0–250.9 range identify diabetes without complication and with specific complications, including:

- Ketoacidosis (250.1)
- Hyperosmolarity (250.2)

type I diabetes
Poor glucose utilization in the cell with juvenile onset.

type II diabetes
Insufficient glucose metabolism that typically begins in adulthood secondary to poor diet and obesity.

- Other causes of coma (250.3)
- Renal manifestations (250.4)
- Ophthalmic manifestations (250.5)
- Neurological manifestations (250.6)
- Peripheral circulatory disorders (250.7)
- Other specified manifestations (250.8)
- Unspecified complications (250.9)

Each of these complications requires one of the four fifth digits listed on page 60.

Many of the codes in category 250 identify specific manifestations with descriptions and diagnosis code numbers. The code(s) from category 250 are listed before the codes identifying the specific manifestations. When multiple specific manifestation codes describe the patient's condition, each is listed following the appropriate code from category 250. When multiple codes from category 250 describe the patient's condition, each is listed with the appropriate manifestation codes immediately following.

All patients with type I diabetes must use insulin to control blood sugar levels. The use of insulin, however, does not mean that the patient has type I diabetes, since some patients with type II diabetes require insulin because they cannot control their blood sugar levels with diet and oral medications alone. If a patient with type II diabetes uses insulin on a routine basis, V58.67 (long-term [current] use of insulin) should also be used as a secondary diagnosis code. The V58.67 code should not be used if insulin is used temporarily to bring a patient's blood sugar under control.

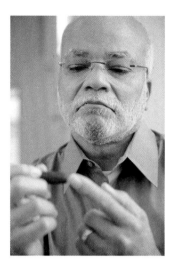

Coding for diabetes requires a careful look at the ICD-9-CM manual's guidelines and instructions.

CODING EXAMPLE

Identify the correct diagnosis codes to describe a patient with primary type II diabetes that is controlled with insulin and complicated by chronic kidney disease requiring dialysis and proliferative diabetic retinopathy.

250.40 Type II diabetes controlled with renal manifestations
585.6 Chronic kidney disease requiring dialysis
250.50 Type II diabetes controlled with ophthalmic manifestations
362.02 Proliferative diabetic retinopathy
V58.67 Long-term (current) use of insulin

Code 250.40 must be followed by code 585.6, and code 250.50 must be followed by code 362.02. The first code in each pair identifies diabetes with certain types of manifestations, and the second code identifies the specific manifestation.

The V-code is added because the patient has type II diabetes and uses insulin to control blood sugars. The V-code is not used to describe patients with type I diabetes controlled with insulin because all type I diabetics use insulin to control blood sugar levels.

Secondary Diabetes Mellitus **Secondary diabetes** mellitus is caused by another primary condition or event, such as cystic fibrosis, pancreatic cancer, pancreatectomy, adverse effects of drugs, or poisoning. Diagnosis codes 249.0–249.9 identify secondary diabetes without complications (249.0) or with specific manifestations (249.1–249.9). Each of these codes describes the same manifestations identified by corresponding category 250 codes. Each code includes a list of manifestations that are the same as those listed under the corresponding code in category 250. The rules for

secondary diabetes
A condition caused by another primary condition or event, such as cystic fibrosis, pancreatic cancer, pancreatectomy, adverse effects of drugs, or poisoning.

sequencing the secondary diabetes with manifestations codes and the specific codes describing those manifestations are the same as the rules for sequencing category 250 codes with the specific manifestation codes.

Each code from category 249 requires the use of a fifth digit, but for this category there are only two recognized digits:

0—Controlled or not identified as uncontrolled

1—Uncontrolled

When sequencing the codes describing secondary diabetes (including any associated manifestations) and codes identifying the cause of the secondary diabetes, the order depends on the reason for the encounter. If the patient is seen to treat the secondary diabetes or any of its manifestations, those codes are reported as the first-listed diagnosis. If the purpose of the encounter is to treat the underlying condition that caused the diabetes, that code is sequenced as the first-listed diagnosis; the secondary diabetes codes, along with codes describing manifestations, are listed as secondary diagnoses.

The V58.67 code (long-term [current] use of insulin) is listed as a secondary diagnosis code to identify patients with secondary diabetes who routinely use insulin to control their blood sugar levels.

EXERCISE 3.1.3

Also available in Mc Graw Hill **connect** (plus+)

Using your ICD-9-CM manual, assign the correct code(s) for each diagnosis.

1. Hypothyroidism _____

(ICD-10-CM: _____)

2. Dyshormonogenic goiter _____

(ICD-10-CM: _____)

3. Diabetes mellitus without mention of complications _____

(ICD-10-CM: _____)

4. Uncontrolled type II diabetes mellitus with unspecified complications _____

(ICD-10-CM: _____)

5. Hypoglycemic coma _____

(ICD-10-CM: _____)

6. Cushing's syndrome _____

(ICD-10-CM: _____)

7. Mineralocorticoid deficiency (hypoaldosteronism) _____

(ICD-10-CM: _____)

8. Other B-complex vitamin deficiency _____

(ICD-10-CM: _____)

9. Late effects of rickets _____

(ICD-10-CM: _____)

10. Vitamin A deficiency with night blindness _____

(ICD-10-CM: _____)

3.2 Coding Diseases and Disorders, Chapters 4–6

Chapter 4: Diseases of the Blood and Blood-Forming Organs (280–289)

Chapter 4 includes 10 code categories (280–289) that describe blood diseases:

- 280 Iron deficiency anemias
- 281 Other deficiency anemias
- 282 Hereditary hemolytic anemias (Figure 3.7)
- 283 Acquired hemolytic anemias
- 284 Aplastic anemia and other bone marrow failure syndromes
- 285 Other and unspecified anemias
- 286 Coagulation defects
- 287 Purpura and other hemorrhagic conditions
- 288 Diseases of white blood cells
- 289 Other diseases of blood and blood-forming organs

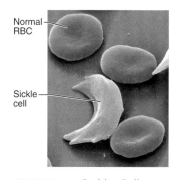

FIGURE 3.7 Sickle Cell Anemia

The only chapter-specific guidelines in Chapter 4 address the selection of codes in subcategory 285.2 (anemia in chronic illness), which includes three specific codes identified by a fifth digit to differentiate between anemia in chronic kidney disease (285.21), anemia in neoplastic disease (285.22), and anemia of other chronic disease (285.29). These codes may be used as the first-listed diagnosis if the reason for the encounter is to treat the anemia. These codes also may be listed as secondary diagnoses when treating the anemia is not the primary reason for the visit.

CODER'S TIP

Codes in category 285 can be used as either the first-listed diagnosis or as secondary diagnosis codes. It is important to refer to the guidance in this section to understand how to report these codes appropriately.

It is necessary to list the underlying cause of the anemia when a code from subcategory 285.2 is reported as the first-listed diagnosis or secondary diagnosis. When reporting code 285.21 (anemia in chronic kidney disease), it also is necessary to report a code from category 585. Similarly, when listing code 285.22 (anemia in neoplastic disease), it also is necessary to list the appropriate code to identify the underlying neoplasm causing the anemia. Code 285.22 is not used when the anemia is caused by the use of antineoplastic chemotherapy; code 285.3 identifies anemia caused by chemotherapy.

From the perspective of the . . .

CODER

Coders must pay attention to details when selecting the correct ICD-9-CM codes to describe a diagnosis or other condition. This will be even more important when ICD-10-CM is implemented in 2013, because selecting the correct code will require more specific anatomical descriptions.

EXERCISE 3.2.1

Also available in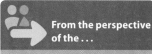

Using your ICD-9-CM manual, assign the correct code(s) for each diagnosis.

1. Pernicious anemia _____
   (ICD-10-CM: _____)

2. Anemia, unspecified _____
   (ICD-10-CM: _____)

(Continued)

3. Congenital factor IX deficiency (hemophilia C) _____

(ICD-10-CM: _____)

4. Anemia in chronic kidney disease _____

(ICD-10-CM: _____)

5. Basophilia _____

(ICD-10-CM: _____)

6. Primary hypercoagulable state _____

(ICD-10-CM: _____)

7. Chronic lymphadenitis _____

(ICD-10-CM: _____)

8. Bandemia _____

(ICD-10-CM: _____)

9. Von Willebrand's disease _____

(ICD-10-CM: _____)

10. Defibrination syndrome _____

(ICD-10-CM: _____)

Chapter 5: Mental Disorders (290–319)

There is no specific guidance regarding this series of codes. This chapter is divided into several subchapters, including:

- Psychoses (290–299)
- Neurotic Disorders, Personality Disorders, and Other Nonpsychotic Mental Disorders (300–316)
- Mental Retardation (317–319)

CODER'S TIP

The *Diagnostic and Statistical Manual of Mental Disorders,* Fourth Edition (DSM-IV), a coding manual of behavioral health diagnoses published by the American Psychiatric Association, provides greater clinical detail for behavioral health specialists. This manual also provides information regarding prognoses for specific diagnoses.

EXERCISE 3.2.2

Also available in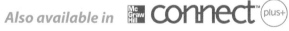

Using your ICD-9-CM manual, assign the correct code(s) for each diagnosis.

1. Alcohol-induced psychotic disorder with hallucinations _____

(ICD-10-CM: _____)

2. Subacute delirium _____

(ICD-10-CM: _____)

3. Anxiety disorder in conditions classified elsewhere _____

(ICD-10-CM: _____)

(Continued)

4. Catatonic schizophrenia _____

    (ICD-10-CM: _____)

5. Manic disorder, recurrent episode _____

    (ICD-10-CM: _____)

6. Major depressive disorder, single episode _____

    (ICD-10-CM: _____)

7. Psychosis, depressive type _____

    (ICD-10-CM: _____)

8. Panic attack _____

    (ICD-10-CM: _____)

9. Social phobia of public speaking _____

    (ICD-10-CM: _____)

10. Continuous opioid dependence _____

    (ICD-10-CM: _____)

Chapter 6: Diseases of the Nervous System and Sense Organs (320–389)

Chapter 6 is divided into subchapters, including:

- Inflammatory Diseases of the Central Nervous System (320–326)
- Organic Sleep Disorders (327)
- Hereditary and Degenerative Diseases of the Central Nervous System (330–337)
- Pain (338)
- Other Headache Syndromes (339)
- Other Disorders of the Central Nervous System (340–349)
- Disorders of the Peripheral Nervous System (350–359)
- Disorders of the Eye and Adnexa (360–379)
- Diseases of the Ear and Mastoid Process (380–389)

Many of these subchapters deal with the central nervous system. Figure 3.8 shows a cross section of the spinal cord, a crucial anatomical section of the nervous system.

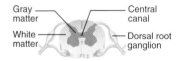

FIGURE 3.8 Cross Section of the Spinal Cord

Only category 338 (Pain) has specific guidelines. Unless specifically not permitted by the guidelines, codes from this category may be used with other diagnosis or condition codes to more fully describe acute pain, chronic pain, or pain related to tumors. To use a code from category 338, the pain must be designated as either acute or chronic. If the pain is not designated as acute or chronic, these codes can only be used to describe post-thoracotomy pain, postoperative pain, neoplasm-related pain, or central pain syndrome.

Category 338 codes may be used as the first-listed diagnosis condition code if pain control or pain management is the main reason for the visit. If the underlying cause of the pain is known, it should be reported as an additional code. Category 338 codes should not be reported if the treatment is for the underlying cause of the pain.

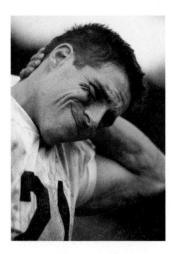

When assigning a code for pain, note whether it is acute or chronic, whether it is the main reason for the visit, and whether its cause is known.

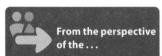

From the perspective of the . . .

CODER

Coders should fully understand when code 338.3 is reported as the first-listed diagnosis and when it is a secondary diagnosis. When code 338.3 is listed as a secondary diagnosis, it is important to correctly identify the neoplasm causing the pain as the first-listed diagnosis.

CODER'S TIP

Codes from category 338 may be reported as the first-listed condition if the main reason for the patient visit is to treat the pain. If the purpose of the visit is to treat the underlying cause of the pain, codes from 338 are not listed; instead diagnosis codes describing the cause of the pain are listed.

For example, if a patient with low back pain and radiculopathy due to a lumbar herniated nucleus pulposus (displaced intervertebral disk) is seen for a spinal steroid injection, the pain may be identified with diagnosis code 338.19 (other acute pain) as the first-listed condition. Diagnosis code 722.10 (displacement of lumbar intervertebral disk without myelopathy) may be listed as a secondary condition to identify the cause of the pain.

If a patient with low back pain and radiculopathy due to a lumbar herniated nucleus pulposus is admitted for surgery to decompress the herniated disk, a diagnosis code from category 338 is not listed. Rather, the reason for the surgical procedure (722.10) is listed as the first-listed condition.

Category 338 codes may be combined with codes from other chapters that identify the site of pain if the combination of codes provides information that neither code describes completely. This includes codes from Chapter 16 (Symptoms, Signs, and Ill-Defined Conditions) if they provide additional information. For example, if another code describes the site of pain but does not describe the pain as either acute or chronic, category 338 codes may be added to characterize the pain.

Subcategories 338.1 (acute pain) and 338.2 (chronic pain) require the use of a fifth digit to delineate the pain as due to trauma (fifth digit 1), post-thoracotomy pain (fifth digit 2), acute postoperative pain (fifth digit 8) or other pain (fifth digit 9). Each of these subcategories has specific exclusions identified by the **Excludes** notation.

If pain is due to a surgically placed device, implant, or graft, the appropriate code from Chapter 17 (Injury and Poisoning) should be listed as the principal diagnosis, with codes from category 338 listed as additional diagnoses.

Postoperative and post-thoracotomy pain may be described with subcategories 338.1 and 338.2, depending on whether the pain is acute or chronic. There is no specific time frame to determine whether the pain is chronic. Rather, documentation should be used to make that determination. These codes may be listed as the first-listed diagnosis if the purpose of the visit is to manage the pain. Otherwise, they may be listed as additional codes.

Code 338.3 describes pain due to either a primary or secondary malignancy. This code may be listed as the first-listed diagnosis if the purpose of the visit is to treat the pain. Diagnosis codes describing the underlying neoplasm may be listed as secondary diagnoses. If the purpose of the visit is to treat the neoplasm, with or without treatment of the associated pain, the neoplasm should be coded as the first-listed diagnosis, with code 338.3 listed as a secondary diagnosis. This code is used regardless of whether the pain related to the neoplasm is acute or chronic.

EXERCISE 3.2.3

Also available in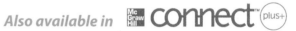

Using your ICD-9-CM manual, assign the correct code(s) for each diagnosis.

1. Meningitis due to mumps _____

   (ICD-10-CM: _____)

2. Other encephalitis due to malaria _____

   (ICD-10-CM: _____)

   (Continued)

3. Parkinson's disease _____

(ICD-10-CM: _____)

4. Schilder's disease _____

(ICD-10-CM: _____)

5. Grand mal epileptic seizure _____

(ICD-10-CM: _____)

6. Facial palsy/Bell's palsy _____

(ICD-10-CM: _____)

7. Polyneuropathy in vascular disease due to rheumatoid arthritis _____

(ICD-10-CM: _____)

8. Diabetic macular edema _____

(ICD-10-CM: _____)

9. Retinal dystrophy due to Bassen-Kornzweig syndrome _____

(ICD-10-CM: _____)

10. Cataract with neovascularization due to iridocyclitis _____

(ICD-10-CM: _____)

3.3 Coding Diseases, Chapters 7–8

Chapter 7: Diseases of the Circulatory System (390–459)

Chapter 7 is divided into a number of subchapters related to specific types of heart disease, including:

- Acute Rheumatic Fever (390–392)
- Chronic Rheumatic Heart Disease (393–398)
- Hypertensive Disease (401–405)
- Ischemic Heart Disease (410–414)
- Diseases of Pulmonary Circulation (415–417)
- Other Forms of Heart Disease (420–429)
- Cerebrovascular Disease (430–438)
- Diseases of Arteries, Arterioles, and Capillaries (440–449)
- Diseases of Veins and Lymphatics, and Other Diseases of Circulatory System (451–459)

Coding from many of these subchapters requires knowledge of circulation. Figure 3.9 provides a diagram of coronary arterial circulation for coders' reference.

Hypertension The Hypertension Table is found under the term "hypertension" in the Alphabetic Index. This table contains a complete list of all conditions that are either due to or associated with hypertension. Hypertension is classified using five categories, including essential hypertension (401), hypertensive heart disease (402), hypertensive chronic kidney disease (403), hypertensive heart and chronic kidney disease (404), and secondary hypertension (405). Each of these has three subcategories designated with a fourth digit, including malignant (fourth digit 0), benign (fourth digit 1), or unspecified (fourth digit 9). Hypertension should not

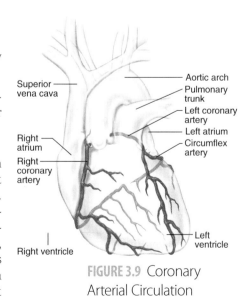

FIGURE 3.9 Coronary Arterial Circulation

TABLE 3.2 Excerpt from the Hypertension Table

Hypertension, hypertensive (*Continued*)	Malignant	Benign	Unspecified
due to			
aldosteronism, primary	405.09	405.19	405.99
brain tumor	405.09	405.19	405.99
bulbar poliomyelitis	405.09	405.19	405.99
calculus			
kidney	405.09	405.19	405.99
ureter	405.09	405.19	405.99
coarctation, aorta	405.09	405.09	405.99
Cushing's disease	405.09	405.19	405.99
glomerulosclerosis (*see also* Hypertension, kidney)	403.00	403.10	403.90
periarteritis nodosa	405.09	405.19	405.99
pheochromocytoma	405.09	405.19	405.99
polycystic kidney(s)	405.09	405.19	405.99
polycythemia	405.09	405.19	405.99
porphyria	405.09	405.19	405.99
pyelonephritis	405.09	405.19	405.99
renal (artery)			
aneurysm	405.01	405.11	405.91
anomaly	405.01	405.11	405.91
embolism	405.01	405.11	405.91
fibromuscular hyperplasia	405.01	405.11	405.91
occlusion	405.01	405.11	405.91
stenosis	405.01	405.11	405.91
thrombosis	405.01	405.11	405.91

be classified as either malignant or benign unless the medical record supports the designation.

Certain heart conditions (425.8, 429.0–429.3, 429.8, and 429.9) are assigned codes from category 402 if there is a causal relationship between the two, either stated or implied. These conditions are identified with a notation that the code **Excludes** hypertension.

One or more additional codes from category 428 are also listed to identify heart failure if it is present. If these heart conditions are not related to hypertension, the underlying heart conditions are identified with individual codes, even if hypertension exists as a separate condition. Unrelated hypertension should be listed as a separate diagnosis code.

If chronic kidney disease and hypertension are both present, codes from category 403 are used to describe those conditions. The relationship between the two diseases is presumed to exist, even if it is not specifically stated in the medical record. Each code in this category should have a fifth digit to differentiate chronic kidney disease stages I–IV (fifth digit 0) from chronic kidney disease stage V or end-stage renal disease (fifth digit 1). The appropriate code from category 585 (chronic kidney disease) should be listed as a secondary code with the code from category 403.

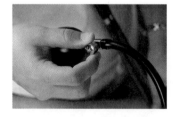

If hypertension is present in addition to chronic kidney disease, use a combination code to report these conditions.

When both hypertensive heart disease and chronic kidney disease are present, the condition should be described with codes from category 404. Codes in this category have a fifth digit that identifies the combination of heart failure and stages of kidney disease:

- Fifth digit 0—without heart failure, with chronic kidney disease stages I–IV
- Fifth digit 1—with heart failure and chronic kidney disease stages I–IV
- Fifth digit 2—without heart failure, with chronic kidney disease stage V or end-stage renal disease
- Fifth digit 3—with heart failure, with chronic kidney disease stage V or end-stage renal disease

Hypertensive cerebrovascular disease is reported with two codes, one code from categories 430–438 and a second code from categories 401–405. Similarly, hypertensive retinopathy is reported with two codes, code 362.11 and a secondary code from categories 401–405 to designate the specific type of hypertension. Secondary hypertension also requires two codes, one to identify the etiology causing the secondary hypertension and the other from category 405 to identify the specific type of hypertension. The order of the two codes depends on the primary purpose of the visit.

Cerebral Infarction/Stroke/Cerebrovascular Accident
The terms *stroke, cerebrovascular accident (CVA),* and *cerebral infarction* are often used interchangeably. These are all cross-referenced in the Alphabetic Index to 434.91 (cerebral artery occlusion, unspecified, with infarction). Category 436 (acute, but ill-defined, cerebrovascular disease) should not be used if the documentation includes the words *stroke* or *CVA.*

If a CVA occurs as a result of medical treatment or a procedure, it is coded as 997.02 (iatrogenic cerebrovascular infarction or hemorrhage). The medical record should document the relationship between the treatment and the stroke. A secondary code from categories 430–432 or from subcategories of 433 or 434 with a fifth digit of 1 should also be listed to identify the type of hemorrhage or infarct.

Late Effects of Cerebrovascular Disease
Category 438 describes late effects of cerebrovascular disease with the specific effect identified by the fourth digit, including cognitive deficits (fourth digit 0), speech and language deficits (fourth digit 1), hemiplegia/hemiparesis (fourth digit 2), monoplegia (fourth digit 3 or 4), other paralytic syndromes (fourth digit 5), alterations of sensation (fourth digit 6), disturbances of vision (fourth digit 7), and other late effects of cerebrovascular disease (fourth digit 8). Codes from category 438 may be reported with codes from categories 430–437 if the patient has a new onset of cerebrovascular accident and deficits from an old CVA.

Code V12.54 (transient ischemic attack [TIA], and cerebral infarction without residual deficits) should be listed as an additional code to indicate a history of cerebrovascular disease when no neurological deficits are present. This should not be reported with codes from category 438.

Acute Myocardial Infarction
An acute myocardial infarction (AMI) is classified as an ST elevation myocardial infarction (STEMI) or a non–ST elevation myocardial infarction (NSTEMI) using category 410 codes. The fourth digit identifies the specific location of a STEMI, including anterolateral wall (fourth digit 0), other anterior wall (fourth digit 1), inferolateral wall (fourth digit 2), inferoposterior wall (fourth digit 3), other inferior wall (fourth digit 4), other lateral wall (fourth digit 5), true posterior wall (fourth digit 6), and other specified sites (fourth digit 8).

Codes from subcategory 410.7 (subendocardial infarction) are used to describe subendocardial infarctions, NSTEMI and non-transmural myocardial infarctions. Codes from subcategory 410.9 identify unspecified acute myocardial infarctions. If a STEMI is documented in the chart but the site is not specified, the coder should try to ascertain the correct anatomical location of the infarct to assign the correct code. If no location can be determined, a code from subcategory 410.9 should be listed.

CODER'S TIP

If a subendocardial infarction or nontransmural infarction is documented with a specific location, it is still coded with the subendocardial infarction codes from subcategory 410.7. If an NSTEMI becomes a STEMI over time, it should be described with the specific STEMI code. If a STEMI becomes an NSTEMI due to treatment, such as thrombolytic therapy, it is still classified as a STEMI.

EXERCISE 3.3.1

Also available in **connect** plus+

Using your ICD-9-CM manual, assign the correct code(s) for each diagnosis.

1. Aortic stenosis due to rheumatic disease _____
   (ICD-10-CM: _____)

2. Rheumatic heart disease, unspecified _____
   (ICD-10-CM: _____)

3. Mitral valve insufficiency and aortic valve stenosis _____
   (ICD-10-CM: _____)

4. Acute myocardial infarction _____
   (ICD-10-CM: _____)

5. Iatrogenic septic pulmonary embolism and infarction _____
   (ICD-10-CM: _____)

6. Subacute interstitial myocarditis _____
   (ICD-10-CM: _____)

7. Cardiac arrest _____
   (ICD-10-CM: _____)

8. Late effect of cerebrovascular disease, facial droop _____
   (ICD-10-CM: _____)

9. Chronic venous embolism and thrombosis of thoracic veins _____
   (ICD-10-CM: _____)

10. Chronic hypotension _____
    (ICD-10-CM: _____)

Chapter 8: Diseases of Respiratory System (460–519)

Chapter 8 consists of several subchapters, including:

- Acute Respiratory Infections (460–466)
- Other Diseases of the Upper Respiratory Tract (470–478)
- Pneumonia and Influenza (480–488)
- Chronic Obstructive Pulmonary Disease and Allied Conditions (490–496)
- Pneumoconioses and Other Lung Diseases Due to External Agents (500–508)
- Other Diseases of Respiratory System (510–519)

The guidelines in this chapter include specific instructions regarding chronic obstructive pulmonary disease (COPD) and asthma, COPD and bronchitis, acute respiratory failure, and influenza due to certain specific viruses.

Chronic Obstructive Pulmonary Disease and Asthma Diseases included under the COPD designation include obstructive chronic bronchitis (subcategory 491.2) and emphysema (category 492). All codes describing asthma are included in category 493 (asthma). The nonspecific code 496 (chronic airway obstruction, not elsewhere classified) should only be used if the medical record does not specify the type of COPD treated.

Codes for obstructive chronic bronchitis and asthma include fifth digits that differentiate uncomplicated cases from acute exacerbations. An acute exacerbation is a worsening of a chronic condition. A chronic condition with a superimposed infection is not an acute exacerbation of the chronic condition.

An acute exacerbation of asthma is a worsening of the asthma symptoms, such as wheezing and shortness of breath. This is identified using codes in category 493 that have the fifth digit 2. Status asthmaticus refers to a patient's failure to respond to treatment. This is life threatening and requires emergency treatment. Status asthmaticus is identified using codes in category 493 with the fifth digit 1. If status asthmaticus is documented in the medical record, this should be listed as the first-listed diagnosis regardless of other COPD diagnoses. Codes with fifth digit 1 (status asthmaticus) should not be reported with codes with fifth digit 2 (with acute exacerbation). Only fifth digit 1 should be used.

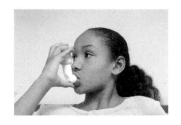

When coding for asthma, note any documented complications. Refer to the ICD-9-CM guidelines for instructions on how to code for these complications.

Chronic Obstructive Pulmonary Disease and Bronchitis Acute bronchitis (code 466.0) is caused by an infection. Acute bronchitis with COPD is reported with code 491.22 (obstructive chronic bronchitis with acute bronchitis). Code 466.0 is not listed as a secondary code because code 491.22 includes acute bronchitis. If the medical record identifies acute bronchitis with COPD with acute exacerbation, only code 491.22 is reported because the acute bronchitis designation takes precedence over the acute exacerbation designation. If acute exacerbation is documented without mentioning the presence of acute bronchitis, code 491.21 (obstructive chronic bronchitis with acute exacerbation) is listed to report the condition.

CODING EXAMPLE

A patient is diagnosed with COPD and asthma. At first it might appear that two codes are necessary to report these diseases. Turn to the Alphabetic Index and look under "asthma" to identify the codes that identify this disease. The first code listed is 493.9 (asthma, unspecified). However, looking farther down the list, you will see code 493.2 (chronic obstructive asthma), which is followed by a notation that it describes asthma with COPD. Since this describes the patient's condition, this would be the correct code.

It is not correct to report 493.2 with 496 (chronic airway obstruction, not elsewhere classified) to report these two diagnoses, because the code descriptor for 493.2 includes COPD. Therefore, a separate code designation is not necessary. A notation under code 496 identifies codes that are excluded, including asthma (493.2).

Acute Respiratory Failure Code 518.81 (acute respiratory failure) may be listed as the first-listed diagnosis or secondary diagnosis, depending on the circumstances. If the acute respiratory failure is the primary reason for treatment, it is identified as the first-listed diagnosis. Code 518.81 may be listed as a secondary diagnosis if respiratory failure was not present initially or if it is not the primary reason for treatment, such as might occur if the underlying condition resulting in acute respiratory failure is the main reason for treatment.

Influenza Due to Certain Identified Viruses Confirmed cases of avian influenza are identified with codes from subcategory 488.0 (influenza due to identified avian influenza virus). Confirmed cases of swine flu are identified

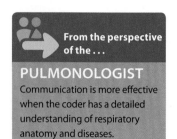
with codes from subcategory 488.1 (influenza due to identified novel H1N1 influenza virus). Each of these subcategories requires the use of a fifth digit to designate specific codes identifying cases of influenza with pneumonia (fifth digit 1), with other respiratory manifestations (fifth digit 2), or with other manifestations (fifth digit 9).

Influenza caused by other unspecified influenza viruses is identified with codes from category 487. Codes in this category describe influenza utilizing a fourth digit to identify influenza with pneumonia (fouth digit 0), with other respiratory manifestations (fourth digit 1), or with other manifestations (fourth digit 8). If the medical record states that avian influenza or swine flu is suspected, possible, or probable, the correct code to designate the condition is one of the codes from category 487. Only confirmed cases of avian influenza or swine flu are designated with codes from subcategories 488.0 or 488.1.

EXERCISE 3.3.2

Also available in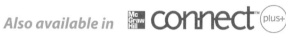

Using your ICD-9-CM manual, assign the correct code(s) for each diagnosis.

1. Acute pharyngitis _____
   (ICD-10-CM: _____)
2. Acute upper respiratory infection _____
   (ICD-10-CM: _____)
3. Acute bronchitis _____
   (ICD-10-CM: _____)
4. Chronic tonsillitis _____
   (ICD-10-CM: _____)
5. Pollinosis _____
   (ICD-10-CM: _____)
6. Pneumonia due to chlamydia _____
   (ICD-10-CM: _____)
7. Childhood asthma _____
   (ICD-10-CM: _____)
8. Chronic obstructive pulmonary disease (COPD) _____
   (ICD-10-CM: _____)
9. Chronic pneumothorax _____
   (ICD-10-CM: _____)
10. Respiratory failure not otherwise specified _____
    (ICD-10-CM: _____)

3.4 Coding Diseases, Chapters 9–10

Chapter 9: Diseases of the Digestive System (520–579)

Chapter 9 is divided into several subchapters:

- Diseases of Oral Cavity, Salivary Glands, and Jaws (520–529)
- Diseases of Esophagus, Stomach, and Duodenum (530–538) (Figures 3.10 and 3.11)

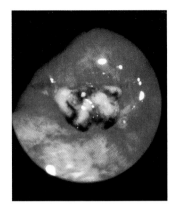

FIGURE 3.10 Bleeding Peptic Ulcer

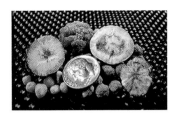

FIGURE 3.11 Gallstones

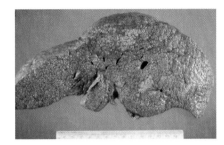

FIGURE 3.12 Cirrhosis of the Liver

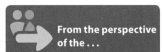

- Appendicitis (540–543)
- Hernias of Abdominal Cavity (550–553)
- Noninfectious Enteritis and Colitis (555–558)
- Other Diseases of Intestines and Peritoneum (560–569)
- Other Diseases of Digestive System (570–579) (Figure 3.12)

There are no specific guidelines associated with this chapter.

EXERCISE 3.4.1

Also available in McGraw Hill **connect** (plus+)

Using your ICD-9-CM manual, assign the correct code(s) for each diagnosis.

1. Dental fluorosis _____
   (ICD-10-CM: _____)

2. Gingival recession, severe _____
   (ICD-10-CM: _____)

3. Nonspecific temporomandibular joint disorders _____
   (ICD-10-CM: _____)

4. Osseointegration failure of dental implant _____
   (ICD-10-CM: _____)

5. Gastric ulcer (peptic), acute with hemorrhage _____
   (ICD-10-CM: _____)

6. Gastrojejunal ulcer, acute with perforation _____
   (ICD-10-CM: _____)

7. Acute appendicitis with peritoneal abscess _____
   (ICD-10-CM: _____)

8. Pylorospasm _____
   (ICD-10-CM: _____)

9. Crohn's disease of rectum _____
   (ICD 10 CM: _____)

10. Calculus of gallbladder with acute cholecystitis with obstruction _____
    (ICD-10-CM: _____)

Chapter 10: Diseases of the Genitourinary System (580 – 629)

Chapter 10 includes several subchapters:

- Nephritis, Nephrotic Syndrome, and Nephrosis (580–589)
- Other Diseases of the Urinary System (590–599)
- Diseases of Male Genital Organs (600–608)
- Disorders of the Breast (610–612)
- Inflammatory Disease of Female Pelvic Organs (614–616)
- Other Disorders of Female Genital Tract (617–629)

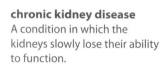

chronic kidney disease
A condition in which the kidneys slowly lose their ability to function.

The only section with chapter-specific guidance is category 585 (**chronic kidney disease [CKD]**), where the use of a fourth digit is required to differentiate the underlying stage of CKD present. The stage of CKD is determined using the glomerular filtration rate (GFR). This is measured in mL/min/1.73 m^2 total body surface area (TBSA), as follows:

- Stage I (585.1):   GFR >90 mL/min/1.73 m^2
- Stage II (585.2):   GFR 60–90 mL/min/1.73 m^2
- Stage III (585.3):   GFR 30–59 mL/min/1.73 m^2
- Stage IV (585.4):   GFR 15–29 mL/min/1.73 m^2
- Stage V (585.5):   GFR <15 mL/min/1.73 m^2
- ESRD (585.6):   GFR <15 mL/min/1.73 m^2 and patient is on dialysis or undergoing kidney transplant

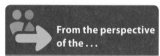

end-stage renal disease (ESRD)
Chronic kidney disease requiring chronic dialysis.

End-stage renal disease (ESRD) is defined as chronic kidney disease requiring chronic dialysis. If the GFR is unknown, but the medical record includes terms describing the severity of CKD, these may be used to infer the corresponding stage of CKD. Stage II equates to mild CKD, stage III equates to moderate CKD, and stage IV equates to severe CKD. The ESRD code is designated if the record documents end-stage renal disease or dialysis treatments.

Patients who have received a kidney transplant may still have reduced GFR because the single transplanted kidney may not function as well as two normal kidneys. This is not a transplant complication. If GFR is reduced, the appropriate CKD stage is identified with the appropriate code from category 585 and code V42.0 (organ or tissue replaced by transplant, kidney) is listed.

Patients with CKD or ESRD also may have other severe diseases. The most common associated diagnoses are diabetes and hypertension.

From the perspective of the . . .

CODER

Be sure to differentiate situations where CKD codes are reported as the first-listed diagnosis from situations where those same codes are reported as a secondary diagnosis. If in doubt, coders should review the guidelines to determine how to report the codes in the particular situation they are reporting.

CODER'S TIP

When CKD is associated with other severe diseases, sequencing of the CKD code and codes describing other contributing conditions depends on the conventions associated with the other conditions.

When CKD is associated with underlying diabetes, the diabetes is reported as the first-listed diagnosis with a code from subcategory 250.4. The appropriate code from category 585 describing the stage of CKD is listed as a secondary condition.

When a patient with CKD and associated anemia receives dialysis treatment, diagnosis code 585.6 (end-stage renal disease) is reported as the first-listed diagnosis, and code 285.21 (anemia in chronic kidney disease) is reported as a secondary condition.

A patient is seen in her physician's office. The coder reviews the medical record to find the diagnosis to report the reason for the visit. The records indicate the patient has moderate renal failure without specific measurements of the glomerular filtration rate.

The Alphabetic Index lists chronic kidney disease under "Disease, kidney, chronic", which identifies several codes, including 585.1–585.9. The Tabular List provides greater detail for each of these codes.

Code 585.3 (chronic kidney disease, stage III [moderate]) accurately describes the patient's diagnosis and should be reported.

EXERCISE 3.4.2

Also available in **Mc Graw Hill connect** (plus+)

Using your ICD-9-CM manual, assign the correct code(s) for each diagnosis.

1. Acute kidney failure _____
   (ICD-10-CM: _____)

2. Renal sclerosis, unspecified _____
   (ICD-10-CM: _____)

3. Acute pyelonephritis _____
   (ICD-10-CM: _____)

4. Chronic interstitial cystitis _____
   (ICD-10-CM: _____)

5. Hypertrophy of prostate, benign, not otherwise specified _____
   (ICD-10-CM: _____)

6. Spermatocele _____
   (ICD-10-CM: _____)

7. Endometrial hyperplasia, unspecified _____
   (ICD-10-CM: _____)

8. Dysplasia of vagina _____
   (ICD-10-CM: _____)

9. Dysmenorrhea, painful menstruation _____
   (ICD-10-CM: _____)

10. Stress incontinence, male _____
   (ICD-10-CM: _____)

Summary

Learning Outcome	Key Concepts/Examples
3.1 Identify the most appropriate diagnosis codes to report infectious and parasitic diseases; neoplasms; endocrine, nutritional, and metabolic diseases; and immune system disorders. **Pages 55–62**	Chapter 1 includes specific diagnoses for infections and parasitic conditions. Specific instructions are included for some conditions, such as when to use diagnosis codes identifying HIV infections or AIDS. Differences between the diagnosis of septicemia and sepsis are included in the guidelines for Chapter 1. Codes in Chapter 2 identify neoplasms, including benign, malignant, in situ, and secondary tumors. Instructions regarding the use of the Neoplasm Table are also provided. The guidelines for Chapter 3 provide specific instructions for reporting diabetes, secondary diabetes, and the presence of any complications or secondary manifestations of diabetes. Chapter 3 includes codes for other metabolic and endocrine disorders.
3.2 Recognize diagnosis codes for diseases of the blood and blood-forming organs; mental disorders; and disorders of the nervous system and sense organs. **Pages 63–66**	Chapter 4 lists codes describing diseases of the blood and/or blood-forming organs, including various types of anemia, clotting deficiencies, bone marrow failure, and specific diseases of the white blood cells. Mental disorders are listed in Chapter 5, including psychoses, neuroses, personality disorders, and mental retardation. The ICD-9-CM does not include any specific guidelines for this chapter. Chapter 6 includes diagnosis codes pertaining to the nervous system and sense organs. The only specific guidelines included in this chapter provide instructions regarding the selection of codes to describe pain. Separate codes describe acute pain and chronic pain. Codes describing pain are usually secondary, following codes that identify the causes of the pain. If the primary reason for the visit is to treat the pain, pain may be reported as the first-listed condition.
3.3 Name the correct diagnosis codes to describe diseases of the circulatory and respiratory systems. **Pages 67–72**	Chapter 7 describes conditions associated with the circulatory system. Specific guidelines provide detailed instructions on the use of the Hypertension Table and codes pertaining to hypertension, including the reporting of hypertension with heart failure and/or associated kidney disease. Specific instructions on the reporting of cerebrovascular accidents (strokes) are provided. These distinguish early and late effects of stroke. Instructions also guide coding of myocardial infarctions (heart attacks) according to which areas of the heart are affected. Chapter 8 includes diagnoses describing conditions of the respiratory system. Specific instructions determine how chronic obstructive pulmonary disease (COPD) is reported, depending on associated conditions such as asthma or bronchitis.
3.4 List diagnosis codes for diseases of the digestive and genitourinary systems. **Pages 72–75**	Diagnosis codes in Chapter 9 describe diseases and conditions of the digestive system. This chapter does not include any specific guidelines. Chapter 10 includes diseases of the genitourinary system. Detailed, specific guidelines provide instructions on the selection of codes describing chronic kidney disease and end-stage renal disease (ESRD).

Using Terminology

Match the key terms with their definitions.

_____ **1.** L03.1 HIV-positive patient

_____ **2.** L03.1 HIV-related condition

_____ **3.** L03.1 Asymptomatic HIV

A. Circulatory failure associated with severe sepsis

B. Does not require documentation of positive serology

C. Septicemia caused by bacteria, viruses, fungi, or other organisms

_____ **4.** L03.1 Septicemia

_____ **5.** L03.1 Sepsis

_____ **6.** L03.1 Septic shock

_____ **7.** L03.1 Systemic inflammatory response syndrome (SIRS)

_____ **8.** L03.1 Methicillin-resistant *Staphylococcus aureus* (MRSA)

_____ **9.** L03.1 Primary malignant tumors

_____ **10.** L03.1 Secondary malignant tumors

_____ **11.** L03.1 Carcinoma in situ

_____ **12.** L03.1 Type I diabetes

_____ **13.** L03.1 Type II diabetes

_____ **14.** L03.1 Secondary diabetes

_____ **15.** L03.1 Chronic kidney disease (CKD)

_____ **16.** L03.1 End-stage renal disease (ESRD)

D. Treatment directed at second site only, this is reported as the first-listed diagnosis.

E. Insufficient glucose metabolism that typically begins in adulthood secondary to poor diet and obesity

F. Assign 585.6 when the provider has documented the disease in the medical record.

G. This disease is designated by stages I–V based upon increasing level of severity. Anemia and/or hypertension can be secondary to this disease.

H. Poor glucose utilization in the cell with juvenile onset. Assign as many codes from category 250.xx as needed to describe the disease.

I. Systemic disease caused by a pathological microorganism or toxins in the blood

J. No signs or symptoms are present or listed in the medical record documentation for V08.

K. Code for personal history of malignancy when this has been previously excised and eradicated, no further treatment is directed at the site, and there is no evidence of disease.

L. Neoplasm at its place of origin

M. Symptoms include fever, tachycardia, tachypnea, and/or leukocytosis

N. Some codes include the infection and the causal organism in a combination code for the condition

O. A condition that can occur during pregnancy, or secondary to some other disease, infection, trauma, or injury

P. Additional diagnosis related to the first-listed diagnosis

Checking Your Understanding

Select the answer that best completes the statement or answers the question.

1. L03.1 HIV should only be coded in which of the following situations?

   a. The physician makes a clinical judgment without further evidence.
   b. Only confirmed cases should be coded.
   c. Two positive serology tests are documented in the medical record.
   d. Only confirmed and documented cases of HIV should be coded.

2. L03.1 Which of the following codes describes a patient with asymptomatic HIV?

   a. V08   **c.** SIRS
   b. AIDS   **d.** 042

3. L03.1 Which of the following is required to code for SIRS?

   a. Underlying etiology
   b. Coding 995.9 first, then the underlying etiology
   c. Two codes
   d. Sepsis and SIRS

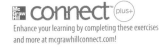

Enhance your learning by completing these exercises and more at mcgrawhillconnect.com!

CHAPTER 3 | ICD-9-CM CHAPTER-SPECIFIC GUIDELINES, PART I: CHAPTERS 1–10   77

4. L03.1 For coding purposes, methicillin-resistant *Staphylococcus aureus* (MRSA) is identified in which of the following ways?

   a. Underlying infection and MRSA are reported with a combination code and/or listed separately.
   b. Underlying infection and MRSA are reported with a combination code.
   c. Only the underlying condition is reported.
   d. Code only for MRSA.

5. L03.1 The correct way to look up a neoplasm code in the ICD-9 manual is to:

   a. Locate the neoplasm in the Neoplasm Table in Volume 1.
   b. Locate the neoplasm in the Neoplasm Table in Volume 2.
   c. Locate the neoplasm by anatomical site in the Neoplasm Table Volume 1.
   d. Look in Volume 2 for the actual type of tumor identified in the medical record.

6. L03.1 Which of the following is correct if a patient has a primary malignancy that has metastasized and treatment is directed at the secondary site?

   a. The primary tumor should be listed as the first-listed diagnosis.
   b. Only the primary tumor is listed.
   c. The secondary tumor should be listed as the first-listed diagnosis.
   d. Both tumors should be listed, with the secondary tumor reported as the first-listed diagnosis.

7. L03.1 Which of the following is the correct way to code for a primary tumor that has been previously excised and is no longer present?

   a. Extensions or metastatic disease may be listed as the first-listed diagnosis.
   b. A secondary tumor may be listed as the first-listed diagnosis code.
   c. A personal history of malignancy code should be used to identify the primary site.
   d. A personal history of malignancy is coded, followed by any extension or metastatic diseases.

8. L03.1 When coding for diabetes, the fifth digit indicates which of the following?

   a. Whether or not the patient has secondary manifestations
   b. That the patient has some complication
   c. Whether the diabetes is controlled or uncontrolled
   d. That no other codes are required to fully explain the diagnosis

9. L03.1 A patient's use of insulin indicates that:

   a. The patient may have either type I or type II diabetes.
   b. The patient has type I insulin-dependent diabetes.
   c. The patient has to use insulin in the long term.
   d. The patient has uncontrolled diabetes.

10. L03.1 Which of the following is reported first when coding for diabetes or any of its manifestations?

   a. Untreated secondary diabetes or its manifestations
   b. An underlying condition that caused the diabetes
   c. Manifestation codes
   d. Long-term use of insulin

11. L03.1 When a patient has anemia secondary to neoplastic disease, the coder must report which of the following?

   a. The underlying neoplasm causing the anemia
   b. Antineoplastic chemotherapy
   c. Chemotherapy, radiation therapy, and/or immunotherapy
   d. The underlying neoplasm causing the anemia in addition to the anemia

12. L03.1 Which of the following statements is correct regarding acute and chronic conditions?

   a. Acute and chronic conditions cannot be coded together.
   b. Chronic conditions are always coded before acute conditions.
   c. Acute conditions are always coded before chronic conditions.
   d. Chronic conditions are coded before acute conditions in some circumstances.

13. L03.1 Given that there are five categories of hypertension, which of the following is not correct?

   a. Hypertension and heart disease need not be related.
   b. Hypertension and heart disease are related.
   c. Hypertension and heart disease are reported with one combination code.
   d. Fifth digits are important for identifying whether or not the patient has heart failure.

14. L03.1 When determining which diagnosis out of many should be listed as the first-listed diagnosis, which of the following factors must be considered?

   a. The treatment provided
   b. The primary reason for the encounter
   c. The chief complaint
   d. All of these factors

15. L03.1 Which of the following codes or code combinations describes a patient with type I diabetes controlled with insulin?

   a. A V-code
   b. A V-code and a category 250.xx code
   c. No V-code
   d. A manifestation code only

16. L03.1 When is it appropriate to use a V-code for reporting diabetes?

   a. When the patient has type II diabetes and uses insulin
   b. When the patient has type I diabetes and uses insulin
   c. Only when manifestations are present
   d. When the patient has type I diabetes and does not use insulin

17. L03.3 What do hypertensive cerebrovascular disease, hypertensive retinopathy, and secondary hypertension share in common?

   a. They are all reported with one code.
   b. They are all reported with two codes.
   c. They are all reported with two codes, and the order of the codes depends on the primary reason for the visit.
   d. They are always secondary to diabetes.

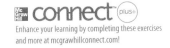

18. L03.3 Which of the following is incorrect regarding cerebrovascular accidents?

    a. Stroke, CVA, and cerebral infarction are often used interchangeably.

    b. Acute but ill-defined cerebrovascular disease should not be used if the documentation includes the words *stroke* or *CVA*.

    c. The medical record need not show a relationship between the treatment and the stroke.

    d. If a CVA occurs secondary to medical treatment or intervention, it is coded with 997.02 and a secondary code from category 430–432.

19. L03.4 Which of the following is not true regarding chronic kidney disease (CKD)?

    a. CKD requires a fourth digit to differentiate the underlying stage of the disease.

    b. CKD is documented in stages I–VI.

    c. CKD is documented in stages I–VI and ESRD.

    d. The stage of CKD is determined by glomerular filtration rate (GFR).

20. L03.4 Which of the following is most commonly associated with CKD and/or ESRD?

    a. Adrenal gland malfunction   **b.** Diabetes and hypertension

    c. Pulmonary disease   **d.** Congestive heart failure

Applying Your Skills

Use the ICD-9-CM manual to assign the correct code(s) for each encounter.

Diagnosis	ICD-9-CM	ICD-10-CM
1. L03.1 Chronic viral hepatitis B without mention of hepatic coma or hepatitis delta	_____	(_____)
2. L03.1 Esophageal malignant neoplasm of the lower third of the esophagus	_____	(_____)
3. L03.1 Skin cancer in situ, scalp	_____	(_____)
4. L03.2 Polycythemia vera	_____	(_____)
5. L03.1 Acquired hypothyroidism	_____	
6. L03.1 Secondary diabetes with ketoacidosis	_____	(_____)
7. L03.1 Septicemia due to MRSA	_____	(_____)
8. L03.2 Occult blood	_____	(_____)
9. L03.2 Nutritional anemia due to poor iron absorption	_____	(_____)
10. L03.2 Secondary acute blood loss anemia	_____	(_____)
11. L03.2 Acute alcoholic intoxication	_____	(_____)
12. L03.2 Gender identity disorder	_____	(_____)
13. L03.2 Amyotrophic lateral sclerosis	_____	(_____)
14. L03.2 Multiple sclerosis	_____	(_____)
15. L03.2 Quadriplegic	_____	(_____)

16. L03.2 Grand mal seizure _____ (_____)

17. L03.3 Mitral stenosis with insufficiency _____ (_____)

18. L03.3 Acute myocardial infarction _____ (_____)

19. L03.3 Angina pectoris _____ (_____)

20. L03.3 Coronary atherosclerosis _____ (_____)

21. L03.3 Cardiomyopathy _____ (_____)

22. L03.4 Acute glomerulonephritis _____ (_____)

23. L03.4 Acute pancreatitis _____ (_____)

24. L03.4 Chronic kidney disease, stage II _____ (_____)

24. L03.4 Mastodynia _____ (_____)

25. L03.4 Gastroesophageal reflux _____ (_____)

26. L03.3 Pneumonia due to respiratory syncytial virus _____ (_____)

27. L03.1 Volume depletion due to dehydration _____ (_____)

28. L03.4 Acute appendicitis _____ (_____)

29. L03.4 Acute pyelonephritis _____ (_____)

30. L03.3 Childhood asthma _____ (_____)

Thinking It Through

Use your critical-thinking skills to answer the questions below.

1. L03.1 When coding for diabetes, what questions should you ask yourself?

_____

_____

2. L03.1 When coding for neoplasms, what questions should you ask yourself?

_____

_____

3. L03.2 When coding for anemia, what questions should you ask yourself?

_____

_____

4. L03.3 When coding for pain, what questions should you ask yourself?

_____

_____

5. L03.4 When coding for chronic kidney disease, what questions should you ask yourself?

_____

_____

connect plus+
Enhance your learning by completing these exercises
and more at mcgrawhillconnect.com!

CHAPTER 3 | ICD-9-CM CHAPTER-SPECIFIC GUIDELINES, PART I: CHAPTERS 1–10   81

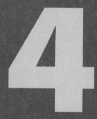

ICD-9-CM CHAPTER-SPECIFIC GUIDELINES, PART II: CHAPTERS 11–19

Learning Outcomes *After completing this chapter, students should be able to:*

4.1 Select appropriate diagnosis codes describing complications of pregnancy, childbirth, and the puerperium.

4.2 Identify codes for diseases of the skin and subcutaneous, musculoskeletal, and connective tissues.

4.3 Identify diagnosis codes describing congenital anomalies; newborn (perinatal) condition guidelines; signs, symptoms, and ill-defined conditions; and injuries and poisonings.

4.4 Describe the uses of E- and V-codes.

Key Terms

Aftercare

Cesarean section

Congenital abnormalities

Ectopic pregnancy

Gestational diabetes

Molar pregnancy

Pathological fractures

Peripartum period

Postpartum period

Prenatal visit

Puerperium

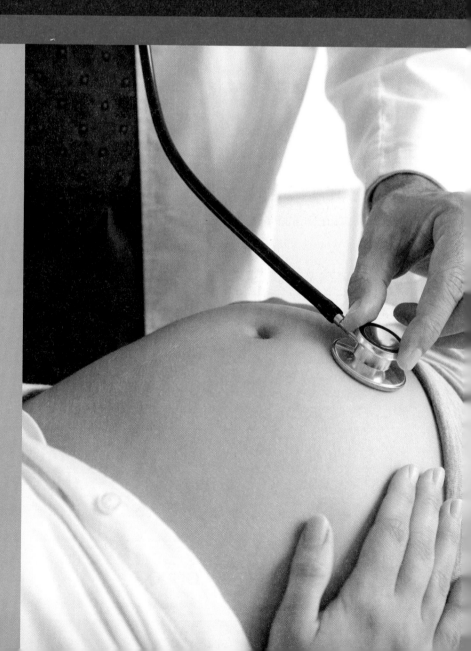

Introduction

This chapter continues the chapter-specific guidelines presentation from the previous chapter, covering Chapters 11–17 of ICD-9-CM, along with the V- and E-code chapters. The specific ICD-9-CM chapters covered in this chapter include:

- Complications of Pregnancy, Childbirth, and the Puerperium (630–679)
- Diseases of the Skin and Subcutaneous Tissue (680–709)
- Diseases of the Musculoskeletal System and Connective Tissue (710–739)
- Congenital Anomalies (740–759)
- Certain Conditions Originating in the Perinatal Period (760–779)
- Symptoms, Signs, and Ill-Defined Conditions (780–799)
- Injury and Poisoning (800–999)
- Supplementary Classification of Factors Influencing Health Status and Contact with Health Services (V01–V91)
- Supplementary Classification of External Causes of Injury and Poisoning (E800–E999)

4.1 Coding Conditions and Complications of Pregnancy, Chapter 11 (630–679)

Chapter 11: Complications of Pregnancy, Childbirth, and the Puerperium

Chapter 11 is devoted exclusively to conditions related to pregnancy and childbirth (Figure 4.1). This chapter is divided into several subchapters, including:

- **Ectopic** and **Molar Pregnancy** (630–633)
- Other Pregnancy with Abortive Outcome (634–639)
- Complications Mainly Related to Pregnancy (640–649)
- Normal Delivery, and Other Indications for Care in Pregnancy, Labor, and Delivery (650–659)
- Complications Occurring Mainly in the Course of Labor and Delivery (660–669)
- Complications of the **Puerperium** (670–677)
- Other Maternal and Fetal Complications (678–679)

Most codes in Chapter 11 require a fourth or fifth digit to identify the diagnosis completely. In some cases, the fourth and fifth digits are listed once but apply to multiple categories and/or subcategories that follow the list of applicable fourth and fifth digits. When that occurs, red parentheses appear after the code descriptor that contain indicators to identify which of the listed fourth or fifth characters can be used with that particular code.

ectopic pregnancy
A pregnancy implanted at a location outside the uterus.

molar pregnancy
A nonviable pregnancy consisting of abnormal cells.

puerperium
The period following childbirth that lasts about six weeks, when the uterus returns to its normal size.

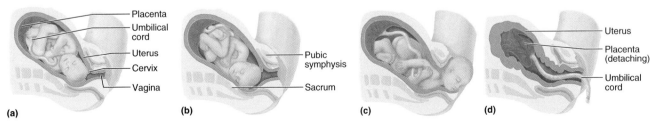

FIGURE 4.1 The Stages of Childbirth (a) First stage: Early dilation; (b) First stage: Late dilation; (c) Second stage: Delivery of the fetus; (d) Third stage: Delivery of the placenta.

General Rules for Obstetric Care Obstetric (OB) cases require diagnosis codes from Chapter 11 (categories 630–679). In most cases, codes from these categories are reported before codes from other chapters. Codes from other chapters may be reported with Chapter 11 codes to provide information regarding other conditions.

If the pregnancy is incidental to the reason for the visit, then the pregnancy may be reported with V22.2 (pregnant state, incidental) as an additional code, with codes describing the primary reason for the encounter reported as the first-listed condition. The medical record should indicate that the condition treated is not affecting the pregnancy. This and other V-codes are discussed in greater detail later in this chapter.

Chapter 11 codes are only reported on the maternal record, never on the newborn record.

prenatal visit
Care encounter occurring before delivery of a pregnancy.

Selection of OB First-Listed Condition Codes Guidance at the beginning of Chapter 11 provides instructions regarding whether to use codes from Chapter 11 or V-codes. For example, routine **prenatal visits** with no complications are reported with V22.0 (supervision of normal first pregnancy) or V22.1 (supervision of other normal pregnancy). Prenatal visits for high-risk pregnancies are reported with a code from category V23. Supervision of high-risk pregnancies should be listed as the first diagnosis code. V-codes are discussed in detail later in this chapter. Other codes from Chapter 11 may be listed to report other conditions if appropriate.

CODER'S TIP

V22.0 describes supervision of the first pregnancy if it is normal. V22.1 is reported for care related to any other normal pregnancy. When pregnant women are seen for conditions that are unrelated to the pregnancy and that are not likely to affect the pregnancy, code V22.2 is reported as a secondary diagnosis code, with a first-listed condition code that describes the reason for the visit.

Codes from category V23 are reported to describe care related to high-risk pregnancies.

CODING EXAMPLE

The following examples illustrate the use of the ICD-9-CM manual to select the appropriate codes to report pregnancy-related conditions:

- A routine prenatal exam during a first pregnancy without complications or other conditions is reported with V22.0. No other codes are necessary.
- A prenatal exam for a woman with mild gestational hypertension (hypertension not present when she is not pregnant) is reported with code 642.33. The fifth character indicates this is an antepartum condition and delivery did not occur during this visit.
- A woman who is 35 weeks pregnant is evaluated for hypertension and mild pre-eclampsia without albuminemia or edema. Due to increasing blood pressure readings over the previous week and an evaluation indicating the fetal lungs are mature enough for a safe delivery, the obstetrician performs a **cesarean section**. The procedure goes well and both mother and baby are fine afterwards. This episode of care is described by code 642.41. The fifth digit indicates that delivery occurred during the current episode of care without postpartum complications.

cesarean section
Delivery of a fetus through an abdominal incision.

For visits in which no delivery occurs, the first-listed diagnosis should be the reason that made the visit necessary. If more than one diagnosis code is appropriate, each may be reported in any order.

Visits that include a delivery should be reported with the first-listed diagnosis that corresponds to the main circumstances or complications of the delivery. If the delivery was accomplished via cesarean section, the first-listed diagnosis should be the condition that resulted in the admission. If the patient was admitted with a condition that resulted in the cesarean section, that condition should be reported as the first-listed diagnosis. If the reason for admission was unrelated to the condition that resulted in the cesarean section, the reason for admission should be listed as the first-listed diagnosis. The reason for the cesarean section is reported as a secondary diagnosis.

Every admission that results in a delivery must include a V-code on the maternal record that describes the outcome of the delivery. These V-codes are discussed later in this chapter.

Fetal Conditions Affecting the Management of the Mother Situations where the condition of the fetus affects the mother should be reported with codes from category 655 (known or suspected fetal abnormality affecting management of the mother) or category 656 (other fetal and placental problems affecting management of the mother). These codes are only reported if the fetal or placental condition is actually responsible for modifying the management of the mother by requiring additional tests, additional observation, special care or procedures, or termination of the pregnancy. The presence of the fetal condition alone is not sufficient to report these codes on the maternal record.

A diagnosis code from category 655 (known or suspected fetal abnormality affecting management of the mother) is reported to identify the specific abnormality when surgery is performed on the fetus in utero. These procedures are reported on the maternal record as an obstetric encounter.

HIV Infection in Pregnancy, Childbirth, and the Puerperium If a patient is admitted during pregnancy, childbirth, or the puerperium for an HIV-related illness, the first-listed diagnosis is a code from subcategory 647.6 (other specified infectious and parasitic diseases in the mother classifiable elsewhere, but complicating the pregnancy, childbirth, or the puerperium) followed by 042 and the code(s) for the HIV-related illnesses.

Current Conditions Complicating Pregnancy Codes from category 648 (other current conditions in the mother classifiable elsewhere, but complicating pregnancy, childbirth, or the puerperium) are reported to indicate that the mother has a condition that affects the management of the pregnancy, childbirth, or puerperium. Category 648 codes are reported as the first-listed diagnosis, with codes from other chapters reported as secondary diagnosis codes to identify the specific conditions.

Diabetes Mellitus in Pregnancy Diabetes may significantly complicate pregnancy. Pregnant women who are diabetic are identified with a diagnosis code from subcategory 648.0 (diabetes mellitus complicating pregnancy) and a secondary code from category 250 (diabetes mellitus) or category 249 (secondary diabetes) to identify the type of diabetes. Code V58.67 (long-term [current] use of insulin) is also reported as a secondary code if the diabetes is treated with insulin.

Gestational diabetes can occur in the second and third trimester in women who were not diabetic prior to becoming pregnant. Gestational diabetes can cause complications similar to those of preexisting diabetes and increase a mother's risk of developing diabetes later. Codes from subcategory 648.8 (abnormal glucose tolerance) are reported to identify this condition. Codes from subcategories 648.0 and 648.8 are never reported together.

gestational diabetes
A form of diabetes that develops during pregnancy.

To report preexisting diabetes in a pregnant woman, it is necessary to report two diagnosis codes. The first is a code from subcategory 648.0 (diabetes mellitus complicating pregnancy), and the second is a code from category 250 (diabetes mellitus).

CODING EXAMPLE

An obstetrician performs a routine prenatal exam on a woman with type II diabetes that is controlled with oral medications but who has no other complications of the diabetes. This encounter is reported with 648.03 and 250.00. The fifth digit in code 648.03 indicates the encounter is an antepartum condition without delivery during the encounter. The fifth digit in code 250.00 indicates that the type II diabetes is controlled.

Normal Delivery Code 650 (normal delivery) does not include any fourth or fifth digits. This code is reported as the first-listed diagnosis when a woman is admitted for a full-term normal delivery and delivers a single healthy infant without any complications during the antepartum period, delivery, or postpartum. This is always the first-listed diagnosis and cannot be reported with any other codes from Chapter 11. Codes from other chapters may be reported to describe other conditions if they are not related to the pregnancy.

Code 650 may be used when a patient had a complicating condition during the antepartum period that has since resolved and is not present at the time of delivery. V27.0 is the only code describing the outcome of the delivery that is appropriate to report with code 650.

The Postpartum and Peripartum Periods The **postpartum period** begins immediately after delivery and ends after six weeks. The **peripartum period** is a six-month period beginning with the last month of pregnancy and continuing for the next five months after delivery. A postpartum complication is one that occurs any time during the six-week postpartum period. Codes from Chapter 11 may be used to describe conditions occurring after the six-week period if the medical record indicates that the condition is related to the pregnancy.

Postpartum complications that occur during the same admission as the delivery are identified by fifth digit 2. A postpartum complication reported during a subsequent visit or admission is identified by fifth digit 4.

Code V24.0 (postpartum care and examination immediately after delivery) is reported as the first-listed diagnosis to identify that a woman who delivered outside the hospital is admitted for routine postpartum care. This code is not reported if the woman who delivered outside the hospital is admitted with a postpartum condition. In that situation, the postpartum conditions are reported.

Code 677 (late effect of complication of pregnancy, childbirth, and the puerperium) identifies cases in which an initial pregnancy-related complication develops sequelae requiring treatment at any time after the postpartum period. This code is listed after the code(s) identifying the sequelae of the pregnancy-related complication.

Abortions Abortions are reported with codes from categories 634 (spontaneous abortion), 635 (legally induced abortion), 636 (illegally induced abortion), and 637

postpartum period
Period that begins immediately after delivery and ends six weeks after delivery.

peripartum period
A six-month period beginning with the last month of pregnancy and continuing for the next five months after delivery.

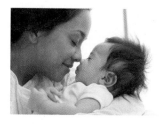

After the postpartum period, codes from ICD-9-CM Chapter 11 may be used to report conditions if the documentation shows that those conditions are related to the pregnancy.

(unspecified abortion). Each code must have a fourth digit to identify any associated complications and a fifth digit to identify whether the abortion is incomplete (fifth digit 1 indicating that all of the products of conception have not been expelled from the uterus) or complete (fifth digit 2 indicating that all the products of conception have been expelled from the uterus). The fifth digit is assigned based on the condition of the patient at the beginning of the visit.

Codes from categories 640–648 and 651–659 may be used in addition to the abortion codes to identify the complication *leading* to the abortion. The only fifth digit that applies to these codes is 3 because the other fifth-digit code definitions would not apply in cases of an abortion.

Complications occurring *after* an abortion are reported with codes from category 639. These codes cannot be reported with codes from categories 634–638.

Several codes are reported if an attempted termination of pregnancy results in the delivery of a live fetus, including diagnosis code 644.21 (early onset of delivery), a code from category V27 (outcome of delivery), and the procedure code for the attempted abortion.

Treatment for retained products of conception after a spontaneous or legally induced abortion is reported with the appropriate code from categories 634 (spontaneous abortion) or 635 (legally induced abortion) with a fifth digit 1 to indicate the previous abortion is incomplete. This fifth digit is reported even if the woman has previously been discharged with a diagnosis of complete abortion.

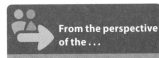

From the perspective of the . . .

CODER

Coders must be able to read and use the lists of fourth and fifth digits that may be added to codes in categories 634–639. Each of these reports greater levels of specificity and must be included to properly report these codes.

EXERCISE 4.1

Also available in connect plus+

Using your ICD-9-CM manual, assign the correct code(s) for each diagnosis.

1. Ovarian pregnancy without intrauterine pregnancy _____
   (ICD-10-CM: _____)

2. Incomplete illegally induced abortion _____
   (ICD-10-CM: _____)

3. Placenta previa without hemorrhage _____
   (ICD-10-CM: _____)

4. Mild hyperemesis gravidarum with metabolic disturbance _____
   (ICD-10-CM: _____)

5. Thyroid dysfunction completing pregnancy _____
   (ICD-10-CM: _____)

6. Pulmonary complication of the administration of anesthetic in delivery _____
   (ICD-10-CM: _____)

7. Acute kidney failure following labor and delivery _____
   (ICD-10-CM: _____)

8. Unspecified infection of the breast and nipple during childbirth _____
   (ICD-10-CM: _____)

9. Fetal conjoined twins _____
   (ICD-10-CM: _____)

10. Complication of in utero procedures _____
    (ICD-10-CM: _____)

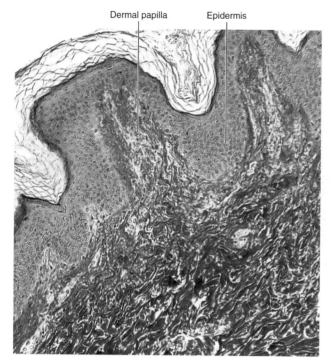

Dermal papilla   Epidermis

FIGURE 4.2 Interlocking Edge of Dermis and Epidermis

4.2 Coding Diseases, Chapters 12–13 (680–739)

Chapter 12: Diseases of the Skin and Subcutaneous Tissue

Chapter 12 includes diseases of the skin and subcutaneous tissues (Figure 4.2) only. This chapter is divided into several sections, including:

- Infections of Skin and Subcutaneous Tissues (680–686)
- Other Inflammatory Conditions of Skin and Subcutaneous Tissues (690–698)
- Other Diseases of Skin and Subcutaneous Tissues (700–709)

The only guidelines in Chapter 12 provide guidance on the coding of pressure ulcers. Category 707 identifies pressure ulcers by site and stage. It is necessary to report two codes to fully describe pressure ulcers (Figure 4.3); one from subcategory 707.0 (pressure ulcer) and the other from subcategory 707.2 (pressure ulcer stages). Codes from subcategory 707.2 are not used as first-listed diagnosis codes, but are only listed as secondary diagnoses with codes from subcategory 707.0.

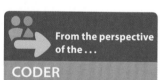

FIGURE 4.3 Decubitus Ulcer on Heel

CODER'S TIP

Pressure ulcer stages are identified with a fifth digit added to subcategory 707.2 as follows:

- Unspecified stage (707.20).
- Stage I (707.21): Skin changes limited to persistent focal erythema.
- Stage II (707.22): Abrasion, blister, partial-thickness skin loss involving epidermis and/or dermis.
- Stage III (707.23): Full-thickness skin loss involving damage or necrosis of subcutaneous tissue.
- Stage IV (707.24): Necrosis of soft tissues to underlying muscle, tendon, or bone.

From the perspective of the . . .

CODER

If sufficient information to accurately report the pressure ulcer stage is not in the medical record, it is important to ask the physician or other provider whether the information is available. Code 707.20 should only be used if it is not possible to obtain the necessary information.

Bilateral pressure ulcers at the same anatomical site and the same stage are reported with one code for the site and one code for the stage. Bilateral pressure ulcers at the same anatomical site but different stages are reported with one code for the site and two codes for the pressure ulcer stages.

Multiple pressure ulcers of different stages present at different anatomical sites are reported with one code for each site and a corresponding code for the ulcer stage. No pressure ulcer codes are assigned if previous pressure ulcers are documented as completely healed.

Pressure ulcers documented as "healing" are reported with the appropriate code designating the site and a second code for the stage of the ulcer at that time. If the record does not provide sufficient information to identify the ulcer stage, it should be reported with 707.20 (pressure ulcer, unspecified stage).

Pressure ulcers documented as progressing to a higher stage are reported with the code that describes the highest stage of the ulcer at that anatomical site.

EXERCISE 4.2.1

Also available in **McGraw Hill connect** plus+

Using your ICD-9-CM manual, assign the correct code(s) for each diagnosis.

1. Cellulitis of axilla _____
   (ICD-10-CM: _____)

2. Acute staphylococcal lymphadenitis _____
   (ICD-10-CM: _____)

3. Diaper rash _____
   (ICD-10-CM: _____)

4. Contact dermatitis due to food contact with skin _____
   (ICD-10-CM: _____)

5. Dermatitis due to adverse effect of medication _____
   (ICD-10-CM: _____)

6. SJS-TEN overlap syndrome _____
   (ICD-10-CM: _____)

7. Actinic keratosis _____
   (ICD-10-CM: _____)

8. Pressure ulcer stage II _____
   (ICD-10-CM: _____)

9. Senile dermatosis not otherwise specified _____
   (ICD-10-CM: _____)

10. Fox-Fordyce disease _____
    (ICD-10-CM: _____)

Chapter 13: Diseases of the Musculoskeletal System and Connective Tissue

Chapter 13 is divided into several sections, including:

- Arthropathies and Related Disorders (710–719)
- Dorsopathies (720–724)
- Rheumatism, Excluding the Back (725–729)
- Osteopathies, Chondropathies, and Acquired Musculoskeletal Deformities (730–739)

The only specific guidelines in Chapter 13 describe coding pathological fractures. A **pathological fracture** is a broken bone caused by weakness of the bone due to disease, such as a tumor or severe osteoporosis. Newly diagnosed pathological fractures are reported with codes from subcategory 733.1. These codes also may

pathological fracture
Broken bone caused by disease leading to a weakness of the bone, such as a tumor or severe osteoporosis.

be used while the patient is receiving active treatment for the fracture. Active treatment includes surgical treatment, emergency department encounter, or treatment by a new physician.

Aftercare of healing pathological and other fractures is reported with codes from category V54. These codes are discussed in more detail below. Care for postoperative complications that occur during the healing phase should be reported with the appropriate complication code.

CODING EXAMPLE

A patient is seen in the emergency department because of increasing pain in his upper arm. The patient reports that he has had osteomyelitis of the humerus for the past five years. An x-ray shows that there is a major osseous defect of this bone.

The Alphabetic Index identifies a number of different types of osteomyelitis. Chronic or old osteomyelitis is listed with code 730.1. The Tabular List indicates that code 730.1 requires a fifth character to identify the infected bone. Fifth digit 2 identifies upper arm. Directions under code 730.1 indicate that additional code 731.3 should be used to identify a major osseous defect if one exists. Therefore, the correct codes to describe this patient's disease are 730.12 and 731.3.

EXERCISE 4.2.2

Also available in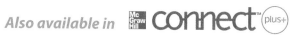

Using your ICD-9-CM manual, assign the correct code(s) for each diagnosis.

1. Arthropathy associated with Reiter's disease and nonspecific urethritis, lower leg _____
   (ICD-10-CM: _____)

2. Osteoarthrosis, localized to the hand, primary _____
   (ICD-10-CM: _____)

3. Chronic rheumatoid arthritis due to myopathy _____
   (ICD-10-CM: _____)

4. Felty's syndrome _____
   (ICD-10-CM: _____)

5. Difficulty in walking _____
   (ICD-10-CM: _____)

6. Postlaminectomy syndrome, thoracic region _____
   (ICD-10-CM: _____)

7. Thoracic radiculitis, unspecified _____
   (ICD-10-CM: _____)

8. Prepatellar bursitis _____
   (ICD-10-CM: _____)

9. Hallux rigidus _____
   (ICD-10-CM: _____)

10. Claw foot, acquired _____
    (ICD-10-CM: _____)

4.3 Coding Abnormalities and Unusual Conditions, Chapters 14–17 (740–799)

Chapter 14: Congenital Anomalies

Congenital abnormalities (Figure 4.4) are reported with codes from categories 740–759. This chapter is not divided into subchapters. Codes from these categories may be reported as a first-listed diagnosis or secondary diagnosis. Manifestations associated with a specific congenital anomaly are considered to be included in the code describing that anomaly and are not reported separately. If no unique code describes the specific anomaly, manifestations associated with that anomaly may be reported separately.

Codes from Chapter 14 may be reported throughout the life of a person with an anomaly. Even though congenital anomalies are present at birth, they may not be identified until later. Therefore, it is appropriate to begin reporting codes from categories 740–759 at any time. If the congenital anomaly has been corrected, a personal history code is reported to indicate the history of the anomaly.

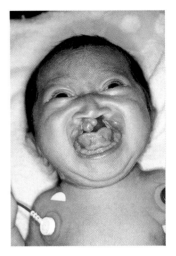

FIGURE 4.4 Infant with Cleft Lip and Palate

congenital abnormalities
Conditions or defects existing at birth.

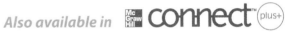

EXERCISE 4.3.1

Also available in **connect** (plus+)

Using your ICD-9-CM manual, assign the correct code(s) for each diagnosis.

1. Congenital hydrocephalus _____
   (ICD-10-CM: _____)

2. Anomalies of the inner ear, congenital _____
   (ICD-10-CM: _____)

3. Renal vessel anomaly _____
   (ICD-10-CM: _____)

4. Cleft palate with cleft lip, unspecified _____
   (ICD-10-CM: _____)

5. Hypospadias _____
   (ICD-10-CM: _____)

6. Congenital ureterocele _____
   (ICD-10-CM: _____)

7. Madelung's deformity _____
   (ICD-10-CM: _____)

8. Osteopoikilosis _____
   (ICD-10-CM: _____)

9. Eagle-Barrett syndrome (prune belly syndrome)
   (ICD-10-CM: _____)

10. Down syndrome, mongolism
    (ICD-10-CM: _____)

Chapter 15: Certain Conditions Originating in the Perinatal Period

Codes from Chapter 15 describe conditions that arise in the perinatal period, which is described as the period from before birth to 28 days of age. Chapter 15 is divided into subchapters to differentiate maternal causes of perinatal conditions from other conditions:

- Maternal Causes of Perinatal Morbidity and Mortality (760–763)
- Other Conditions Originating in the Perinatal Period (764–779)

> ### CODER'S TIP
>
> Codes from Chapter 15 are never reported on the maternal record. They may be used to report congenital anomalies throughout the life of the individual if the condition is still present. Codes from categories 760–763 (maternal causes of perinatal morbidity and mortality) are only reported if the maternal condition actually affects the newborn. The presence of a maternal condition that does not affect the newborn is not sufficient to report the code on the newborn record.

Chapter 15 codes are generally reported as the first-listed condition on the newborn record. Under some circumstances, however, some newborn conditions are also described with V-codes. These are discussed in detail later in this chapter along with examples of the use of Chapter 15 codes and V-codes together.

All clinically significant conditions should be reported on the newborn record. A condition is clinically significant if it requires clinical evaluation, treatment, diagnostic procedures, increased length of hospital stay, increased nursing care, or has implications for future healthcare needs.

If it is not clear whether a condition is due to the birth process or is community acquired, it is considered to be due to the birth process by default, and a Chapter 15 code is used to describe the condition. If the condition is known to be community acquired, Chapter 15 codes are not used to identify the condition.

Newborn sepsis is reported with code 771.81 (septicemia [sepsis] of the newborn) with a secondary diagnosis code from category 041 (bacterial infections in conditions classified elsewhere and of unspecified site) to identify the organism. Newborn sepsis is not reported with codes from category 038 (septicemia). Also, code 995.91 (sepsis) is not used to report newborn sepsis because code 771.81 includes the term *sepsis*. However, code 995.92 (severe sepsis) and any appropriate additional codes to identify associated organ dysfunction may be used to report those conditions.

EXERCISE 4.3.2

Also available in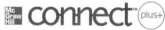

Using your ICD-9-CM manual, assign the correct code(s) for each diagnosis.

1. Newborn affected by amniocentesis _____
   (ICD-10-CM: _____)

2. Polyhydramnios _____
   (ICD-10-CM: _____)

3. Multiple pregnancy _____
   (ICD-10-CM: _____)

(Continued)

4. Cesarean delivery _____

(ICD-10-CM: _____)

5. Fetal distress first noted during labor and delivery, with a liveborn infant _____

(ICD-10-CM: _____)

6. Neonatal hypoglycemia _____

(ICD-10-CM: _____)

7. Neonatal bradycardia _____

(ICD-10-CM: _____)

8. Cardiac arrest of newborn _____

(ICD-10-CM: _____)

9. Fetal alcohol syndrome _____

(ICD-10-CM: _____)

10. Necrotizing enterocolitis in newborn, unspecified _____

(ICD-10-CM: _____)

Chapter 16: Symptoms, Signs, and Ill-Defined Conditions

Chapter 16 contains codes for symptoms, signs, and conditions that are not well defined. The chapter is divided into three subchapters:

- Symptoms (780–789)
- Nonspecific Abnormal Findings (790–796)
- Ill-Defined and Unknown Causes of Morbidity and Mortality (797–799)

There is no specific guidance associated with this chapter.

CODING EXAMPLE

The Alphabetic Index lists signs and symptoms under numerous entries. Painful urination can be found in several parts of the index, including "painful urination" or "dysuria," which is the medical term describing painful urination. Each of these terms refers to code 788.1.

EXERCISE 4.3.3

Also available in **McGraw Hill connect** plus+

Using your ICD-9-CM manual, assign the correct code(s) for each diagnosis.

1. Insomnia, unspecified _____

(ICD-10-CM: _____)

2. Fever with chills _____

(ICD-10-CM: _____)

3. Memory loss _____

(ICD-10-CM: _____)

4. Headache _____

(ICD-10-CM: _____)

(Continued)

5. Postnasal drip _____

(ICD-10-CM: _____)

6. Dysuria _____

(ICD-10-CM: _____)

7. Nausea and vomiting _____

(ICD-10-CM: _____)

8. Abnormal mammogram, unspecified _____

(ICD-10-CM: _____)

9. Senility without mention of psychosis _____

(ICD-10-CM: _____)

10. Decreased libido _____

(ICD-10-CM: _____)

Chapter 17: Injury and Poisoning

This chapter is divided into multiple subchapters of diagnostic codes describing different types of injuries, including:

- Fractures (800–829)
- Dislocation (830–839)
- Sprains and Strains of Joints and Adjacent Muscles (840–848)
- Intracranial Injury, Excluding Those with Skull Fracture (850–854)
- Internal Injury of Thorax, Abdomen, and Pelvis (860–869)
- Open Wounds (870–897)
- Injury to Blood Vessels (900–904)
- Late Effects of Injuries, Poisonings, Toxic Effects, and Other External Causes (905–909)
- Superficial Injury (910–919)
- Contusion with Intact Skin Surface (920–924)
- Crushing Injury (925–929)
- Effects of Foreign Body Entering through Orifice (930–939)
- Burns (940–949)
- Injuries to Nerves and Spinal Cord (950–957)
- Certain Traumatic Complications and Unspecified Injuries (958–959)
- Poisoning by Drugs, Medicinal and Biological Substances (960–979)
- Toxic Effects of Substances Chiefly Nonmedicinal as to Source (980–989)
- Other and Unspecified Effects of External Causes (990–995)
- Complications of Surgical and Medical Care, Not Elsewhere Classified (996–999)

Injuries When multiple injuries are present, each injury is reported separately. Categories describing combinations of injuries are reported when there is insufficient information to report the individual injuries. Traumatic injury codes are not used to report normal healing surgical wounds or to describe complications of surgical wounds.

The code for the most serious injury is reported as the first-listed diagnosis. Superficial injuries (e.g., abrasions or contusions) that are associated with more serious injuries at the same site are not reported separately. If an injury causes damage to nerves or blood vessels, the code describing that injury is the first-listed diagnosis, with codes from categories 950–957 (injury to nerves and spinal cord) or 900–904 (injury to blood vessels) reported as secondary diagnoses. If the primary injury is to the nerves or blood vessels, those codes are reported as the first-listed diagnosis.

Traumatic Fractures Fractures of specific sites are reported with codes from categories 800–829. These codes report acute traumatic fractures under active treatment, such as surgical treatment, emergency department encounter, and evaluation and treatment by a new physician. The most severe fracture as determined by the provider should be reported as the first-listed diagnosis, with other fractures reported as secondary diagnoses. Aftercare of a healing fracture is reported with V-codes, as discussed later in this chapter.

Multiple fractures of the same limb that are classified to the same three- or four-digit category are coded to that category. Multiple unilateral or bilateral fractures of the same bone that are classified to different four-digit subcategories within the same three-digit category are reported individually by site. Multiple fracture categories 819 (multiple fractures involving both upper limbs) and 828 (multiple fractures involving both lower limbs) are reported when more specific details of the fractures are unknown.

Burns Burns are classified by depth, extent, and cause; they are assigned a code for the burn itself and another code (an E-code) for the cause of the burn. The depth of a burn (Figure 4.5) is described as first degree (erythema), second degree (blistering) or third degree (full-thickness involvement). The code that describes the highest degree of burn is assigned first, followed by codes describing burns of lesser degree. If burns of different degrees are present at the same site, the code describing the highest degree is reported. Nonhealing burns, including necrosis of burned tissue, are reported as acute burns.

Burns at multiple sites are reported with separate codes. Category 946 (burns of multiple specified sites) is only used if the actual locations of the burns are not documented. Category 949 (burn, unspecified) is very vague and should rarely be used to report burns.

Codes from category 948 (burns classified according to extent of body surface involved) are reported with other codes from categories 940–947 to describe the extent of body surface involved or when there is not sufficient information to report a more specific code. Fourth digits describe the total extent of the burn, whereas fifth digits describe the extent of third-degree burns.

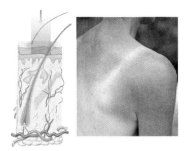
(a) First degree (superficial)

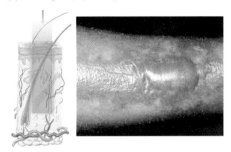
(b) Second degree (partial thickness)

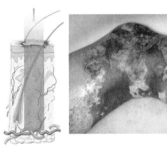
(c) Third degree (full thickness)

FIGURE 4.5 First-, Second-, and Third-Degree Burns

CODER'S TIP

The total body surface area (BSA) involved is determined through conventions, called the Rule of Nines (Figure 4.6), that assign percentages of body surface area to various body parts. For adults, the usual percentages are head (9 percent), anterior thorax and abdomen (18 percent), upper and lower back (18 percent), lower extremities (18 percent each), upper extremities (9 percent each), and groin (1 percent).

In infants and young children, these percentages are slightly different due to the increased head size in relation to the rest of the body: head (18 percent), anterior thorax and abdomen (18 percent), upper and lower back (18 percent), lower extremities (14 percent each), upper extremities (9 percent each), and groin (1 percent).

It is important for coders to review the records to determine the total body surface area involved in burns of all degrees (fourth digit) and separately determine the extent of third-degree burns by total body surface area (fifth digit). If no part of the burn is third degree, the fifth digit is reported as 0 (less than 10 percent or unspecified).

FIGURE 4.6 Rule of Nines

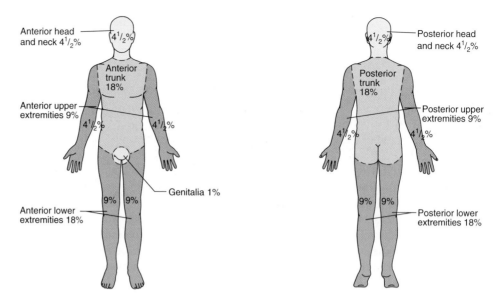

When patients are seen for the late effects or sequelae of a burn, the residual condition should be reported using the appropriate code, followed by the code describing the late effect (906.5–906.9). If a patient is treated for both the late effects of a previous burn and a current burn, codes describing both conditions should be reported.

Adverse Effects, Poisoning, and Toxic Effects Use and misuse of medications that result in adverse effects are reported as poisoning with categories 960–979. Medication poisoning may include several different mishaps:

- Errors in prescribing or administration of a drug by a physician, nurse, patient, or other person.
- Intentional overdose resulting in drug toxicity.
- A nonprescribed drug taken in combination with a correctly prescribed and administered drug, resulting in drug toxicity due to the interaction of the two drugs.
- Interactions of drugs and alcohol.

When reporting codes to describe a medication poisoning, the poisoning code is reported first, followed by a code or codes describing manifestations due to the poisoning. If there is a history of drug abuse or drug dependence, codes describing those conditions also are reported.

Toxic effects may occur with exposure to or ingestion of harmful, nonmedicinal substances. Toxic effects are reported with codes from categories 980–989. Codes describing toxic effects are listed first, followed by codes describing the results of the toxic effect. Toxic effects also may include codes to describe their external cause, including codes from categories E860–E869 (accidental exposure), codes E950.6 or E950.7 (intentional self-harm), category E962 (assault), or categories E980–D982 (undetermined).

Sepsis, Severe Sepsis, Septicemia, and Systemic Inflammatory Response Syndrome Infectious or noninfectious processes may cause a systemic inflammatory response syndrome (SIRS). These are reported with codes from subcategory 995.9, which include a fifth digit. These codes are distinguished from one another according to whether SIRS is due to an infectious or noninfectious process and whether there is associated organ dysfunction.

ICD-9-CM code 995.91 (sepsis) describes SIRS due to an infectious process without acute organ dysfunction, and code 995.92 (severe sepsis) describes SIRS with acute organ dysfunction or multiple organ dysfunctions. Code 995.93 identifies SIRS due to a noninfectious process without acute organ dysfunction, and 995.94 describes SIRS due to a noninfectious process with acute organ dysfunction. Each of these codes

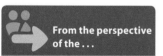

From the perspective of the . . .

CODER

It is important to understand the Rule of Nines to accurately report burn codes. It is useful to have an illustration of the Rule nearby for reference when coding.

includes an instruction to code first for the underlying infection or condition. In addition, codes 995.92 and 995.94 include instructions to use additional codes to specify the associated acute organ dysfunction.

Complications of Care Complications and rejections of transplanted organs are reported with codes under subcategory 996.8 (complications of transplanted organs). The fifth digit identifies the specific organ involved in the transplant. A transplant complication code is only reported if the complication affects the function of the transplanted organ. Two codes are reported to fully describe complications of transplants, one from subcategory 996.8 and a second code that identifies the complication.

Some patients do not have normal kidney function following a kidney transplant because the transplanted kidney may not fully replace two normal functioning kidneys. This is not considered a transplant complication, and code 996.81 (complications of transplanted organ, kidney) is not reported to describe the presence of some degree of chronic kidney disease. This code is reported to describe transplant failure or rejection.

Code 997.31 (ventilator-associated pneumonia) is reported when the medical record documents this diagnosis. A second code describing the organism causing this disorder, such as a code from category 041 (bacterial infections in conditions classified elsewhere) is also reported to describe ventilator-associated pneumonia. The type of pneumonia is not reported with codes from categories 480–484. If a patient is admitted with pneumonia and subsequently develops ventilator-associated pneumonia, the original pneumonia is reported with the appropriate code from categories 480–484, followed by code 997.31 as a secondary diagnosis.

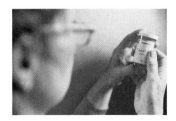

When coding a medication poisoning, report the poisoning code first, then a code or codes to describe manifestations of the poisoning.

EXERCISE 4.3.4

Also available in **McGraw Hill connect** plus+

Using your ICD-9-CM manual, assign the correct code(s) for each diagnosis.

1. Fracture, neck of humerus, not otherwise specified _____
   (ICD-10-CM: _____)

2. Open fracture of the metacarpal bone, base of thumb _____
   (ICD-10-CM: _____)

3. Closed fracture of the lower end of the femur, condyle, femoral _____
   (ICD-10-CM: _____)

4. Dislocation of the jaw, closed _____
   (ICD-10-CM: _____)

5. Whiplash injury, neck sprain _____
   (ICD-10-CM: _____)

6. Injury to the ascending colon _____
   (ICD-10-CM: _____)

7. Injury to the bladder and urethra, open cavity wound _____
   (ICD-10-CM: _____)

8. Second-degree burn of the right lower leg _____
   (ICD-10-CM: _____)

9. Third-degree burn of the left forearm _____
   (ICD-10-CM: _____)

10. Disruption of closure of muscle flap surgical wound _____
    (ICD-10-CM: _____)

4.4 V-Codes and E-Codes, Chapters 18–19 (V01–V91, E000–E030, E800–E999)

Chapter 18: Supplemental Classification of Factors Influencing Health Status and Contact with Health Services

Patients may encounter the healthcare system for reasons other than treating a disease or injury. Codes from categories V01–V91 describe these circumstances, including:

- When a person who is not currently sick uses health services for some specific reason (e.g., acting as an organ donor, receiving prophylactic care, or obtaining counseling regarding a health condition).
- A person receives aftercare for a chronic condition or a resolving disease/injury that requires ongoing care (e.g., renal dialysis for end-stage renal disease, chemotherapy for a malignancy, or cast changes for aftercare of a fracture).
- Factors influencing a person's health status that are not a current disease or injury.
- Circumstances surrounding a newborn's birth.

V-codes may be used in any healthcare setting, and most may be used as either a first-listed condition or as a secondary diagnosis code, depending on the actual circumstances. Certain V-codes may only be used as a first-listed condition, while others may only be reported as secondary conditions.

V-codes are used to report factors that influence a patient's health status or contact with health services. One example of this is an encounter to provide cast changes for aftercare of a fracture.

CODER'S TIP

The Chapter 18 guidelines at the front of the ICD-9-CM manual include a list of V-codes that may only be reported as first-listed diagnoses. Coders should review this list when reporting a series of codes that includes one or more V-codes to determine which code should be listed first.

Chapter 18 is divided into sections with similar V-codes grouped together:

- Persons with Potential Health Hazards Related to Communicable Diseases (V01–V06)
- Persons with Need for Isolation, Other Potential Health Hazards and Prophylactic Measures (V07–V09)
- Persons with Potential Health Hazards Related to Personal and Family History (V10–V19)
- Persons Encountering Health Services in Circumstances Related to Reproduction and Development (V20–V29)
- Liveborn Infants according to Type of Birth (V30–V39)
- Persons with a Condition Influencing Their Health Status (V40–V49)
- Persons Encountering Health Services for Specific Procedures and Aftercare (V50–V59)
- Persons Encountering Health Services in Other Circumstances (V60–V69)
- Persons without Reported Diagnosis Encountered during Examination and Investigation of Individuals and Populations (V70–V82)
- Genetics (V83–V84)
- Body Mass Index (V85)
- Estrogen Receptor Status (V86)
- Other Specified Personal Exposures and History Presenting Hazards to Health (V87)
- Acquired Absence of Other Organs and Tissue (V88)

- Other Suspected Conditions Not Found (V89)
- Retained Foreign Body (V90)
- Multiple Gestation Placenta Status (V91)

V-codes are used for multiple purposes, which are listed in the chapter guidelines. Coders should review these purposes when selecting V-codes.

Some of the major reasons or purposes to report V-codes include:

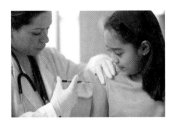

V-codes can be used to describe an encounter at which a vaccination or inoculation is received. If the vaccine is part of a preventative care examination, list the V-code as a secondary code.

- Codes from category V01 describe contact with or exposure to communicable diseases. Codes from category V01 are only used for patients who do not show any signs or symptoms of the disease, but have been exposed to it by close contact with an infected individual.
- Codes from categories V03–V06 describe situations where a patient is seen to be given a vaccination or inoculation. This may also be listed as a secondary code if the vaccine is given as part of a preventive care examination.
- Status codes indicate that the patient is a carrier of a disease or has residual effects from a past disease or condition. The guidelines include a long list of status codes describing a broad range of residual effects from prior diseases. A few examples include prophylactic use of agents affecting estrogen receptors (V07.5); asymptomatic HIV infection (V08); infection with a drug-resistant organism (V09); transplant recipient (V42); upper limb amputee (V49.6); lower limb amputee (V49.7); awaiting organ transplant (49.83); or BMI (V85).
- V-codes that describe a "history of" a condition refer to a personal history of a past medical condition that no longer exists and is not being treated. These codes are included in categories V10–V15. Similar "history of" V-codes describe a family history of a disease to indicate that the patient may have an increased risk of developing the disease. Most of these codes are in categories V16–V19.
- Screening V-codes describe testing for diseases in apparently healthy individuals. Most of the screening V-codes are located in categories V73–V82. Antenatal screening is described by codes in category V28.
- **Aftercare** codes describe situations in which the initial treatment of a disease or injury has been provided but the patient requires continued care through the recovery or healing phases. These V-codes are not reported if treatment for an acute disease or injury is still needed. Aftercare codes are found in categories V51–V59.

aftercare
Continued care through the recovery or healing phases that follow the initial treatment of a disease or injury.

- Aftercare of fractures is reported with the appropriate codes from subcategories V54.0 (aftercare involving internal fixation device), V54.2 (aftercare for healing pathologic fracture), V54.8 (other orthopedic aftercare), or V54.9 (unspecified orthopedic aftercare). Aftercare includes cast change or removal, removal of external or internal fixation devices, medication changes, and follow-up visits.
- Obstetric and related conditions are reported with codes from V22–V28, including supervision of normal pregnancies, high-risk pregnancies, postpartum care, outcome of deliveries, and antenatal screening. Every admission resulting in a delivery must include a code from category V27 (outcome of delivery) on the maternal record. These codes are not reported on subsequent maternal records or on the newborn record.
- Liveborn infants according to type of birth are reported with codes from categories V30–V39 (liveborn infants according to type of birth). These may be reported as the first-listed diagnosis once at the time of birth with codes from Chapter 14 (Congenital Anomalies) and Chapter 15 (Certain Conditions Originating in the Perinatal Period) listed as secondary diagnoses, if they exist.
- If a healthy newborn is evaluated for a suspected condition that, after evaluation, is found not to be present, that evaluation is reported with codes from category V29 (observation and evaluation of newborns and infants for suspected condition not found). Codes from V29 are only reported for healthy newborns when studies

determine that no abnormal conditions are present. These codes are not reported if the infant has signs or symptoms of a condition; instead the codes for those signs or symptoms are reported. Category V29 codes may be reported as the first-listed diagnosis on a readmission when the V30–V39 codes are no longer listed.

CODING EXAMPLE

V-codes may be used to identify a personal history of a particular disease or a family history of a disease. These are reported with separate codes. For example, a woman who has had a previous mastectomy for breast cancer who is not currently under treatment for this disease is identified with code V10.3. If a woman has no personal history of breast cancer, but has family members (e.g., mother, sister, or aunt) with breast cancer, she would be identified with code V16.3.

EXERCISE 4.4.1

Also available in **McGraw Hill connect** (plus+)

Using your ICD-9-CM manual, assign the correct code(s) for each diagnosis.

1. Encounter for the removal of an intrauterine device _____
   (ICD-10-CM: _____)
2. Sperm count for fertility testing _____
   (ICD-10-CM: _____)
3. Outcome of delivery of twins, both liveborn _____
   (ICD-10-CM: _____)
4. Prophylactic removal of the breast _____
   (ICD-10-CM: _____)
5. Aftercare during the healing of a traumatic fracture of the lower leg _____
   (ICD-10-CM: _____)
6. Orthopedic training _____
   (ICD-10-CM: _____)
7. Encounter for insulin pump training _____
   (ICD-10-CM: _____)
8. General psychiatric examination requested by the authority _____
   (ICD-10-CM: _____)
9. Observation for a specified mental, adult antisocial behavior _____
   (ICD-10-CM: _____)
10. Estrogen receptor–positive status [ER+] _____
    (ICD-10-CM: _____)

Chapter 19: Supplemental Classification of External Causes of Injury and Poisoning

E-codes describe the circumstances causing injuries and poisonings. These codes are not used to describe disease processes. E-codes denote how the injury, poisoning, or adverse effect happened (cause), the intent (unintentional or intentional), the person's status, the associated activity, and the place where the injury occurred.

E-codes are divided into broad categories, including:

- External Cause Status (E000)
- Activity (E001–E030)
- Railway Accidents (E800–E807)
- Motor Vehicle Traffic Accidents (E810–E819)
- Motor Vehicle Nontraffic Accidents (E820–E825)
- Other Road Vehicle Accidents (E826–E829)
- Water Transport Accidents (E830–E838)
- Air and Space Transport Accidents (E840–E845)
- Vehicle Accidents, Not Elsewhere Classifiable (E846–E849)
- Accidental Poisoning by Drugs, Medicinal Substances, and Biologicals (E850–E858)
- Accidental Poisoning by Other Solid and Liquid Substances, Gases, and Vapors (E860–E869)
- Misadventures to Patients during Surgical and Medical Care (E870–E876)
- Surgical and Medical Procedures as the Cause of Abnormal Reaction of Patient or Later Complication, without Mention of Misadventure at the Time of Procedure (E878–E879)
- Accidental Falls (E880–E888)
- Accidents Caused by Fire and Flames (E890–E899)
- Accidents Due to Natural and Environmental Factors (E900–E909)
- Accidents Caused by Submersion, Suffocation, and Foreign Bodies (E910–E915)
- Other Accidents (E916–E928)
- Late Effects of Accidental Injury (E929)
- Drugs, Medicinal, and Biological Substances Causing Adverse Effects in Therapeutic Use (E930–E949)
- Suicide and Self-Inflicted Injury (E950–E959)
- Homicide and Injury Purposely Inflicted by Other Persons (E960–E969)
- Legal Intervention (E970–E978)
- Injury Undetermined Whether Accidentally or Purposely Inflicted (E980–E989)
- Injury Resulting from Operations of War (E990–E999)

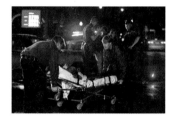

Use E-codes to report the circumstances of a patient's injury, such as a car accident.

E-codes from categories E800–E999 may be used with any code from categories V01–V91 to indicate that an injury, poisoning, or adverse effect may be due to an external cause. E-codes describing activities (E001–E030) may be reported with any code from categories V01–V91 to indicate that an injury or other health condition resulted from that activity or that the activity contributed to the condition.

E-codes may never be used as the first-listed condition. E-codes should be reported for the initial visit to treat an injury, poisoning, or adverse effect of drugs, but they should not be included on visits for subsequent treatment. When reporting fracture care, the E-code may be included on every visit reported with an acute fracture code, but not for aftercare when the fracture is healing.

Multiple E-codes are reported to completely describe the circumstances or cause of an injury, poisoning, or adverse effect. These codes may be selected from different sections of the E-code chapter. The Index to External Causes, located after the Alphabetical Index to Diseases in Volume 2, and the Inclusion/Exclusion notations in the Tabular List of Diseases are used to select the appropriate E-codes to describe the specific injury, poisoning, or adverse effect.

When multiple E-codes describe the circumstances surrounding an injury, poisoning, or adverse effect, these are listed in a specific hierarchy as follows:

1. Codes describing child and adult abuse;
2. Codes describing terrorism events;
3. Codes describing cataclysmic events;

4. Codes describing transport accidents;

5. Codes describing intentional acts;

6. Codes describing activity and external cause status.

If multiple E-codes are reported for one or more of the categories identified in the hierarchy above, the first-listed E-code in each hierarchy should identify the cause of the most serious injury caused by that event, followed by additional appropriate E-codes. After all codes for one hierarchy category are listed, additional codes describing injuries in lower hierarchy categories are listed.

In cases of intentional child and adult abuse, the first-listed E-code should be from categories E960–E968 (homicide and injury purposely inflicted by other persons), with the exception of codes from E967 (child and adult battering and other maltreatment). An E-code from category E967 is listed as an additional code to identify the perpetrator if that individual is known.

If the neglect is determined to be accidental, E904.0 (abandonment or neglect of infant and helpless person) should be reported as the first-listed E-code.

If the federal government identifies the cause of an injury as terrorism, the first-listed E-code should be a code from category E979 (terrorism). The terrorism E-code should be the only E-code reported. Additional E-codes from the assault category are not reported.

Codes from category E979 are not reported in cases of suspected terrorism. If an incident is suspected to be due to terrorism, E-codes should be listed based on the circumstances documented in the medical record regarding the mechanism of injury and intent. If the patient's condition is a secondary effect due to a previous act of terrorism, it is reported with E979.9.

Additional E-codes are listed to identify the place of occurrence when it is known. E849.9 (unspecified place) is not reported when the record does not indicate where the event occurred. That code is used when the event occurred at an identified place for which no specific place of occurrence code exists.

CODER'S TIP

In addition to the general Alphabetic Index in ICD-9-CM, there is a separate Index to External Causes. This is useful for identifying appropriate E-codes to describe the causes of injury and poisoning.

In addition, a separate Table of Drugs and Chemicals appears in the Volume 2 Alphabetic Index to Diseases. This table (see excerpt in Table 4.1) lists substances that may cause adverse events and the corresponding codes describing those events. Poisonings are identified with codes from categories 960–989. The table also lists E-codes describing adverse events associated with external causes such as accident, therapeutic use, suicide attempt, assault, and undetermined cause.

TABLE 4.1 Excerpt from the Table of Drugs and Chemicals

	External Cause (E Code)					
Substance	**Poisoning**	**Accident**	**Therapeutic Use**	**Suicide Attempt**	**Assault**	**Undetermined**
Baking soda	963.3	E858.1	E933.3	E950.4	E962.0	E980.4
BAL	963.8	E858.1	E933.3	E950.4	E962.0	E980.4
Bamethan (sulfate)	972.5	E858.3	E942.3	E950.4	E962.0	E980.4
Bamipine	963.0	E858.1	E933.0	E950.4	E962.0	E980.4
Baneberry	988.2	E865.4		E950.9	E962.1	E980.9

TABLE 4.1 *(Continued)*

Banewort	988.2	E865.4		E950.9	E962.1	E980.9
Barbenyl	967.0	E851	E937.0	E950.1	E962.0	E980.1
Barbital, barbitone	967.0	E851	E937.0	E950.1	E962.0	E980.1
Barbiturates, barbituric acid	967.0	E851	E937.0	E950.1	E962.0	E980.1
anesthetic (intravenous)	968.3	E855.1	E938.3	E950.4	E950.4	E980.4
Barium (carbonate) (chloride) (sulfate)	958.8	E866.4		E950.9	E962.1	E980.9
diagnostic agent	977.8	E858.8	E947.8	E950.4	E962.0	E980.4
pesticide	985.8	E863.4		E950.6	E962.1	E980.7
rodenticide	985.8	E863.7		E950.6	E962.1	E980.7
Barrier cream	976.3	E858.7	E946.3	E950.4	E962.0	E980.4
Battery acid or fluid	983.1	E864.1		E950.7	E962.1	E980.6
Bay rum	980.8	E860.8		E950.9	E962.1	E980.9
BCG vaccine	978.0	E858.8	E948.0	E950.4	E962.0	E980.4

EXERCISE 4.4.2

Also available in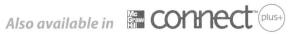

Using your ICD-9-CM manual, assign the correct code(s) for each diagnosis.

1. Injury sustained during a motor vehicle accident with another car; patient is the passenger in the car _____
   (ICD-10-CM: _____)

2. Animal-drawn vehicle accident _____
   (ICD-10-CM: _____)

3. Accident by powered household blender _____
   (ICD-10-CM: _____)

4. Adverse effect of Vitamin A used therapeutically _____
   (ICD-10-CM: _____)

5. Suicide by hanging _____
   (ICD-10-CM: _____)

6. War injury from gasoline bomb (incendiary bomb) _____
   (ICD-10-CM: _____)

7. Unarmed fight or brawl _____
   (ICD-10-CM: _____)

8. Accidental drowning by scuba diving not otherwise specified _____
   (ICD-10-CM: _____)

9. Accident due to lightning _____
   (ICD-10-CM: _____)

10. Exposure to radiofrequency radiation _____
    (ICD-10-CM: _____)

CHAPTER **4** REVIEW

Summary

Learning Outcome	Key Concepts/Examples
4.1 Select appropriate diagnosis codes describing complications of pregnancy, childbirth, and the puerperium. **Pages 83–87**	Codes from Chapter 11 describe conditions related to pregnancy and childbirth. In most cases, these codes are reported as first-listed conditions, with other codes reported as additional diagnoses. When delivery occurs by cesarean section, the first-listed diagnosis should be the reason the patient was admitted, even if that condition is not the reason that the cesarean section was performed. When a pregnant patient has other conditions that could complicate the pregnancy or childbirth, the appropriate code from category 648 is the first-listed condition, with additional codes listed as secondary diagnoses to identify the other conditions. Code 650 is reported when a pregnant patient delivers a healthy baby without any complications. Abortions are reported with codes from categories 634, 635, 636, or 637 with appropriate fourth and fifth digits to describe the exact circumstances.
4.2 Identify codes for diseases of the skin and subcutaneous, musculoskeletal, and connective tissues. **Pages 88–90**	Chapter 12 describes diseases of the skin and subcutaneous tissues. Most conditions are reported with a single code. Pressure ulcers are reported with two codes. The first-listed code is from subcategory 707.0, while the secondary condition is reported with a code from subcategory 707.2 that describes the stage of the pressure ulcer with a fifth digit of 0–4. Chapter 13 includes codes that describe diseases of the musculoskeletal system. Pathological fractures are reported with codes from subcategory 733.1. Active fracture care includes surgical treatment, emergency department treatment, or assumption of care by a new physician. These codes are not used to report aftercare during the healing process, including cast changes, removal of internal or external fixation devices, or follow-up visits. Aftercare is reported with the appropriate V-code.
4.3 Identify diagnosis codes describing congenital anomalies; newborn (perinatal) condition guidelines; signs, symptoms, and ill-defined conditions; and injuries and poisonings. **Pages 91–97**	Chapter 14 includes codes that describe congenital anomalies. These codes may be reported throughout the lifetime of the individual born with a congenital anomaly. If the anomaly has been corrected, a V-code indicating a personal history of the anomaly may be reported. Chapter 15 describes conditions arising during the perinatal period. These are reported with codes from categories 760–763 if the condition arises from a maternal cause or from categories 764–779 if it has other causes. Codes describing symptoms, signs, and ill-defined conditions are listed in Chapter 16. These may be used as first-listed diagnosis codes when the specific diagnosis causing the symptoms is unknown. Injuries and poisonings are listed in Chapter 17, including injuries, traumatic fractures, burns, adverse effects, poisoning, toxic effects, and complications of care. These have specific guidance associated with them, which should be reviewed when using these codes. Injuries are reported with codes from categories 800–999, with separate codes reported for each injury. The most serious injury is usually the first-listed diagnosis. Burns are reported with codes that indicate the degree of the burn and the extent of the burn described by the total body surface area burned. These codes are used to report medication errors, adverse effects of medications taken or given correctly, and interactions between medications and other drugs and alcohol. Other codes describe toxic effects of other substances.

4.4 Describe the uses of E- and V-codes. **Pages 98–103**	Chapter 18 outlines the V-codes, which describe factors that influence a patient's health status, including past history or family history of certain conditions. These codes also describe reasons that the patient encountered the health system other than for the diagnosis or treatment of a disease. Chapter 19 identifies E-codes used to identify the types of activities a patient was engaged in at the time of injury. These codes also identify specific types of accidents that cause injuries or poisonings.

Using Terminology

Match the key terms with their definitions.

_____ **1.** L04.1 Ectopic pregnancy

_____ **2.** L04.1 Molar pregnancy

_____ **3.** L04.1 Prenatal visits

_____ **4.** L04.1 Cesarean section

_____ **5.** L04.1 Gestational diabetes

_____ **6.** L04.1 Postpartum period

_____ **7.** L04.1 Peripartum period

_____ **8.** L04.2 Pathological fracture

_____ **9.** L04.3 Congenital abnormalities

A. From delivery until six weeks following delivery

B. A nonviable pregnancy consisting of abnormal cells

C. A broken bone caused by an underlying disease

D. Manifested by high blood sugar during pregnancy

E. From one month before delivery until five months following delivery

F. A pregnancy implanted at a location outside the uterus

G. Delivery of a fetus through an abdominal incision

H. A condition existing at birth

I. Care encounters that occur before delivery of a pregnancy

Checking Your Understanding

Select the answer that best completes the statement or answers the question.

1. L04.1 V22.0 would be appropriate to use for _____.

  a. A woman who sees her doctor and has a positive pregnancy test performed

  b. A woman with a high-risk pregnancy seeing her doctor for a routine prenatal check

  c. A first-time pregnant woman seeing her doctor for a refill on her thyroid medication

  d. A first-time pregnant woman seeing her doctor for a routine prenatal check

2. L04.1 Codes from ICD-9 Chapter 11 (630–677) may not be reported on the record for _____.

  a. A woman in active labor

  b. A pregnant woman

  c. A newborn

  d. A postpartum woman

3. L04.1 A code from the V30–V39 category may be used on the record for _____.

  a. An unborn fetus in a hospitalized pregnant woman

  b. A newborn baby still in the hospital where it was delivered

  c. A transferred newborn baby

  d. A seven-day-old infant at a clinic visit

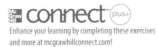

Enhance your learning by completing these exercises
and more at mcgrawhillconnect.com!

4. L04.1 The record for a woman with diabetes that has worsened due to pregnancy who is being seen for a prenatal visit should be coded as _____.

   a. 648.01
   b. 648.03, V22.2
   c. V22.2, 250.00
   d. 648.03

5. L04.1 The record for a woman who develops a breast abscess on postpartum day 2 after a home birth should be coded as _____.

   a. 611.0, 675.14
   b. 771.5
   c. 675.14
   d. 675.11

6. L04.1 The record for a woman being treated with dilatation and curettage for a missed abortion should be coded as _____.

   a. A failed attempted abortion without complication.
   b. A successful legal abortion with complication.
   c. An early fetal demise.
   d. An incomplete spontaneous abortion.

7. L04.2 Multiple pressure ulcers of different stages are reported using codes for _____.

   a. The site and stage of the most advanced ulcer only
   b. The sites and stages of all ulcers
   c. The sites of all ulcers and the highest-stage ulcer present among them
   d. The stages of all ulcers present and the site of the most advanced ulcer

8. L04.2 Dermatitis caused by taking penicillin for a strep throat infection, where the throat is now cured, would be coded as _____.

   a. 034.1, 693.0
   b. 693.0, E930.0
   c. 639.0, V14.0
   d. V14.0, E930.0

9. L04.2 When a patient with osteoporosis slips and falls on level ground and fractures her patella, you would code her encounter as _____.

   a. 822.0, 733.19, 733.00
   b. 733.19, 733.00
   c. 733.00, 733.19, E885.9
   d. 822.0, E885.9, 733.00

10. L04.3 Using codes V30.00 and 745.5 is appropriate when _____.

   a. A fetus is diagnosed with atrial septal defect (ASD) in utero.
   b. A newborn is diagnosed with ASD in the hospital the day of her delivery.
   c. A newborn is being seen by a cardiologist in the office for an ASD.
   d. A one-month-old is being seen for follow-up after surgery to close an ASD.

11. L04.3 A malnourished mother who gave birth to a full-term, 2,690-gram infant is coded as _____.

   a. 764.29   **b.** 263.9

   c. 760.4   **d.** 648.92

12. L04.3 Nausea and vomiting would be coded as _____.

   a. 787.03

   b. 787.02, 787.03

   c. 536.2

   d. 787.01

13. L04.4 The traumatic injury code for a fracture should be included in each of these instances except _____.

   a. The emergency department visit in which the fracture is diagnosed

   b. The orthopedist office visit to discuss treatment options for the fracture

   c. The hospital admission for surgical fixation of the fracture

   d. The hospital admission for removal of the fixation plate after the fracture has healed

14. L04.1 Codes from ICD-9 Chapter 15 in the range 760–763 may be reported on the record for _____.

   a. A pregnant woman

   b. A postpartum woman

   c. A newborn

   d. A two-month-old baby

15. L04.4 A patient with second- and third-degree burns of both the feet and hands is assigned the code _____.

   a. 946.3, 946.2

   b. 945.32, 944.30

   c. 945.32, 945.22, 944.30, 944.20

   d. 945.42, 944.40

16. L04.4 An E-code would be assigned in each of the following circumstances except _____.

   a. A fracture sustained in a fall

   b. An adverse reaction to a pain medication

   c. A history of a fall

   d. A complication of orthopedic fixation implants

17. L04.4 Which of the following can be reported as a first-listed diagnosis?

   a. E-codes

   b. V-codes

   c. Both E-codes and V-codes

   d. Neither E-codes nor V-codes

18. L04.4 All of the following would be assigned codes within the 800–829 range except _____.

   a. A compression fracture of the T12 vertebra

   b. A torus fracture of the radius

   c. An impacted fracture of the humerus

   d. An epiphyseal fracture of the tibia

connect plus+

Enhance your learning by completing these exercises
and more at mcgrawhillconnect.com!   CHAPTER 4 | ICD-9-CM CHAPTER-SPECIFIC GUIDELINES, PART II: CHAPTERS 11–19   107

19. L04.4 E-codes may be used to describe each of the following circumstances in an accident, injury, or poisoning, except _____.

    a. Where it occurred

    b. What the patient was doing when it occurred

    c. What time of day it occurred

    d. What caused it to occur

20. L04.4 When coding burns, the coder must be certain to determine all of the following except _____.

    a. The location of the burn on the body

    b. The laterality of the burn on the body

    c. The body surface area burned

    d. The depth or degree of the burn

Applying Your Skills

Using your ICD-9-CM manual, assign the correct code(s) for each encounter.

Diagnosis	ICD-9-CM	ICD-10-CM
1. L04.1 Missed abortion	_____	(_____)
2. L04.1 Placenta previa without hemorrhage, present antepartum, not delivered	_____	(_____)
3. L04.1 Transient hypertension of pregnancy, present antepartum, delivered this episode	_____	(_____)
4. L04.1 Early onset of delivery, delivered this care episode	_____	(_____)
5. L04.1 Retained placenta, delivered this care episode	_____	(_____)
6. L04.1 Obstetrical air embolism, occurring 3 days postpartum, after patient originally had been discharged after delivery	_____	(_____)
7. L04.1 Eclampsia, prenatal, resolved with delivery this care episode	_____	(_____)
8. L04.2 Cellulitis of the neck	_____	(_____)
9. L04.2 Acute dermatitis due to solar radiation	_____	(_____)
10. L04.2 Pressure ulcer of heel, stage 3	_____	(_____)

Diagnosis	ICD-9-CM	ICD-10-CM
11. L04.2 Chronic urticaria	_____	(_____)
12. L04.2 Sjögren's disease	_____	(_____)
13. L04.2 Psoriatic arthritis of the shoulders and hands	_____	(_____)
14. L04.4 Fell down stairs, lacerated wrist with tendon injury	_____	(_____)
15. L04.2 Trigger thumb	_____	(_____)
16. L04.2 Sequestrum of the fifth metatarsal	_____	(_____)
17. L04.3 Dislocation of the right hip, congenital	_____	(_____)
18. L04.2 Deformity of hip, acquired	_____	(_____)
19. L04.2 Compression fracture of L1 vertebra due to senile osteoporosis	_____	(_____)
20. L04.2 Claw foot	_____	(_____)
21. L04.3 Clubfoot	_____	(_____)
22. L04.3 Colon malrotation	_____	(_____)
23. L04.4 Fell off of horse, contused knee	_____	(_____)
24. L04.3 Complete unilateral cleft palate	_____	(_____)
25. L04.3 Placenta previa (baby's chart)	_____	(_____)
26. L04.4 Fracture base of thumb metacarpal	_____	(_____)
27. L04.4 Traumatic rupture of Achilles tendon	_____	(_____)
28. L04.4 Private (noncommercial) pilot, aircraft caught fire upon landing, third-degree burn of foot	_____	(_____)
29. L04.4 Follow-up after chemotherapy	_____	(_____)
30. L04.4 Status after kidney transplant	_____	(_____)

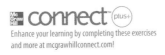
Enhance your learning by completing these exercises and more at mcgrawhillconnect.com!

CHAPTER 4 | ICD-9-CM CHAPTER-SPECIFIC GUIDELINES, PART II: CHAPTERS 11–19   109

Thinking It Through

Use your critical-thinking skills to answer the questions below.

1. LO4.1 Describe the significance of the fifth digit of the "complications of pregnancy" codes in ICD-9 Chapter 11.

   _____

   _____

2. LO4.1 What should prompt the coder to consider a given condition or diagnosis in a pregnant patient to be a "complication of pregnancy" in order to justify assigning a diagnosis code from ICD-9 Chapter 11, rather than using a standard diagnosis code?

   _____

   _____

3. LO4.2 Define the number of codes needed to fully describe a diagnosis of pressure ulcers. What is their significance?

   _____

   _____

4. LO4.2 Describe the significance of the fourth digit on the code for cellulitis (other than finger and toe). What, if any, additional codes might be needed when coding for cellulitis?

   _____

   _____

5. LO4.3 Which codes would a coder assign when a condition originates in the perinatal period, before birth through the first 28 days after birth, even though death or morbidity occurs later?

   _____

   _____

6. LO4.4 When coding for injury and poisoning (codes 800–999), what codes must the coder assign? Why?

   _____

   _____

7. LO4.4 Describe the distinction between a "poisoning" and an "adverse effect" of a medication. What is the difference between how each of these instances is coded?

   _____

   _____

INTRODUCTION TO ICD-10-CM AND ICD-10-PCS

5

Learning Outcomes *After completing this chapter, students should be able to:*

5.1 Describe the upcoming transition to ICD-10-CM.

5.2 Discuss the basic structure of ICD-10-CM diagnosis codes.

5.3 Explain the structure of the ICD-10-CM manual.

5.4 Compare ICD-10-CM general guidelines with ICD-9-CM guidelines.

5.5 Discuss the structure of the ICD-10-PCS system for procedure codes.

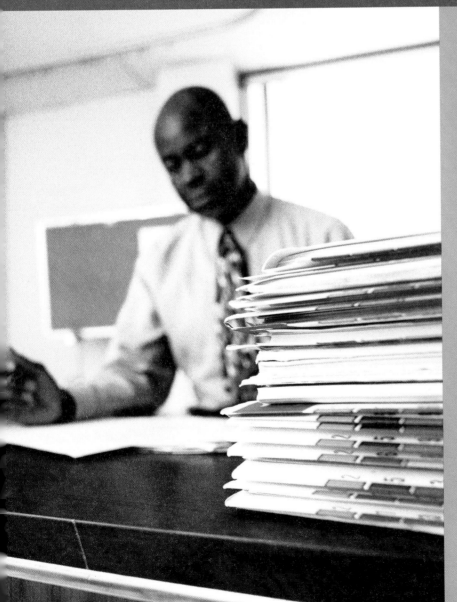

Key Terms

Conventions
Etiology
Excludes1
Excludes2
General Equivalence Mappings (GEMs)
General guidelines
ICD-10-PCS
Includes
Initial treatment
Laterality
Manifestations
Placeholder
Sequelae
Subsequent encounter

Introduction

On October 1, 2013, the U.S. healthcare system will undergo a massive change. Entities that share information involving diagnosis codes must convert from the 30-year-old ICD-9-CM diagnosis coding system (Volumes 1 and 2) to ICD-10-CM diagnosis codes. The World Health Organization (WHO) developed ICD-10 many years ago, and many countries adopted it and have used it for a number of years.

In the United States, the Centers for Medicare and Medicaid Services (CMS) and the Centers for Disease Control and Prevention (CDC) have adapted the international edition of the ICD-10 for use in the United States. The U.S. version of ICD-10, called ICD-10-CM (Clinical Modification), contains diagnosis codes. There are a number of reasons for the change from ICD-9-CM diagnosis codes to ICD-10-CM, including the following shortcomings of the current ICD-9-CM coding system:

- Lack of ability to expand for all necessary coding information.
- Lack of code granularity to describe diagnoses to the greatest possible detail.
- Lack of lateral specificity to distinguish right from left.
- Lack of ability to differentiate between care for initial injury or aftercare.

Hospitals also must convert from using ICD-9-CM procedure codes (Volume 3) to ICD-10-PCS codes to report procedures. ICD-10-PCS will be discussed later in this chapter.

General Equivalence Mappings (GEMs)
System developed to help identify potential ICD-10-CM codes, which are sometimes mapped from multiple ICD-9-CM codes.

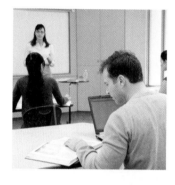

GEMs can help identify potential ICD-10-CM codes that correspond to ICD-9-CM codes. However, they do not replace a coder's thorough knowledge of ICD-10-CM itself. Rather than rely on GEMs entirely, coders must become familiar with ICD-10-CM in preparation for the transition in 2013.

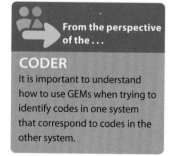

From the perspective of the . . .

CODER
It is important to understand how to use GEMs when trying to identify codes in one system that correspond to codes in the other system.

5.1 Transitioning to the ICD-10-CM Coding System

The ICD-9-CM diagnosis coding system includes approximately 14,000 codes. The structure of the ICD-9-CM system was discussed in detail in Chapters 2–4. Some code sections have few, if any, available unused code numbers because essentially all available codes have been assigned. New diseases or other diagnoses cannot be assigned to codes that are sequenced logically, but instead must be assigned to other sections.

In contrast, ICD-10-CM currently has more than 69,000 codes, with the capacity to expand to several hundred thousand codes if necessary. Thus, ICD-10-CM includes more than enough codes to accommodate the description of diseases and injuries to significantly greater specificity than they are currently described, with a sufficient number of unassigned codes to accommodate future expansions. However, even though ICD-10-CM is significantly larger and contains much more detail than ICD-9-CM, its basic structure retains enough similarity to ICD-9-CM that coders should be able to adapt to this new system.

General Equivalence Mapping

No universal mapping of ICD-9-CM codes to ICD-10-CM codes exists. A single ICD-9-CM code may correspond to many ICD-10-CM codes or to only a single ICD-10-CM code. Occasionally, multiple ICD-9-CM codes map to a single ICD-10-CM code. **General Equivalence Mappings (GEMs)** have been developed to help identify potential ICD-10-CM codes. These do not replace proper use of the ICD-10-CM code set.

There are two sets of GEMs—one mapping from ICD-9-CM to ICD-10-CM (forward mapping) and another mapping from ICD-10-CM to ICD-9-CM (backward mapping). The GEM sets consist of code pairs and a flag indicator. The flag indicators provide information to assist in converting from one system to the other. Flags consist of five digits.

The first digit is the "approximate" flag, which is either a "0" or "1." A 0 indicates that there is a direct match between the two coding systems. The GEM file maps to a single code. A 1 indicates that one code in the first system maps to more than one code in the other system.

A coder is converting from ICD-9-CM diagnosis code 711.05 (pyogenic arthritis, pelvic region and thigh) to ICD-10-CM codes to report the same condition. Looking up ICD-9-CM code 711.05 in the GEMs shows the following:

71105	M00059	10000
71105	M00159	10000
71105	M00259	10000
71105	M00859	10000

These entries indicate that ICD-9-CM code 711.05 maps to four separate ICD-10-CM codes—M00059, M00159, M00259, and M00859.

The second digit in the flag is the "no map" indicator. A 0 appears when there is at least one match between the two code sets. In situations where no match exists, a 1 appears in the second position of the flag, and a notation of "NoDx" appears in the second column of the GEMs file.

The third digit in the flag is the "combination" indicator. This signifies whether a combination of codes is necessary to fully translate from one system to the other. A 0 indicates that it is not necessary to use a combination of codes from the second system to indicate the equivalent diagnosis. A 1 indicates that a combination of codes is necessary.

The fourth and fifth digits of the flag are the "scenario" and "choice list" indicators. Some codes cross to more than one combination of codes in the other system. The scenario indicator identifies each separate combination. The first combination has a 1 in the fourth flag position of each code. If other combinations may be used, these are identified with a 2, 3, or other digit in the fourth flag position. The choice indicator provides information regarding each combination of codes that can be used.

This chapter is an optional study section. It will be left to course instructors to decide whether students should review this material. Most students will not have an ICD-10-CM manual, but these codes and GEMs may be found online at the official CDC and CMS websites.

CODER'S TIP

Coders who are familiar with ICD-9-CM coding should be able to adapt to the new ICD-10-CM system with a modest degree of training and practice. Although the new ICD-10-CM system has a different structure than the existing ICD-9-CM system, the rationale behind choosing the correct code to describe a particular condition is similar enough that it will be relatively familiar to experienced coders.

EXERCISE 5.1

Also available in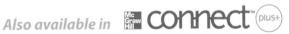

Fill in the word(s) to complete each statement.

1. ICD-10-CM will be implemented in _____.

2. In ICD-9-CM, some conditions cannot be assigned codes in logical sequence because _____
_____.

3. If necessary, ICD-10-CM can be expanded to include over _____ codes.

4. GEM is an abbreviation for _____.

5. How many digits appear in the GEM flag? Name them. _____

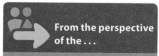
5.2 Diagnosis Code Structure

ICD-9-CM codes consist of three, four, or five digits. The codes in Chapters 1–17 of ICD-9-CM include three numerical digits, followed by a decimal point and up to two digits after the decimal point. The supplemental classification codes begin with a letter (E or V), followed by up to four digits. The ICD-9-CM manual is divided into 19 chapters, including E- and V-codes.

In contrast, ICD-10-CM codes consist of 3–7 digits. The first digit is always an alpha character (A–Z). The second digit is always numeric. The third digit is either alpha or numeric. If the code consists of more than three digits, a decimal point always follows the third digit, with the remaining 1–4 digits following the decimal point. The digits to the right of the decimal point may be alpha or numeric digits. Examples of three-, four-, five-, six-, and seven-digit codes include:

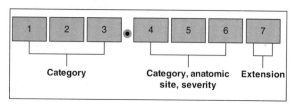

J36	Peritonsillar abscess
J38.6	Stenosis of larynx
J95.81	Postprocedural pneumothorax
L89.321	Pressure ulcer of left buttock, stage 1
S72.031A	Displaced midcervical fracture right femur, initial encounter for closed fracture

The first digit of an ICD-10-CM code is always an alpha character. The second digit is always a numeric character. Digits 3–7 may each be either alpha or numeric characters.

The additional code-level specificity available with ICD-10-CM codes has several advantages, including individual codes that indicate:

- Laterality.
- Trimesters during pregnancy.
- Whether a patient was seen for initial treatment, follow-up care, or treatment of sequelae.

Laterality

laterality
Refers to one side of the body (right or left).

Laterality is indicated by the code itself, usually with a specific number in the fifth or sixth digit. For example, in some code series, the right side is indicated with the number 1, left with the number 2, and bilateral with the number 3. If the side is unspecified, it is indicated with either the number 0 or 9, depending on whether it is the fifth or sixth digit. For example:

S42.201	Unspecified fracture of upper end of right humerus
S42.202	Unspecified fracture of upper end of left humerus
S42.209	Unspecified fracture of upper end of unspecified humerus (9 in sixth digit)
M75.50	Bursitis of unspecified shoulder (0 in fifth digit)
M75.51	Bursitis of right shoulder
M75.52	Bursitis of left shoulder

Some code groups include two related, but slightly different, injuries, each of which requires right, left, and unspecified designations. In many of those sections, laterality is indicated with numbers 1–6 in the sixth position. For example, the following group of codes describes fractures of the midsection of the femoral neck:

S72.031	Displaced midcervical fracture of right femur
S72.032	Displaced midcervical fracture of left femur
S72.033	Displaced midcervical fracture of unspecified femur
S72.034	Nondisplaced midcervical fracture of right femur
S72.035	Nondisplaced midcervical fracture of left femur
S72.036	Nondisplaced midcervical fracture of unspecified femur

Some code sequences contain an individual code indicating a bilateral condition. If no specific bilateral code exists, codes indicating both right and left are listed.

Trimesters

During pregnancy, the digits 1, 2, or 3 within the code indicate the trimester. The first trimester is defined as up to 14 weeks 0 days, the second trimester is 14 weeks 0 days to less than 28 weeks 0 days, and the third trimester is from 28 weeks 0 days through delivery. If the trimester is undetermined, the numbers 0 or 9 are used, depending on whether it is in the fifth- or sixth-digit location. Examples of pregnancy-related codes include:

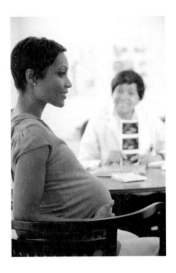

ICD-10-CM's greater specificity includes codes to indicate the trimester of a patient's pregnancy. This allows for more detailed health management and data collection.

O09.211	Supervision of pregnancy with history of preterm labor, first trimester
O09.212	Supervision of pregnancy with history of preterm labor, second trimester
O09.213	Supervision of pregnancy with history of preterm labor, third trimester
O09.219	Supervision of pregnancy with history of preterm labor, unspecified trimester (9 in sixth position)
Z34.00	Encounter for supervision of normal first pregnancy, unspecified trimester (0 in fifth position)
Z34.01	Encounter for supervision of normal first pregnancy, first trimester
Z34.02	Encounter for supervision of normal first pregnancy, second trimester
Z34.03	Encounter for supervision of normal first pregnancy, third trimester

Initial Treatment, Subsequent Encounter, and Sequelae

The ICD-10-CM codes also indicate whether the encounter is for the **initial treatment** of the injury, **subsequent encounter,** or to treat **sequelae** of the injury. The simplest indicators of these encounters are the alpha characters *A, D,* and *S* in the seventh position. Aftercare of an injury is indicated by using the code describing the injury and D in the seventh position. Examples of these indicators include:

initial treatment
Primary treatment for an injury.

subsequent encounter
Care and/or treatment following the initial treatment of an injury.

sequelae
Term used in coding to refer to late effects.

S73.011A	Posterior subluxation of right hip, initial encounter
S73.011D	Posterior subluxation of right hip, subsequent encounter
S73.011S	Posterior subluxation of right hip, sequelae

In some cases, the choice of possible seventh digits is more expansive, including additional indicators of initial encounters and subsequent encounters. For example, the possible choices for the seventh-digit indicator of the initial treatment of a fracture include A for closed fractures, B for type I and II open fractures, and C for type IIIA, IIIB, and IIIC open fractures. Choices for seventh digit indicators of subsequent encounters include D–H, J–N, and P–R (the letters *I* and *O* are not used to avoid confusion with the numbers 1 and 0). These indicators are used to identify routine healing, delayed healing, nonunions, and malunions. Encounters involving sequelae are identified with an S in the seventh position.

When a code of less than six digits requires the use of a seventh digit to convey specific information, a **placeholder** is inserted for the unused digits. Placeholders are indicated with an "x" in the unused place. For example, if a code has only five digits but requires a specific seventh digit, an "x" is placed in the sixth position. An example of this is code S70.11 (contusion of right thigh), which requires a seventh digit to indicate whether the encounter is for the initial injury (A), aftercare (D), or sequelae (S):

placeholder
The character "x" inserted to hold the place of unused digits when a code of less than six digits requires the use of a seventh digit to convey specific information.

S70.11xA	Contusion of right thigh, initial treatment
S70.11xD	Contusion of right thigh, subsequent encounter
S70.11xS	Sequelae

CODER'S TIP

The codes in ICD-9-CM and ICD-10-CM can appear identical but never have the same meaning. Both systems have E-codes, but they have entirely different meanings. Examples include:

Code	Meaning in ICD-9-CM	Meaning in ICD-10-CM
E8021	Railway accident involving derailment without antecedent collision injuring passenger	Acute intermittent (hepatic) porphyria
E8300	Accident to watercraft causing submersion, injuring occupant of small boat unpowered	Disorder of copper metabolism unspecified
E8301	Accident to watercraft causing submersion, injuring occupant of small boat powered	Wilson's disease

EXERCISE 5.2

Also available in **McGraw Hill connect** plus+

Fill in the word(s) to complete each statement.

1. The right side is often designated with _____ as the fifth or sixth character.

2. During the course of a pregnancy, a specific trimester may be indicated with the character _____.

3. An "x" in the fifth or sixth position is used to indicate _____.

5.3 Structure of the ICD-10-CM Manual

Similar to ICD-9-CM, the ICD-10-CM manual is divided into an Alphabetic Index and Tabular List of codes. Both volumes are much longer in ICD-10-CM to accommodate the total number of codes. The Alphabetic Index is arranged in alphabetical order with several possible listings for each code.

The Tabular List is divided into 21 chapters, two more than the ICD-9-CM. The two new chapters are Chapter 7, Diseases of the Eye and Adnexa, and Chapter 8, Diseases of the Ear and Mastoid Process. The ICD-10-CM includes the chapters shown in Table 5.1.

CODER'S TIP

Coders should note that the chapters in ICD-10-CM have been reorganized to group similar conditions together. For example, the conditions identified in Chapters 15 (Pregnancy, Childbirth, and the Puerperium), 16 (Certain Conditions Originating in the Perinatal Period), and 17 (Congenital Malformations, Deformations, and Chromosomal Abnormalities) are grouped together in ICD-10-CM, whereas these conditions did not appear in contiguous chapters in ICD-9-CM.

TABLE 5.1 Organization of ICD-10-CM

Chapter	Title	Categories
1	Certain Infectious and Parasitic Diseases	A00–B99
2	Neoplasms	C00–D49
3	Diseases of the Blood and Blood-Forming Organs and Certain Disorders Involving the Immune Mechanism	D50–D89
4	Endocrine, Nutritional, and Metabolic Diseases	E00–E89
5	Mental and Behavioral Disorders	F01–F99
6	Diseases of the Nervous System and Sense Organs	G00–G99
7	Diseases of the Eye and Adnexa	H00–H59
8	Diseases of the Ear and Mastoid Process	H60–H95
9	Diseases of the Circulatory System	I00–I99
10	Diseases of the Respiratory System	J00–J99
11	Diseases of the Digestive System	K00–K94
12	Diseases of the Skin and Subcutaneous Tissue	L00–L99
13	Diseases of the Musculoskeletal System and Connective Tissue	M00–M99
14	Diseases of the Genitourinary System	N00–N99
15	Pregnancy, Childbirth, and the Puerperium	O00–O99
16	Certain Conditions Originating in the Perinatal Period	P00–P96
17	Congenital Malformations, Deformations, and Chromosomal Abnormalities	Q00–Q99
18	Symptoms, Signs, and Abnormal Clinical and Laboratory Findings, Not Elsewhere Classified	R00–R99
19	Injury, Poisoning, and Certain Other Consequences of External Causes	S00–T88
20	External Causes of Morbidity	V00–Y99
21	Factors Influencing Health Status and Contact with Health Services	Z00–Z99

EXERCISE 5.3

Also available in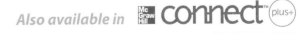

Identify the ICD-10-CM chapter in which each disease will be located.

1. Diabetes mellitus _____

2. Hypertension _____

3. Cholecystitis _____

4. Breast cancer _____

5. Fractures _____

5.4 ICD-10-CM Conventions and General Guidelines

conventions
Standards or rules within the coding systems.

general guidelines
Overall instructions to follow within the coding systems.

Many of the **conventions** and **general guidelines** in ICD-10-CM are very similar to those in ICD-9-CM. However, some new notes and instructions have been introduced to guide code selection in ICD-10-CM.

Conventions

Similar to ICD-9-CM Volumes 1 and 2, ICD-10-CM is divided into an Alphabetic Index and Tabular List. The Alphabetic Index includes four parts: Index of Diseases and Injuries, Index of External Causes of Injuries, Table of Neoplasms, and Table of Drugs and Chemicals.

The Tabular List includes categories, subcategories, and codes. Characters for categories, subcategories, and codes may be either letters or numbers. Categories have three-digit designations. A category that has only three digits without further subdivision is also a code. Subcategories may be four or five characters, and codes may be three, four, five, six, or seven characters. Each level of division beyond a category is a subcategory. The final subdivision is the code, regardless of the number of characters in the final subdivision. Final subdivisions with six characters are considered codes even if they require a seventh character. A six-character code with an applicable seventh character is considered an invalid code without the seventh character.

Some codes include a placeholder in a position other than the last position of the code. This is to allow for future expansions of these categories and subcategories. Examples of the use of these placeholders can be found in categories T36–T50, with numerous six-character codes that have an "x" as the fifth character and specific numbers as the sixth character.

When a code of less than six characters requires the use of a seventh character, the intervening places have an "x" inserted. Common examples include five-character codes that require an applicable seventh character. In those cases, the sixth position is designated with an "x."

CODER'S TIP

Some codes have placeholders as part of the full code and include the "x" indicator in the Tabular List. Other codes, such as five-digit codes requiring a seventh character, will not include the "x" in the Tabular List, listing only the five-digit codes. Coders must place the "x" in the sixth position before adding the seventh character.

Abbreviations, Punctuation, and Notes Two common abbreviations appear in both the Alphabetic Index and Tabular List. Not elsewhere classifiable (NEC) indicates that a specific condition exists but there is no specific code designating that known condition. Not otherwise specified (NOS) is used when no specific condition is specified.

Common punctuation includes the use of brackets [ ], parentheses ( ) and a colon (:) as part of the Alphabetic Index and Tabular List. Brackets in the Tabular List enclose synonyms, alternative wording, or explanations. Brackets in the Alphabetic Index indicate manifestation codes. Parentheses are used in both the Alphabetic Index and Tabular List to identify words that may be part of the descriptive term that do not affect code selection. These are also termed *nonessential modifiers*. Colons are used after an incomplete term to indicate that one or more modifiers after the colon are necessary to assign a specific code.

Some categories have an **Includes** indicator under the category title to further define the contents of the category. Specific codes may also have an Includes notation that lists specific conditions for which that code is used. When this appears after an "other specified" code, it indicates a list of conditions that may be indicated with that particular code. These lists are not necessarily exhaustive of all conditions included with the code.

Some categories, subcategories, and codes have exclusion notations. ICD-10-CM has two different exclusion notations: **Excludes1** and **Excludes2**. These exclusion notations have different definitions, but both mean that the excluded codes are independent of one another. Excludes1 means the excluded code is never used with the code above the Excludes1 note. The two codes are mutually exclusive, such as congenital and acquired forms of a condition. Excludes2 means the condition described by the excluded code is not generally part of the condition described by the code above the Excludes2 note, but under some circumstances a particular individual may have both conditions, in which case both codes may be reported together.

Manifestations Some conditions have an underlying **etiology** and one or more systemic **manifestations** due to the underlying etiology. For those conditions, the code describing the etiology is listed first, followed by the codes describing the manifestations. In such cases, the etiology code often contains a notation to "use additional code," and the manifestation code has a "code first" instruction.

Many of the manifestation codes include the designation "in diseases classified elsewhere" in the code descriptor. Such codes cannot be listed as the first-listed diagnosis, but must instead follow another code that designates the etiology of the condition.

The code listed next to a main term in the Alphabetic Index is referred to as a default code. The default code represents the condition that is most commonly associated with the main term or is the unspecified code for that condition. In the absence of additional information in the medical record to indicate the selection of a more specific code, the default code is selected.

The Alphabetic List identifies syndromes, which often have multiple manifestations. Some listings include specific guidance regarding the coding of the syndrome. In the absence of such guidance, the manifestations associated with the syndrome should be listed separately.

The terms *and, with, see,* and *see also* have the same meanings and uses described in Chapter 2 for the use of terms in ICD-9-CM.

General Guidelines

Similar to using Volume 2 followed by Volume 1 in ICD-9-CM, coders should use the Alphabetic Index followed by the Tabular List in ICD-10-CM. Often, the Alphabetic Index does not provide the full code. A dash (-) following an Alphabetic Index listing indicates that the code is not complete and additional characters are required. For example, characters indicating laterality and the seventh characters are not listed in the Alphabetic Index and can only be determined by using the Tabular List.

ICD-10-CM diagnosis codes may be three, four, five, six, or seven characters. Diagnosis codes must be reported to the greatest level of specificity possible (i.e., with the highest number of characters available). A code is not valid if it is not reported with the highest number of characters available, including a seventh character if applicable.

The main reason for the visit or encounter is most often the first-listed diagnosis. Other conditions may be listed as secondary diagnoses. Codes describing signs and symptoms, as opposed to specific diagnoses, may be the first-listed diagnosis if the provider has not confirmed any specific diagnoses. Chapter 18 (Symptoms, Signs, and Abnormal Clinical and Laboratory Findings, Not Elsewhere Classified), consisting of categories R00–R99, includes many, but not all codes describing symptoms. Once the actual diagnosis is known, codes for that diagnosis should be listed and the signs and symptoms codes no longer used.

Includes
A term that indicates some specific conditions described by the code under which it is listed.

Excludes1
A term unique to ICD-10-CM that is used to indicate that the excluded code should not be assigned in conjunction with the code under which it is listed, as the two conditions do not occur together.

Excludes2
A term unique to ICD-10-CM that is used to indicate that the condition being excluded is not considered to be part of the condition for the code under which it is listed, but rather another code should also be assigned.

etiology
The cause of a disease.

manifestation
A symptom or sign of a disease.

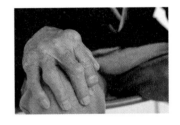

Some diseases, such as arthritis and pneumonia, have one or more systemic manifestations. In these cases, refer to the code for the disease's etiology, then choose the code that describes the particular manifestation. Follow the relevant sequencing guidelines.

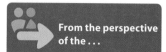

From the perspective of the . . .

CODER

ICD-10-CM codes allow the coder to extract more information from medical records and report the information in much greater detail than before.

PAYER

The increased information embedded in the ICD-10-CM diagnosis codes allows payers to process claims more efficiently and pay those claims more quickly than they could under the old system.

CODER'S TIP

Signs and symptoms that are commonly associated with a condition are not listed as additional codes with the diagnosis code describing that condition unless there are instructions to do so. Signs and symptoms not commonly associated with a condition should be listed separately when present.

If a condition is documented to be both acute and chronic, and separate codes exist in the Alphabetic Index at the same indentation level for the two conditions, the code describing the acute condition should be listed first.

Combination codes identify two diagnoses, a diagnosis and manifestation, or a diagnosis and complication. Combination codes can be identified by referring to subcategories in the Alphabetic Index and the inclusion and exclusion notations in the Tabular List. Only the combination code is used if it describes all the associated conditions. Additional codes are used if the combination code does not fully describe associated conditions, signs, and symptoms.

EXERCISE 5.4

Also available in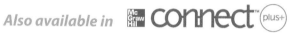

Fill in the word(s) to complete each statement.

1. Categories always begin with a _____ and have _____ characters.
2. Valid codes may have the following number of characters _____.
3. Codes identified with the Excludes2 designation may both be listed if _____.
4. A code that includes the term "in diseases classified elsewhere" cannot be listed as _____.
5. Codes describing signs and symptoms may be listed if _____.

5.5 Introduction to ICD-10-PCS

ICD-10-PCS

A coding system dedicated to coding procedures.

Unlike ICD-9-CM, which includes procedure codes in Volume 3, the ICD-10-CM does not include any procedure codes. Instead, a separate coding system, the ICD-10 Procedure Coding System (**ICD-10-PCS**), is dedicated to coding procedures. The ICD-10-PCS was developed by the 3M Company for CMS, which will maintain this code set. Whereas ICD-9-CM Volume 3 only includes about 3,000 procedure codes, ICD-10-PCS contains over 87,000 procedure codes.

The structure of ICD-10-PCS codes is very different than those of ICD-9-CM and ICD-10-CM. ICD-10-PCS codes are seven digits, each of which may be chosen from 34 different values—10 digits and 24 letters. The letters *O* and *I* are not used to avoid confusion with digits 0 and 1.

Breakdown of Sections

ICD-10-PCS is divided into 16 sections. The first digit of the seven-digit procedure code identifies the section. The ICD-10-PCS sections include:

0   Medical and Surgical
1   Obstetrics
2   Placement
3   Administration
4   Measurement and Monitoring
5   Extracorporeal Assistance and Performance
6   Extracorporeal Therapies
7   Osteopathic

8   Other Procedures

9   Chiropractic

B   Imaging

C   Nuclear Medicine

D   Radiation Oncology

F   Physical Rehabilitation and Diagnostic Audiology

G   Mental Health

H   Substance Abuse Treatment

Characters 2–7 of the ICD-10-PCS code have standard meanings within each section. These characters may, however, have different meanings from one section to another. For example, the seven characters of ICD-10-PCS codes in the Medical and Surgical section are:

1   Section (Section 0, Medical and Surgical)

2   Body System

3   Root Operation

4   Body Part

5   Approach

6   Device

7   Qualifier

For the Extracorporeal Assistance and Performance Measurement section, characters 2–7 have slightly different meanings:

1   Section (Section 5, Extracorporeal Assistance and Performance Measurement)

2   Physiological System

3   Root Operation

4   Body System

5   Duration

6   Function

7   Qualifier

Like ICD-9-CM Volume 3 codes, the codes in ICD-10-PCS are only used to report inpatient hospital services.

CODER'S TIP

Unlike ICD-10-CM, which is very similar to ICD-9-CM Volumes 1 and 2, ICD-10-PCS has a completely different code structure than its corresponding ICD-9-CM Volume 3 code. Rather than look up codes, coders must build ICD-10-PCS codes digit by digit.

EXERCISE 5.5

Also available in **McGraw Hill connect** (plus+)

Fill in the word(s) to complete each statement.

1. ICD-10-PCS codes consist of _____ characters, each of which can be either a _____ or a _____.

2. The letters _____ and _____ are never used as part of ICD-10-PCS codes, in order to avoid confusion with the characters _____ and _____.

3. In all procedure codes, the _____ character has the same designated meaning.

4. ICD-10-PCS will only be used by _____ to report _____ procedures.

5. ICD-9-CM Volume 3 codes will be used until _____, when ICD-10-PCS will be implemented.

CHAPTER **5** REVIEW

Summary

Learning Outcome	Key Concepts/Examples
5.1 Describe the upcoming transition to ICD-10-CM. **Pages 112–113**	The 30-year-old ICD-9-CM code system is inadequate to convey all the diagnosis information currently available. In 2013, a new coding system, the ICD-10-CM, will be implemented. ICD-10-CM will include approximately five times the number of diagnosis codes as ICD-9-CM. Each code has more information embedded in the code itself.
	There is no universal mapping system to convert ICD-9-CM codes to ICD-10-CM codes. General Equivalence Mappings (GEMs) help coders identify new codes that describe the same conditions as the older codes.
5.2 Discuss the basic structure of ICD-10-CM diagnosis codes. **Pages 114–116**	ICD-10-CM codes consist of 3–7 digits. The first digit is always an alpha character (A–Z). The second digit is always numeric. The third digit is either alpha or numeric. If the code consists of more than three digits, a decimal point always follows the third digit, with the remaining 1–4 digits following the decimal point. The digits to the right of the decimal point may be alpha or numeric digits.
	ICD-10-CM codes contain information embedded in the code that is not available in ICD-9-CM codes, including information regarding laterality, pregnancy trimester, and whether the encounter is for the initial treatment of an injury, subsequent visits, or to treat sequelae of the injury.
5.3 Explain the structure of the ICD-10-CM manual. **Pages 116–117**	The ICD-10-CM includes an Alphabetic Index and Tabular List to help coders select the most appropriate code to describe conditions. The Tabular List is divided into 21 chapters listing more than 69,000 codes.
	Coders should use the Alphabetic Index and Tabular List in the same manner as they currently use the Volume 2 followed by Volume 1 of the ICD-9-CM manual
5.4 Compare ICD-10-CM general guidelines with ICD-9-CM guidelines. **Pages 118–120**	The ICD-10-CM conventions and general guidelines are very similar to those in ICD-9-CM. The differences that do exist are not very difficult for coders to understand and adopt.
5.5 Discuss the structure of the ICD-10-PCS system for procedure codes. **Pages 120–121**	ICD-9-CM Volume 3 procedure codes will not be part of the ICD-10-CM system. Instead, a completely new procedure code system, ICD-10-PCS, has been developed. It includes approximately 87,000 codes that will be adopted at the same time that ICD-10-CM is implemented in 2013.
	ICD-10-PCS codes are also seven characters in length, but they have rules of construction that are significantly different than those governing ICD-10-CM Volume 3 procedure code construction. Coders will need to devote time to mastering the format and selection of these codes.

Using Terminology

Match the key terms with their definitions.

_____ **1.** L05.1 General Equivalence Mappings (GEMs)

_____ **2.** L05.2 Laterality

_____ **3.** L05.2 Initial treatment

A. Signifies a combination of related or similar codes that might be reported together

B. The underlying cause of a condition or manifestation

C. Distinction between left or right

____ **4.** L05.2 Subsequent encounter
____ **5.** L05.2 Sequelae
____ **6.** L05.2 Placeholder
____ **7.** L05.4 Conventions
____ **8.** L05.4 General guidelines
____ **9.** L05.4 Excludes1
____ **10.** L05.4 Excludes2
____ **11.** L05.4 Etiology

D. Tool to help identify ICD-10 codes that correspond to ICD-9 codes
E. First care encounter for a diagnosis or problem
F. Care encounter after the initial care event
G. A condition that persists after the causative condition has resolved
H. A character inserted into an unused position of a code to preserve code length
I. Describes the structure and organization of codes and code sets
J. Describes the methodology of finding and correctly applying codes
K. Signifies a combination of codes that are never reported together

Checking Your Understanding

Select the answer that best completes the statement or answers the question.

1. L05.1 An ICD-10-CM code will _____ describe a disease or condition exactly corresponding to that described by an ICD-9-CM code.

  a. Never
  b. Always
  c. Randomly
  d. Sometimes

2. L05.2 The ICD-10-CM code structure allows the potential capability to specify each of the following details about a condition except _____.

  a. Laterality
  b. Episode of care
  c. Gender of patient
  d. Trimester of pregnancy

3. L05.1 ICD-10-CM will be implemented _____.

  a. After all available ICD-9-CM codes have been utilized
  b. On October 1, 2013
  c. On January 1, 2013
  d. Once all WHO member countries have prepared for the transition

4. L05.1 After the date of transition, the use of ICD-10-CM codes will be mandatory _____.

  a. By state departments of health
  b. by presidential decree
  c. For providers who accept Medicare
  d. For entities that share information involving diagnosis codes

5. L05.1 In comparison with ICD-9-CM, ICD-10-CM _____.

  a. Has a one-to-one code equivalency plus many additional codes for detail
  b. Reuses ICD-9 codes but adds additional digits for greater specificity
  c. Has additional digits and a different structure for greater granularity of detail
  d. Has many more codes but cannot be expanded to include new codes

connect plus+
Enhance your learning by completing these exercises and more at mcgrawhillconnect.com!

CHAPTER 5 | INTRODUCTION TO ICD-10-CM AND ICD-10-PCS   123

6. L05.2 Which of the following statements is true about the ICD-10-CM code structure?

   a. All codes have seven digits.
   b. Placeholder character "x" should be used as the final digit.
   c. The first digit is always an alphabetic character.
   d. The third digit is always numeric.

7. L05.2 All of the following are valid characters for specifying the encounter (initial, subsequent, sequela) except:

   a. A   **c.** D
   b. I   **d.** S

8. L05.2 Which of the following is a valid character for indicating laterality?

   a. R   **c.** B
   b. 2   **d.** 8

9. L05.3 Which of the following statements is true about the ICD-10-CM Alphabetic Index?

   a. It is ordered alphabetically by the first digit of the ICD-10-CM code.
   b. It is ordered alphabetically by the chapter title.
   c. Each alphabetic entry corresponds to one ICD-10-CM code.
   d. It is ordered alphabetically by clinical term.

10. L05.3 Which of the following statements is true regarding the first digit of an ICD-10-CM code and its location in the Tabular Index?

   a. The first digit is the same as the chapter number.
   b. The first digit is determined by the code category.
   c. The first digit is the same as the letter that begins the name of the organ system involved.
   d. Only one particular first digit is valid for each chapter number.

11. L05.4 Which of the following numbers is in the correct format for an ICD-10-CM code?

   a. A12.345x
   b. A1234x5
   c. A12.34x5
   d. A123.4x5

12. L05.4 Which of the following conditions would most likely be assigned a code with an NEC indicator?

   a. A dysfunction of the thyroid gland, not further described
   b. A throat infection with no other stated details
   c. A thermal burn without qualification of the location or severity
   d. A specific lung infection caused by a newly discovered and named virus

13. L05.4 Which of the following conditions would most likely be assigned a code with an NOS indicator?

   a. Acute methicillin-resistant *Staphylococcus aureus* septic arthritis of the left knee
   b. Open fracture of the midshaft right tibia
   c. Lung infection, unspecified organism
   d. Chronic hepatic failure caused by hepatitis B virus

14. L05.4 Under which of the following circumstances might a coder find an Excludes2 notation for one code under the other in the Tabular List?

   a. Surgical absence of a kidney and surgical absence of the gallbladder
   b. Congenital absence of the uterus and surgical absence of the uterus
   c. Congenital absence of one ovary and surgical absence of one ovary
   d. Congenital absence of part of the tongue and congenital absence of the whole tongue

15. L05.4 Which of the following combination of conditions would be the most likely to have an Includes indicator?

   a. Pharyngitis and pneumonia
   b. Cystitis and urinary tract infection
   c. Femur fracture and lower leg laceration
   d. Hepatitis as a result of generalized malaria infection

16. L05.4 Which of the following is an example of an etiology plus a manifestation code combination?

   a. A fall down stairs causing a fracture
   b. AIDS with a superimposed pneumonia
   c. Cirrhosis causing esophageal varices
   d. A laceration that has become infected

17. L05.4 Which of the following could be coded as a principal (first-listed) diagnosis?

   a. Dementia in a condition classified elsewhere
   b. Myocardial infarction, third episode of care
   c. Nausea as a symptom of acute gastritis
   d. A traffic accident as an external cause of morbidity

18. L05.5 Which of the following statements is true about ICD-10-PCS?

   a. The first digit always indicates the body system.
   b. Each digit position always has the same meaning across all sections of ICD-10-PCS.
   c. ICD-10-PCS codes use existing ICD-9-PCS codes with expansion using additional digits.
   d. Every ICD-10-PCS code is comprised of seven digits.

19. L05.5 Which of the following numbers is in the correct format for an ICD-10-PCS code?

   a. A1B2Cx4
   b. A1B.2C3D
   c. A1B2C3D
   d. A1B2C3O

20. L05.5 Within each section of ICD-10-PCS, there is a specific designation for each digit position. Which of the following is not a valid digit designation in ICD-10-PCS section 0?

   a. Body system
   b. Physiological system
   c. Body part
   d. Root operation

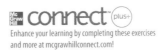
Enhance your learning by completing these exercises and more at mcgrawhillconnect.com!

CHAPTER 5 | INTRODUCTION TO ICD-10-CM AND ICD-10-PCS   125

Applying Your Skills

Using an official source for ICD-10-CM codes, assign the correct code(s) to each diagnosis.

Encounter   **Codes**

1. L05.4 Amebic infection of appendix   _____

2. L05.4 Tuberculous pleurisy   _____

3. L05.4 Listeriosis with meningitis   _____

4. L05.4 Methicillin-resistant *Staphylococcus aureus*   _____

5. L05.4 Acute nonparalytic poliomyelitis   _____

6. L05.4 *H. pylori* as the cause of a disease classified elsewhere   _____

7. L05.4 Human immunodeficiency virus (HIV) infection   _____

8. L05.4 Trench fever   _____

9. L05.4 Malignant neoplasm, base of the tongue   _____

10. L05.4 Prostate cancer   _____

11. L05.4 Cancer of the temporal lobe of the brain   _____

12. L05.4 Benign carcinoid tumor of the ascending colon   _____

13. L05.4 Hemangioma of the skin of the newborn's right arm   _____

14. L05.4 Intraductal carcinoma in situ, right breast   _____

15. L05.4 Neoplasm of uncertain behavior of the bone   _____

16. L05.4 Type II diabetes mellitus treated with insulin,
    complicated by gastroparesis   _____

17. L05.4 Amyotrophic lateral sclerosis   _____

18. L05.4 Chronic atherosclerotic heart disease without
    angina pectoris   _____

19. L05.4 Impacted gallstones with obstruction, without
    acute cholecystitis   _____

20. L05.4 Spinal stenosis, L1–S1   _____

21. L05.4 Kidney stones with one or more ureteral stones   _____

22. L05.4 Supervision of normal first pregnancy, third trimester   _____

23. L05.4 Newborn suspected of being affected by maternal
    periodontal disease   _____

24. L05.4 Midline cleft lip without cleft palate   _____

25. L05.4 Initial treatment of closed midshaft fracture of the
    right clavicle with 1 cm. of displacement   _____

26. L05.4 Traumatic amputation of the right big toe,
    follow-up visit to assess healing   _____

Encounter	Codes
27. L05.4 Initial treatment for second-degree burn of the chest wall caused by house fire	_____
28. L05.4 Evaluation of loosening of left artificial hip prosthesis without evidence of infection	_____
29. L05.4 Initial treatment for injury to a car driver involved in a collision with another car	_____
30. L05.4 Encounter for routine gynecological exam with Pap smear and no abnormal findings	_____

Thinking It Through

Use your critical-thinking skills to answer the questions below.

1. L05.1 Discuss three advantages ICD-10-CM has over ICD-9-CM.

_____

_____

2. L05.2 What type of character is the first digit of every ICD-10-CM code? What does it always indicate?

_____

_____

3. L05.2 Describe the function of the seventh digit of an ICD-10-CM code.

_____

_____

4. L05.3 What are the two divisions of the ICD-10-CM manual? How is each organized?

_____

_____

5. L05.4 In ICD-10-CM, what is the difference between an Excludes1 notation and an Excludes2 notation?

_____

_____

6. L05.4 How is the character "x" properly used in an ICD-10-CM code?

_____

_____

7. L05.5 Describe how many digits comprise a valid ICD-10-PCS code. Explain the significance of each digit position for all the codes within a given section of the ICD-10-PCS code set.

_____

_____

Enhance your learning by completing these exercises and more at mcgrawhillconnect.com!

CHAPTER 5 | INTRODUCTION TO ICD-10-CM AND ICD-10-PCS   127

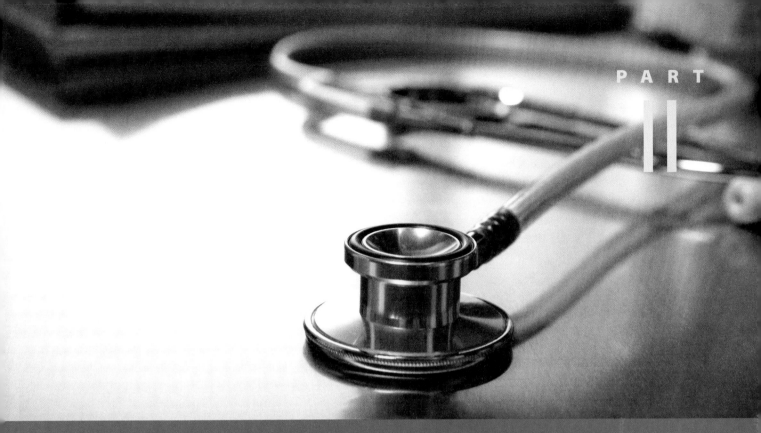

PART II

CPT AND HCPCS

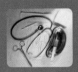 6 Introduction to CPT

 7 Modifiers

 8 Evaluation and Management Services, Part I: Structure and Guidance

 9 Evaluation and Management Services, Part II: Code Selection

 10 Anesthesia Services

 11 Radiology Services

 12 Surgery Codes: Coding for Surgical Procedures on Specific Organ Systems

 13 Pathology and Laboratory Services

 14 Medicine Services

 15 Introduction to the Healthcare Common Procedure Coding System (HCPCS)

6 INTRODUCTION TO CPT

Learning Outcomes *After completing this chapter, students should be able to:*

6.1 Explain the structure of the CPT manual.

6.2 Identify the information contained within each code section.

6.3 Describe the functions of the index, appendices, and additional information in the CPT manual.

6.4 Describe the uses of Category II CPT codes.

6.5 Differentiate the uses of Category III codes from those of Category I and Category II codes.

Key Terms

Add-on code
Appendices
Category I
Category II
Category III
Code sections
CPT manual
Emerging technology
Guidelines
Index
Main terms
Modifier
Modifier 51 exempt
Modifying terms
Parent code
Parenthetical note
Performance measurement
    exclusion modifiers
Performance measures
Place of service
Separate procedure
Symbols
Unlisted procedure

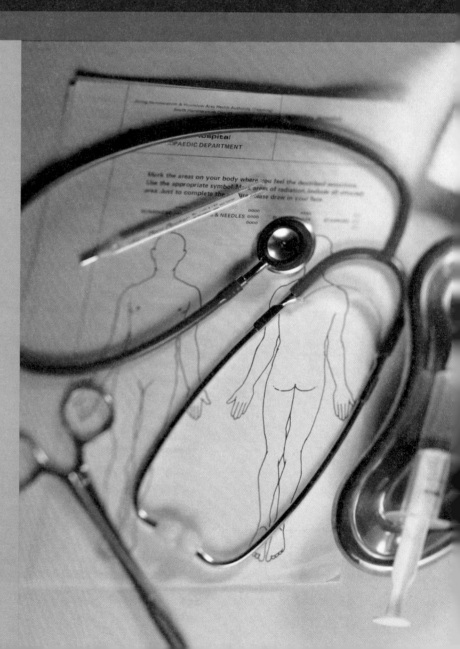

Introduction

The American Medical Association (AMA) maintains the Current Procedural Terminology (CPT), Fourth Edition, code set to describe services generally provided by physicians and other healthcare professionals to individual patients. The CPT manual was first published in 1966 as a set of four-digit codes describing surgical procedures. In 1970, the AMA expanded the codes to five digits and increased the number of codes to describe a larger group of services and procedures. Use of the CPT codes is intended to accurately describe those services and provide a convenient method of communicating this information among providers, payers, administrators, and regulators. The codes are shorthand notations that, when used properly, provide essential data to all those providing care, paying for care, and overseeing the quality of care.

This chapter provides a high-level overview of the structure and functions of the CPT manual and is not intended to provide detailed instructions for students. Chapters 7–14 provide detailed information about each section of CPT codes. This chapter can be thought of as a map of the entire United States, whereas Chapters 7–14 are like detailed city maps showing individual streets. Both are necessary to understand the relationships between the different parts of the CPT manual and how to connect information from these parts to report medical services.

6.1 Structure of the CPT Manual

The **CPT manual** includes three categories of codes. **Category I** codes describe services that are generally acceptable in the current practice of medicine and are performed by many physicians in clinical practice in multiple clinical locations. These procedures are generally considered to be within standard medical practice, but the existence of a code does not indicate that the particular procedure is considered the standard of care. The existence of a Category I code is not an endorsement by the American Medical Association of any particular procedure described by that code. Category I codes are five-digit numerical codes.

> ### CODER'S TIP
>
> Although payment issues are beyond the scope of this course, it is important for students to understand that inclusion as a Category I code does not imply coverage of the procedure for payment purposes by Medicare, Medicaid, or commercial insurance plans.

Category II codes are used primarily as performance measures. Medicare uses these codes to document the quality of services provided to individual patients and to the patient population under the care of individual providers, groups of providers, or a healthcare system. Widespread use of these codes and adoption of electronic data systems may reduce the manual efforts currently necessary to document provider performance through chart reviews. Other payers may also use these codes to assess the quality of care. Category II codes are four numeric digits followed by the letter *F*.

Category III codes are a set of temporary codes used to designate emerging technologies, services, and procedures. Category III codes help document the extent to which these services are provided in terms of the number of providers and how geographically widespread they are. The AMA and the CPT Editorial Panel will consider this, as well as other information, when deciding whether a Category I code will be adopted to describe a service. Category III codes consist of four numeric digits followed by the letter *T*.

CPT° manual
Code set to describe services generally provided by physicians and other healthcare professionals to individual patients.

Category I
Category of codes in the CPT manual that describe services that are generally acceptable in the current practice of medicine and are performed by many physicians in clinical practice in multiple clinical locations.

Category II
Category of codes in the CPT manual used primarily as performance measures.

Category III
Category of codes in the CPT manual that include a set of temporary codes used to designate emerging technologies, services, and procedures.

The CPT Editorial Panel, consisting of physicians from many specialties, recommends changes to the CPT code set, including the addition of new codes, deletion of codes that are no longer necessary, and revisions to the code descriptors. The Category I code set is revised annually, with new editions of the CPT manual published in the fall of each year with the latest revisions. Revisions may include code additions, code deletions, and editorial changes to code descriptors. The new code set becomes effective the following January 1st. The time between publication and January 1st is the implementation period during which providers, payers, and vendors incorporate the changes into their systems. Category II, Category III, and vaccine codes may be updated more frequently.

Code Sections

Category I CPT codes are organized by **code sections,** each of which designates a specific grouping of codes. Codes are placed in numerical order within the manual, with the exception of the evaluation and management codes (99201–99499), which appear in the first section at the beginning of the manual because these codes are used by almost all providers to report a large number of services.

In general, CPT codes are divided into sections as follows:

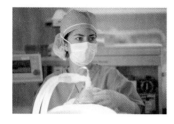

Anesthesia procedures are reported using codes 00100–01999 from the CPT manual.

Evaluation and Management	99201–99499
Anesthesia	00100–01999
Surgery	10021–69990
Radiology	70010–79999
Pathology and Laboratory	80047–89356
Medicine	90281–99199 and 99500–99607

Placement of a procedure within one code section does not indicate which providers may perform the service. Providers may perform services within the scope of their licenses regardless of the placement of the code that describes the particular service within the CPT manual. Each of the above sections may be further divided. For example, the Surgery section codes are generally divided as follows:

Integumentary System	10021–19499
Musculoskeletal System	20100–29999
Respiratory System	30000–32999
Cardiovascular System	33010–37799
Hemic and Lymphatic Systems	38100–38999
Mediastinum and Diaphragm	39000–39599
Digestive System	40490–49999
Urinary and Genital Systems	50010–58999
Maternity Care and Delivery	59000–59899
Endocrine System	60000–60699
Nervous System	61000–64999
Ocular System	65091–68899
Auditory System	69000–69979
Operating Microscope Use	69990

Coders must select the CPT codes that most accurately describe the services provided. If a specific code accurately describes the actual services provided, it is improper to utilize a more general code or an **unlisted procedure** code. Unlisted procedure codes can only be used when no specific code exists that describes the service provided.

Each of the six main sections and most of the surgical subsections listed above include specific **guidelines.** These guidelines provide information necessary to correctly report procedures listed in each section, including definitions of terms unique to that section. For example, guidelines at the beginning of the Radiology section define the term *radiological supervision and interpretation*. Guidelines in the Anesthesia code section discuss how time is reported with regard to anesthesia codes.

Use the CPT manual to complete each statement.

1. The CPT codes are owned and maintained by the _____.
2. When did the American Medical Association first publish the CPT manual? _____
3. What are guidelines? _____

6.2 Code Format and Additional Information

Indented Code Structure

Each code is a stand-alone descriptor of a medical procedure. However, in some code sections, multiple sequential codes have the same initial descriptors. These common descriptor elements are not repeated in each code. Instead, the common portion of a code series appears in the description of the first code of the series, followed by a semicolon (;) and the unique portion of that code. Subsequent codes do not include the common portion, but are indented with only the unique portion of those codes printed.

Some examples of CPT code series include:

61680	Surgery of intracranial arteriovenous malformation; supratentorial, simple
61682	supratentorial, complex
61684	infratentorial, simple
61686	infratentorial, complex
61690	dural, simple
61692	dural, complex

or

27560	Closed treatment of patellar dislocation; without anesthesia
27562	requiring anesthesia

In both of the examples above, the first code in the series includes a portion of the descriptor followed by a semicolon. This portion of the code is presumed to be included in each of the codes indented under the main code. The first code has a second portion of the code descriptor following the semicolon. That portion is unique to that code. In each of the following codes, the printed portion of the descriptor would appear to the right of the semicolon if the common portion were printed in each code. If the codes were printed in their entirety, they would appear as follows:

61680	Surgery of intracranial arteriovenous malformation; supratentorial, simple
61682	Surgery of intracranial arteriovenous malformation; supratentorial, complex
61684	Surgery of intracranial arteriovenous malformation; infratentorial, simple
61686	Surgery of intracranial arteriovenous malformation; infratentorial, complex
61690	Surgery of intracranial arteriovenous malformation; dural, simple
61692	Surgery of intracranial arteriovenous malformation; dural, complex

or

27560	Closed treatment of patellar dislocation; without anesthesia
27562	Closed treatment of patellar dislocation; requiring anesthesia

Symbols

symbols
Representations attached to specific CPT codes to designate information relevant to the particular codes.

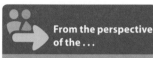

From the perspective of the . . .

CODER

Coding symbols and their meanings convey important information regarding codes. Coders must determine whether this information affects the selection of the appropriate code to report the services provided.

add-on code
Codes identified with the plus sign, indicating they cannot be reported alone.

parent code
The primary code associated with a procedure, sometimes accompanied by an additional code, sometimes accompanied by an add-on code.

modifier 51 exempt
Describes codes that cannot have modifier 51 added to them, represented by the circle-slash symbol (⊘).

parenthetical note
Message included with individual or groups of codes that provides specific instructions unique to those codes, commonly directing the use of specific codes for some services or prohibiting the use of certain code combinations; notes always have parentheses around the instructions.

One or more **symbols** may be attached to specific CPT codes to designate information relevant to that particular code. These symbols include the following:

- ● Indicates a new procedure. This symbol appears for only one year after a new code is added to the CPT manual.
- ▲ Designates code descriptors that have been substantially altered.
- ►◄ Indicates new and revised text such as parenthetical notes and guidelines.
- ✛ Designates add-on codes, which also are listed in Appendix D.
- ⊘ Designates codes that are exempt from the use of modifier 51 but are not add-on codes. These also are listed in Appendix E.
- ⊙ Designates codes that include conscious sedation as an inherent part of the procedure. These also are listed in Appendix G.
- ✗ Designates vaccine codes pending approval from the Food and Drug Administration (FDA). These also are listed in Appendix K.
- # Designates a code that is out of numerical sequence. This allows codes to be placed with a family of related codes even when code numbers are not available for sequential numbering. Out-of-sequence codes are listed in Appendix N.

Several symbols indicate that the codes marked with those symbols are different from most other codes. Coders must be familiar with those differences and how they affect coding. For example, codes identified with the plus sign (✛) as add-on codes cannot be reported alone. If an **add-on code** is reported, the **parent code** for that add-on code also must be reported. It is incorrect to report an add-on code unless the parent code is also reported. Add-on codes may include phrases such as "each additional" or "(List separately in addition to code for primary procedure)" as part of the descriptor.

The circle-slash symbol (⊘) indicates that modifier 51 cannot be added to the code. These codes are designated as **modifier 51 exempt.** Add-on codes are also automatically exempt from modifier 51, but that exemption is understood whenever a code is identified with a plus sign. Add-on codes do not have the circle-slash identifier.

The above descriptions of several symbols indicate that codes identified with those symbols are listed in one of the appendices that appear in the back of the CPT manual. The appendices will be discussed in greater detail later in this chapter.

Parenthetical Notes

Individual codes or groups of codes may include **parenthetical notes** that provide specific instructions unique to those codes. These notes always have parentheses around the instructions. Parenthetical notes commonly direct the use of specific codes for some services or prohibit the use of certain code combinations. Coders must understand how to apply parenthetical notes when reporting codes associated with those notes.

For example, CPT codes 11010, 11011, and 11012 describe debridement at the site of an open fracture, with each code describing an increasing amount of tissue. Code 11010 includes skin and subcutaneous tissue only. Code 11011 includes skin, subcutaneous tissue, muscle fascia, and muscle. Code 11012 includes skin, subcutaneous tissue, muscle fascia, muscle, and bone. Three parenthetical notes follow code 11012 that apply to all three codes:

(For debridement of skin, i.e., epidermis and/or dermis only, see 97597, 97598.)

(For active wound care management, see 97597, 97598.)

(For debridement of burn wounds, see 16020–16030.)

CPT codes 64479–64495 describe certain unilateral spinal injections. Each of these requires the use of image guidance (defined as fluoroscopy or computed tomography [CT]). Parenthetical notes provide instructions to coders, including the following:

- The correct parent code to report with add-on codes.
- Instructions to report bilateral procedures with modifier 50.
- The use of ultrasound does not meet the image guidance requirement for these codes. Injections with ultrasound guidance must be reported with specific Category III codes.
- If procedures described by CPT codes 64490–64495 are performed without the required fluoroscopy or CT guidance, the injections should be reported as trigger point injections using CPT codes 20552–20553.

Modifiers

A **modifier** may be added to a code to indicate that a procedure has been altered by specific circumstances but the code still describes the service provided. Some modifiers provide specific information that is necessary for payers to accurately process the claim. Each modifier conveys specific information, such as whether:

- The service or procedure was increased or reduced.
- Only part of a service was performed.
- An additional or adjunctive service was performed.
- The procedure was performed bilaterally.
- The service was provided more than once.
- The service included both a professional and technical component.
- More than one physician performed the procedure.
- The procedure was repeated a second time on the same day.

Separate Procedure

Numerous codes include the designation **(separate procedure)** in the code descriptor. Students, as well as some experienced coders, sometimes misunderstand this, thinking it means that these codes may be billed separately no matter what other procedures are performed during the same setting. That is an incorrect interpretation. These codes are used when the procedure described by the code is performed alone. If the procedure is performed as part of another procedure or in addition to other procedures, then separate reporting of the separate procedure code is incorrect.

In some cases, the code descriptors make it obvious that one procedure is inherently a part of another procedure and cannot be reported separately, even though the code descriptor includes the (separate procedure) designation. For example, the following CPT codes cannot be reported together:

47425 (Choledochotomy or choledochostomy with exploration, drainage, or removal of calculus, with or without cholecystotomy; with transduodenal sphincterotomy or sphincteroplasty)

47460 (Transduodenal sphincterotomy or sphincteroplasty, with or without transduodenal extraction of calculus [separate procedure])

Even though CPT code 47460 is designated as a separate procedure, the description of that procedure is inherent in the description of CPT code 47425. Therefore, only

modifier
An addition to a code to indicate that a procedure has been altered by specific circumstances, but the code still describes the service provided.

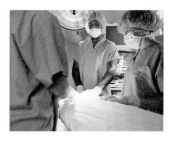

If more than one physician performed a procedure, the code for that procedure must contain a modifier that reflects this fact.

separate procedure
Term used in the code descriptor when the procedure described by the code is performed alone.

47425 is used to report these procedures. CPT code 47460 is only reported as a separate procedure if it is the only procedure performed.

In other situations, it is not obvious that a procedure designated as a separate procedure is part of one or more other procedures. For example, CPT code 49000 describes an exploratory laparotomy and includes the (separate procedure) designation. This code is used when an exploratory laparotomy is the only intra-abdominal procedure provided. If another intra-abdominal procedure is performed during the same operation, this code is not listed because the other procedure includes the exploratory laparotomy.

EXERCISE 6.2

Also available in **McGraw Hill connect** plus+

Use the CPT manual to answer the questions below.

1. What is the significance of an indented code? _____

2. What symbol indicates that the coder should verify whether a vaccine has received FDA approval since the CPT manual was published? _____

3. What instruction does the parenthetical note below CPT code 37761 provide regarding bilateral procedures?
_____

6.3 Other Information Included in the CPT Manual

In addition to the list of codes, descriptors, symbols, parenthetical notes, and modifiers, the CPT manual includes significant additional information. This additional information is included in sections of the CPT manual other than the code lists and guidelines associated with the code sections. Most of this information is provided in the index, appendices, introductory pages, and the inside front and back covers. Each of these is described below.

Index

index
Section of the CPT manual used to identify all possible codes that describe a procedure, organized alphabetically by main terms.

The **index** is an essential part of the CPT manual. Students should routinely use the index to identify all possible codes that describe a procedure before selecting the single code that best describes the procedure or service provided. Even experienced coders should routinely refer to the index when selecting codes they do not use on an everyday basis.

main terms
Key terms organized alphabetically in the index of the CPT manual that can stand alone or be followed by one to three indented modifying terms, of which there are four primary types: procedure or service; organ or other anatomical site; condition; and synonyms, eponyms, and abbreviations.

The index is organized alphabetically by **main terms**. There are four primary types of main terms:

- Procedure or service
  Examples: Laparoscopy; repair; incision
- Organ or other anatomical site
  Examples: Esophagus; femur; heart
- Condition
  Examples: Abscess; dislocation; fistula
- Synonyms, eponyms, and abbreviations
  Examples: EKG; Ilizarov procedure; Latzko operation

modifying terms
Indented terms listed under a main term in the index that alter or add to that main term's conditions.

Each main term can stand alone or be followed by one to three indented **modifying terms** that have an effect on code selection. Coders should consider modifying terms when determining the codes they should review as part of their code-selection process.

If only one code applies to an index entry, it is listed on its own. If more than one code applies, these codes are listed as a code range. If the code range includes nonsequential codes, commas are used to separate them. If two or more sequential codes apply to the entry, a hyphen is used. Both commas and hyphens may be used in the same entry, as in the examples below.

Myelography
    Brain   70010
Orbit
    Exploration   61332, 67400, 67450
Mastectomy
    Radical   19303–19306
Metacarpophalangeal Joint
    Fusion   26516–26518, 26850–26852

To save space and avoid unnecessary words, the index infers the use of some words, such as "of" or other commonly used words. The common term used in almost every anesthesia code, "for procedures on," is also inferred when the term *anesthesia* appears, as in the example below.

Elbow
    Anesthesia (for procedures on)   00400, 01710–01782
    Incision and drainage (of)   24000

In the examples in this section, the words in parentheses are not included in the index entry.

CODER'S TIP

The use of the CPT index does not substitute for the main text in the list of CPT codes. Even if only one code is listed in the index, coders must refer to the actual code and descriptor to confirm that the code identified in the index appropriately describes the procedure or service provided.

Appendices

The CPT manual includes a number of **appendices** that contain essential information for complete and accurate coding. These include:

- Appendix A: Modifiers
- Appendix B: Summary of Additions, Deletions, and Revisions
- Appendix C: Clinical Examples
- Appendix D: Summary of CPT Add-on Codes
- Appendix E: Summary of CPT Codes Exempt from Modifier 51
- Appendix F: Summary of CPT Codes Exempt from Modifier 63
- Appendix G: Summary of Codes That Include Moderate Sedation
- Appendix H: Alphabetical Clinical Topics Listing (no longer used)
- Appendix I: Genetic Testing Code Modifiers
- Appendix J: Electrodiagnostic Medicine Listing of Sensory, Motor, and Mixed Nerves
- Appendix K: Product Pending FDA Approval
- Appendix L: Vascular Families
- Appendix M: Deleted CPT Codes with Crosswalks to New Codes
- Appendix N: Summary of Resequenced CPT Codes

appendices
Sections of the CPT manual that contain different areas of essential information for complete and accurate coding.

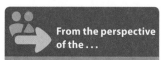

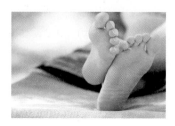

From the perspective of the ...

CODER

It is important to understand what information is included in each appendix. Consider this information when determining which codes to report for a specific service, including adding modifiers and using conscious sedation procedure codes.

Modifiers from Appendix A are used to indicate that the provider performed a bilateral procedure, such as a procedure that involved both of a patient's feet.

The information contained in the appendices is discussed briefly in this chapter. How coders should use this information is presented in detail in subsequent chapters. This chapter provides an overview of the CPT appendices.

Appendix A This is a list of CPT modifiers that often are added to CPT codes. Examples of the use of these modifiers include clinical situations where:

- The same provider performed multiple procedures on the same date.
- The provider performed bilateral procedures.
- One procedure is not part of other procedures reported on the same date of service by the same provider.
- One provider performed only the professional or technical component of the procedure, but not both.
- The surgical care is divided among two or more providers.
- One surgeon assisted another during a procedure.

A series of anatomical modifiers identify specific fingers, toes, eyelids, and coronary arteries. Some modifiers are only used with anesthesia codes to indicate the physical status of the patient. These are discussed in detail in the Modifier chapter.

Appendix B This appendix lists all new, deleted, and revised codes in numerical order. New codes are identified with the "new code" symbol (red bullet). Deleted codes are identified with strikethroughs of the entire code number and descriptor. Revised codes are identified with the "revised code" symbol (blue triangle), and a combination of strikethroughs of deleted language and underlining of new language is added to the code.

Appendix C This appendix includes numerous clinical examples of many of the CPT evaluation and management (E/M) codes. These examples are meant as a guide to help coders select the most appropriate E/M codes. Appendix C includes clinical examples of office or other outpatient services; hospital inpatient services; consultations; emergency department services; critical care services; prolonged services; and care plan oversight services. E/M code selection in these areas and others is discussed in detail in Chapters 8 and 9. Once coders understand how E/M codes are selected, they may use this appendix as a reference to help their selection in particular instances.

Appendix D This appendix lists add-on codes in numerical order. These codes are identified with a plus sign (✚) in the CPT manual. These codes cannot be reported without the parent code. Payment methodologies are beyond the scope of this course, but add-on codes are treated similarly to the modifier 51 exempt codes listed in Appendix E and identified by the circle-slash symbol (⊘).

Appendix E This appendix identifies CPT codes that do not have modifier 51 added to the code even when they are performed with other procedures. Although payment methodologies are beyond the scope of this course, the use of modifier 51 affects payment for the additional procedures when more than one service is provided. This is commonly referred to as the Multiple Procedure Reduction rules. Those payment rules are not applied to procedures that are modifier 51 exempt. The additional procedure payment rules also do not apply to add-on codes listed in Appendix D, but it is not necessary to add the circle-slash symbol (⊘) to those codes, as that is inferred from the plus sign (✚).

Appendix F This appendix lists procedures to which it is improper to add modifier 63, which identifies procedures performed on infants weighing less than 4 kg. These procedures entail more surgical difficulty and risks than do the same procedures on larger infants, children, or adults. Some CPT codes specifically identify procedures that are almost always performed on infants weighing less than 4 kg, so modifier 63 is unnecessary, as the information is inherent in the code itself. Those procedure codes are listed in Appendix F.

Appendix G This appendix identifies procedures that include moderate (conscious) sedation as part of the work of performing those procedures, even though the code descriptors do not explicitly state that sedation is included. Because sedation is included with these codes, physicians performing these services cannot also report CPT codes 99143–99145 (conscious sedation by the same physician) with these codes.

CODER'S TIP

Inclusion of a code in Appendix G does not preclude reporting anesthesia codes (00100–01999) when a provider other than the one performing the underlying procedure listed in Appendix G performs anesthesia services. The provider of anesthesia services must be present to continuously monitor the patient and cannot act as a surgical assistant to the provider performing the underlying procedure.

Appendix H Clinical topics were previously listed alphabetically in this appendix. This list is constantly changing, rapidly expanding, and is used to link Category II codes, clinical conditions, and explanations of the performance measures. Annual updates are not adequate, so updates now are available on the AMA website at www.ama-assn.org/go/cpt.

Appendix I This appendix includes more than 100 modifiers that identify specific genetic tests. These modifiers are added to CPT codes that identify laboratory procedures related to genetic tests to provide diagnostic specificity to those laboratory procedure codes. Without these modifiers, it would be necessary to include hundreds of individual CPT codes in the laboratory section to identify the specific tests. The modifiers are two digits, with the first character (numeric) identifying the disease category and the second character (alpha) indicating the specific gene type. This appendix groups genetic tests into 11 disease categories.

Appendix J This appendix assigns each motor, sensory, and mixed nerve to a specific nerve conduction study code to accurately report CPT codes 95900, 95903, and 95904. Each test performed on a listed nerve is one unit of service for the nerve conduction test code.

Appendix K This is a list of codes that identify products that have not yet received FDA approval, such as the newest vaccines, when approval is expected shortly after publication. This makes it easier for coders to identify the appropriate code to report these services after the FDA approves those products.

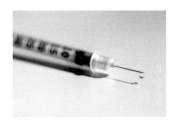

Appendix L This appendix graphically identifies vascular families with assignment of the first-, second-, and third-order arterial vessels in each family. This information is essential to correctly report CPT codes describing angiography procedures when more than one artery is included in the procedure.

Codes listed in Appendix K identify products that have not received FDA approval yet but are expected to be approved shortly after the CPT codes for that year will be published. These products include new vaccines.

Appendix M This appendix identifies CPT codes that were deleted and renumbered between 2007 and 2009. This appendix will not be updated, as the methodology of deleting and renumbering CPT codes is no longer being utilized during updates of the CPT code set.

Appendix N This appendix is a list of CPT codes that appear out of sequence in the code set. Allowing codes to be relocated out of sequence to group them with other appropriate services avoids the necessity of deleting and renumbering those codes.

Introductory Pages

place of service
The location in which services are provided, identified by specific codes listed in the introductory pages of the CPT manual.

The first pages of the CPT manual list all **place of service** codes, place of service names, and place of service descriptions in a table. When coders report procedures and services, it is often necessary to identify the location in which those services were provided. Coders use the place of service codes to link the procedure with the place where the service was provided.

Information Listed on the Inside Front and Back Covers

The inside front and back covers of the CPT manual include information useful to coders reporting services with CPT codes. In most editions of the CPT manual, the inside front cover identifies commonly used symbols and a list of most (but not all) modifiers that are commonly added to CPT codes. The inside back cover lists common abbreviations encountered by coders reporting healthcare services. This is not an exhaustive list of all abbreviations.

EXERCISE 6.3

Also available in **McGraw Hill connect** (plus+)

Use the CPT manual to answer each question.

1. What does the ⊘ symbol mean when it is attached to a CPT code? _____
2. There are five places within the CPT manual where modifiers are listed. Name two. _____
3. What does the # symbol indicate when it is attached to a code? _____

6.4 Reporting Category II Codes and Using Category II Modifiers

performance measures
Tools that Medicare and other insurance programs use to document the quality of care provided by individual providers and healthcare systems, identified by supplementary tracking codes, or Category II codes.

Category II codes are supplementary tracking codes that are used as **performance measures** by the Medicare program and other insurance programs. Reporting Category II codes can replace extensive manual chart reviews and record abstraction to document the quality of care provided by individual providers and healthcare systems. These codes facilitate quality measurements by documenting certain services and/or test results that contribute to quality patient care.

The use of Category II codes is optional at this time, but in the future Medicare may institute penalties for not reporting these codes. Reporting Category II codes is not a substitute for reporting Category I codes. Category II codes describe components that are often performed as part of an E/M service. There are no additional or independent fees associated with these codes because they do not reflect additional services provided.

The Performance Measures Advisory Group (PMAG) reviews new Category II codes. This is an advisory panel of performance measurement experts that represent a number of other healthcare organizations, such as the Agency for Healthcare Research and Quality (AHRQ), the American Medical Association (AMA), the Centers for Medicare and Medicaid Services (CMS), The Joint Commission (TJC), and the Physician Consortium for Performance Improvement (PCPI). The PMAG may seek additional expert opinions from other national healthcare organizations.

Format of Category II Codes

Category II codes consist of four numeric characters followed by the letter *F*. These numbers are not related to placement of these services in the Category I section of the CPT manual. The Alphabetical Clinical Topics Listing includes information about these performance measures, exclusion modifiers associated with the measures, and the source of the measurement.

Each Category II code includes an acronym at the end of the code to identify the disease or clinical condition with which the measurement is associated. The Alphabetical Clinical Topics Listing includes a complete list of these conditions and their acronyms. The Alphabetical Clinical Topics Listing can be found on the web at www.ama-assn.org under the Category II link. Each Category II code includes a footnote number at the end of the code descriptor that refers to a footnote identifying the name of the organization that developed and promoted that particular measure.

Category II codes are updated more often than Category I codes. New Category II codes may be added throughout the year. The most up-to-date list of Category II codes is located on the AMA website.

There are three **performance measurement exclusion modifiers** and one reporting modifier associated with some Category II codes. The modifiers indicate that the provider considered providing a service associated with the performance measure, but because of a medical, patient, or system reason did not provide the service. These modifiers exclude that patient from the denominator of the performance measure calculation.

> **performance measurement exclusion modifiers**
> Modifiers used to exclude a patient from the denominator of the performance measure calculation, which can only be added to certain Category II codes.

CODER'S TIP

Excluding a patient from the denominator of the calculation has a significant effect on the calculated performance measure. The formula for the performance measure percentage calculation is:

$$\frac{\text{Number of patients receiving the required service}}{\text{Number of patients eligible to receive the required service}} \times 100\%$$

The performance measure percentage increases as the numerator increases, the denominator decreases, or both occur simultaneously. Excluding individual patients from the denominator improves the performance measure percentage even if no additional patients receive the required service. Category II modifiers identify patients who should be excluded from the denominator.

Exclusion modifiers cannot be added to all Category II codes. The list of measures to which these modifiers may be attached can be found on the AMA website using the Alphabetical Clinical Topics Listing.

Category II modifiers include:

1P—Performance Measure Exclusion Modifier due to Medical Reasons

   Reasons include:

- Not indicated (absence of organ/limb, already received/performed, other).
- Contraindicated (patient allergic history, potential adverse drug interaction, other).
- Other medical reasons.

2P—Performance Measure Exclusion Modifier due to Patient Reason

   Reasons include:

- Patient declined.
- Economic, social, or religious reasons.
- Other patient reasons.

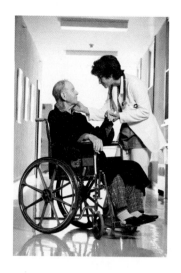

Category II codes make it easier to measure the quality of patient care by documenting services and test results that contribute to this care.

3P—Performance Measure Exclusion Modifier due to System Reason
Reasons include:

- Resources needed to perform the services are not available.
- Insurance coverage/payer-related limitations.
- Other reasons attributable to healthcare delivery system.

8P—Performance Measure Reporting Modifier

- The indicated action was not performed, but the reason is not specified.

Modifier 8P is a "reporting modifier" that indicates that an action described in the numerator of a performance measurement was not performed, but the reason for this is not specified. This differs from the other exclusion modifiers listed, which do provide a reason for not performing the action described in the performance measure.

Types of Category II Performance Measurement Codes

Category II performance measurement codes are divided into the following sections:

- Composite Measures codes (0001F–0015F) combine several measures into a single code descriptor. These codes are only reported if all of the included components are provided. If only some components are provided, they should be identified with the individual Category II codes associated with those components. If additional services are provided in addition to the composite code services, those additional services should be identified with individual Category II codes.
- Patient Management codes (0500F–0575F) describe utilization measures or patient care provided for specific purposes, such as prenatal care or preoperative/postoperative surgical care.
- Patient History codes (1000F–1494F) describe specific aspects of patient history or review of systems.
- Physical Examination codes (2000F–2060F) describe specific aspects of the physical examination or clinical assessment.
- Diagnostic/Screening Processes or Results codes (3006F–3725F) describe the results of tests ordered as part of an examination, including laboratory tests, radiological or other procedural examinations, and conclusions of medical decision making.
- Therapeutic, Preventive, or Other Interventions Codes (4000F–4526F) describe pharmacological, procedural, or behavioral therapies. These include preventive services such as patient education and counseling.
- Follow-up or Other Outcomes codes (5005F–5250F) describe the review and communication of test results to patients, patient satisfaction, patient functional status, and patient morbidity and mortality.
- Patient Safety codes (6005F–6110F) describe processes related to patient safety.
- Structural Measures codes (7010F–7025F) identify measures addressing the setting or system in which the care was delivered, including the capabilities of the organization or professional providing the care.

EXERCISE 6.4

Also available in **McGraw Hill connect** plus+

Use the CPT manual to answer the following questions.

1. What is the main purpose of Category II codes? _____

2. Category II codes always end in which character? _____

3. What are composite codes? _____

6.5 Reporting Category III Codes

The Category III section consists of temporary codes that identify **emerging technology,** services, and procedures. Emerging technologies include new technologies and new uses for existing technologies. The Category III codes allow data collection regarding the use of these services and procedures, which would be difficult if the services were reported with unlisted codes. It is incorrect to report a service with a Category I unlisted code if a Category III code describes the service provided. Use of the Category III codes allows healthcare professionals, insurers, health services researchers, and health policy experts to measure the use of emerging technologies and services.

Assigning a Category III code to a particular technology, service, or procedure does not imply that the AMA endorses its use or applicability to clinical practice. Category III codes may not satisfy the requirements of a Category I code—such as FDA approval and geographically widespread use by many healthcare professionals.

Category III codes differ from Category I codes in that they have four numeric characters followed by a letter *T* as the fifth character. The numeric digits do not correspond to Category I code sections. There is no inherent structure to this code section or the division of these codes into categories. Category III codes are assigned in numerical order. When it is necessary and logical to include a new Category III code with an existing Category III code assigned earlier, the codes may be placed out of sequence and noted with the resequenced symbol (#) to indicate that the codes are out of numerical order.

> **emerging technology**
> New technologies and new uses for existing technologies identified by temporary codes in the Category III section of the CPT manual.

CODER'S TIP

Because Category III codes are not organized into well-defined groups, coders must use the index to determine whether there is a Category III code that describes the service provided. It also is important to determine that there is no Category I code that describes the service or procedure.

For example, some spinal blocks must be performed with image guidance, which is defined as fluoroscopy or CT. These procedures are identified using Category I codes (e.g., codes 64479–64495). If ultrasound is used as image guidance, the Category I codes may not be reported. Instead, Category III codes are used to describe the services (e.g., codes 0213T–0218T or 0228T–0231T). Parenthetical notes with the Category I codes identify Category III codes that should be reported if ultrasound is used.

A Category III code usually remains in the CPT manual for five years, after which time it is deleted (or archived) unless the temporary code continues to be needed. Category III codes that have been deleted are identified by parenthetical notes at the appropriate location in the Category III section of the CPT manual. If the Category III code is archived without creating an equivalent Category I code, the service described by the archived code can be reported with a Category I unlisted procedure code. If the Category III code is converted to an equivalent new Category I code, the service is then reported with the new code.

New Category III codes are released semiannually, with new codes appearing on the web at www.ama-assn.org/go/cpt and in the next regularly published CPT manual.

EXERCISE 6.5

Also available in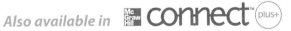

Use the CPT manual to answer the following questions.

1. What types of services do Category III codes describe? _____

2. In general, how long is a Category III code valid from the time it is first released? _____

3. How are add-on Category III codes identified? _____

CHAPTER 6 REVIEW

Summary

Learning Outcome	Key Concepts/Examples
6.1 Explain the structure of the CPT manual. **Pages 131–132**	The CPT manual is divided into three separate categories describing Category I, II, and III codes. Category I is divided into six main sections. Some of these sections are further divided into smaller sections. Each section includes guidelines that provide instructions for selecting codes from that section.
	Coders should select the code that corresponds most accurately to the service provided. If no code describes the service, an unlisted procedure code may be reported.
6.2 Identify the information contained within each code section. **Pages 133–136**	CPT codes include information essential to determining which code should be selected to report services, including indented formats in the code descriptors, symbols, parenthetical notes, modifiers, and identification of separate procedures.
6.3 Describe the functions of the index, appendices, and additional information in the CPT manual. **Pages 136–140**	The CPT manual includes information other than that provided with the individual codes, including the index, appendices, place of service codes, and lists of common abbreviations found in healthcare records.
6.4 Describe the uses of Category II CPT codes. **Pages 140–142**	Category II codes identify performance measures that may be used to measure the quality of services provided by individual providers, large groups of providers, or healthcare systems.
	These codes are organized according to the types of services measured. Several modifiers may be attached to Category II codes to indicate that the provider did not provide the measured service for a reason that allows exclusion from the denominator of the measurement calculations.
6.5 Differentiate between the Category III CPT codes and the Category I and II codes. **Page 143**	Category III codes identify emerging technologies, which are defined as new devices, services, and procedures, or new applications of existing technologies. These codes usually are added in numerical order without any particular organization. It is improper coding to report a service with an unlisted Category I code if a Category III code describes the service.
	Category III codes usually remain in effect for five years. After that time, the utilization of these services is analyzed to determine whether the technology has been sufficiently adopted by medical providers. If so, a new Category I code may be adopted to describe that service. If the Category III code is deleted without a new Category I code, the service may continue to be reported with an unlisted Category I code.

Using Terminology

Match the key terms with their definitions.

_____ **1.** L06.1 CPT manual
_____ **2.** L06.1 Category I
_____ **3.** L06.4 Category II
_____ **4.** L06.5 Category III
_____ **5.** L06.1 Code sections
_____ **6.** L06.1 Unlisted procedure
_____ **7.** L06.2 Add-on code
_____ **8.** L06.2 Parent code
_____ **9.** L06.2 Modifier 51 exempt
_____ **10.** L06.2 Parenthetical note
_____ **11.** L06.1 Modifier
_____ **12.** L06.3 Appendices
_____ **13.** L06.3 Place of service

A. Procedures not designated as additional or multiple procedures

B. Sections of the CPT manual that contain essential information beyond that provided by the code lists and guidance to enable complete and accurate coding

C. Used primarily as performances measures; comprised of four numeric digits followed by the letter *F*

D. Codes that are never reported alone; may include phrases such as "each additional"

E. Can be considered a primary code; an add-on code can be used with it, but an add-on code cannot be reported without it

F. Can only be used when no specific code exists that describes the service provided

G. Set of temporary codes used to designate emerging technologies, services, and procedures; comprised of four numeric digits followed by the letter *T*

H. Services that are generally acceptable in the current practice of medicine and are performed by many physicians in multiple locations

I. Code set to describe services and procedures generally provided to patients by physicians and other healthcare professionals

J. Indicates that a procedure has been altered by specific circumstances but the code still describes the service provided

K. One factor that determines which code series is used to report E/M services

L. Organized components of Category I CPT codes, each of which designates a specific grouping of codes

M. Commonly directs the use of specific codes for some services or prohibits the use of certain code combinations; provides specific information unique to codes

McGraw Hill connect (plus+)
Enhance your learning by completing these exercises and more at mcgrawhillconnect.com!

CHAPTER 6 | INTRODUCTION TO CPT   145

Checking Your Understanding

Select the letter that best describes the statement or answers the question.

1. L06.4 The modifier that indicates that the provider considered providing a service associated with the performance measure, but because of a medical, patient, or system reason did not provide the service, is best described as a(n) _____.

   a. Performance measurement exclusion modifier
   b. HCPCS modifier
   c. Performance measure modifier
   d. Category I modifier

2. L06.1 Category I is divided into _____ main sections.

   a. Two
   b. Four
   c. Six
   d. Eight

3. L06.1 Each section in the CPT manual provides instructions for selecting codes. This section includes _____.

   a. Modifiers only
   b. Performance measures
   c. Appendices
   d. Guidelines

4. L06.5 Category III codes describe _____.

   a. Emerging technologies
   b. Codes that include four numeric digits followed by the letter *F*
   c. Codes that are exempt from modifier 63
   d. Genetic testing

5. L06.1 Mandated reporting of CPT codes for Medicare began in _____.

   a. 1966
   b. 1983
   c. 1965
   d. 1986

6. L06.2 The CPT index is organized by alphabetical terms printed in _____.

   a. Small alphabetical letters
   b. Large alphabetical letters
   c. Boldface
   d. Italics

7. L06.2 What is reported when another procedure is performed in addition to the primary procedure during the same operative session?

   a. Separate procedure
   b. Add-on codes
   c. Modifying terms
   d. Unlisted procedure

8. L06.1 Which type of code is used when no specific code describes the services provided?

    a. Separate procedure
    b. Add-on code
    c. Modifying term
    d. Unlisted procedure

9. L06.3 What place of service code identifies an urgent care facility?

    a. 20
    b. 23
    c. 22
    d. 24

10. L06.5 The following is true regarding Category III codes:

    a. Category III codes are not endorsed.
    b. Category III codes represent services and procedures that are performed by many healthcare professionals across the country.
    c. If a Category III code is available, it must be reported instead of a Category I unlisted code.
    d. Unlike Category I codes, Category III codes are updated once every two years.

11. L06.2 According to the CPT guidelines, the designation (separate procedure) as part of the code descriptors identifies _____.

    a. Procedures that are always reported on their own
    b. Procedures that are never coded, as they are part of another, larger procedure
    c. Procedures that are never reported with modifiers
    d. Procedures that may be reported by themselves when they are the only service provided and are not reported when they are provided as part of a larger service or procedure

12. L06.2 CPT codes identified by a + sign indicate _____.

    a. Codes that are always reported first
    b. Codes that are reported in addition to a primary procedure code
    c. Codes that designate new and revised text
    d. Codes that designate vaccine codes

13. L06.2 CPT codes identified with a full code description are called _____.

    a. Indented codes
    b. Stand-alone codes
    c. Complete codes
    d. FDA-approved codes

14. L06.2 In a CPT code descriptor, what symbol indicates that indented codes appear below that describe services that are partially the same and partially different from the code in question?

    a. Semicolon (;)
    b. Plus symbol (+)
    c. Bullet symbol (●)
    d. Number or pound symbol (#)

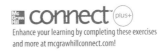
Enhance your learning by completing these exercises and more at mcgrawhillconnect.com!

CHAPTER 6 | INTRODUCTION TO CPT   147

15. L06.1 The CPT manual includes three categories. Which of the following best describes Category I?

    a. It includes codes that describe generally accepted procedures.
    b. It contains performance measures.
    c. It includes codes that describe new technologies.
    d. It contains appendices.

16. L06.3 Place of service codes are located _____.

    a. In the back of the CPT manual
    b. On the first and second pages of the CPT manual
    c. After the guidelines for the Surgery section
    d. Not in the CPT manual but in ICD-9-CM

17. L06.5 When a specific Category I CPT code does not describe the procedure or service provided, coders should _____.

    a. Select the CPT code whose descriptor comes the closest to the procedure or service performed
    b. Select the CPT code whose descriptor comes the closest to the procedure or service performed and append a modifier to indicate no specific CPT code is listed in the CPT manual
    c. Select the appropriate unlisted CPT code if a Category III code does not describe the procedure or service
    d. Select the appropriate unlisted CPT code

18. L06.3 Genetic testing code modifiers are located in _____.

    a. Appendix A
    b. The Surgery section guidelines
    c. Appendix I
    d. The front flap of the CPT manual

19. L06.1 A code set that is revised annually, with new editions of the CPT manual published in the fall of each year containing the latest revisions, is _____.

    a. FDA-approved list
    b. Category I
    c. Category II
    d. Category III

20. L06.2 If an add-on code is reported, then _____.

    a. The parent code also must be reported
    b. Modifier 51 must be attached
    c. A parenthetical note will follow the code
    d. The separate procedure rule applies

Applying Your Skills

Fill in the blank with the appropriate answer(s).

1. L06.3 The emergency room place of service code for a healthcare facility is _____.

2. L06.3 This appendix includes numerous clinical examples for a number of CPT evaluation and management codes. This appendix is identified as _____.

3. L06.4 Category II codes are supplementary tracking codes that are used as _____.

4. L06.4 Modifiers that identify patients who should be excluded from the performance measure denominator are _____.

5. L06.1 Category I is divided into _____ main sections.

6. L06.1 The _____ include specific information for each section and some subsections of CPT codes. They most often appear at the beginning of a section, but they also may be located at the beginning of a subsection of codes.

7. L06.5 Codes that remain in the CPT manual for 5 years are found in _____.

8. L06.3 A summary of CPT codes that include moderate sedation is found in Appendix _____.

9. L06.5 Category III codes describe _____.

10. L06.1 The Current Procedural Terminology (CPT), Fourth Edition, code set used to describe services generally provided to patients by physicians and other healthcare professionals is maintained by the _____.

11. L06.3 Modifiers are located in Appendix _____.

12. L06.3 Appendix _____ contains the Electrodiagnostic Medicine Listing of Sensory, Motor, and Mixed Nerves.

13. L06.5 Category III codes have four numeric characters, followed by the letter _____.

14. L06.5 Code modifiers that are listed in Appendix I are for _____ _____.

15. L0 6.2 The symbol that identifies add-on codes is _____.

16. L0 6.2 Within a code series, parenthetical notes provide information about _____ codes.

17. L0 6.2 A procedure that includes moderate sedation is identified by the symbol _____.

18. L0 6.2 A modifier is not added to codes identified with a + symbol because payers discount reimbursement for add-on codes. This modifier is _____.

19. L0 6.2 A code that is placed out of numerical sequence is represented by the symbol _____.

20. L06.5 Codes that include four numeric digits followed by the letter T are called _____.

21. L06.1 Anesthesia CPT codes are located between code _____ and _____.

22. L06.1 Use of the operating microscope is identified using code number _____.

23. L06.3 The index is organized alphabetically by _____ _____.

24. L0 6.2 New codes are identified with the symbol _____ _____.

25. L0 6.2 New and revised text, such as parenthetical notes and guidelines, are identified by the symbol _____.

26. L0 6.2 The inside front and back covers of the CPT manual include information useful to coders reporting services with CPT codes. The inside front cover identifies _____ and _____.

27. L0 6.2 Whenever a semicolon appears in a code descriptor, it indicates that indented codes will be listed _____ the code with the semicolon.

Enhance your learning by completing these exercises and more at mcgrawhillconnect.com!

CHAPTER 6 | INTRODUCTION TO CPT   149

28. L06.4 Codes organized according to the types of services measured are found in Category _____.

29. L06.1 Codes that appear at the beginning of the code series because almost all providers report a large number of these services are called _____ and _____ codes.

30. L06.3 Clinical examples are found in Appendix _____.

Thinking It Through

Use your critical-thinking skills to answer the questions below.

1. L06.5 What happens to Category III codes after they have remained in effect for five years?

_____

_____

2. L06.1 Refer to the Office or Outpatient Services category of E/M and note that it contains two subcategories. Explain the two subcategories, the codes for each, and how the E/M code service is ranked.

_____

_____

3. L06.1 Explain when an unlisted procedure code can be used.

_____

_____

4. L06.1, L06.2 Where can guidelines be found within the CPT coding manual? What kind of guidance do they offer?

_____

_____

5. L06.1 How many systems are described in the Surgery section of CPT codes? Identify each one.

_____

_____

MODIFIERS

7

Learning Outcomes *After completing this chapter, students should be able to:*

7.1 Explain the functions and uses of modifiers.

7.2 Discuss modifiers used to indicate services provided during a procedure's global period.

7.3 Use modifiers to report components of procedures or services.

7.4 Explain bilateral, multiple, repeat, or additional procedures performed on the same date of service.

7.5 Cite appropriate modifiers to identify individuals who assist the primary provider during procedures.

7.6 Discuss circumstances where the amount of work necessary to perform the service differs significantly from the amount typically necessary.

7.7 Define modifiers describing mandatory services, physical status, and genetic tests.

7.8 Define HCPCS modifiers to primary codes.

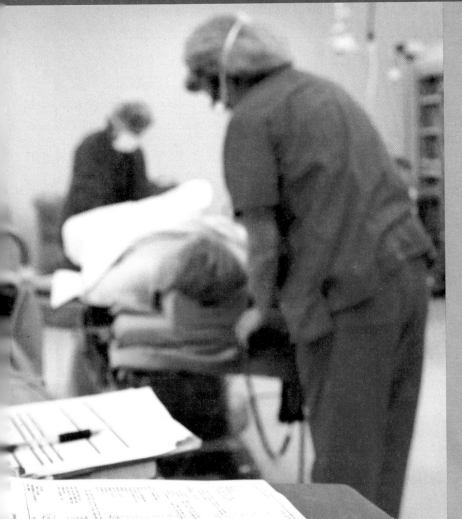

Key Terms

Ambulance trip
Anesthesia
Assistant surgeon
Bilateral procedure
Co-surgeons
Decision to perform surgery
Distinct procedure
Global period
Multiple procedures
Physical status modifiers
Professional component
Resident physician
Staged procedure
Surgical team
Technical component

Introduction

CPT and Healthcare Common Procedure Coding System (HCPCS) codes do not always describe services provided with as much detail as is available in the medical record. Some of this additional information is important for coding or payment purposes. When available, coders should provide this additional information through the use of modifiers. Modifiers are two-digit alphanumeric characters that are added to CPT or HCPCS codes to provide the additional information necessary to fully describe the services provided. Coders must understand how to use modifiers as precisely as they use specific CPT codes. Pay as much attention to selecting the correct modifiers as to selecting correct codes.

7.1 The Function and Use of Modifiers

There are two major types of modifiers: payment modifiers and informational modifiers. Payment modifiers almost always affect the amount of payment for the services described by the codes to which the modifiers are attached. Informational modifiers, on the other hand, provide specific additional information about the services provided, but they do not automatically affect payment for those services. Informational modifiers can affect payment, but this is not always the case. Coders must learn how to use both types of modifiers. Some of the material below describes how a modifier affects payments. This information is provided to illustrate why it is important to select the correct modifier.

Examples of modifiers include those that identify:

- Evaluation and management (E/M) services provided during the global period following a surgical procedure.
- A separate E/M service provided on the same day as another service.
- Procedures with both professional and technical components, but only one component is being reported.
- When more than one provider performed all or part of a procedure.
- Bilateral procedures, which are defined as the same procedure performed on both sides of the body.
- Multiple procedures performed during the same session.
- A single procedure performed more than once during the same session.
- When an assistant participated in performing all or part of a procedure.
- Situations where the procedure was much more difficult than usual.
- Procedures that were increased or decreased from the usual procedure definition, but no other procedure code correctly identifies the modified procedure.
- The physical status of a patient undergoing anesthesia.
- Specific anatomical sites, right and left side of the body, specific digits (fingers and toes), or particular cardiac arteries.
- Where an ambulance trip began and ended.

Table 7.1 shows a list of modifiers and their meanings.

Most modifiers may be used on codes from several, but not necessarily all, CPT code sections. Modifiers are often presented in numerical order. This chapter takes a different approach, grouping modifiers according to their function.

Coders should understand which modifiers can be used with various CPT codes and be able to apply the modifiers to all appropriate codes. Coders must understand the use of modifiers and be able to apply them to CPT codes identified as correct under the circumstances. It is equally important that coders be able to identify incorrect uses of modifiers.

TABLE 7.1 Numerical List of Modifiers

Modifier	Description
22	Increased services
24	Unrelated E/M service by the same physician during the postoperative global period
25	Significant, separately identifiable E/M service by the same physician on the same day as another procedure or service
26	Professional component
32	Mandatory services
47	Anesthesia performed by a surgeon
50	Bilateral procedure
51	Multiple procedures
52	Reduced services
53	Discontinued procedure
54	Surgical care only
55	Postoperative management only
56	Preoperative management only
57	Decision for surgery
58	Staged or related procedure or service by the same physician during the postoperative global period
59	Distinct procedure or service
62	Co-surgeons
63	Procedure performed on an infant less than 4 kg
66	Surgical team
76	Repeat procedure or service by the same physician
77	Repeat procedure or service by another physician
78	Unplanned return to the operating room or procedure room by the same physician for a related procedure during the global period
79	Unrelated procedure or service by the same physician during the global period
80	Assistant surgeon
81	Minimum assistant surgeon
82	Assistant surgeon when a qualified resident is not available
91	Repeat clinical diagnostic laboratory test
TC	Technical Component
P1–P6	Physical status modifiers describing the condition of a patient undergoing anesthesia
E1–E4	Eyelids: upper left (E1); lower left (E2); upper right (E3); lower right (E4)

(Continued)

TABLE 7.1 *(Continued)*

Modifier	Description
FA, F1–F9	Fingers: left thumb (FA); left index (F1); left long (F2); left ring (F3); left small (F4); right thumb (F5); right index (F6); right long (F7); right ring (F8); right small (F9)
TA, T1–T9	Toes: left great toe (TA); left 2nd digit (T1); left 3rd digit (T2); left 4th digit (T3); left 5th digit (T4); right great toe (T5); right 2nd digit (T6); right 3rd digit (T7); right 4th digit (T8); right 5th digit (T9)
LT	Left side (identifies procedures performed on the left side of the body)
RT	Right side (identifies procedures performed on the right side of the body)
RC	Right coronary artery
LC	Left coronary artery
LD	Left anterior descending coronary artery
NU	Equipment new when provided to the patient
UE	Equipment used when provided to the patient
RR	Equipment rented
Ambulance pickup and delivery codes	Diagnostic or therapeutic site other than a hospital or physician office (D); hospital (H); end-stage renal disease facility (J); skilled nursing facility (N); physician office (P); residence (R); scene of accident (S)

Many modifiers affect payments for services. Even before determining reimbursement implications, coders must be able to correctly determine which modifier should be added to a code based on the specific circumstances.

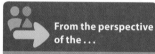

From the perspective of the . . .

CODER

Some modifiers are informational only, while others affect payment. Coders must understand how the correct use of modifiers affects payments.

CODER'S TIP

Selecting the correct modifier can be almost as complex as selecting the correct code. Each modifier has very specific uses and rules governing its appropriate use. These modifiers allow coders to report services to a greater level of specificity.

EXERCISE 7.1

Also available in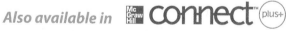

1. In your own words, describe the function of a modifier. _____
2. Which modifiers describe the patient's health condition prior to the induction of anesthesia? _____
   _____
3. Modifiers that specify specific sites of the body are called _____ modifiers.

global period
Period of time after initial procedure is performed during which related follow-up procedures are considered part of the initial procedure.

7.2 Services Provided during the Global Period

Many services require follow-up visits. For example, major surgery usually requires postoperative hospital and office visits. Payment for services that require follow-up services usually includes payment for follow-up services provided during a period of time known as the **global period.**

At times, a provider may provide services during the global period that should not be considered part of the original procedure. Several modifiers may be used to indicate that services provided should be considered separate from the original procedure. These modifiers may affect whether the services are paid for separately.

Modifier 24

Many surgical procedures have a period of time, called the global period, during which E/M services provided by the physician who performed the original procedure are considered to be related to that procedure. On occasion, a surgeon may perform E/M services during the global period that are unrelated to the original procedure. Modifier 24 is used to report those unrelated E/M services. It is important to note that modifier 24 may only be added to CPT codes 99201–99499 and 92012–92014.

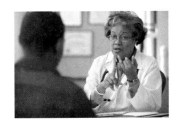

Many services and procedures require follow-up visits, such as postoperative hospital and office visits.

CODING EXAMPLE

A surgeon performs a hip procedure. During the postoperative global period, the surgeon sees the patient, who now complains of knee pain, which is unrelated to the hip surgery. The coder adds modifier 24 to the appropriate E/M code describing the visit to indicate that this visit is unrelated to the previous surgical procedure.

CODING EXAMPLE

An ophthalmologist performs a cataract extraction on a patient's right eye. During the global period, the ophthalmologist examines the patient's left eye to determine whether a similar procedure is necessary. Modifier 24 is added to an ophthalmology E/M code describing services for an established patient.

CODING EXAMPLE

A surgeon admits a postoperative patient to a skilled nursing facility (SNF) during the global period for reasons unrelated to the original surgical procedure. Modifier 24 is attached to a code that describes the SNF admission E/M services.

Coders should not:

- Add modifier 24 to any CPT code other than 99201–99499 or 92012–92014.
- Add modifier 24 for hospital visits by the surgeon during the initial postoperative period, unless the physician is providing one of the following services:
  - Immunosuppressive therapy
  - Chemotherapy
  - Critical care services unrelated to the original surgery

- Add modifier 24 to office visits during the global period when the major purpose of the visit is to follow up on the original surgery. For example:
  - A patient returns for a postoperative office visit during the global period to discuss increasing pain at the operative site. Modifier 24 should not be added to the office E/M code.
  - A patient is admitted to a SNF during the global period for postoperative care related to the surgery. Modifier 24 should not be added to the SNF admission E/M code.

CODER'S TIP

Modifier 24 is only used on codes describing E/M services. Several other modifiers identify non-E/M services provided during the global period. Modifiers 58, 78, and 79 identify procedures performed during the global period. Which modifier is the correct one to use depends on whether the additional procedure is related or unrelated to the previous procedure (see modifiers 58, 78, and 79).

Modifier 25

Modifier 25 identifies significant, separately identifiable E/M services provided by the same physician on the same day as another procedure or other service. Routine preoperative and postoperative care associated with a procedure does not substantiate the use of modifier 25 with an E/M code.

When using modifier 25, the required elements of E/M services (history, physical exam, and medical decision making) should be well documented and show that the E/M service has been provided in addition to the other procedure. Examples of using Modifier 25 include:

- Use modifier 25 to describe an E/M visit on the same day as a surgical procedure if the purpose of the E/M service is unrelated to the surgical procedure itself.
- Use modifier 25 when a significant, separately identifiable E/M service is performed on the same day as a preventive care visit. The E/M service must be performed for a nonpreventive reason (e.g., to evaluate specific complaints or symptoms separate from the preventive exam). The need for the separate E/M service must be clearly documented.
- Modifier 25 may be used even in those instances where the diagnosis for the E/M service is the same as the diagnosis for the other procedure or service. It is important to note, however, that documentation should reflect the necessity of the separately identifiable E/M service.

Coders should not use modifier 25:

- To identify E/M services that result in a decision to perform surgery (see modifier 57).
- With a surgical procedure code (10021–69990). It is only added to the E/M code when both are performed together.
- With an office visit E/M code when the primary purpose of the visit is to perform a minor surgical procedure. In that instance, only the minor surgical procedure is reported.

CODING EXAMPLE

A patient comes to her physician's office for a procedure to remove skin tags. Before the procedure, the patient complains of ear pain. The physician performs the skin tag removal procedure and examines the patient's ear to determine whether she also has an ear infection. The correct modifier to add to the office visit code is modifier 25 to designate the visit as a significant, separately identifiable service.

A patient is scheduled to undergo arthroscopy of her left knee. When the surgeon arrives for the procedure, the patient reports that she also is having shoulder pain. The surgeon takes a history and performs an exam of the patient's shoulder, then proceeds with the scheduled surgical procedure. The E/M code should be reported with modifier 25 to indicate that this is a significant, separately identifiable E/M service provided on the same day as another procedure.

Modifier 57

Modifier 57 is used to report that the **decision to perform surgery** was made during an E/M service occurring during the global period. For major surgeries, the global period begins the day before surgery. For minor surgeries, the global period begins the day of surgery. Medicare does not recognize the use of modifier 57 with minor surgeries (those with 0- and 10-day global periods), but other payers might. When the decision to perform surgery is made earlier than the beginning of the global period, that visit would be coded with the appropriate E/M code but without the modifier. For example:

decision to perform surgery
Decision made during an E/M service in the global period, reported by adding modifier 57 to the E/M code.

- Attach modifier 57 to an E/M code to report that the surgeon made the decision to perform surgery if that visit occurred the day of or the day before surgery.
- When the decision to perform a subsequent surgery occurs during the global period of a previous procedure, add modifiers 24 and 57 to the appropriate E/M code. (Refer to the discussion of the proper uses of modifier 24.)

Coders should not use modifier 57:

- To report the decision to perform a minor surgical procedure (0- or 10-day global period) for Medicare patients.
- With an E/M code on the day of surgery when the actual decision to perform surgery was made in advance.
- With a procedure code. Modifier 57 is only added to E/M codes.

CODER'S TIP

The decision to perform surgery should be well documented in the patient's medical record. Coders should review all records to determine when the surgeon made the actual decision to operate and only add modifier 57 to the E/M code for that visit if it occurred on the day of or day before surgery.

CODING EXAMPLE

A surgeon is called to the emergency department at 10 p.m. to evaluate a patient with right upper quadrant pain. After taking a history, performing a physical exam, and reviewing laboratory tests, the surgeon determines the patient should have her gallbladder removed. He schedules the surgery for 8 a.m. the following morning. The surgeon reports the E/M service with the appropriate code and attaches modifier 57 to indicate that he made the decision to perform surgery as part of this E/M service, which occurred during the global period one day prior to surgery.

CODING EXAMPLE

An orthopedic surgeon examines a patient and schedules him for knee surgery in one week. On the day of surgery, the surgeon reexamines the patient to make sure that surgery is still indicated and proceeds to perform the surgical procedure. The surgeon reports the E/M code for the visit one week before surgery, but he does not add modifier 57 to that code because it is more than one day prior to surgery. He also reports the E/M service on the day of surgery, but he does not add modifier 57 to this code either, because the decision to perform surgery had been made earlier. Neither visit is reported with modifier 57.

Modifier 58

staged procedure
Subsequent procedure(s) commonly performed during the global period under one of three circumstances: planned staged procedure anticipated prior to the first procedure, more extensive procedure needed than originally planned, or a therapeutic procedure performed following a diagnostic procedure.

Modifier 58 is used when a procedure is performed over two or more operative sessions, known as a **staged procedure.** The subsequent procedures commonly occur during the global period. Staged procedures may occur under several circumstances, including:

- For planned staged procedures (anticipated prior to the first procedure).
- When a more extensive procedure is needed than originally planned, requiring a second procedure that was not necessarily planned prior to the first procedure.
- For a therapeutic procedure performed following a diagnostic procedure.

CODING EXAMPLE

A surgeon performs a mastectomy on a patient who indicates that she wants a prosthesis implanted as part of the reconstruction. The surgeon performs the reconstructive procedure after the original mastectomy has healed. Modifier 58 is added to the second procedure to indicate that it was planned as part of the original procedure.

CODING EXAMPLE

A patient undergoes a complex abdominal procedure and the wound cannot be closed at the end of the procedure. The surgeon leaves the wound open and documents that she plans to close the wound after several days. When the wound closure is performed, it is coded with modifier 58 to indicate that this second procedure was planned.

Coders should not use modifier 58 to indicate that it was necessary to perform a second procedure due to a complication. For example:

- A patient with postoperative bleeding is taken back to the operating room to explore the surgical site. This is coded with modifier 78 (see modifier 78), not as a staged procedure.

Modifiers 76 and 77

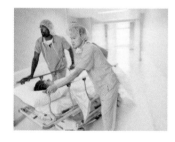

Modifiers often are used to describe characteristics of surgeries, such as the number of surgeons who performed a procedure.

Modifier 76 indicates that the provider who performed a procedure repeated that same procedure during the global period of the original procedure. Modifier 77 is used to identify that a second provider repeated the same procedure during the global period of the original procedure. These modifiers indicate that the exact same procedure was performed at the same anatomical site, not that the same procedure was performed at a different anatomical site. The reasons for repeating the procedure should be documented by the provider. Modifiers 76 and 77 may be used for surgical procedures and diagnostic test procedures, but they may not be used for laboratory tests.

Procedures may be repeated for a number of reasons. For example, a surgical procedure may be performed and then may need to be repeated during the global period. Another example is when x-rays or electrocardiograms (EKGs) are performed before and after treatment to assess whether the treatment has been successful. Modifiers 76 and 77 are not used to identify laboratory tests that are repeated. Repeated laboratory tests are reported with modifier 91 (see modifier 91).

CODING EXAMPLE

A surgeon performs an exploratory laparotomy to correct a perforated intestine secondary to diverticulitis. Several days later, another perforation may occur, making it necessary for the same surgeon or another surgeon to repeat the exploratory laparotomy. The second procedure would be reported with either modifier 76 (same surgeon) or 77 (different surgeon).

CODING EXAMPLE

An initial x-ray shows that a patient has a broken leg. The physician sets the fracture and places the leg in a cast. The x-ray is repeated to make sure the leg is in the correct position. The second x-ray is reported with modifier 76.

CODING EXAMPLE

A physician places a chest tube after an x-ray shows a pneumothorax. She repeats the chest x-ray to show whether the lung has expanded. The second x-ray is reported with modifier 76 added to the code.

CODING EXAMPLE

An EKG shows that a patient in the hospital has a cardiac arrhythmia. The physician treats the arrhythmia and repeats the EKG. The repeat EKG is reported with modifier 76. Later the same day, the nurse is concerned because it appears the arrhythmia may be recurring. She calls the on-call cardiologist, who is not the physician who treated the patient earlier. The on-call cardiologist sees the patient and repeats the EKG. This EKG is reported with modifier 77 added to the code.

Coders should not use modifier 76 or 77:

- To identify the same procedure performed on another body part, such as when a surgeon performs an open reduction and internal fixation on a fractured metacarpal and then performs the same procedure on a second metacarpal. The second procedure should be reported as an additional procedure with modifier 51.
- To identify laboratory tests that are repeated to assess the condition of patients during or after treatment (see modifier 91).

Modifier 78

Modifier 78 indicates that a patient returned to the operating room for an unplanned second procedure by the same provider during the global period of an earlier procedure. In this situation, the term *operating room* is defined broadly and includes locations such as the cardiac catheterization suite, ambulatory surgical center (ASC), endoscopy suite, or laser treatment room.

Modifier 78 is only used when the second procedure is related to the original procedure. This modifier is most often used to describe circumstances when a complication makes the second procedure necessary, not to describe staged procedures (see modifier 58). The second procedure is reported with the appropriate CPT code with modifier 78 added to the code. The second procedure does not typically initiate a new global period. Rather, the global period of the original procedure remains in place. Modifier 78 is only used when the patient returns to an operating room for the second procedure.

CODING EXAMPLE

A patient who recently had a cholecystectomy develops peritonitis and requires an exploratory laparotomy. The second procedure would be coded with the appropriate CPT code (49000) with modifier 78.

CODING EXAMPLE

A patient undergoes an open reduction and internal fixation of a tibial fracture. The next day, an x-ray shows that one of the screws holding the fracture pieces in place has pulled loose. The surgeon takes the patient to the operating room and replaces the loose screw with two others to hold the fracture together. Modifier 78 is added to the code that describes the procedure to replace the loose screw. In addition, either the RT or LT modifier should be added to the procedure code to indicate the affected knee.

Coders should not use modifier 78:

- If the treatment of the complication did not require that the patient be brought to the operating room or its equivalent for the second procedure. Procedures performed in the office during the postoperative period are not identified with modifier 78.

Modifier 79

Modifier 79 identifies an unrelated surgical procedure performed during the global period of an earlier procedure performed by the same surgeon. The second procedure identified with modifier 79 is not usually performed to treat a complication of the first procedure (see modifier 78). The second procedure may be the same as the original procedure, but performed on a different body part.

CODING EXAMPLE

A surgeon performs a total knee arthroplasty on a patient's right knee (CPT code 27447). This procedure has a 90-day global period. After six weeks, the surgeon performs a total knee arthroplasty on the left knee. The second procedure is reported with CPT code 27447 with modifier 79.

CODING EXAMPLE

A trauma patient undergoes surgical treatment for fractures of her lower extremities. Several days later, she is taken back to the operating room for skin grafting procedures that are unrelated to the previous surgical procedures. Modifier 79 is added to the codes that describe the skin graft procedures.

Coders should not use modifier 79 when:

- The second procedure is related to the first procedure (see modifier 78).
- A different provider performs the second procedure.
- The second surgical procedure is performed during the same operative session as the first procedure.

From the perspective of the . . .

CODER

When a second procedure is performed during the global period of another procedure, it is important to know whether the second procedure was planned or staged, related to a complication of the first procedure, or unrelated to the first procedure. This determines which modifier should be selected.

CODER'S TIP

Coders should never try to be mind readers. When the reason is not clear for a second procedure performed during the global period of an original procedure, the coder should discuss the situation with the provider who performed the procedures to determine which is the correct modifier to describe those circumstances.

EXERCISE 7.2

Also available in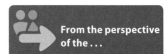

Using your CPT manual, answer each of the following questions.

1. A patient is badly burned and requires multiple surgeries, some of which are performed during the global period of the initial procedure. What modifier would be appended to the CPT codes describing the subsequent procedures? _____

2. A patient goes to see her orthopedic surgeon two weeks after hip replacement surgery complaining of shoulder pain. Which modifier would be required to appropriately report the visit to the doctor? _____

3. Which modifier is appended to an office visit code to show that it was separately identifiable from a procedure performed during the same visit? _____

4. A surgeon performs a procedure on a patient and takes the patient back to the operating room to repeat the same procedure several days later. Assuming the procedure has a global period associated with it and the second procedure is performed during the global period, what modifier should be used to report the second surgical service? _____

5. If a surgeon performs a procedure during the global period of the same procedure previously performed by a different surgeon, which modifier would be reported? _____

6. A surgeon is asked to consult on a patient with abdominal pain in the emergency room. The surgeon examines the patient and determines she has gallstones and requires surgery. Which modifier, if any, would be appropriate to add to the exam code? _____

7. A patient is returned to the operating room for a complication that arose during the global period of an earlier procedure. What modifier would be appropriate to add to the CPT code describing the second procedure? _____

8. A patient who underwent surgical correction of a fractured metacarpal bone falls, injures her metatarsal bone, and requires surgery during the global period of the first procedure. The same surgeon performs the surgery for this injury. What modifier would be appropriate to append to the second procedure? _____

7.3 Reporting Portions of a Procedure or Service

CPT codes commonly include an array of services under a single procedure code number. Reporting a code implies that the provider performed all the services included in the code descriptor. Under some circumstances, different providers may perform various aspects of the total service described by the code. In those cases, modifiers are attached to the code to indicate which services each provider performed.

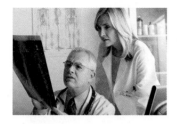

Modifiers 26 and TC describe the professional and technical components of a service, such as equipment used to generate x-rays or the expertise of a physician to read the x-rays.

professional component
The portion of a procedure that is performed by a physician that does not include the equipment necessary to perform the procedure, such as the interpretation of x-rays by a radiologist.

technical component
The portion of a procedure that requires the use of special equipment, such as imaging equipment.

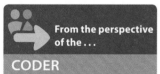

From the perspective of the . . .

CODER

It is important to know which CPT codes allow use of the professional and technical components (modifiers 26 and TC).

Professional and Technical Components

Modifier 26 Some procedures, such as x-rays and other imaging techniques, require the use of complex equipment to perform the tests and physician expertise to interpret the meaning of those tests. These two functions may be provided by separate entities. For example, a hospital or outpatient imaging center may provide the equipment to take the x-ray, and a radiologist may review the film to render a professional opinion regarding what the x-ray shows. The same is true of other imaging techniques, such as CT scans, magnetic resonance imaging (MRI) scans, and positron emission tomography (PET) scans. Modifier 26 identifies the **professional component** of a procedure.

CODING EXAMPLE

A patient is sent to the hospital for a CT scan. A radiologist comes to the hospital to interpret the scan and prepares a report of her interpretation. She reports the service with the appropriate CPT code and modifier 26.

CODING EXAMPLE

A patient has an x-ray at an imaging center. A radiologist not employed by the center interprets the film and reports that service with the appropriate CPT code and modifier 26.

Physicians should only report professional services when they interpret tests and prepare written reports of their interpretations for others to use. Modifier 26 should not be used:

- To report the professional and technical components provided by a single provider. If the same provider performs both the professional and technical components, no modifier is attached to the code.
- When a provider reads the radiologist's interpretation and uses that information to form a diagnosis or determine further treatments. In this situation, the provider is not performing a formal interpretation and preparing a report for others to use.

Modifier TC The TC modifier identifies the **technical component** of a procedure that has both a professional and technical component. This modifier is most often used by hospitals, imaging centers, and other entities that have the equipment to perform the imaging procedure when that entity is not also performing the associated professional services.

Coders should not report both modifier 26 and TC together to report the professional and technical components by a single provider. If the same provider performs both the professional and technical components, no modifier is attached to the code.

CODING EXAMPLE

A patient is sent to the hospital for a CT scan. A radiologist comes to the hospital to interpret the scan. The hospital reports the service with the appropriate CPT code and TC modifier. The radiologist reports the same code with modifier 26 added to it.

CODING EXAMPLE

A patient is seen in a freestanding imaging center for an MRI scan ordered by her primary care physician. The scan is performed and read by a radiologist employed by the imaging center. The imaging center reports both the technical and professional services with the code describing the particular scan. No modifiers are attached to the code.

Surgical Procedure Components

Surgical procedures can be divided into three separate components—preoperative, intraoperative, and postoperative services. Modifiers 54, 55, and 56 are added to procedures to indicate that different physicians provided the preoperative, intraoperative and postoperative services.

- Modifier 54 identifies the intraoperative surgical component.
- Modifier 55 identifies the postoperative management component.
- Modifier 56 identifies the preoperative management component.

These modifiers are only attached to codes that have a 10-day or 90-day global period. For procedures with a 0-day global period, the preoperative and postoperative services are reported with E/M codes, not with the surgical code and modifiers. These modifiers may be used to report various combinations of these three services.

Coders should not add modifiers 54, 55, or 56 to:

- CPT codes with a 0-day global period.
- E/M codes. (These modifiers are only used with procedure codes.)

Coders also should not use modifier 55 to identify inpatient postoperative visits by another physician. Those visits should be identified by hospital visit E/M codes (99231–99233).

EXERCISE 7.3

Also available in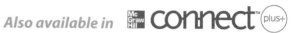

Using your CPT manual, answer each of the following questions.

1. A hospital provides equipment for tests performed in the facility. What modifier, if any, is attached to the CPT code to report the use of equipment for an EKG or x-ray if a physician reports the professional service separately? _____

2. If a physician renders only the preoperative care of a patient prior to transferring care to a surgeon, what modifier would be appended to the procedure code? _____

3. A physician interprets an x-ray of the hand. Which modifier, if any, is attached to the CPT code describing a hand x-ray? _____

4. A physician refers her patient to a surgeon with the understanding that she will provide the postoperative care. When she sees the patient postoperatively, what modifier must be attached to the surgical code to indicate the services provided? _____

5. Which modifier is added to a surgical code to report that the physician provided only the intraoperative surgical care and no preoperative or postoperative services? _____

7.4 Reporting Multiple Services on the Same Date

Physicians often perform more than one procedure on a patient during a single operative session. It usually is not necessary for the physician to repeat all the components of the primary procedure to perform the additional procedures. For example, a surgeon would not perform separate preoperative evaluations for each procedure. Also, when the patient returns for postoperative follow-up visits, the surgeon does not schedule separate visits for each surgical procedure.

Medicare and other payers usually reduce the fees they allow for additional procedures to account for the services that are provided with the first procedure but not repeated for subsequent procedures. Modifiers are used to identify the additional procedures.

Modifier 50

bilateral procedure
Identical procedures performed on both sides of the body (bilaterally) during the same operative session.

Modifier 50 designates **bilateral procedures,** identical procedures performed on both sides of the body (bilaterally) during the same operative session. This modifier is only used when the same procedure is performed on both sides of the body, not just to indicate that the surgeon operated on both sides of the body.

CODING EXAMPLE

An orthopedic surgeon performs diagnostic arthroscopy on both knees of a patient. The coder would report CPT code 27373 with modifier 50.

Not all procedures can be reported with modifier 50. Some code definitions specifically state that the code applies only to bilateral procedures. Other code definitions include the statement "unilateral or bilateral," "one or both," or similar language indicating that the code is used only once without modifier 50 even if the procedure is performed on both sides. Other procedures cannot be performed bilaterally due to anatomical considerations, and modifier 50 should not be added to those codes.

Coders should not add modifier 50 to codes when:

- The same procedure is performed on different right and left body parts.
- Different procedures are performed on the same right and left body parts.
- A code is identified as a bilateral procedure.
- A code is identified as either unilateral or bilateral, such as:
  - CPT code 69210 (Removal impacted cerumen (separate procedure), one or both ears). It is inappropriate to add modifier 50 to this code to indicate that the procedure was performed on both ears since the code indicates that it is only reported once for both ears.

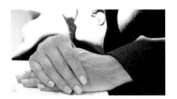

Modifier 50 reports laterality of a procedure, such as a surgery on both of a patient's hands. However, if a code is already identified as unilateral or bilateral, modifier 50 should not be used.

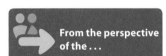

From the perspective of the . . .

CODER

Be aware of how each payer wants bilateral procedures to be reported. There are at least three methods commonly used: (1) the code is listed on one line with modifier 50 added; (2) the code is listed twice with modifier 50 added on both lines; and (3) the code is listed twice with anatomical modifiers indicating right and left procedures on each line.

Modifier 51

When providers perform **multiple procedures** on the same date of service, modifier 51 is added to the secondary procedures. Coders should recognize when this modifier is correctly used to report additional procedures. Modifier 51 can be used to:

- Identify additional procedures performed during the same operative session. For example:
  - Reporting the delivery of twins.
  - Indicating multiple instances of the same service.

multiple procedures
Two or more procedures performed.

A surgeon performs an open reduction and internal fixation of a metacarpal fracture (26615) and a distal phalangeal fracture (26765). Assuming the metacarpal fracture repair is primary, these services would be reported with CPT codes 26615 and 26765-51.

A surgeon performs arthroplasties of the metacarpophalangeal joints with prosthetic implants (26531) on two fingers. This would be reported with CPT codes 26531 and 26531-51.

Some CPT codes are never reported with modifier 51, including those designated as add-on codes. Add-on codes are always secondary to the code describing the primary procedure and usually designate that the provider performed the same procedure at multiple sites. Add-on codes are identified with a plus sign (+) in the CPT manual and are listed in Appendix D.

There are a few other codes that should not be reported with modifier 51, even when they are performed as additional procedures. These codes are designated as modifier 51 exempt and are identified with the ⊘ symbol in the CPT manual. They also are listed in Appendix E of the CPT manual. Coders should not:

- Separate or unbundle a procedure into its components and add modifier 51 to one or more components.
- Add modifier 51 to E/M codes.
- Add modifier 51 to add-on codes or to codes that are modifier 51 exempt. For example:
  - An interventional pain specialist treating a patient with chronic back pain injects medications into two separate transforaminal epidural spaces of the lumbar spine, both on the same side of the body. Modifier 51 is not added to the add-on code designating the additional level (64484). These injections are coded with CPT codes 64483 (first level) and 64484 (additional level).

CODER'S TIP

Coders should always use the most recent CPT manual and other coding information. The list of modifier 51 exempt codes changes frequently, and coders need to know which codes can be reported with this modifier. The Medicare Physician Fee Schedule also indicates which procedure codes cannot be reported with modifier 51.

Modifier 59

distinct procedure
A procedure that is not usually reported separately from another procedure, but under certain circumstances may be reported separately.

Modifier 59 identifies services that are not usually reported together, but which may, under certain circumstances, be reported together as **distinct procedures.** The Correct Coding Initiative (CCI) identifies pairs of codes that are not usually reported together. This includes code pairs that can never be provided together under any circumstances, as well as other code pairs where circumstances might allow both codes to be reported separately. Modifier 59 can be used when services that would normally be inclusive of one another are performed:

- On another body part;
- Through a separate incision; or
- During a different session as the primary service.

Modifier 59 may be used in combination with other modifiers to indicate why the services are distinct. Other modifiers include the HCPCS anatomical modifiers. When appropriate, add both modifier 59 and the anatomical modifiers to the second code of the CCI code pair. Anatomical modifiers without modifier 59 should be added to the primary code of the CCI code pair. This makes it clear that the two procedures were performed on separate anatomical sites.

Coders should not use modifier 59:

- With E/M codes.
- With a code pair that does not permit the use of modifier 59.
- Unless documentation shows that the services were separate and distinct.
- If another modifier can be used to indicate that the service is separate and distinct.
- To indicate a separate anatomical site if it is a body area that is contiguous with the body part involved in the other procedure. For example, the fingernail and cuticle of the same finger are not separate anatomical sites for purposes of modifier 59.

HCPCS anatomical modifiers (see section 7.8) may be used to indicate that procedures were performed on separate anatomical sites. Each procedure would include an anatomical modifier, and the secondary procedure(s) would also include modifier 59.

Inaccurate or inappropriate use of modifier 59 is a common coding error. Coders should be familiar with CCI edits and the circumstances that permit the use of modifier 59, such as surgery at a different site, through a separate incision, or performed at a different time. Coders also should be familiar with the structure of the CCI tables and how to determine which codes may be reported together under appropriate circumstances and which cannot be reported together under any circumstances. Codes usually are designated as Column 1 and Column 2 codes. A Column 2 code usually cannot be reported with a Column 1 code. If a modifier is allowed (modifier indicator = 1), then a modifier can override the CCI edit. If a modifier is not allowed (modifier indicator = 0), then a modifier cannot override the CCI edit and the two codes cannot be reported together under any circumstances.

Table 7.2 is a sample from a CCI table showing Column 1 and 2 codes, begin date, end date, and modifier indicator. Two code pairs are no longer CCI edits (entries in the end

TABLE 7.2 Sample of a CCI Table

Column 1	Column 2	Begin Date	End Date	Modifier Indicator
20900	64445	20090401	*	0
20900	64446	20090401	*	0
20900	64447	20090401	*	0
20900	64448	20090401	*	0
20900	64449	20090401	*	0
20900	64450	20021001	*	1
20900	64470	20021001	20091231	0
20900	64475	20021001	20091231	0
20900	64479	20090401	*	0
20900	64483	20090401	*	0
20900	64490	20100101	*	0
20900	64493	20100101	*	0

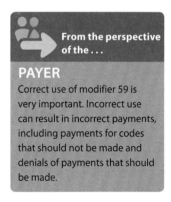

From the perspective of the . . .

PAYER

Correct use of modifier 59 is very important. Incorrect use can result in incorrect payments, including payments for codes that should not be made and denials of payments that should be made.

date column show when the code pairs were deleted). One code pair (20900 and 64450) allows the use of a modifier to override the CCI edit.

Modifier 91

Modifier 91 is used to indicate that it was necessary to repeat a laboratory test on the same day for treatment purposes. This modifier indicates that the repeat test is medically necessary to manage the patient. It is not used if the test is repeated due to problems with the first specimen or to confirm the results of the first test.

CODING EXAMPLE

A patient with a low potassium level is treated with IV solutions containing extra potassium. Several hours later, the patient's potassium level is rechecked to ascertain the adequacy of the treatment. Modifier 91 is attached to the CPT code reporting the second potassium test.

CODING EXAMPLE

A patient in respiratory distress and experiencing an inadequate arterial blood oxygen level has a breathing tube inserted and is placed on a ventilator to manage the respiratory distress. After stabilizing the ventilator settings, a repeat arterial blood gas test is performed to assess the arterial oxygen level. Modifier 91 is added to the CPT code identifying the second arterial blood gas test.

Modifier 91 is not used when multiple lab tests are performed on separate samples rather than to recheck the value of the same test. For example:

- Cultures are performed on different wounds to determine whether any of them are infected. These are identified with modifier 59 to indicate that they are distinct procedures. These are not repeat procedures performed to assess treatment, and modifier 91 should not be used.
- Multiple blood cultures are performed as part of the workup for sepsis. Multiple blood cultures are typically performed together, and the additional cultures are identified with modifier 59, not modifier 91.

EXERCISE 7.4

Also available in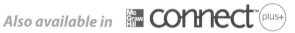

Using your CPT manual, answer each of the following questions.

1. A surgeon performs several procedures during the same operative session. Assuming that the primary procedure is identified, what modifier would be appended to the other procedures if they are not listed in Appendix D or E of the CPT manual? _____

2. A provider performs identical procedures on both sides of a patient. The CPT code describing that particular procedure does not indicate that it describes a bilateral procedure. What modifier is reported with the CPT code to indicate that identical services were performed on both sides of the body? _____

3. A physician orders a laboratory test that indicates the patient needs medication. After treatment, the physician repeats the lab test to see if the patient's condition has improved. What modifier would be used to show the lab test was repeated? _____

4. A provider performs two procedures that usually cannot be reported together, but in this particular instance the provider performs the second procedure during a separate session from the primary procedure. What modifier, if any, is added to the CPT code describing the second procedure? _____

7.5 Identifying Additional Providers Involved in Procedures

Multiple providers sometimes are needed to perform complex procedures. These additional professionals report their contributions to the procedure by adding modifiers to the same procedure codes reported by the primary surgeon.

Modifiers 80, 81, and 82

Modifiers 80, 81, and 82 identify assistant surgeons under differing circumstances:

- Modifier 80 identifies an **assistant surgeon** who provides services throughout the procedure.
- Modifier 81 identifies an assistant surgeon who only helps during a portion of the procedure.
- Modifier 82 is used to identify situations in a teaching institution where **resident physicians** typically act as surgical assistants, but no resident was available at the time of surgery. In such cases, another surgeon who is not a resident may provide those services.

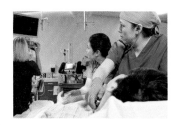

Modifiers 80, 81, and 82 identify the assistance of surgeons in a procedure.

assistant surgeon
Aide to a surgeon who provides services throughout the procedure.

resident physician
A medical school graduate in training to be a specific medical specialist who may assist surgeons during surgical procedures.

CODER'S TIP

Not all procedures require the use of an assistant. Medicare identifies procedures for which it permits an assistant surgeon on the Medicare Physician Fee Schedule. Other payers may have different rules regarding procedures for which they will pay for an assistant surgeon. Coders must know the assistant surgeon rules for each payer to which they report services.

CODER'S TIP

Medicare expects teaching programs to utilize residents as assistant surgeons in most cases, but it does not directly pay professional fees for services provided by a resident. Modifier 82 is used to identify situations in which a resident was not available to assist in a procedure and another professional performed these services.

CODING EXAMPLE

A provider assists the surgeon during a procedure identified as one for which an assistant surgeon is permitted. To report the assistant surgeon's services, the coder would add modifier 80 to the CPT code that identifies the surgical procedure.

CODING EXAMPLE

An assistant surgeon is present during only a portion of a surgical procedure. This service is reported by adding modifier 81 to the CPT code that describes the surgical procedure.

These modifiers cannot be used in all situations. For example, not all procedures require an assistant. Additionally, many payers, including Medicare, only pay for an assistant when the procedure is complex enough to require an assistant.

Modifier 62

co-surgeons
Two surgeons who operate together and perform distinct parts of a single procedure.

Modifier 62 is used to designate situations where two surgeons perform distinct parts of a single procedure. In such cases, the two surgeons are sometimes referred to as **co-surgeons.** This must be differentiated from situations in which one surgeon is assisting the other (see modifier 80). Modifier 62 also may be used with add-on codes that designate additional procedures that the two surgeons perform together. For example:

- Two surgeons operate together to perform an anterior spinal fusion at L3–L4 and L4–L5. One surgeon performs the anterior surgical approach, while the other performs the spinal fusion. Each surgeon reports CPT codes 22558 and 22585 (primary code and add-on code) with modifier 62.

Modifier 62 cannot be used:

- When one surgeon assists another surgeon during a procedure. (See modifiers 80, 81, and 82.)
- With E/M, anesthesia, radiology, laboratory, or medicine codes.

Modifier 66

surgical team
Group of healthcare providers that performs a surgical procedure together.

Modifier 66 is used when a **surgical team** of three or more surgeons, often from different specialties, is necessary to perform a complex surgical procedure. For example:

- A kidney transplant from a living donor usually requires one team of surgeons to remove the kidney from the donor and a second team of surgeons to implant the kidney into the recipient.
- A double lung transplant with cardiopulmonary bypass may require a team of surgeons to put the patient on bypass and a second team to implant the lungs into the recipient.
- Separating conjoined twins often requires separate surgical teams to perform the necessary procedures on each twin.

Modifier 66 is not used when only two surgeons perform different parts of a procedure.

CODING EXAMPLE

Two surgeons work together to perform an anterior spinal fusion of the lumbar spine. One surgeon performs the anterior approach through the abdomen to expose the lumbar vertebral bodies. The other surgeon performs the spinal fusion. Both surgeons report the same CPT code to describe the surgery, and each attaches modifier 62 to the code.

Using your CPT manual, answer each of the following questions.

1. What modifier would be reported when there is a team of surgeons from four different specialties working to-gether to perform the separation of conjoined twins? _____

2. A provider assists a surgeon during a procedure that Medicare recognizes as one for which an assistant surgeon is permitted. When the coder reports the assistant surgeon's services, what modifier, if any, would be added to the CPT code describing the surgical procedure to indicate that the provider assisted the surgeon?

   _____

3. When two surgeons perform distinct parts of a single surgical procedure, what modifier is attached to the CPT code to indicate the role of each surgeon? _____

4. A surgeon has an assistant help him while performing a procedure that is on the list of those for which an assistant is permitted. When the coder reports the surgeon's services, what modifier, if any, would be added to the CPT code describing the surgical procedure to indicate that the surgeon utilized the services of an assistant? _____

7.6 Reporting Procedures Involving Significantly More or Less Work than Is Typical

Occasionally a procedure requires significantly more or less work than is typically necessary for that procedure, the circumstances of which should be reported by providers. Several modifiers are used for this purpose.

Reporting Procedures Involving More Work than Is Typical

Modifier 22 Modifier 22 is used to identify those circumstances when the amount of work necessary to perform a procedure is significantly more than is typically necessary. Providers should be prepared to submit documentation supporting the use of this modifier. Modifier 22 may be used when anatomical variations or intraoperative complications beyond those that typically occur make the procedure more difficult.

CODING EXAMPLE

When Blake was a child, he was involved in a car accident that shattered his knee. After multiple unsuccessful surgeries, it is determined that Blake requires a total knee replacement. Due to the injury and damage caused by the previous unsuccessful surgeries, the orthopedic surgeon spends more than twice the amount of time normally necessary to perform the surgery, which is much more difficult than usual. In this instance, it may be appropriate for the coder to add modifier 22 to the CPT code describing the total knee replacement.

Modifier 22 is not used whenever a procedure takes longer than typical. For example, modifier 22 would not be used when:

- The increased time to perform a procedure is due to variations in provider practice or minor anatomical variation.
- Another code exists that describes the increased work.

Modifier 47 Attaching modifier 47 to a surgical code indicates that the surgeon also provided regional or general **anesthesia.**

anesthesia
Total or partial loss of sensation or awareness caused by disease, injury, or an anesthetic drug.

CODING EXAMPLE

The surgeon performing surgery on a patient's hand administers a Bier block (a form of regional anesthesia) prior to performing the procedure. The coder selects the most appropriate code to describe the surgery and adds modifier 47.

Modifier 47 is not used in cases where the surgeon provides local anesthesia for the procedure. Local anesthesia is considered to be a part of the surgical procedure. This modifier is not added to the surgical code when an anesthesiologist or certified registered nurse anesthetist (CRNA) provides the anesthesia services. In those cases, the anesthesiologist or CRNA reports his or her services separately from those of the surgeon. Modifier 47 also is not added when the surgeon provides conscious sedation during a surgical procedure. Examples of situations where modifier 47 is not reported include the following:

- Prior to performing surgery, the surgeon infiltrates the area with local anesthesia to provide a pain-free area. This is considered part of the surgical procedure.
- The surgeon supervises a CRNA providing general anesthesia for the procedure.
- A physician provides conscious sedation during a procedure.

Modifier 63 Performing surgical procedures on neonates and infants up to 4 kg is technically more challenging. Adding modifier 63 to the CPT code that describes the surgical procedure indicates that the patient was less than 4 kg at the time of surgery. This modifier can only be added to surgical codes in the (20000–69999) range.

Some CPT codes describe procedures that are commonly performed on infants and neonates. It is inappropriate to add modifier 63 to those codes because the additional work involved in those surgeries is already included in the code. Each of those CPT codes is identified with a parenthetical note not to report modifier 63 in conjunction with that code. In addition, these procedures are listed in Appendix F.

CODING EXAMPLE

A surgeon repairs an incarcerated inguinal hernia in a newborn infant who weighs slightly less than 4 kg. This procedure is reported with CPT code 49492. The coder must decide whether to add modifier 63 to identify the infant as less than 4 kg. Looking in the CPT manual, however, she finds that this code is listed in Appendix F and has a parenthetical note that modifier 63 is not reported in conjunction with CPT code 49492.

Reporting Procedures Involving Less Work than Is Typical

Modifier 52 Modifier 52 indicates that the services provided involved significantly less work than usually required for that procedure, but no other CPT code describes the actual services provided. For example, modifier 52 can be reported when:

- The physician reduced or eliminated some services usually associated with the code to which the modifier is attached, but there is no other code that describes those lesser services.
- A planned procedure is terminated prior to the induction of anesthesia.

Modifier 52 is not used:

- To indicate that the procedure was terminated after the induction of anesthesia but before the surgery started (see modifier 53 below).
- With E/M services.
- With time-based services, such as psychotherapy, anesthesia, or critical care services, to indicate that the services involved a shorter time period than indicated in the code descriptor or required by the guidance associated with the code.

Modifier 53 Modifier 53 identifies procedures that are terminated after the induction of anesthesia, usually due to the patient's condition. The procedure may be terminated at any time after the induction of anesthesia, either before or after the surgeon begins the procedure. For example:

- Modifier 53 is added to the code if the surgeon begins surgery but discontinues the procedure due to:
  - Uncontrollable bleeding, hypotension, or physiologic changes.
  - Unexpected findings during surgery that make continuing surgery unnecessary or ill advised.
  - Anesthesia complications.
- Modifier 53 may be used to report terminated procedures in the office setting.

Modifier 53 is not used to:

- Identify procedures that are canceled prior to the induction of anesthesia (see modifier 52 above).
- Indicate that the physician reduced or eliminated some services usually associated with the code to which the modifier is attached (see modifier 52).

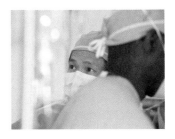

Modifier 53 describes procedures that are terminated after the induction of anesthesia. This termination usually results from a change in the circumstances of the procedure (e.g., anesthesia complications, change in patient status, or unexpected findings during surgery).

CODER'S TIP

Only professionals use modifiers 52 and 53 to report procedures that are canceled before or after anesthesia induction. Hospitals and other facilities use other modifiers to identify procedures that are canceled before or after the induction of anesthesia. Hospital coding is beyond the scope of this course.

CODING EXAMPLE

A surgeon schedules emergency surgery to reduce an incarcerated hernia. The patient is taken to the preoperative area to prepare for the procedure. The surgeon reexamines the patient and finds that the incarcerated hernia has spontaneously reduced during preparation for surgery. The surgeon cancels the procedure before the patient is anesthetized. The surgeon reports the code that describes the intended hernia repair with modifier 52.

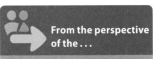

From the perspective of the ...

CODER

To determine whether to add modifier 52 or 53 in situations where a surgical procedure is canceled, determine whether anesthesia was already administered when the procedure was canceled. If cancellation occurs before the induction of anesthesia, modifier 52 is reported; after anesthesia induction, modifier 53 is reported.

EXERCISE 7.6

Also available in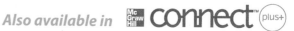

Using your CPT manual, answer each of the following questions.

1. A surgeon performs a procedure that was more extensive than usual because the patient was obese. What modifier, if any, is added to the surgical code to indicate that the work was greater than usual?
   _____

2. A hand surgeon performs a regional block for anesthesia and then performs a carpal tunnel release. When the coder reports these services, what modifier, if any, does she use to indicate that the same physician performed the surgery and administered the anesthetic? _____

3. A pediatric surgeon performs a surgical procedure on a baby that weighs less than 4 kg. What modifier, if any, would be added to the surgical code to report this service? _____

4. A surgeon performs a procedure that is not described by any CPT code, but another code exists that describes a more complex procedure that includes the procedure actually performed. What modifier, if any, is added to the more complex surgical code to indicate that the surgery performed is less than the procedure described by the code? _____

5. After a surgeon starts a procedure, the patient starts to bleed uncontrollably and the surgeon decides to discontinue the procedure. What modifier, if any, is added to the CPT code that describes the surgery to report the discontinued surgery? _____

7.7 Reporting Mandatory Services, Preventive Services, Physical Status, and Genetic Tests

Mandatory Services

Modifier 32 is added to a code to indicate that the government, a third-party payer, or another entity with the authority to do so mandated the physician to perform a particular service. This modifier is not used when the physician would have performed the service even if not required to do so. For example, modifier 32 is used:

- To report blood alcohol or other tests required by police or courts when someone in custody is brought to the emergency room.
- When an insurance company or other payer requires a specific test prior to approving a request for a surgical procedure.
- When a second opinion is required prior to performing a procedure or providing other therapeutic modalities.

Modifier 32 is not used:

- To report a medical service that typically would have been performed in the absence of a requirement to do so. In such cases, the coder reports the service using the appropriate CPT code without this modifier.
- When a patient or family members request a medical service or a second opinion.

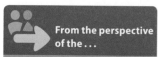

From the perspective of the . . .

CODER

Understand how to report mandated services, including what services are mandated by each payer or government entity.

Preventive Services

Modifier 33 should be added to a code when the primary purpose of the service is the delivery of a recommended preventive service. Modifier 33 is used when:

- The service provided is recommended as a preventive service by the US Preventive Services Task Force (USPSTF) and has an A or B rating on the USPSTF list posted on the Agency for Healthcare Research and Quality website: (www.uspreventiveservicestaskforce.org/uspstf/uspsabrecs.htm)
- An immunization is recommended for routine use in children, adolescents, and adults as recommended by the Advisory Committee on Immunization Practices of the Center for Disease Control and Prevention.

Modifier 33 is not added to codes when the code specifically identifies the service as preventive.

Physical Status Modifiers P1 through P6

Modifiers P1–P6 are **physical status modifiers** to identify how healthy or sick a particular patient is before undergoing anesthesia. Only anesthesia providers use these modifiers. These modifiers are only added to the anesthesia CPT codes (00100–01999):

physical status modifiers
Modifiers attached to CPT codes 00100-01999 by anesthesia providers to identify how healthy or sick a particular patient is before undergoing anesthesia.

P1   A normal healthy patient.

P2   A patient with mild systemic disease.

P3   A patient with severe systemic disease.

P4   A patient with severe systemic disease that is a constant threat to life.

P5   A moribund patient who is not expected to survive without the operation.

P6   A brain-dead patient whose organs are being removed for donor purposes.

Anesthesiologists or other providers reporting services with anesthesia codes use the physical status modifiers to describe the patient's preanesthetic health status.

CODING EXAMPLE

A previously healthy patient is scheduled for surgery on her knee. The anesthesiologist adds the P1 modifier to the appropriate anesthesia code.

CODING EXAMPLE

An elderly patient with stable diabetes, heart disease, and high blood pressure is scheduled for abdominal surgery. The anesthesiologist adds the P3 modifier to the anesthesia code.

CODING EXAMPLE

An anesthesiologist provides services to a patient with mild systemic disease. The anesthesiologist adds the P2 modifier to the anesthesia code.

It is inappropriate to add the P1–P6 modifiers to surgical procedure codes or E/M codes to indicate the patient's state of health.

Genetic Modifiers

Rather than identify individual genetic tests, CPT codes identify general molecular diagnostic procedures and cytogenetic studies. Modifiers are added to these general codes to identify the specific disease for which the tests were performed. There are numerous modifiers, and the list constantly increases as new tests are developed. These modifiers, located in Appendix I of the CPT manual, are organized into 10 major groupings, each identified by the first numerical digit of a two-digit alphanumeric code. The 10 major groupings are:

0	Neoplasia (Solid Tumor, Excluding Sarcoma and Lymphoma)
1	Neoplasia (Sarcoma)
2	Neoplasia (Lymphoid/Hematopoietic)
3	Non-Neoplastic Hematology/Coagulation
4	Histocompatibility/Blood Typing/Identity/Microsatellite
5	Neurologic, Non-Neoplastic
6	Muscular, Non-Neoplastic
7	Metabolic, Other
8	Metabolic, Transport
9	Metabolic—Pharmacogenetics/Dysmorphology

The modifiers designating the specific diseases for which a test is performed are added to the genetic test code. For example:

- Modifiers 0A and 0B are added to the genetic test code to indicate that the test was performed to identify the BRCA1 and BRCA2 genes associated with certain breast cancers.
- Modifier 1G is added to the genetic test code to indicate that the test was performed to identify a neuroblastoma.
- Modifier 5D is added to the genetic test code to indicate that the test was performed to determine whether a patient has inherited the gene that causes Huntington's disease.

These modifiers are not added to codes describing procedures for the treatment of an inherited disease.

EXERCISE 7.7

Also available in **connect** plus+

Using your CPT manual, answer each of the following questions.

1. An insurance company requires a patient to have an EKG prior to surgery, even though the surgeon knows the patient has no history of cardiac disease. What modifier, if any, would the coder add to the code for the EKG when reporting this service? _____

2. An otherwise healthy patient is undergoing a complicated incision and drainage procedure under anesthesia. What modifier would the coder add to the anesthesia code to describe this patient's physical status? _____

3. An organ donation procedure involving a brain-dead patient is performed under anesthesia. What modifier does the coder add to the anesthesia code? _____

4. What modifier identifies a genetic test for Niemann-Pick disease? _____

5. What modifier identifies a genetic test for factor VIII hemophilia? _____

7.8 HCPCS Modifiers

In addition to CPT modifiers (those listed in the CPT manual), coders must be familiar with HCPCS modifiers (additional modifiers listed in the HCPCS Level II manual). These modifiers may be added to both Level I (CPT) and Level II (HCPCS) codes. As with CPT modifiers, HCPCS modifiers are used to further define services without changing the definition of the code.

Anatomical Modifiers

HCPCS modifiers are used to provide additional information related to the specific anatomical site of the procedure. They may be used with a single code to indicate the specific anatomical structure. They also may be used in combination with modifier 59 to identify that the second procedure was performed on a separate anatomical site (refer to the discussion of the use of modifier 59). The anatomical modifiers include:

E1–E4	Used to identify specific eyelids.
FA, F1–F9	Used to identify specific fingers.
TA, T1–T9	Used to identify specific toes.
RC, LC, and LD	Used to identify specific coronary arteries.
LT and RT	Used to identify left and right.

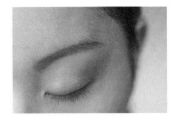

Modifiers E1–E4 identify the specific eyelids on which a procedure was performed.

CODER'S TIP

Coders should be familiar with the appropriate use of HCPCS anatomical modifiers and where they can be found in the HCPCS manual. To be sure that the correct modifiers are used, confirm the proper modifiers each time they are used.

CODING EXAMPLE

A surgeon performs a procedure on the middle finger of the patient's right hand. When reporting this procedure, the coder adds modifier F7 to the surgical code to indicate the specific finger.

CODING EXAMPLE

A surgeon performs a procedure on the patient's right upper eyelid and a second procedure on the left lower lid. These two procedures typically are not reported together. In this case, the surgeon adds modifier E3 to the code describing the right eyelid procedure and E2 to the left lower lid procedure to indicate these were performed on different anatomical locations.

Ambulance Modifiers

When ambulance services are reported, special modifiers must be used to identify the pickup point and destination of the **ambulance trip.** Single-digit characters identify each of these locations and are combined into a two-digit code to accurately describe the two location points. The most common locations are:

D   Diagnostic or therapeutic site other than a hospital or physician's office

H   Hospital

J   Freestanding end-stage renal disease (ESRD) facility

N   Skilled nursing facility (SNF)

ambulance trip
Transportation of a patient from the pickup point to the destination of the ambulance.

P   Physician's office
R   Residence
S   Scene of an accident

For example, when the ambulance transports an injured individual from the scene of an accident to the hospital after a severe automobile accident, the coder would report HCPCS code A0427 with modifier SH. This indicates the trip started at the accident scene and ended at the hospital. Additional codes may be used to indicate the number of miles and equipment utilized during the transport. It is possible that an ambulance modifier could be the same as another HCPCS modifier. The meaning of the modifier depends on the code to which it is attached.

CODING EXAMPLE

An ambulance arrives at the scene of an accident and transports an injured patient to the hospital emergency department. When the ambulance provider submits a claim for that trip, the modifier SH is added to the code to indicate that the transportation occurred between the scene of the accident and the hospital.

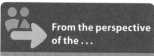

From the perspective of the . . .

CODER

It is important to know whether the equipment provided to a patient was purchased new, purchased used, or rented for the patient.

Equipment Modifiers

Durable medical equipment (DME) and other medical equipment may be purchased or rented. Purchased equipment may be new or refurbished and reused by more than one patient. Modifiers are used to identify these equipment-related options.

NU   Equipment is new.
UE   Equipment is used.
RR   Equipment is rented.
LL   Equipment is leased; lease payments are applied to purchase price.

EXERCISE 7.8

Also available in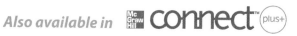

Using your CPT manual, answer each of the following questions.

1. What modifier is reported to show that a power wheelchair has been rented? _____

2. An ambulance is called to the mall, where a shooting has taken place. The ambulance transports a patient to the emergency room. What modifier is used with the ambulance code to report the beginning and ending points of this trip? _____

3. A patient is having a blepharoplasty of the right upper eyelid. What modifier would be reported with the surgical code? _____

4. What modifier is used with the surgical code to indicate that a patient is having surgery on her right knee? _____

5. What modifier is used to indicate that a patient is being transported by ambulance from a skilled nursing facility to the hospital? _____

6. A physician gives a patient with a fractured ankle a set of crutches. What modifier would be reported with the code for the new crutches? _____

Summary

Learning Outcome	Key Concepts/Examples
7.1 Explain the functions and uses of modifiers. **Pages 152–154**	Modifiers may be added to CPT or HCPCS codes that do not completely describe the actual services provided. Modifiers may be used to indicate: • E/M services provided during the global period. • Separate E/M services provided on the same day as another service. • Professional and technical components when these are provided by different providers. • When more than one provider performed all or part of a procedure. • Bilateral procedures. • Multiple procedures. • A single procedure performed more than once during the same session. • Work done by an assistant surgeon. • When a procedure is more difficult than usual. • Procedures that are increased or decreased from the usual procedure definition. • Physical status of a patient undergoing anesthesia. • Anatomical sites to differentiate surgical site. • Beginning and ending points of an ambulance trip. Most modifiers may be used on codes from multiple sections of CPT codes. Many modifiers affect payments.
7.2 Discuss modifiers to indicate services provided during a procedure's global period. **Pages 154–161**	A number of modifiers describe services provided during the global period, including: • Modifier 24—Identifies E/M procedures that are unrelated to the original procedure. • Modifier 25—Describes a significant, separately identifiable E/M service provided on the same day as another procedure or service. • Modifier 57—Signifies that the decision to perform surgery was made during an E/M visit that occurred during the global period. • Modifier 58—Describes staged procedures when the second procedure occurs during the global period of the first procedure. • Modifier 76—Identifies situations where the provider repeated the same procedure during the global period. • Modifier 77—Indicates that another provider performed the same procedure during the global period of the first procedure. • Modifier 78—Indicates that the patient returned to the operating room for an unplanned procedure that is related to the first procedure during the global period of the first procedure. • Modifier 79—Identifies an unrelated surgical procedure performed during the global period of the first procedure.
7.3 Use modifiers to report components of procedures or services. **Pages 161–164**	Modifiers are used to identify situations where providers perform only part of the procedure described by the code. There are two main situations where this occurs. The first is when different providers perform the professional and technical components of services. Modifier 26 identifies the professional component, and modifier TC identifies the technical component. The second situation is when different providers perform the preoperative, intraoperative and postoperative services. Modifiers 54, 55, and 56 identify these surgical components.

(Continued)

Learning Outcome	Key Concepts/Examples
7.4 Explain bilateral, multiple, repeat, or additional procedures performed on the same date of service. **Pages 164–168**	Modifiers identify situations when providers perform more than one procedure during a single operative session. These include the following modifiers: • Modifier 50—Identifies bilateral procedures in which the same procedure is performed on the same body part on each side of the body. • Modifier 51—Indicates that the provider performed multiple procedures during the same session. • Modifier 59—Identifies services that usually are not reported with another service, but in this particular situation should be considered a separate and distinct procedure. This usually occurs when the procedure is performed on a different body part, through a separate incision, or during a different session on the same day. • Modifier 91 indicates that it was necessary to repeat a laboratory test on the same day as the original test.
7.5 Cite appropriate modifiers to identify individuals who assist the primary provider during procedures. **Pages 169–170**	Modifiers are used to identify additional providers involved in procedures, including: • Modifier 80—Indicates the procedure involved an assistant surgeon throughout the procedure. • Modifier 81—Indicates the procedure involved an assistant surgeon during part of the procedure. • Modifier 82—Indicates the procedure involved an assistant surgeon who provided services when a resident physician was unavailable to assist. • Modifier 62—Identifies situations where two surgeons performed distinct parts of a single procedure. • Modifier 66—Indicates that a team of three or more surgeons performed a complex procedure.
7.6 Discuss circumstances where the amount of work necessary to perform the service differs significantly from the amount typically necessary. **Pages 171–174**	Modifiers may be added to CPT codes to indicate that the procedure involved significantly more or less work than usual, including: • Modifier 22—Indicates that the procedure involved significantly more work, which may occur due to significant anatomical variation or intraoperative complications. • Modifier 47—Identifies situations where the surgeon provided general or regional anesthesia for the procedure. This is not used when the surgeon provides local anesthesia. • Modifier 63—Designates procedures performed on an infant that is less than 4 kg in weight at the time of surgery. • Modifier 52—Indicates that the procedure involved significantly less work than is typical. This may be due to eliminating some services usually performed or when the procedure is terminated prior to the induction of anesthesia. • Modifier 53—Designates procedures terminated after the induction of anesthesia, which is usually due to patient condition.
7.7 Define modifiers describing mandatory services, physical status, and genetic tests. **Pages 174–176**	Modifiers may designate mandatory services, the physical status of a patient undergoing anesthesia, or the specific genetic test performed, including: • Modifier 32—Indicates that the services provided were mandated by the government or a third-party payer. • Modifiers P1–P6—Designate the physical status of a patient undergoing anesthesia. • Modifiers listed in Appendix I—A series of over 100 modifiers that identify specific diseases for which genetic tests may be performed.

Learning Outcome	Key Concepts/Examples
7.8 Define HCPCS modifiers to primary codes. **Pages 176–178**	HCPCS modifiers may be used to identify anatomical locations, ambulance begin and end locations, and whether durable medical equipment or other medical equipment is new, used, or rented. These modifiers include: • Anatomical modifiers to identify specific eyelids, fingers, toes, coronary arteries, and right and left sides. • Ambulance pickup and destination locations identified with individual alpha characters that are combined into two-character modifiers. • Modifiers NU, UE, and RR to indicate that DME or other medical equipment is new, used, or rented.

Using Terminology

Match the key terms with their definitions.

_____ **1.** L07.1 Ambulance trip

_____ **2.** L07.1 Anesthesia

_____ **3.** L07.5 Assistant surgeon

_____ **4.** L07.1 Bilateral procedure

_____ **5.** L07.5 Co-surgeons

_____ **6.** L07.2 Decision to perform surgery

_____ **7.** L07.4 Distinct procedure

_____ **8.** L07.1 Global period

_____ **9.** L07.1 Multiple procedures

_____ **10.** L07.7 Physical status modifier

_____ **11.** L07.3 Professional component

_____ **12.** L07.5 Resident physician

_____ **13.** L07.2 Staged procedure

_____ **14.** L07.5 Surgical team

_____ **15.** L07.3 Technical component

A. Period of time after an initial procedure was performed, in which follow-up procedures may be billed as such

B. A portion of a procedure that is completed by a separate specialist, such as the interpretation of x-rays by a radiologist

C. A portion of a procedure that requires the use of special equipment

D. Aide to a surgeon who provides services throughout the procedure

E. Resident surgeon who assists the main physician during a procedure

F. Two surgeons who operate together and perform distinct parts of a single procedure

G. Group of healthcare providers performing a surgery together

H. Identical procedures performed on both sides of the body during the same operative session

I. Two or more procedures performed

J. Partial or complete loss of sensation as a result of disease, injury, or administration of an anesthetic agent

K. Modifiers used to identify how healthy or sick a particular patient is before undergoing anesthesia

L. Transportation of a patient from the pickup point to the ambulance's destination

M. Decision made during an E/M service in the global period, reported by adding modifier 57 to the E/M code

N. Subsequent procedure(s) commonly performed during the global period under one of three circumstances: planned staged procedure anticipated prior to the first procedure, more extensive procedure needed than originally planned, or a therapeutic procedure performed following a diagnostic procedure

O. Procedure that is not usually reported with another procedure but can be reported together under certain circumstances

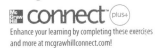

Enhance your learning by completing these exercises and more at mcgrawhillconnect.com!

CHAPTER 7 | MODIFIERS   181

Checking Your Understanding

Match each modifier with its definition.

_____ **1.** L07.2 25
_____ **2.** L07.3 26
_____ **3.** L07.4 76
_____ **4.** L07.5 62
_____ **5.** L07.6 52
_____ **6.** L07.7 32
_____ **7.** L07.8 FA
_____ **8.** L07.2 79
_____ **9.** L07.3 54
_____ **10.** L07.4 50
_____ **11.** L07.5 66
_____ **12.** L07.6 22
_____ **13.** L07.9 NU
_____ **14.** L07.8 T9
_____ **15.** L07.8 E1

A. Example of an eyelid anatomical modifier
B. Reduced services
C. Co-surgeons
D. Separately identifiable E/M service provided on the same day as another service
E. Repeat procedure by same physician
F. Professional component (e.g., interpreting fluoroscopy during surgery)
G. Unrelated service by the same physician during the global period
H. Example of a toe anatomical modifier
I. Surgical care only
J. Surgical team
K. Increased services
L. Mandatory services
M. New equipment issued
N. Bilateral procedure
O. Example of a finger anatomical modifier

Select the letter that best describes the statement or answers the question.

1. L07.3 Which type of office visit does not require a modifier?
   a. Preoperative management office visit
   b. Office visit with decision to perform surgery
   c. Regular office visit for illness
   d. Postoperative management office visit

2. L07.4 Which scenario requires the use of modifier 51?
   a. Draining and then redraining an abscess on the same day
   b. Bilateral knee replacement
   c. Suture repair of a laceration and removal of a mole in a separate location, also requiring suture closure
   d. Normal vaginal delivery of twins

3. L07.8 A modifier is not used to indicate durable medical equipment that is _____.
   a. Provided in used condition
   b. Provided on the same day as surgery
   c. Rented to the patient
   d. Provided in new condition

4. L07.5 A modifier is not required for which of the following situations where there is an assistant during surgery?
   a. A physician assistant (PA) assists the surgeon
   b. A surgeon assists another surgeon in a procedure
   c. A surgeon provides minimum assistance to the main surgeon
   d. A surgeon assists another surgeon in a university hospital where no resident is available

5. L07.8 It is necessary to append a modifier to the base transportation code to describe which of the following about an ambulance transport of a patient?

    a. If the patient was ambulatory when picked up

    b. When the patient was picked up

    c. Whether a family member rode with the patient

    d. Where the patient was delivered

6. L07.2 Which of these situations requires using modifier 32 for a service?

    a. An insurance company requires a second opinion before an operation.

    b. An emergency department patient asks for a routine INR blood test.

    c. A surgeon removes a skin tag from a patient who is undergoing an appendectomy.

    d. A 15-year-old patient's mother demands a urine drug screen for her son.

7. L07.4 Which of the following situations requires the use of modifier 51?

    a. Primary laminotomy with a second-level laminotomy

    b. Cholecystectomy done at the same time as a required (not incidental) appendectomy

    c. Return to the operating room for the second stage of an abscess drainage

    d. Foraminal epidural injection of steroid done at one main level and two additional levels

8. L07.5 Modifier 62 should be used when _____.

    a. Two surgeons work together, each performing a separate part of the surgery

    b. A surgeon assists the primary surgeon in performing the surgery

    c. A surgeon performs the second stage of a surgery at a later date

    d. A physician provides the postoperative care in the hospital

9. L07.8 Which of the following HCPCS codes cannot accept modifiers?

    a. Surgical HCPCS codes

    b. E/M HCPCS codes

    c. Dental codes

    d. DME HCPCS codes

10. L07.1 Which of the following situations does not require a modifier?

    a. Blood CK-MB levels repeated 3 times in one day to rule out myocardial infarction

    b. Colonoscopy with snare polypectomy and separate biopsy of colon

    c. Lumbar epidural injection at the primary level with additional injection at two other levels

    d. Cholecystectomy and routine follow-up clinic visit

11. L07.3 Which of the following modifiers would only be used with a procedure code for a surgery (not E/M)?

    a. 54

    b. 55

    c. 56

    d. 57

Mc Graw Hill connect (plus+)

Enhance your learning by completing these exercises and more at mcgrawhillconnect.com!

CHAPTER 7 | MODIFIERS   183

12. L07.2 Which of the following scenarios requires using modifier 24 for the E/M code?

    a. A surgeon sees a patient in the office for a wound check 5 days after appendectomy.

    b. A surgeon sees a patient in the office for staple removal 10 days after heart surgery.

    c. A surgeon sees a patient in the hospital the day after surgery for routine postoperative care

    d. A surgeon sees a patient in the office for abdominal pain the day after throat surgery.

13. L07.2 An emergency physician comprehensively cares for a patient who has been in a car accident and has several minor injuries. The physician also sutures a facial laceration sustained in the accident. Which modifier would be used to distinguish between the overall evaluation and management of the patient and the actual suturing procedure?

    a. 22

    b. 23

    c. 25

    d. 26

14. L07.4 Which of the following scenarios would require modifier 50 on the CPT code when all care is performed at one episode?

    a. A physician excises moles from the skin of the left arm and the skin of the right arm.

    b. A physician removes cataracts from the left eye and right eye.

    c. A physician injects the left knee with steroid and arthroscopes the right knee.

    d. A physician removes both lobes of the thyroid gland.

15. L07.5 Which of the following scenarios would require modifier 62 on the surgical CPT code?

    a. A surgeon performs the careful dissection through the brain to the tumor while a second surgeon actually excises the tumor.

    b. A surgeon manipulates the left knee for the duration of the case while a second surgeon performs a left knee joint replacement.

    c. A surgeon is called in to briefly inspect the neck lymph nodes where a second surgeon has performed a total thyroidectomy.

    d. A surgeon performs an appendectomy while a second surgeon performs an incidental excision of a skin cancer on the face.

16. L07.6 A surgeon performs an excision of a ganglion cyst from a patient's wrist. This is normally a simple procedure, but in this case, the cyst is enveloped in nerves and blood vessels, requiring careful dissection and taking three times as long as usual. Which modifier should be applied to the CPT code for the ganglion excision to best describe this situation?

    a. 24

    b. 52

    c. 22

    d. 51

17. L07.2 Which of the following scenarios would require use of modifier 76?

    a. An EKG done by the same physician who performed an echocardiogram on a patient

    b. A repeat EKG done by a different physician on the same day for a patient with chest pain

    c. A repeat EKG done by the same physician on a different day for a patient with chest pain

    d. A repeat EKG done by the same physician on the same day for a patient with chest pain

18. L07.4 Which of the following scenarios would require the use of modifier 91 on at least one of the lab CPT codes?
    a. A patient being retested for blood potassium level after the first sample hemolyzed and became invalid
    b. A pregnant patient who has serial quantitative beta-HCG levels done every two days for a week
    c. A patient with anemia who has a complete blood count (CBC) performed and a hemoglobin level taken later the same day after transfusion
    d. A patient with chest pain who has three repeat troponin I blood tests to rule out myocardial infarction

19. L07.2 A surgeon is performing a lengthy excision procedure on a very large pancreatic cancer and must complete the excision in two different surgeries a day apart. Which modifier should be used for the CPT code on the second procedure?
    a. 58
    b. 78
    c. 79
    d. 76

20. L07.8 A patient has a trigger finger release done on the right ring finger (fourth digit). Which modifier should be used to indicate the anatomical site of the procedure?
    a. RT
    b. RF
    c. F8
    d. T8

Applying Your Skills

Using your CPT manual, answer the questions below.

1. L07.1 A physician orders a CBC more than once in a given day. What is the correct modifier code to append to the appropriate laboratory code for this test? _____

2. L07.2 A provider performs an unrelated separate E/M service on the same day she performs a procedure. Which modifier, if any, is used to report this situation? If a modifier is used, to which code is it appended?
   _____

3. L07.2 A surgeon performs an E/M service and determines that a patient requires a surgical procedure that has a 90-day global period. If the E/M procedure occurred the day before surgery, which modifier, if any, is added to the E/M visit code? _____

4. L07.2 A surgeon performs an E/M service and determines that a patient requires a surgical procedure that has a 90-day global period. Which modifier, if any, would be added to the E/M visit code if the visit occurred a week before surgery? _____

5. L07.3 Which modifier identifies the technical component, as in the use of x-rays and other imaging?
   _____

6. L07.3 A radiologist interprets x-rays in the hospital several days a week. He is not employed by the hospital. Which modifier, if any, does the radiologist add to the CPT codes that describes the x-ray codes to report those interpretations? _____

7. L07.3 When coding for the supervision and interpretation of a chest x-ray, which modifier, if any, should be appended to the CPT code describing the x-ray? _____

8. L07.4 A surgeon performs identical procedures on both sides of the patient's body. Which modifier does the coder attach to the CPT code describing the procedure? _____

connect plus+
Enhance your learning by completing these exercises
and more at mcgrawhillconnect.com!   CHAPTER 7 | MODIFIERS   185

9. L07.4 Which modifier or code would be reported when a repeat surgical procedure is performed on one patient by a different surgeon on the same day? _____

10. L07.4 Which modifier code(s) would be reported when a patient returns to the operating room on the same day for a similar or related procedure performed by the same surgeon? _____

11. L07.4 Which modifier indicates that a service that is usually considered part of another procedure performed on the same day was performed on a different body part? _____

12. L07.4 When the code descriptor includes the word "unilateral" and the procedure is done bilaterally, which modifier should be appended to the CPT code? _____

13. L07.5 Which modifier code(s) may be reported when there is an assistant surgeon? _____

14. L07.5 A team of four surgeons performs complex procedures on a patient during a single surgical session. Which modifier would the surgeons add to the surgical code to report their participation on the surgical team? _____

15. L07.5 When two surgeons of different specialties perform different parts of a complex surgical procedure, which modifier is added to the surgical code to report their services? _____

16. L07.6 A surgeon discontinues a surgical procedure after the induction of anesthesia due to complications affecting the patient. Which modifier is added to the surgical code to report this occurrence? _____

17. L07.6 A surgeon only performs part of a procedure, but no other code exists to describe what she actually did. There is a code that describes a more comprehensive procedure that includes the procedure performed. Which modifier, if any, is added to the existing code to report that not all the services included in the descriptor were performed? _____

18. L07.6 Which modifier code would be reported when a patient undergoes local anesthesia? _____

19. L07.7 A physician performs a service required by court order. Which modifier, if any, is added to the CPT code to indicate this situation? _____

20. L07.7 An 85-year-old patient undergoes anesthesia for chronic kidney disease and is not expected to survive unless she has the operation. What is the correct modifier to append to the anesthesia code? _____

21. L07.8 An ambulance picks up a drowning victim at a lake and takes him to the hospital. Which modifier would be used to indicate these locations? _____

22. L07.8 Which modifier is used to report that a set of crutches was purchased new? _____

23. L07.8 Which modifier reports that a procedure was performed on the right coronary artery? _____

24. L07.8 Which modifier is used to report the rental of a wheelchair? _____

25. L07.8 A patient is having a blepharoplasty of the right upper eyelid. Which modifier would be reported with the surgical code? _____

Thinking It Through

Use your critical-thinking skills to answer the questions below.

1. L07.8 An ambulance is called from the hospital to the mall, where a shooting of an adult male has taken place at 11:00 a.m. on a Saturday. The ambulance picks up the patient and takes him to the hospital. What about the nature of this ambulance call demands a modifier? Which modifier should the coder use?

   _____

   _____

2. L07.2 A patient presents to his physician's office for removal of skin tags. He informs the physician that he also has a significant amount of shoulder pain. The physician surgically removes the skin tags from the patient's back and right leg. The physician then examines the patient for shoulder pain. What modifier, if any, should be appended to the office visit E/M code? Explain your answer.

   _____

   _____

3. L07.4 A surgeon performs an umbilical hernia repair and an excision of a facial mole during the same operative session. What modifier, if any, is reported with the CPT code that describes the second surgical procedure and why?

   _____

   _____

4. L07.5 A surgeon assists another surgeon during a coronary bypass graft procedure by harvesting the saphenous vein graft and then holding the heart while the primary surgeon sutures the grafts. What modifier, if any, does the assistant surgeon add to the CPT code to report the service?

   _____

   _____

5. L07.8 A surgeon performs multiple, identical tendon repairs of the right index, ring, and little fingers. What modifiers are used to distinguish multiple iterations of the CPT procedure code in this case?

   _____

   _____

6. L07.4 A physician performs a colonoscopy and removes one polyp with snare electrocautery but also performs a biopsy of a different part of the colon and an injection in yet another part of the colon. What modifier, if any, is needed to qualify each of these colonoscopic procedures done at the same time and why?

   _____

   _____

McGraw Hill connect (plus+)

Enhance your learning by completing these exercises
and more at mcgrawhillconnect.com!

CHAPTER 7 | MODIFIERS   187

8

EVALUATION AND MANAGEMENT SERVICES, PART I: STRUCTURE AND GUIDANCE

Learning Outcomes

After completing this chapter, students should be able to:

8.1 Explain the breakdown of E/M services into categories and subcategories.

8.2 Define key terms related to E/M coding.

8.3 Determine the level of various E/M codes based on primary and secondary components.

8.4 Differentiate among the four types of histories.

8.5 Contrast the four types of physical examination.

8.6 Differentiate among the four types of medical decision making.

8.7 Explain how the key components determine the level of E/M services provided.

Key Terms

Care coordination

Chief complaint

Comprehensive history

Concurrent care

Consultation

Contributory components

Counseling

Critical care

Detailed history

Established patient

Evaluation and management services

Expanded problem-focused history

Family history

History of present illness

Key components

Medical decision making

New patient

Past, family, and social history (PFSH)

Past medical history

Physical examination

Problem-focused history

Review of systems

Social history

Time

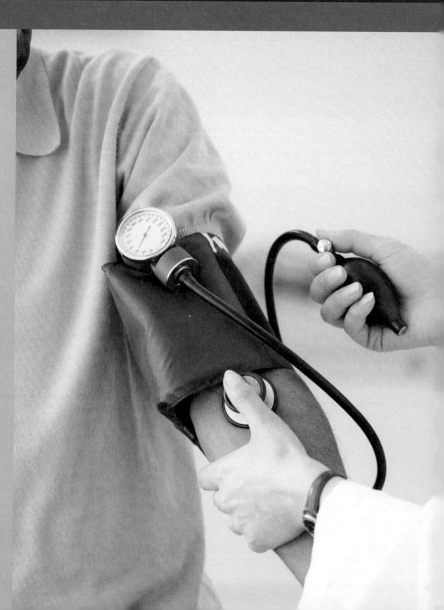

Introduction

Evaluation and management (E/M) codes (99201–99499) describe a broad range of physician services. These codes do not describe procedures; instead, they describe services commonly associated with a "doctor visit," in which a physician takes the patient's history, performs a physical examination, determines the cause of the patient's medical condition, orders and interprets appropriate tests, decides on necessary treatments, and monitors the patient for changes in his or her health status.

Selecting the most appropriate E/M code to describe these services is more complex than determining the correct code to describe surgical procedures. The CPT manual includes guidance to help coders identify the multiple elements associated with the code selection process. This chapter provides coders with the background to identify these elements, determine the level to which each element is performed during the E/M visit, and determine the E/M code that describes that visit based on those performance levels.

8.1 Categories and Subcategories of E/M Services

Categories of E/M Services

Evaluation and management services are divided into multiple categories. The categories are primarily based on the setting in which the services are provided. Therefore, the initial question that the coder must ask when reporting E/M services is, "Where were the services provided?"

Broad categories of E/M services include:

- Office or Other Outpatient Services (99201–99215)
- Hospital Observation Services (99217–99226)
- Hospital Inpatient Services (99221–99239)
- Consultations (99241–99255)
- Emergency Department Services (99281–99288)
- Critical Care Services (99291–99292)
- Nursing Facility Services (99304–99318)
- Domiciliary, Rest Home, or Custodial Care Services (99324–99337)
- Domiciliary, Rest Home, or Home Care Plan Oversight Services (99339–99340)
- Home Services (99341–99350)
- Prolonged Services (99354–99360)
- Case Management Services (99363–99368)
- Care Plan Oversight (99374–99380)
- Preventive Medicine Services (99381–99429)
- Non–Face-to-Face Physician Services (99441–99444)
- Special E/M Services (99450–99456)
- Newborn Care Services (99460–99465)
- Inpatient Neonatal Intensive Care Services and Pediatric/Neonatal Critical Care Services (99466–99480)
- Other E/M Services (99499)

Several categories of E/M codes are commonly provided in the same setting. Criteria used to determine the appropriate level of E/M code that should be reported for services are often similar among these categories. It may be helpful to consider the categories of E/M codes in groups that are treated similarly for the purpose of determining levels of service.

Evaluation and Management services
Physician services commonly associated with "doctor visits," in which the physician takes the patient's history, performs a physical examination, determines the cause of the patient's problem, orders and interprets appropriate tests, decides on necessary treatments, and monitors the patient for changes in his or her health status.

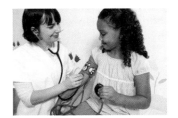

Evaluation and management services include a broad range of services typically associated with doctor's office visits, including routine checkups.

consultation
Type of service by a physician whose opinion or advice is requested by another physician.

critical care
Delivery of medical care to a patient who is critically ill or injured.

E/M services primarily provided in the office setting include office or other outpatient services, office or other outpatient **consultations,** some prolonged services, preventive services, and special E/M services. E/M services primarily provided in the hospital setting include hospital observation services, hospital inpatient services, inpatient consultations, emergency department services, **critical care** services, some prolonged services, newborn care services, inpatient neonatal intensive care services, and pediatric/neonatal critical care services. Some E/M services are provided in settings other than physician offices or hospitals, including a nursing facility, domiciliary, rest home, or in the patient's own home.

CODER'S TIP

Not all of the above categories of E/M services identify particular settings in which the services are provided. For example, prolonged services, case management, care plan oversight, preventive medicine services, non–face-to-face physician services, special E/M services, newborn services, and other E/M services may be provided in more than one location. Coders must initially determine the place the E/M services were provided to determine the correct code to describe those services.

At first glance, it appears that there may be some overlap between codes in some of the above categories (e.g., Hospital Observation Services [99217–99226] and Hospital Inpatient Services [99221–99239]), but this is due to recently added codes being "out of sequence," where some codes in numerical order in one section actually describe services from another section.

Subcategories of E/M Services

Within each category, secondary factors divide E/M services into subcategories. These secondary factors vary depending on the setting in which the services are provided. The specific secondary factors will be discussed in each section below, but the most common secondary factors include the following:

1. Is the patient a new or established patient?
2. Is the visit an initial or subsequent visit in this setting?
3. What is the patient's age?

Not all secondary factors apply in each setting. Usually only one or two secondary factors determine the correct subcategory. Each subcategory includes a number of codes that differ from one another in terms of the level of services provided or the difficulty of providing those services. The factors differentiating the codes in each subcategory will be discussed in detail below.

Most E/M codes have a similar format, including:

- A unique CPT code number.
- The type of service or place in which the service is provided.
- The content of the service (e.g., level of history, examination, and decision making, including the number of factors that must be met or exceeded to report that code).
- The type of presenting problem usually associated with that particular code.
- The time typically required to provide the particular service.

How these elements determine the correct CPT code to describe particular E/M services varies between categories and subcategories. The code levels in one category are not the same as the levels in another category.

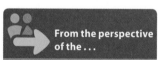

From the perspective of the . . .

CODER

Several questions determine which category of E/M codes describes the services provided, including:

1. Where was the service provided?
2. Is it a new or established patient? (Or, is it an initial or subsequent visit?)
3. What is the patient's age?

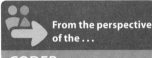
Answer each of the following questions.

1. Identify at least five separate locations that primarily determine which section of E/M codes is used to identify E/M services. _____

2. What other secondary factors may determine which section of E/M codes describes the services provided? _____

3. Which categories of E/M codes are not primarily determined by the location in which the services were provided? _____

8.2 Defining Key Terms in E/M Coding

To select the correct E/M code, it is essential to understand the terms that determine the selection of those codes.

New vs. Established Patient

A **new patient** is one who has not been seen by the physician or another physician of the same specialty within the same group practice during the previous three years.

An **established patient** is one who has been seen by the physician or another physician of the same specialty within the same group practice during the previous three years.

If one physician is on call or covering for another physician, determining whether patients are new or established is based on their history with the physician who is not available.

Chief Complaint

The **chief complaint** is a brief statement, usually in the patient's own words, that describes the reason the patient is seeing the physician. This may be a symptom, condition, problem, diagnosis, or other medical reason.

Concurrent Care and Transfer of Care

Concurrent care occurs when two or more physicians provide care to the same patient on the same day. Each physician may report the CPT codes that describe the care he or she provided to the patient.

Transfer of care occurs when one physician who is managing all or some of the patient's medical conditions gives that care to another physician who agrees to accept responsibility for providing care for those conditions. The physician transferring care no longer provides services for the conditions transferred to the other physician, but may continue to provide services for other medical problems. The physician to whom the care is transferred may not report the services with E/M codes describing consultations. However, if necessary, a physician may provide consultation services to determine whether it is appropriate to transfer the care for some or all of the patient's medical conditions. Once the patient is accepted in transfer, consultation E/M codes may no longer be used to report services.

Counseling

For purposes of E/M coding, the term **counseling** does not refer to psychotherapy or similar treatments, which have their own set of codes (90804–90857). When used in the context of E/M coding, *counseling* describes discussions with a patient and/or family regarding any of the following aspects of the patient's medical situation:

• Diagnostic tests and their results.

• Patient prognosis.

From the perspective of the ...

CODER

A patient can only be a new patient if he or she has not been seen for at least three years by that physician or another physician of the same specialty within the same group practice.

new patient
Patient who has not been seen by a particular physician or another physician of the same specialty within the same group practice during the previous three years.

established patient
Patient who has been seen by a particular physician or another physician of the same specialty within the same group practice during the previous three years.

chief complaint
A brief statement, usually in the patient's own words, that describes the reason the patient is seeing the physician.

concurrent care
When two or more physicians provide care to the same patient on the same day.

counseling
Discussions with a patient and/or family regarding aspects of the patient's medical situation.

- Treatment options, including risks and benefits.
- Patient instructions regarding compliance with treatment.
- Risk factors for disease and reducing those risks.
- Education of the patient and/or family.

Family History

The **family history** is a review of the medical histories of family members (parents, siblings, and children) that includes their health status or cause of death. It also includes diseases in family members related to the patient's chief complaint, present illness, or system review. Additionally, it includes diseases present in family members that may place the patient at risk, such as hereditary conditions.

History of Present Illness (HPI)

The **history of present illness** is a chronological description of the patient's present illness from onset to the present that includes factors describing the medical reason for the encounter with the physician. This description usually includes the signs and symptoms associated with the patient's condition, including some or all of the following elements:

- Location
- Quality
- Severity
- Duration
- Timing
- Context
- Modifying factors
- Associated signs and symptoms

Nature of the Presenting Problem

The presenting problem is the disease, illness, injury, complaint, sign, symptom, or other reason for the encounter, with or without a definitive diagnosis. Five types of presenting problems are associated with E/M coding:

- Minimal—A problem that usually does not require the presence of a physician, but services are provided under physician supervision.
- Self-limited or minor—A problem that usually runs a prescribed course, is short lived, and does not usually permanently change the patient's health status. Alternatively, a problem that has a good prognosis with treatment.
- Low severity—A problem where lack of treatment presents low risk of morbidity, little risk of mortality, and full recovery is likely without functional impairment.
- Moderate severity—A problem where lack of treatment presents moderate risk of morbidity or mortality, an uncertain prognosis, or a probability of prolonged functional impairment.
- High severity—A problem where the lack of treatment presents a high to extreme risk of morbidity, moderate to high risk of mortality, or high probability of severe prolonged functional impairment.

Past History

A review of the patient's **past medical history** includes major illnesses, injuries, operations, hospitalizations, medications, allergies, immunizations, and dietary status.

Review of Systems

The **review of systems** (ROS) is a series of questions regarding body and organ systems designed to identify signs and symptoms that the patient is experiencing or has experienced, including:

- Constitutional symptoms (fever, weight gain, weight loss, etc.)
- Eyes
- Ears, nose, mouth, and throat
- Cardiovascular
- Respiratory
- Gastrointestinal
- Genitourinary
- Musculoskeletal
- Integumentary (skin and breasts)
- Neurological
- Psychiatric
- Endocrine
- Hematologic and lymphatic
- Allergies and immunologic

Physical Examination

The **physical examination** is the process by which a physician or other healthcare provider assesses a patient for the presence or extent of an illness or injury. The provider uses his own senses of touch, sight, and hearing as well as instruments designed to assist in this process, such as stethoscopes, ophthalmoscopes, or otoscopes.

Medical Decision Making

Medical decision making involves a physician's consideration of all available information, including history, physical exam, diagnostic laboratory tests, imaging studies, and other individualized information regarding the patient to determine possible diagnoses and treatment options for the patient's medical condition. The complexity of this process is determined by the number of possible conditions, the amount of information reviewed, and the risks to the patient or complications that may result from these decisions.

Social History

The **social history** is a review of the patient's nonmedical information, including current employment, occupational history, marital status, education, sexual history, and use of alcohol, tobacco, and drugs. Any other relevant data also may be recorded as part of the social history.

Time

Time is an explicit component of most E/M services. Each E/M code that includes time specifies an average time associated with that service. Because this is an average time, the actual times associated with the service span a range that includes more or less time than specified. If the E/M service provided to a particular patient involves significantly longer time than the average time specified in the code descriptor, add-on codes describing those prolonged services are reported in addition to the underlying E/M code. The use of the prolonged services add-on codes is discussed in detail in Chapter 9. Note that E/M services provided in the emergency department do not include a time component.

review of systems
A series of questions regarding body and organ systems designed to identify signs and symptoms that the patient is experiencing or has experienced.

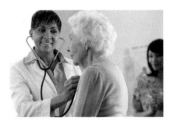

When selecting an E/M code, consider every aspect of the service provided, including the physical examination and history taking.

physical examination
The process by which a physician or other healthcare provider assesses a patient for the presence or extent of an illness or injury.

medical decision making
Involves consideration of all available information, including history, physical exam, diagnostic laboratory tests, imaging studies, and other individualized information regarding the patient to determine possible diagnoses and treatment options for the patient's medical condition.

social history
A review of the patient's nonmedical information.

time
An explicit component of most E/M services. Each E/M code that includes time specifies an average time associated with that service.

The total time to provide a service includes preservice time, intraservice time, and postservice time. It is difficult to estimate the total amount of time it takes to provide all the components associated with an E/M service. It is much easier to estimate intraservice time associated with an E/M service. Studies have shown that the intraservice time closely correlates with the total time and work associated with a particular E/M service. Therefore, intraservice time is used as the typical time associated with each E/M code.

In the office or other outpatient setting, intraservice time is defined as face-to-face time. Most of the work associated with an office or outpatient visit is performed during the time the physician spends face to face with the patient taking a history, performing a physical examination, and counseling the patient regarding his or her medical condition.

For hospital and other inpatient settings (hospital observation services, inpatient hospital care, inpatient hospital consultations, and nursing facilities), intraservice time is defined as the total time the physician spends on the unit or floor. This includes time spent at the patient's bedside examining the patient; time reviewing charts; writing; and communicating with other professionals and the patient's family. Preservice and postservice time includes time spent off the patient's unit reviewing x-rays, imaging studies, laboratory results, and other services provided in other units of the hospital. Similar to the office and other outpatient settings, the intraservice time correlates well with the total time and the intensity of work involved in providing E/M services in the inpatient setting.

Unlisted Services

Two codes are used to report E/M services that are not identified by a specific CPT code. These codes are 99429 (Unlisted preventive medicine service) and 99499 (Unlisted evaluation and management service). If these codes are used to report a service, it may be necessary to include a special report to explain the nature of the service provided and why no other code adequately describes the services provided.

Special Report

A special report may be used to demonstrate the medical appropriateness of an E/M service, especially for unlisted services. Information in the special report should include an adequate definition of the services provided; the time, effort, and equipment needed to perform the service; and pertinent information regarding the complexity of the symptoms, diagnosis, physical findings, associated procedures, concurrent problems, and follow-up care.

EXERCISE 8.2

Also available in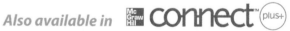

In your own words, give brief definitions of the following terms:

1. Chief complaint _____

2. History of present illness _____

3. Past medical history _____

4. Family history _____

5. Social history _____

6. Review of systems _____

7. Physical examination _____

8. Medical decision making _____

8.3 Selecting the Level of E/M Service

The category of E/M services usually is designated by the location of the patient when the services were provided. In turn, each category includes three to five levels for reporting purposes. Selecting the most appropriate level to report E/M services is one of the more difficult tasks coders perform. Selection of E/M levels is also one of the more subjective decisions made by coders when reporting professional services, even though objective criteria are used to make these selections.

E/M code descriptors include up to seven components used to define the level of E/M services provided:

- History
- Physical exam
- Medical decision making
- Counseling
- Coordination of care
- Nature of the presenting problem
- Time

The first three components (history, physical examination, and medical decision making) are **key components** used to determine the E/M level. The next three components (counseling, **care coordination**, and the nature of the presenting problem) are **contributory components** to the determination of the level of E/M services. These three components contribute to E/M services, but they are not necessarily provided during every E/M encounter.

The last component (time) is variable during E/M services. Most E/M code descriptors include an average length of time necessary to provide that level of E/M service, but it is not necessary that the time meet this average. The time necessary to provide E/M services may result in the use of add-on E/M codes for "prolonged services" if significantly greater than the average time for a given level of E/M code. Use of these add-on codes will be discussed in detail in Chapter 9.

key components
Three components of E/M code descriptors—history, physical examination, and medical decision making—used to define the level of E/M services provided.

care coordination
Organizing a patient's care with other healthcare providers.

contributory components
Counseling, care coordination, and the nature of the presenting problem as they relate to E/M.

CODER'S TIP

Specific procedures identified with CPT codes may be reported separately when provided on the same day as an E/M service. No specific modifiers need to be added to either the procedure code or the E/M code. If a patient's condition makes it necessary to provide separate E/M services at the time of a procedure that is described by a CPT code that goes beyond the usual services provided as part of that procedure, the E/M service may be reported separately. In this case, modifier 25 is added to the E/M code describing the level of E/M services provided.

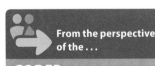

From the perspective of the . . .

CODER
Evaluating key components and contributory components to determine the level of code that describes the services provided requires an in-depth understanding of these components and how to determine the level of each component.

Once a coder determines the main category or subcategory of E/M services provided according to the primary and secondary factors (e.g., the setting in which the services were provided, new vs. established patient, initial vs. subsequent visit, or patient age), he or she will need to review all special instructions applicable to that category or subcategory of codes. At that point, the coder must determine the particular code within that category of E/M services that correctly describes the level of E/M services provided.

In most cases, the key components (history, physical examination, and medical decision making) determine the correct level of E/M services. Each of these key components is divided into four types. The combination of the three key component types determines the actual level of E/M services provided.

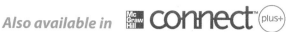
Answer each of the following questions.

1. What element typically designates each CPT evaluation and management category (or code series)?
_____

2. What are the three key components of every E/M code? _____

3. Name three of the four contributory components to an E/M code. _____

8.4 Working with Histories

There are four types of patient history. Each type has its own requirements that differentiate it from the others. The requirements for each type of history are as follows:

1. **Problem-focused history:** Chief complaint; brief history of present illness.
2. **Expanded problem-focused history:** Chief complaint; brief history of present illness; review of systems pertinent to the problem.
3. **Detailed history:** Chief complaint; extended history of present illness; extended review of systems including pertinent systems and a limited number of additional systems; pertinent past, family, and social history directly related to the patient's problems.
4. **Comprehensive history:** Chief complaint; extended history of present illness; complete review of systems related to the problems identified in the history of present illness, plus a review of all additional systems; complete past, family, and social history.

Table 8.1 includes the elements of each of the four types of history with respect to E/M coding. To qualify for any type of history, all three elements must meet or exceed the requirements for that history type.

All four types of history require documentation of the chief complaint. This documentation does not determine or contribute to the selection of the type of history.

Elements of History

The history of present illness (HPI) is a chronological description of the development of the patient's current problem, including some or all of the elements listed in the definition at the beginning of this chapter. A brief HPI differs from an extended HPI by the number of elements necessary to characterize the clinical problem. A brief HPI usually includes one to three elements. An extended HPI requires four or more elements.

problem-focused history
Consists of a limited exam of the affected body area or organ system.

expanded problem-focused history
A limited exam of the affected body areas or organ systems and other related systems.

detailed history
An extended exam of the affected body areas or organ systems and other related systems.

comprehensive history
A general multisystem exam or a complete exam of a single body area or organ system.

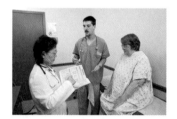

E/M services include taking a patient's history. This history always includes the chief complaint and a brief history of the present illness, but it often includes more information about the patient.

TABLE 8.1 Elements of Four Types of E/M History

Type of History	History of Present Illness (HPI)	Review of Systems (ROS)	Past, Family, and/or Social History (PFSH)
Problem focused	Brief	N/A	N/A
Expanded problem focused	Brief	Problem pertinent	N/A
Detailed	Extended	Extended	Pertinent
Comprehensive	Extended	Complete	Complete

The review of systems (ROS) results from a series of questions that identify the signs and/or symptoms that the patient may be experiencing. There are three different types of ROS:

- A problem-pertinent ROS addresses the system directly related to the problem identified in the chief complaint and/or HPI. Usually only one system is addressed.
- An extended ROS inquires about the system directly related to the problem identified in the HPI and a limited number of additional systems. Usually two to nine additional systems are addressed and documented.
- A complete ROS addresses the system directly related to the problem identified in the HPI plus all other systems. Ten or more systems must be addressed and documented.

The **past, family, and social history (PFSH)** group includes information regarding all three of these areas. A pertinent PFSH includes at least one specific item from any one of the three history areas. A complete PFSH must include at least one specific item from either two or three of these history areas, depending on the category of E/M services provided.

The following categories of E/M services only require that one specific item from two out of three history areas be documented for a complete PFSH: office or other outpatient services, established patient; hospital observation services, subsequent care; hospital inpatient services, subsequent care; emergency department services; subsequent nursing facility care; domiciliary care, established patient; and home care, established patient.

The following categories of E/M services require that at least one specific item from all three history areas must be documented for a complete PFSH: office or other outpatient services, new patient; hospital observation services, initial care; hospital inpatient services, initial care; consultations; comprehensive nursing facility assessments; domiciliary care, new patient; and home care, new patient.

In general, categories of E/M services that include comprehensive levels of service require that the PFSH include at least one specific item from all three areas of the history, while other categories of E/M services only require a specific item from two of the three history areas.

past, family, and social history (PFSH)
A patient history that includes information regarding the patient's past, family, and social history and is a factor in E/M coding.

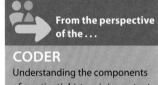

From the perspective of the . . .

CODER
Understanding the components of a patient's history is important when differentiating among the four types of patient history.

EXERCISE 8.4

Also available in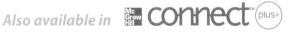

Answer each of the following questions.

1. Identify the three components included in the patient history. _____
2. List the four types of history. _____
3. When determining the type of history involved in the E/M visit, how many of the elements that determine history must be met or exceeded to assign it that type? _____

8.5 The Physical Examination

There are four types of physical examinations, based on the number of body areas or organ systems examined or the extent of the exam of a single body area or organ system.

The following are distinct body areas recognized for E/M coding purposes:

- Head and/or face
- Neck
- Chest, including breast and axilla
- Abdomen
- Genitalia, groin, and buttocks
- Back
- Each extremity

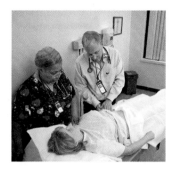

For E/M coding, the level of physical exam is determined by how many body areas or organ systems are examined. If only one body area or organ system is examined, then the degree of that exam is the basis for selecting an E/M code.

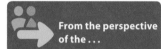

From the perspective of the . . .

CODER
Recognizing how many elements of the physical exam were performed during the E/M visit is essential to determining the type of physical exam that occurred during the visit.

The generally recognized organ systems include:

- Constitutional (e.g., vital signs, general appearance, etc.)
- Eyes
- Ears, nose, mouth, and throat
- Cardiovascular
- Respiratory
- Gastrointestinal
- Genitourinary
- Musculoskeletal
- Skin
- Neurologic
- Psychiatric
- Hematologic, lymphatic, and immunologic

For the purposes of E/M coding, physical exams are classified into four types:

- A problem-focused physical exam consists of a limited exam of the affected body area or organ system. This typically only requires an exam of a single system.
- An expanded problem-focused exam is a limited exam of the affected body areas or organ systems and other related systems.
- A detailed exam is an extended exam of the affected body areas or organ systems and other related systems.
- A comprehensive exam is a general multisystem exam or a complete exam of a single body area or organ system. A general multisystem exam usually includes documentation regarding findings from at least 8 of the 12 organ systems.

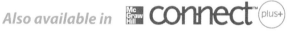

EXERCISE 8.5   *Also available in*

Answer each of the following questions.

1. For any given chief complaint, an exam of the affected body area and other related systems describes what type of physical exam? _____

2. A general multisystem exam usually involves how many organ systems? _____

3. An extended exam of an affected body area combined with other related systems describes what type of physical exam? _____

8.6 The Complexity of Medical Decision Making

Medical decision making includes establishing a diagnosis and/or selecting from among treatment or management options. The four types of medical decision making are *straightforward*, *low complexity*, *moderate complexity*, and *high complexity*. The type of decision making depends on the following elements:

- The number of possible diagnoses or treatment options that must be considered.
- The amount and complexity of medical records, diagnostic tests, and other information that must be reviewed and analyzed.

TABLE 8.2 Requirements for Levels of Medical Decision Making

Type of Medical Decision Making	Number of Diagnoses or Treatment Options	Amount and/or Complexity of Data Reviewed	Risk of Complications or Morbidity/Mortality
Straightforward	Minimal	Minimal or none	Minimal
Low complexity	Limited	Limited	Low
Moderate complexity	Multiple	Moderate	Moderate
High complexity	Extensive	Extensive	High

- The risks of complications, morbidity/mortality, or comorbidities associated with the patient's chief complaint, diagnostic tests, and/or treatment options.

Each of these elements has four levels of increasing complexity. The correct type of decision making is the highest one that meets or exceeds the requirements for two out of three of these elements.

Table 8.2 identifies the requirements for each level of the decision-making elements. Coders should use this table to correctly identify the complexity of decision making for purposes of selecting the correct level of E/M services.

CODING EXAMPLE

A patient is seen for a chief complaint for which a limited number of diagnoses or treatments (low complexity) exist; the data is of moderate complexity/amount (moderate complexity); and there is a moderate risk of complications (moderate complexity). The appropriate type of decision making is moderate complexity because two out of three of the elements meet that level (data and risk).

CODING EXAMPLE

A patient is evaluated for a problem that has multiple diagnoses and treatment options (moderate complexity), a limited amount of data to review (low complexity), and a low risk of complications (low complexity). The correct type of decision making in this example is low complexity because at least two out of three elements meet that level (all three elements actually meet that level). Only one element meets the requirements for moderate complexity (number of diagnoses/treatments), and none meet the requirements for high complexity.

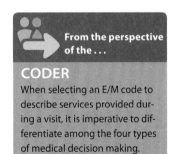

From the perspective of the . . .

CODER

When selecting an E/M code to describe services provided during a visit, it is imperative to differentiate among the four types of medical decision making.

EXERCISE 8.6

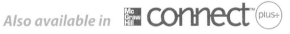

Also available in **connect** (plus+)

Answer each of the following questions.

1. Identify the three elements that determine the type of decision-making complexity.

   _____

2. How many decision-making elements must meet or exceed the requirements to assign a type of decision-making complexity? _____

3. Identify the types of medical decision-making complexity. _____

8.7 Selecting the Correct Level of E/M Services

After determining the extent of the history, physical examination, and medical decision-making complexity, coders must select the correct level of E/M services provided. Each section or subsection of E/M codes has different requirements for the levels of E/M codes in that section. Some sections require that all three key components meet or exceed the requirements for the level of E/M services selected. Other sections only require that two out of three key components meet or exceed the level of E/M services selected.

Determining Coding Requirements

The following categories of E/M services require that all three key components meet or exceed the requirements of the selected level of E/M service:

- Office, new patient.
- Initial hospital observation care.
- Initial hospital care.
- Office consultations.
- Initial inpatient consultations.
- Emergency department services.
- Initial nursing facility care.
- Domiciliary care, new patient.
- Home, new patient.

The following categories of E/M services only require that two out of three key components meet or exceed the requirements for the selected level of E/M service:

- Office, established patient.
- Subsequent hospital observation care.
- Subsequent hospital care.
- Subsequent nursing facility care.
- Domiciliary care, established patient.
- Home, established patient.

In general, the first time a healthcare provider sees a patient (new patient or initial day of service), all three key components must meet or exceed the requirements for the selected level of E/M service. For established patients or subsequent days of service, only two out of three key components must meet or exceed the requirements for the selected level of service.

When patients are seen in the emergency department, all three key components must meet or exceed the requirements of the E/M code selected, because these patients are considered "new" patients each time they are seen (regardless of how often they visit the emergency department).

Each category and subcategory of E/M codes identifies how many key components must meet or exceed the requirements for the levels of E/M services in that section. This is just one reason coders must review the specific instructions included with each category or subcategory of E/M codes. Once the coder determines which category or subcategory of E/M services describes the actual services provided, the coder should review the CPT manual to identify how many key components must be met for the levels of E/M services in that section. Then the coder should examine the medical records to assess the levels of each key component to determine the correct level of E/M service provided.

Table 8.3 summarizes the four levels of each key component. Each key component has its own requirements to determine these levels.

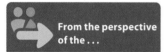

From the perspective of the . . .

CODER

Keep track of which categories of E/M codes require that two of three components meet or exceed the requirements of the individual codes, as well as which categories require that all three meet or exceed the individual code requirements.

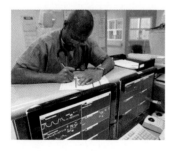

When coding for a visit to the emergency department, ensure that all three key components—history, examination, and medical decision making—meet or exceed the requirements of the code.

TABLE 8.3 Levels of Key Components Needed for E/M Code Selection

History	Physical Examination	Complexity of Medical Decision Making
Problem focused	Problem focused	Straightforward
Expanded problem focused	Expanded problem focused	Low complexity
Detailed	Detailed	Moderate complexity
Comprehensive	Comprehensive	High complexity

CODER'S TIP

There is no single progression of requirements that applies to all sections of E/M services. Each section has its own progression pattern. Some sections have more than one subsection (e.g., new vs. established patients), and there is sometimes a different progression pattern in each of the subsections.

For categories or subcategories of E/M services requiring that all three key components meet or exceed the requirements for the level of E/M services code used to report the services, coders should select the *lowest* level of E/M service that matches the type of any of the three key components. By selecting the lowest level that satisfies any one of the key components, the other key components will meet or exceed that level.

For categories or subcategories of E/M services requiring that two out of three key components meet or exceed the requirements for the level of E/M services code used to report the services, selecting the correct level of E/M code is a little more difficult. Coders should select the *highest* level of E/M service for which at least two key components meet or exceed the requirements.

Special Situations

In some instances, counseling or care coordination is the major service provided during an E/M visit. If one or both of these contributing factors comprises more than 50 percent of the services provided during the E/M visit, then time determines the level of E/M services, rather than the more commonly used key components. Face-to-face time defines this component in the office or other outpatient setting, whereas unit or floor time is used in the hospital or nursing facility setting. This includes time spent with other individuals responsible for the care of the patient or those having decision-making authority, whether or not those others are family members.

The time spent providing these services must be documented in the medical record. In these cases, the E/M level is determined by comparing the documented time with the average time in the code descriptor. If the total time exceeds the average time of the highest level of E/M services in that category, the additional time may be reported with the prolonged services add-on codes as discussed in the next chapter.

EXERCISE 8.7

Also available in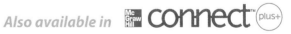

Answer each of the following questions.

1. How many key components must meet or exceed the key component requirements to select the E/M code level for a patient being seen in the office for the first time? _____

2. How many key components must meet or exceed the key component requirements of an E/M code describing a hospital visit on a subsequent day? _____

3. If the major service provided during an E/M visit is counseling, how is the level of E/M code selected?

_____

Summary

Learning Outcome	Key Concepts/Examples
8.1 Explain the breakdown of E/M services into categories and subcategories. **Pages 189–190**	In most cases, the primary factor that determines the category of E/M services is the location of the patient when those services are provided. Secondary factors that determine subcategories of E/M services include new vs. established patients, initial vs. subsequent days of service, and the patient's age.
8.2 Define key terms related to E/M coding. **Pages 191–194**	Review the definitions of important terms and concepts provided in this section and explain how each of these is relevant to determining the correct E/M service provided.
8.3 Determine the level of various E/M codes based on primary and secondary components. **Pages 195–196**	The key components that determine the level of E/M services provided include history, physical exam, and complexity of medical decision making. Secondary components include counseling, care coordination, the nature of the presenting problem, and time.
8.4 Differentiate among the four types of histories. **Pages 196–197**	The four types of history are problem focused, expanded problem focused, detailed, and comprehensive. The elements that differentiate these are the history of present illness (HPI); review of systems (ROS); and the past, family, and social history (PFSH).
8.5 Contrast the four types of physical examination. **Pages 197–198**	The four types of physical examination are problem focused, expanded problem focused, detailed, and comprehensive.
8.6 Differentiate among the four types of medical decision making. **Pages 198–199**	The four types of complexity of medical decision making are straightforward, low complexity, moderate complexity, and high complexity. These are differentiated by the number of diagnoses or treatment options; the complexity or amount of data that must be reviewed; and the risks of complications, morbidity, or mortality that may result from those decisions.
8.7 Explain how the key components determine the level of E/M services provided. **Pages 200–201**	The types of the three key components determine the level of E/M services provided. Usually all three key components must meet or exceed the requirements listed in the code descriptor for new patients or initial days of service. In contrast, usually only two out of three key components must meet or exceed the requirements listed in the code descriptor for established patients or subsequent days of service.

Using Terminology

Match each key term with its definition.

_____ **1.** LO 8.1 Evaluation and management

_____ **2.** LO 8.2 New patient

_____ **3.** LO 8.2 Established patient

_____ **4.** LO 8.2 History of present illness

_____ **5.** LO 8.2 Medical decision making

A. Delivery of medical care to a patient who is critically ill or injured

B. Series of questions regarding body and organ systems to identify signs/symptoms a patient is experiencing

C. Patient has received services from a particular physician or group within three years

_____ **6.** LO 8.2 Review of systems
_____ **7.** LO 8.2 Critical care
_____ **8.** LO 8.2 Concurrent care
_____ **9.** LO 8.3 Comprehensive history
_____ **10.** LO 8.3 Detailed history
_____ **11.** LO 8.2 Family history
_____ **12.** LO 8.2 Chief complaint
_____ **13.** LO 8.2 Past medical history
_____ **14.** LO 8.2 Social history
_____ **15.** LO 8.3 Care coordination

D. Chronological description of patient's illness from onset to present

E. Patient has not received services from a particular physician or group within three years

F. Office visits, hospital services, nursing home visits

G. Number of diagnoses/management options, amount of data reviewed, and risk factors are elements of this key component

H. When two or more physicians provide care to the same patient on the same day

I. A general multisystem exam or a complete exam of a single body area or organ system

J. A review of the patient's nonmedical information

K. A review of the medical histories of family members

L. An extended exam of the affected body areas or organ systems and other related systems

M. A brief statement that describes the reason the patient is seeing the physician

N. Includes major illnesses, injuries, operations, hospitalizations, medications, allergies, immunizations, and dietary status

O. Organizing a patient's care with other healthcare providers

Checking Your Understanding

Select the letter that best describes the statement or answers the question.

1. LO 8.3 What is the main determining factor for a critical care code?

    a. Whether a patient is inpatient or outpatient
    b. Length of time spent by the physician
    c. Whether a patient is new or established
    d. Level of history, exam, and medical decision making performed

2. LO 8.5 Which of the following would be considered a body area as part the physical exam?

    a. Respiratory
    b. Neck
    c. Constitutional
    d. Eyes

3. LO 8.3 Under organ systems in the physical exam, *constitutional* refers to _____.

    a. Signs and symptoms
    b. Vital signs
    c. General appearance
    d. Both vital signs and general appearance

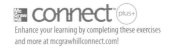
Enhance your learning by completing these exercises and more at mcgrawhillconnect.com!

CHAPTER 8 | EVALUATION AND MANAGEMENT SERVICES, PART I: STRUCTURE AND GUIDANCE   203

4. LO 8.2 Counseling can consist of the following elements:

   a. Discussing the health status or cause of death of parents

   b. Reviewing the history of present illness and family history

   c. Risks benefits, prognosis, patient family education

   d. Identifying whether the patient is a new or established patient

5. LO 8.2 The chief complaint is described as:

   a. The issue bothering the patient most, such as an argument with her spouse

   b. The symptom, problem, condition, diagnosis or other factor that is the reason for the encounter

   c. Dissatisfaction with previous treatment by other providers

   d. An outline of medical conditions affecting the patient over the last five years

6. LO 8.2 One element of the patient's social history is:

   a. The date the patient had last week

   b. The movie the patient saw yesterday

   c. The patient's marital status

   d. The last time the patient saw the dentist

7. LO 8.3 What modifier would be used to report a significant, separately identifiable E/M service by the same physician on the same day of a procedure or other service?

   a. 24

   b. 25

   c. 51

   d. 59

8. LO 8.7 The following service only requires that two out of three key components meet or exceed the requirements for the level of E/M service selected:

   a. Emergency department services

   b. Office visit, new patient

   c. Office visit, established patient

   d. Initial nursing facility care

9. LO 8.2 Time may become the determining factor for each of the following E/M codes, except for:

   a. Established patients

   b. New patients

   c. Nursing home visits

   d. Emergency room visits

10. LO 8.2 How many unlisted service codes are included in the full list of E/M codes?

   a. 2

   b. 3

   c. 5

   d. 4

11. LO 8.4 A brief statement in the patient's own words that describes the reason he has presented for treatment and that must be included in the documentation of every encounter is labeled a _____.

    a. History of present illness

    b. Review of systems

    c. Chief complaint

    d. First-listed diagnosis

12. LO 8.2 An 11-year-old patient presents to the office with a rash. A diagnosis of poison ivy is made. This is an example of which type of presenting problem?

    a. Low severity

    b. Moderate severity

    c. Self-limited or minor

    d. Minimal

13. LO 8.3 Which of the following is not a key component for determining an E/M level of service?

    a. History

    b. Exam

    c. Time

    d. Medical decision making

14. LO 8.2 Robert sees his family physician complaining of chest pain. The physician cannot determine whether the pain is gastric or cardiac in nature and requests that Dr. G., a cardiologist, see Robert to render an opinion on the nature of Robert's chest pain. Dr. G. examines Robert and sends a written report back to the requesting physician. What type of visit would this be considered?

    a. Transfer of care /new patient

    b. Consultation

    c. Preventive medicine

    d. Second opinion

15. LO 8.7 Critical care codes require how many key components to meet or exceed the requirements of the specific level code chosen?

    a. All three key components

    b. Two of the key components

    c. One key component

    d. None, because time is one of the contributing factors for these codes

16. LO 8.4 Which categories of E/M services only require that one specific item from two out of three history areas be documented for a complete PFSH?

    a. Office or other outpatient services, new patient

    b. Office or other outpatient services, established patient

    c. Hospital observation services, initial services

    d. Consultations

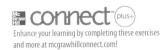
Enhance your learning by completing these exercises and more at mcgrawhillconnect.com!

CHAPTER 8 | EVALUATION AND MANAGEMENT SERVICES, PART I: STRUCTURE AND GUIDANCE   205

17. LO 8.4 Which type of ROS inquires about the system directly related to the problem identified in the chief complaint and/or HPI (history of present illness)?

　　a. Complete ROS
　　b. Problem-pertinent ROS
　　c. Extended ROS
　　d. Problem-focused ROS

18. LO 8.5 A notation in Erika Young's progress note states that there were abnormal bowel sounds upon examination. Within a physical examination, which organ system would be identified for this note?

　　a. Abdomen
　　b. Gastrointestinal
　　c. Genitourinary
　　d. Constitutional

19. LO 8.1 Levels of evaluation and management codes are based upon _____.

　　a. Key components
　　b. Documentation
　　c. Contributing factors
　　d. All of the above

20. LO 8.4 Olivia, a 34-year-old female, presents to the emergency department with cough, fever, and overall malaise. The emergency department physician performs an extended HPI, an extended ROS, and a pertinent PFSH. The correct level of history is _____.

　　a. Problem focused
　　b. Expanded problem focused
　　c. Detailed
　　d. Comprehensive

Applying Your Skills

Fill in the word(s) to complete each statement.

1. LO 8.3 Office visit E/M codes include two types of components. These are _____ and _____.

2. LO 8.1 To select the correct E/M code for a preventive medicine exam, coders must know two factors about the patient: whether she is _____ and her _____.

3. LO 8.3 _____ key components must be known to select the correct E/M code for new patients seen in the office. They are _____, _____, and _____.

4. LO 8.4 In order to determine in which code section an E/M code would likely be found, it is necessary to know _____ the service was provided.

5. LO 8.6 The four types of medical decision making are _____, _____, _____, and _____ complexity.

6. LO 8.2 A 43-year-old woman presents to her physician's office complaining of sore throat, tightness in the chest that "feels like something is sitting on my chest," and a runny nose with a yellowish-green discharge. She states she has had a low-grade fever for the past three days. Her physician orders a chest x-ray and a throat culture, performs a problem-focused history and expanded problem-focused exam, and the medical decision making is of straightforward complexity. In this scenario, the patient's _____ is her sore throat, chest tightness, runny nose, and fever.

7. LO 8.1 The three key components of E/M service are _____, _____, and _____.

8. LO 8.4 ROS is an acronym for _____. It includes up to _____ body systems.

9. LO 8.4 PFSH is an acronym for _____.

10. LO 8.3 Unless time is the determining factor for the selection of the CPT code, it is usually a(n) _____ component.

11. LO 8.2 When one physician who is managing all or some of the patient's medical conditions gives that care to another physician who agrees to accept responsibility for providing care for those conditions, it is referred to as _____.

12. LO 8.3 Rather than depending on whether the patient is new or established, E/M code selection for inpatient hospital services is based on whether the service was provided on the _____ or on _____.

13. LO 8.4 HPI is an acronym for _____.

14. LO 8.2 A condition that usually runs a prescribed course, is short lived, and does not usually permanently change the patient's health status is a(n) _____ presenting problem.

15. LO 8.3 A review of a patient's nonmedical information such as employment, marital status, etc., is a(n) _____ history.

16. LO 8.3 In the office or outpatient setting, intraservice time is also defined as _____.

17. LO 8.3 In the hospital or inpatient setting, _____ time is defined as the total time the physician spends on the floor.

18. LO 8.4 All four types of history—problem focused, expanded focused, detailed, and comprehensive—require documentation of the patient's _____.

19. LO 8.5 The four types of physical exam are based on the numbers of _____ and/or _____ examined.

20. LO 8.6 _____, a key component of E/M services, depends on the number of diagnoses or treatment options, the amount and complexity of data reviewed, and risk factors.

21. LO 8.7 An established patient E/M code requires _____ of _____ key components to meet or exceed the requirements for the level of service.

22. LO 8.1 Codes from the range _____ are used to identify office or other outpatient services.

23. LO 8.1 Before Mika moved to Florida five years ago, she had been a patient of Dr. Green's. She recently moved back to the area and presented to Dr. Green's office for treatment of a cough. Dr. Green would code her visit as a _____ patient.

Enhance your learning by completing these exercises and more at mcgrawhillconnect.com!

CHAPTER 8 | EVALUATION AND MANAGEMENT SERVICES, PART I: STRUCTURE AND GUIDANCE   207

24. LO 8.2 When two or more physicians provide care to the same patient on the same day, this is labeled as _____ _____.

25. LO 8.4 A detailed history requires a(n) _____ level of review of systems.

26. LO 8.4 Problem-focused and expanded problem-focused histories do not require a _____.

27. LO 8.2 The two codes _____ and _____ are used to report E/M services that are not identified by a specific CPT code.

28. LO 8.2, LO 8.4 Philip Ross presents as a patient at Greater Sacandaga Clinic. Kira, a medical assistant at the clinic, interviews Philip and documents that he has had ocular migraines in the past. There is no history of seizure disorder. Eye examination and neurological examination are normal. For the purposes of E/M coding, this type of history is known as a(n) _____.

29. LO 8.2, LO 8.4 Allen Thomas denies smoking cigarettes and drinking alcohol. He also denies sexual promiscuity that could be a health risk. For the purposes of E/M coding, this type of history is known as a(n) _____.

30. LO 8.2, LO 8.5 Vital signs are documented in Alexandra Prose's medical record as follows: *HT 66; WT 180; no fever; Pulse 72; RR 12; BP 120/80.* For the purposes of E/M coding, these signs are also known as _____.

31. LO 8.2, LO 8.5 Aichiko Troy's medical record contains the following segment: *HEENT, Chest, CV, GI, Neuro, GU.* With respect to E/M coding, this segment is also known as the _____.

32. LO 8.6 Felicia Brown's primary care physician assesses her and determines a plan of action as follows: *CXR for SOA and a Prescription for Medrol Dose Pack.* A referral is made to see a pulmonologist. The component of E/M coding that this segment relates closest to is _____.

Thinking It Through

Use your critical-thinking skills to answer the questions below.

1. LO 8.1 For each of the five types of presenting problems listed below, give the definition in your own words. Then list an example of the type of presenting problem.

   a. Minimal _____

   _____

   _____

   b. Self-limited or minor _____

   _____

   _____

   c. Low severity _____

   _____

   _____

    d. Moderate severity _____

_____

_____

    e. High severity _____

_____

_____

2. LO 8.1 When determining the level of E/M services provided to a patient, why don't coders just use the clinical examples of a presenting problem? Why are other factors, such as time and level of decision making, also considered?

_____

_____

3. LO 8.2 What information should be included in a special report to demonstrate medical appropriateness of an E/M service, such as an unlisted service?

_____

_____

connect plus+

Enhance your learning by completing these exercises and more at mcgrawhillconnect.com!

CHAPTER 8 | EVALUATION AND MANAGEMENT SERVICES, PART I: STRUCTURE AND GUIDANCE   209

9 EVALUATION AND MANAGEMENT SERVICES, PART II: CODE SELECTION

Learning Outcomes *After completing this chapter, students should be able to:*

9.1 Explain how differences between new and established patients affect E/M code selection in outpatient settings.

9.2 Differentiate among various categories and subcategories of hospital services.

9.3 Describe how consultation codes are different from other E/M services.

9.4 Identify factors of E/M codes for emergency services.

9.5 Explain how critical care services are reported.

9.6 Describe factors that determine subcategories of E/M services in special settings.

9.7 Explain how time is calculated and used to report prolonged services.

9.8 Identify the factors that determine which E/M codes are reported for case management and care plan oversight services.

9.9 Describe preventive medicine services.

9.10 Identify elements of telephone, online, and special E/M services.

9.11 Contrast E/M coding standards for various newborn services.

Key Terms

Admit/discharge codes
Hospital inpatient services
Hospital observation services
Newborn services
Preventive medicine services
Prolonged services

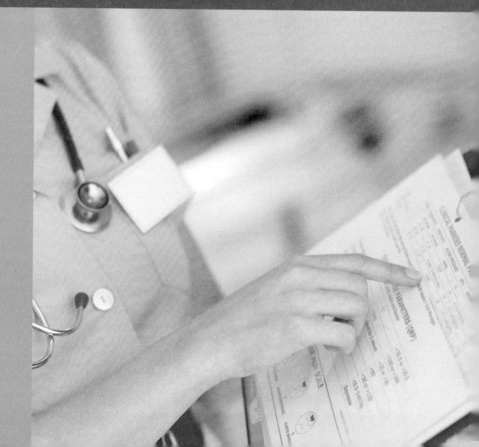

Introduction

Now that the different types of E/M services have been discussed, along with the factors used to assign their codes, E/M code selection can begin. In this chapter, the types of history and physical examination (problem focused, expanded problem focused, detailed, and comprehensive) and the types of medical decision making (straightforward, low complexity, moderate complexity, and high complexity) will be compared for the various E/M code levels. In categories with multiple subcategories, differences between the subcategories will be discussed. Table 9.1 outlines the four types of history, physical exam, and medical decision-making key components.

E/M services that are not otherwise described by any of the specific CPT codes in this section (99201–99480) may be reported with CPT code 99499 (Unlisted evaluation and management service). It should be rare that the specific E/M codes do not describe the services provided. In such circumstances, providers may report those services with CPT code 99499, but they should provide documentation of the particular E/M services provided and explain why no existing specific code describes those services.

TABLE 9.1 Levels of Key Components in E/M Coding

History	Physical Examination	Complexity of Medical Decision Making
Problem focused	Problem focused	Straightforward
Expanded problem focused	Expanded problem focused	Low complexity
Detailed	Detailed	Moderate complexity
Comprehensive	Comprehensive	High complexity

9.1 Outpatient Services Coding for New or Established Patients (99201–99215)

This section of codes describes E/M services provided in the office or other ambulatory settings, with the exception of services provided in an emergency department or hospital observation area, both of which are commonly considered outpatient settings. Services in those settings are described by other sections of E/M codes.

This category of codes is divided into two subcategories based on whether the patient is a new or established patient. Five CPT codes describe E/M services in each subcategory. Each code includes a different combination of the types of history, physical exam, and medical decision-making complexity. It is important to note that the progressions of requirements for key component types are not the same in these two subcategories.

Each code descriptor includes a description of the nature of the presenting problem and the typical face-to-face time the physician spends with the patient and/or family. These contributing factors do not determine the level of E/M code selected. The typical time associated with each E/M code is used to determine whether a prolonged services add-on code may be reported. How these add-on codes are used is discussed later in this chapter.

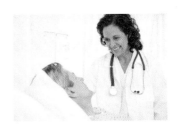

Outpatient consultation codes are classified by whether the patient is new or established.

New Patient

A new patient is one who has not had any professional medical services provided by a particular provider or another provider of the same specialty or subspecialty in the same group practice within the previous three years. New patient codes require that all three key components meet or exceed the requirements listed in the code descriptors, as shown in Table 9.2.

TABLE 9.2 Requirements for New Patient E/M Codes

Code	History	Examination	Decision Making	Presenting Problem	Typical Time (minutes)
99201	Problem focused	Problem focused	Straightforward	Self-limited or minor	10
99202	Expanded problem focused	Expanded problem focused	Straightforward	Low to moderate severity	20
99203	Detailed	Detailed	Low complexity	Moderate severity	30
99204	Comprehensive	Comprehensive	Moderate complexity	Moderate to high severity	45
99205	Comprehensive	Comprehensive	High complexity	High severity	60

CODING EXAMPLE

A physician sees a patient he has not treated for approximately five years. The patient presents with symptoms of sinus congestion and earache. Because of the length of time since he has seen this patient, the physician performs a comprehensive history and examination. The decision making is low complexity. What code would be reported to describe this E/M service?

Even though the history and examination are comprehensive and would meet the requirements of code 99204 or 99205, the medical decision making only meets the requirement of code 99203. Because all three elements must meet or exceed the code requirements for a new patient, the highest-level code that can be reported for this visit is 99203.

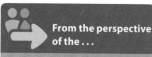

From the perspective of the . . .

CODER

It is imperative to know the location where the E/M services were provided—office, home, hospital, nursing facility, etc. This is necessary to select the correct type of code to describe the E/M service.

Established Patient

An established patient is one who has received professional services from a particular physician or another physician of the same specialty who belongs to the same group practice within the previous three years. With the exception of CPT code 99211, established patient codes require that two out of three key components meet or exceed the requirements listed in the code descriptor. Code 99211 should be assigned when a service does not need to meet the requirements for the key components; may not require the presence of a physician; the presenting problem is minimal; and the typical service time is five minutes. Examples might include a nurse visit for a blood pressure check. Table 9.3 describes requirements for additional established patient E/M codes.

TABLE 9.3 Requirements for Established Patient E/M Codes

Code	History	Examination	Decision Making	Presenting Problem	Typical Time (minutes)
99212	Problem focused	Problem focused	Straightforward	Self-limited or minor	10
99213	Expanded problem focused	Expanded problem focused	Low complexity	Low to moderate severity	15
99214	Detailed	Detailed	Moderate complexity	Moderate to high severity	25
99215	Comprehensive	Comprehensive	High complexity	Moderate to high severity	40

CODING EXAMPLE

A patient returns to see her physician after a two-year absence. The physician performs a detailed history and physical exam. The medical decision making is of low complexity. How would this service be reported?

An E/M outpatient service for an established patient need only meet or exceed two out of three of the requirements to report a particular code. In this case, the history and exam meet the requirements for 99214, so this is the proper code, regardless of the level of medical decision making.

CODER'S TIP

A patient can only be "new" once every three years. If a provider has seen the patient within a three-year period, she is an established patient for purposes of reporting E/M services.

EXERCISE 9.1

Also available in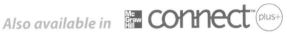

Use the CPT manual to select the E/M code for each of the following scenarios.

1. A 35-year-old female presents to her physician's office for the first time. She complains of shortness of breath, cough, difficulty breathing, and tightness in her chest. She also states that when she coughs, the sputum is "yellow in color." The doctor orders a chest x-ray and performs a detailed history and examination. The medical decision making is of moderate complexity. _____

2. A 55-year-old man presents to his urologist's office for a follow-up to last week's visit. He is complaining of urinary frequency and pain and burning during urination. The medical assistant collects a urine specimen and takes the patient's vital signs. The physician performs an expanded problem-focused history and exam. The medical decision making is of low complexity. _____

3. A four-year-old child presents to his pediatrician's office. His mother states that he is pulling his left ear and crying. She also reports that he has had a low-grade fever for two days that goes away with acetaminophen. The physician performs a detailed history and an expanded problem-focused exam, and the medical decision making is of low complexity. _____

9.2 Categories and Subcategories of Hospital Services (99217–99239)

Codes describing hospital services are divided into four main groups, depending on whether the patient is under observation, admitted as an inpatient, admitted and discharged on the same day (**admit/discharge codes**), or discharged one or more days after admission. Some groups are subdivided into codes that describe E/M services on the initial day of hospitalization, with other codes describing services on subsequent days. Each of these code groups, except hospital discharge services, includes several codes describing levels of E/M services based on the types of key components performed as part of the E/M service. Hospital discharge codes are based on the length of time the discharge services require to be completed.

admit/discharge codes
Set of codes that describe services when a patient is admitted and discharged on the same date.

Hospital Observation Services

Hospital observation services are provided when it is unclear whether it is medically necessary to admit the patient to the hospital as an inpatient. It is not necessary that the patient stay in an area of the hospital designated as an observation area.

hospital observation services
Services provided when it is unclear whether it is medically necessary to admit the patient to the hospital as an inpatient.

However, if an observation area of the hospital exists, these codes must be utilized for patients admitted to that area.

Observation Care Discharge Services

CPT code 99217 identifies services provided by physicians discharging patients from observation when the discharge occurs subsequent to the initial date of observation. If admission and discharge from observation occur on the same date, the combined services are reported with CPT codes 99234–99236. Discharge services include a physical exam, discussions with the patient and/or family, instructions for continuing care, and all discharge records.

Initial Observation Care

CPT codes 99218–99220 describe observation services by physicians admitting patients to observation status, including initiation of observation, supervision of the care plan, and periodic reassessment. Initial observation services are reported with three separate levels of E/M codes. Observation codes are not used to report postoperative recovery for surgical procedures. If additional physicians evaluate an observation patient, those services are reported with the office or other outpatient consultation codes (99241–99245) or the subsequent observation care codes (99224–99226).

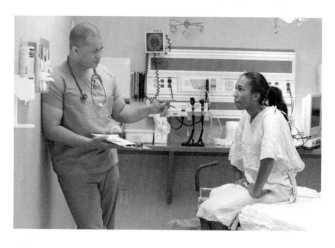

Observation codes are not used to report postoperative recovery for surgical procedures.

If a patient admitted for observation services is subsequently admitted to the hospital as an inpatient on the same date of service, all E/M services during the observation period are considered to be part of the initial hospital care and are reported with codes describing the initial hospital E/M inpatient care. Observation E/M codes are not reported on the same date of service as a hospital admission.

When observation is initiated as part of the services provided in another location such as a physician's office, emergency department, or nursing facility, all E/M services provided in the other location are part of the initial observation care E/M services and are not reported with separate E/M codes.

Initial observation codes differentiate between three levels of E/M services. Each code requires that all three key components meet or exceed the requirements in the code descriptor. Each physician may only report one E/M code describing initial observation care per day, even if the physician provides services multiple times during that day. Time is not a factor in selecting observation E/M codes. Table 9.4 describes requirements for selecting observation E/M codes.

Subsequent Observation Care

Subsequent observation care is reported with three levels of E/M codes. Each level includes reviewing medical records, test results, and changes in the patient's history, exam, and responses to management that have occurred since the last assessment by that physician. Each code only requires that two out of three key components meet or exceed the requirements in the code descriptor. Each physician may only report one E/M code describing subsequent

TABLE 9.4 Requirements for Initial Observation E/M Codes

Code	History	Examination	Decision Making
99218	Detailed or comprehensive	Detailed or comprehensive	Straightforward or low complexity
99219	Comprehensive	Comprehensive	Moderate complexity
99220	Comprehensive	Comprehensive	High complexity

TABLE 9.5 Requirements for Subsequent Observation Care Codes

Code	Interval History	Examination	Decision Making
99224	Problem focused	Problem focused	Straightforward or low complexity
99225	Expanded problem focused	Expanded problem focused	Moderate complexity
99226	Detailed	Detailed	High complexity

observation care per day, even if the physician provides services multiple times during the day. Table 9.5 shows requirements for assigning subsequent observation care codes.

Note that the CPT codes describing subsequent observation care are out of sequence. These have been added recently to the CPT manual, and code numbers following the initial observation care codes were already in use describing other E/M services.

CODING EXAMPLE

A patient is admitted to the observation unit of the hospital at 10:00 p.m. and is seen at 11:45 p.m. by his physician, who performs a comprehensive history and exam and medical decision making of low complexity. What code would appropriately report this service?

The visit is described by an initial observation care code. The components must meet or exceed three out of three requirements listed in the code descriptor. The only code for which all three components meet or exceed the listed requirements is 99218.

Hospital Inpatient Services

Hospital inpatient services are divided into two subcategories of codes: initial hospital care and subsequent hospital care. No distinction is made between new and established patients. Each code includes key component requirements; the nature of the problem usually associated with that code level; and the typical time the physician spends providing those services.

Unlike in office and other outpatient settings, where time is defined as face-to-face time with the patient or family members, time is defined differently in the inpatient hospital or other facility setting. For these settings, time is defined as the time the physician spends on the unit or floor. Some of the physician's time may be spent at the patient's bedside, but additional time on the unit also counts when determining the level of E/M services provided to inpatients. Time spent off the unit in the hospital, such as in the radiology or laboratory areas, does not count as total time for purposes of level of E/M selection.

hospital inpatient services E/M services provided to hospital inpatients that are divided into two subcategories of codes: initial hospital care and subsequent hospital care.

Initial Hospital Care The initial hospital care E/M codes are only reported by the admitting physician and only for the first inpatient day. Other physicians who see the patient in the hospital but who are not the admitting physician report their initial hospital encounters with initial inpatient consultation codes (99251–99255) or subsequent hospital care codes (99231–99233). If a patient is admitted and discharged from the hospital on the same date of service, the E/M services are reported with CPT codes 99234–99236.

When the physician initially treats a patient in another location such as the emergency department, observation, or office setting, and then admits the patient as an inpatient on the same date of service, E/M services provided in the other location are considered part of the initial hospital care. The level of initial hospital care reported by the admitting physician should include all the services provided in the other location. Services provided in the other location on the date of admission are not reported separately.

TABLE 9.6 Requirements for Initial Hospital Care E/M Codes

Code	History	Examination	Decision Making	Presenting Problem	Typical Time (minutes)
99221	Detailed or comprehensive	Detailed or comprehensive	Straightforward or low complexity	Low severity	30
99222	Comprehensive	Comprehensive	Moderate complexity	Moderate severity	50
99223	Comprehensive	Comprehensive	High complexity	High severity	70

Initial hospital care E/M codes are reported only once on the date of admission, even if the admitting physician sees the patient more than once during that day. Each code requires that all three key components meet or exceed the requirements in the code descriptor. Each code also includes the level of severity of the problem and the typical time the physician spends on the floor providing services to the patient, although these factors do not directly affect the level of E/M code selected. Table 9.6 depicts the requirements for assigning initial hospital care E/M codes.

CODER'S TIP

It is important for the coder to report only one initial hospital care code per admission. This code should only be reported for services provided on the initial hospital day by the admitting physician.

Subsequent Hospital Care Physicians providing subsequent hospital inpatient care may report one E/M code per day to describe the appropriate level of care. Each level includes reviewing medical records, results of diagnostic tests, and changes in the patient's history, exam, and responses to treatment since the last assessment. These codes only require that two out of three of the key elements meet or exceed the requirements in the code descriptor. Typical time the physician spends on the floor or unit is included. However, these codes do not describe the nature of the patient's problem, because that was included in the initial hospital care code. Rather, these codes include a description of the condition of the typical patient described by the code. Table 9.7 shows the requirements for assigning subsequent hospital care E/M codes.

TABLE 9.7 Requirements for Subsequent Hospital Care E/M Codes

Code	Interval History	Examination	Decision Making	Patient Condition	Typical Time (minutes)
99231	Problem focused	Problem focused	Straightforward or low complexity	Stable, recovering or improving	15
99232	Expanded problem focused	Expanded problem focused	Moderate complexity	Inadequate response to treatment or has developed a minor complication	25
99233	Detailed	Detailed	High complexity	Unstable, has developed a significant complication or a new problem	35

A patient who was playing baseball is admitted to the hospital with a spiral fracture to his right humerus. The admitting physician performs a comprehensive history and exam, and the medical decision making is of high complexity. On the second day, the physician performs a detailed exam, medical decision making of moderate complexity, and a problem-focused interval history. What codes would be reported on each day?

On the first day, all three key components must meet or exceed the requirements in the code descriptor for initial hospital care. The components meet all three requirements of code 99223. On the second day, the key components must meet or exceed two out of three requirements in the code descriptor for subsequent hospital care codes. This situation meets two out of three key component requirements of code 99232. The reported codes would be 99223 and 99232.

Observation or Inpatient Care Services (Including Admission and Discharge)

This category of E/M codes describes inpatient hospital care or observation services when the patient is admitted and discharged on the same day. These codes require that all three key components meet or exceed the requirements in the code descriptor. These codes include the nature of the typical presenting problem, but they do not include a time component. Only one of these codes may be reported for the date of service. Table 9.8 describes the requirements for assigning these codes.

For observation or inpatient admissions that do not result in a discharge on the same day, the appropriate inpatient hospital E/M codes or observation E/M codes should be used to report those services.

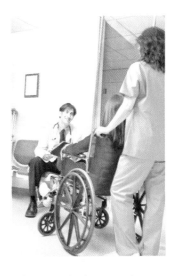

Admission/discharge codes describe services provided when a patient is admitted and discharged on the same day.

The physician examines a patient in the observation area of the hospital. The patient was admitted earlier that day and is complaining of right upper quadrant abdominal pain. After a series of tests, the physician determines that the patient is suffering from gallstones. The physician reviews the test results and performs a comprehensive history and exam. The medical decision making is of moderate complexity. The physician reviews the plan of treatment and is ready to discharge the patient on the same day as admission. What code would report this service?

For admission and discharge services on the same day, all three components must meet or exceed the requirements in the code descriptor. In this case, the services meet or exceed all the requirements of code 99235.

TABLE 9.8 Requirements for Hospital Admission/Discharge Codes

Code	History	Examination	Decision Making	Presenting Problem
99234	Detailed or comprehensive	Detailed or comprehensive	Straightforward or low complexity	Low severity
99235	Comprehensive	Comprehensive	Moderate complexity	Moderate severity
99236	Comprehensive	Comprehensive	High complexity	High severity

Hospital Discharge Services

Hospital discharge E/M codes 99238 and 99239 describe the total time the physician spends discharging a hospital inpatient, provided that the admission and discharge do not occur on the same date. This time includes services provided by the discharging physician on the discharge day, such as a final physical examination, instructions for continuing care, and preparation of discharge records, prescriptions, and referral forms. The time need not be continuous but should be documented in the medical record.

Other physicians who provide services on the discharge day but who are not discharging the patient should report those services with the subsequent hospital care services codes (99231–99233). CPT code 99217 is used to report observation care discharge services. If the patient is admitted and discharged on the same date, the services should be reported with CPT codes 99234–99236.

CPT code 99238 is used to report discharge day management time of 30 minutes or less. CPT code 99239 describes discharge day management time greater than 30 minutes. If the discharge day management time is not recorded in the medical record, code 99238 is reported to describe the hospital discharge services.

CODING EXAMPLE

The physician discharges the patient and spends 45 minutes between examining the patient and unit time at the nurses' station. He does not document the start and stop times. What discharge code should be reported when the time is not documented in the medical record?

Even though the physician spent 45 minutes on the hospital floor, which would qualify for code 99239, the times are not recorded in the medical record. Therefore, these services should be reported with code 99238.

EXERCISE 9.2

Also available in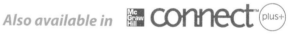

Use the CPT manual to answer the following questions.

1. A patient is admitted to the observation unit of the hospital. The staff physician sees the patient each day for three consecutive days. On the first day, the physician performs a comprehensive history and exam, and the medical decision making is of moderate complexity. On day two, the physician performs an expanded problem-focused interval history and exam, and the medical decision making is of moderate complexity. On day three, the physician performs a problem-focused interval history and exam, and the medical decision making is of moderate complexity. What code would be reported for each of the three days? _____

2. What code is reported when a physician performs a problem-focused exam and history and discharges the patient from observation status to home? _____

3. A patient is admitted to the hospital with breast cancer. The physician performs a comprehensive history and exam, and the medical decision making is of high complexity. On the second day, he performs a detailed interval history and exam, and the medical decision making is of high complexity. On day three, he performs an expanded problem-focused interval history and exam, and the medical decision making is of high complexity. What codes would the physician report for each day? _____

4. A patient is admitted to the hospital with diabetes and elevated blood glucose levels. On day one, the physician performs a comprehensive history and exam, and the medical decision making is of moderate complexity. On day two, the physician performs a problem-focused interval history and exam with medical decision making of moderate complexity. What is the correct code to report services provided on days one and two? _____

5. A physician is preparing to discharge his patient today. This patient has been in the hospital for five days. On the final day, the physician spends about 20 minutes with the patient, performing a final exam, discussing the hospital treatment, and providing instructions for postdischarge follow-up. He also spends another 20 minutes at the nursing station writing orders and reviewing the patient's chart. The physician documents the start and stop times on the discharge of this patient. What code would be reported for the patient's discharge? _____

9.3 Consultation Services (99241–99255)

A consultation is a specific type of E/M service that is provided by one physician at the request of another physician or provider. The purpose of the consultation is either to recommend care for a specific condition that would then be managed by the requesting physician or to determine whether to accept the responsibility of providing care for all or some of the patient's ongoing medical problems.

If the request for evaluation is initiated by either the patient or a family member, the evaluation should not be reported with a consultation E/M code. Rather, those E/M services should be reported with other appropriate codes, such as those used to report E/M services in an office, hospital, or nursing home.

Consultation E/M services require more extensive documentation than many other services. The request for the consult may be documented in the medical record or other written document by either the requesting physician or consultant. The consulting physician must document findings and the results of any diagnostic procedures in the records, as well as communicate those findings in a written report to the requesting provider. Consultations require three basic elements: request, render, and respond.

If the consulting physician assumes responsibility for some or all of the patient's care after completing the consultation, further services are reported with E/M codes that are appropriate for the place in which the physician provides those services, such as an office or hospital. The initial consultation still may be reported using the consultation E/M codes.

Consultants may order or perform diagnostic procedures as part of their consulting services. If these procedures are identified with CPT codes, they may be reported separately.

Office or Other Outpatient Consultations

Five E/M codes describe consultation services in office and other outpatient settings. This includes services provided in hospital observation areas and emergency departments, which are considered outpatient settings. No distinction is made between new and established patients.

If the consulting physician provides follow-up services, those services are reported with the appropriate E/M codes for established patients. If a different referring physician requests a new consultation regarding the same problem or a different problem, the office or other outpatient consultation codes may be used again.

Consultation codes are not reported when patient care is transferred from one physician to another. Those services are reported with the new or established patient E/M codes that are appropriate for the location in which the services are provided. Transfer of care occurs when one physician agrees to take responsibility for the care of all or some of a patient's medical problems and the transferring physician agrees to relinquish that responsibility. In some cases, a physician cannot make the decision to accept the responsibility for care until a consultation has been completed. In those cases, it is appropriate to report the initial services with the consult codes.

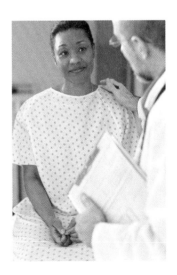

When coding for consultations provided in outpatient settings, no distinction is made between new and established patients.

TABLE 9.9 Requirements for Consultation E/M Codes

Code	History	Examination	Decision Making	Presenting Problem	Typical Time (minutes)
99241	Problem focused	Problem focused	Straightforward	Self-limited or minor	15
99242	Expanded problem focused	Expanded problem focused	Straightforward	Low severity	30
99243	Detailed	Detailed	Low complexity	Moderate severity	40
99244	Comprehensive	Comprehensive	Moderate complexity	Moderate to high severity	60
99245	Comprehensive	Comprehensive	High complexity	Moderate to high severity	80

The office or other outpatient consultation codes require that all three key components meet or exceed the requirements in the code descriptor, as shown in Table 9.9.

CODING EXAMPLE

A primary care physician requests a consultation from a urologist regarding a patient who presented with low back pain on the right side. The urologist performs an expanded problem-focused history and exam. The medical decision making is straightforward. The urologist collects a urine specimen and determines that the patient has a bladder infection. The urologist then dictates a letter back to the primary care physician outlining his findings. What code would report this service?

The appropriate code to report this service is 99242. All three components meet the requirements listed in the code descriptor.

Inpatient Consultations

Five E/M codes describe consultations provided to hospital inpatients or residents of a nursing facility. No distinction is made between new and established patients. Consultants should only report one consultation E/M code during the admission. Other services are reported with subsequent hospital care codes or subsequent nursing facility care codes, including follow-up care, completion of the consultation services, revising recommendations, addressing new problems, or accepting the patient in transfer for all or some of the patient's medical problems.

If the consultant sees an inpatient on the day of admission, all E/M services provided by the consultant that are related to the admission are reported with the appropriate inpatient consultation code. If a patient is admitted after an outpatient consultation and the consultant does not see the patient in the inpatient setting on the date of admission, the consultation is reported with the appropriate office or outpatient consultation code. If a patient is admitted after an outpatient consultation and the consultant does see the patient in the inpatient setting on the date of admission, all E/M services related to the admission are reported with either an inpatient consultation code or initial inpatient admission service code. Outpatient and inpatient consultation codes are not reported for services related to a single inpatient stay. The inpatient consultation codes require that all three key components meet or exceed the requirements in the code descriptor. Table 9.10 describes the requirements for assigning inpatient consultation codes.

TABLE 9.10 Requirements for Inpatient Consultation Codes

Code	History	Examination	Decision Making	Presenting Problem	Typical Time (minutes)
99251	Problem focused	Problem focused	Straightforward	Self-limited or minor	20
99252	Expanded problem focused	Expanded problem focused	Straightforward	Low severity	40
99253	Detailed	Detailed	Low complexity	Moderate severity	55
99254	Comprehensive	Comprehensive	Moderate complexity	Moderate to high severity	80
99255	Comprehensive	Comprehensive	High complexity	High severity	110

CODING EXAMPLE

A four-year-old child is admitted to the hospital by his pediatrician because of an exacerbation of his asthma. The pediatrician requests a consultation by a pulmonologist to assess the severity of his condition. The pulmonologist performs a detailed history, a comprehensive exam, and straightforward medical decision making. What code describes the pulmonologist's services?

All three components meet or exceed the requirements of code 99252.

CODER'S TIP

Medicare no longer covers consultations. Instead, Medicare now instructs providers to report these services with the appropriate level of office or inpatient E/M codes.

EXERCISE 9.3

Also available in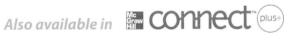

Use the CPT manual to answer the following questions.

1. A 43-year-old female presents to her primary care physician's office complaining of chest pain that radiates to her left arm after the patient walks for a long period. The primary care physician believes this warrants the opinion of a cardiologist and requests a consultation. The cardiologist examines the patient, documents a problem-focused exam and history, and the medical decision making is documented as straightforward. A letter is sent back to the requesting primary care physician to share his findings and recommendations. What code should the consulting physician use to report the service? _____

2. A patient presents to a podiatrist's office for the first time. She is complaining of a very painful ingrown toenail. She did not have a referral from her primary care physician and has her toenail treated. The physician performs an expanded problem-focused history and exam, and the medical decision making is of straightforward complexity. What code would be reported for this service? _____

3. A patient has been admitted to the hospital with severe pain in the right femur. The primary care provider suspects that the patient has a pathological fracture and requests a consultation from an orthopedic surgeon. The orthopedic surgeon examines the patient and orders a CT scan to determine whether a fracture exists that will require further care. He performs a detailed history and exam and medical decision making of low complexity. The orthopedic surgeon documents his findings and sends them back to the requesting physician. What code would be reported for this service? _____

(Continued)

4. During surgery on the patient in the previous scenario, the patient's blood pressure begins to drop and the surgeon aborts the procedure. The orthopedic surgeon requests the consultation of a cardiologist before proceeding with the surgery. The cardiologist performs a comprehensive exam, a detailed history, and medical decision making of moderate complexity. On day two, the cardiologist performs a problem-focused history and exam and medical decision making of moderate complexity. What codes describe the services of the cardiologist? _____

9.4 Emergency Department Services (99281–99285, 99288)

Services provided in an emergency department (ED) are considered outpatient services. Patients seen in the ED are either sent home or admitted to the hospital as inpatients. For some patients, it is not immediately clear whether the patient needs to be admitted or can safely be discharged. In those cases, the patient may be kept under observation to determine whether he or she needs to be admitted.

E/M Services for New or Established Patients

Five CPT codes describe E/M services provided in the emergency department. There is no distinction between new and established patients in the ED. If critical care services are provided in the ED, they are reported with the critical care codes (see below). These codes are not used to report observation services provided in the ED, which are reported with the appropriate observation E/M codes instead.

Time is not a contributing factor for E/M services provided in the ED. The emergency department E/M codes require that all three key components meet or exceed the requirements in the code descriptor. Table 9.11 showcases the requirements for assigning E/M codes for services provided in the ED.

CODER'S TIP

The components of emergency department E/M services must always meet or exceed three out of three requirements listed in the code descriptors.

Other Emergency Services

Code 99288 describes situations where the physician is located in the hospital emergency department or critical care area and is directing emergency care in a remote location via two-way communication with rescue personnel located outside the

TABLE 9.11 Requirements for E/M Codes for ED Services

Code	History	Examination	Decision Making	Presenting Problem
99281	Problem focused	Problem focused	Straightforward	Self-limited or minor
99282	Expanded problem focused	Expanded problem focused	Low complexity	Low to moderate severity
99283	Expanded problem focused	Expanded problem focused	Moderate complexity	Moderate severity
99284	Detailed	Detailed	Moderate complexity	High severity
99285	Comprehensive	Comprehensive	High complexity	High severity

hospital. In these situations, the physician directs necessary medical procedures, such as cardiopulmonary resuscitation, electrical conversion of cardiac arrhythmias, airway management, fluid administration, and administration of necessary drugs. Like emergency department E/M codes, code 99288 is not time based.

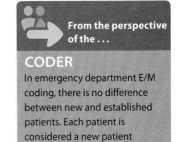

CODING EXAMPLE

A patient is seen in the emergency department after sustaining a fall while hiking and fracturing her ankle. The ED physician performs an expanded problem-focused history, a detailed exam, and medical decision making of moderate complexity. What E/M code would be reported to describe these services?

Three out of three components must meet or exceed the requirements of the CPT code descriptor. The components meet or exceed the requirements for code 99283.

EXERCISE 9.4

Also available in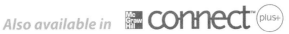

Use the CPT manual to answer the following questions.

1. A patient is brought to the emergency room by ambulance after sustaining lacerations to his forehead and left arm in a motor vehicle accident. The head laceration is 2.2 cm, and the laceration on his arm is 7.2 cm. The emergency room physician performs an expanded problem-focused history and exam, and the medical decision making is of moderate complexity. What code would be reported? _____

2. A 77-year-old male is brought to the emergency room by ambulance complaining of chest pain radiating to his left arm. The emergency room physician performs a comprehensive history and exam and medical decision making of high complexity. What code would be reported? _____

3. A patient presents to the emergency room complaining of tightness in her chest, shortness of breath, abdominal pain, and a deep cough. The emergency room physician performs a detailed history and exam. He orders laboratory tests and a chest x-ray to determine whether the patient has pneumonia. The medical decision making is of moderate complexity. What codes would be reported? _____

9.5 Reporting Critical Care Services (99291–99292)

Physicians providing critical care services to critically ill or injured patients report those services with two time-based codes. CPT code 99291 is used to report the first 30–74 minutes of critical care services on any given day. Add-on code 99292 is used to report each additional 30 minutes or portion thereof. These codes report the total critical care time, even if that time is not continuous. Critical care services may be provided on multiple days if necessary. Critical care services of less than 30 minutes' duration on any given day are not reported as critical care, but rather with the appropriate E/M codes.

Most often, critical care services are provided in a critical care unit, such as an intensive care unit (ICU), cardiac care unit, pediatric intensive care unit, or the emergency department, but this is not required. Critical care services are defined by the care provided, not where it is provided. Even if care is provided in a critical care location, it can only be reported with critical care codes if the conditions and treatments meet the requirements for critical care.

A critical illness or injury is one that significantly impairs one or more vital organ systems to a sufficient degree that there is a high probability of life-threatening deterioration of the patient. Critical care services involve high-complexity medical decision making to diagnose and treat failure of one or more organ systems, such as the cardiovascular, central nervous, hepatic, renal, respiratory, or metabolic systems.

TABLE 9.12 E/M Codes for Critical Care Time

Time	E/M Code
Less than 30 minutes	Appropriate E/M codes
30–74 minutes	99291 X 1
75–104 minutes	99291 X 1 and 99292 X 1
105–134 minutes	99291 X 1 and 99292 X 2
135–164 minutes	99291 X 1 and 99292 X 3
165–194 minutes	99291 X 1 and 99292 X 4

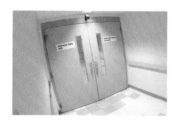

Unlike most other E/M codes, critical care services are defined by the care provided, not where it is provided.

Critical care codes are not used to report services to patients in a critical care unit if the patient's condition does not meet the requirements for critical care. In those cases, the services are reported with other appropriate E/M codes. Physicians may report both E/M and critical care codes for a single patient on the same date.

Services Included in Critical Care

Certain services and procedures commonly performed as part of critical care services are included in the critical care codes and cannot be reported separately. These include the interpretation of commonly used diagnostic tests or physiological measures such as cardiac output measurements (93561, 93562); chest x-rays (71010, 71015, 71020); pulse oximetry (94760, 94761, 94762); blood gases, and information stored in a computer (99090). Critical care codes also include certain procedures such as gastric intubation (43752, 45753); temporary transcutaneous pacing (92953); ventilator management (94002, 94003, 94004, 94660, 94662); and vascular access (36000, 36410, 36415, 36591, 36600). Other services may be reported separately with the appropriate CPT codes. Table 9.12 presents examples of using CPT codes 99291 and 99292 to report critical care time.

Guidance included in the critical care section of the CPT manual provides instructions on reporting critical care services to neonates and infants, including services in a neonatal or pediatric intensive care unit. These services are not time based and are reported with different codes. Coders should review this section whenever they report intensive care or critical care services provided to neonates, infants, and young children.

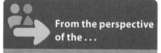

From the perspective of the . . .

CODER

Because critical care services are always time based, the medical record should document the beginning and ending time of critical care services. These times need not be continuous. The times are totaled for each day for reporting purposes.

CODER'S TIP

Longer times may be reported with 99291 X 1 and 99292 with sufficient units to account for each 30-minute block of time, including any partial time.

CODING EXAMPLE

A patient is admitted to the ICU in multiple system failure. The critical care physician performs several procedures, including placement of an endotracheal tube (31500), ventilator management (94002), placement of an IV catheter (36000), and arterial puncture for blood gas measurements (36600). The physician spends a total of 145 minutes performing these procedures and providing critical care services. How are these services reported?

The critical care services are reported based on 145 minutes total time. This would be reported with codes 99291 X 1 and 99292 X 3. In addition, endotracheal intubation (31500) is not included in the critical care codes and may be reported separately.

Also available in 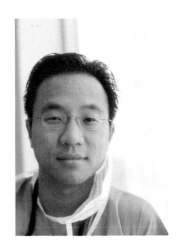 **Mc Graw Hill** CONNECT™ (plus+)

9.6 Reporting E/M Codes in Other Settings (99304–99350)

Patients may need to stay in facilities other than hospitals either for a short-term recovery or on a long-term basis. These settings may include a nursing facility, domiciliary, rest home, or custodial care setting. Some patients are able to stay in their own homes but require ongoing care.

Physicians and other professionals provide E/M services to patients in these settings. Several series of codes describe these E/M services. Most code groups are divided into subgroups depending on whether a patient's initial visit or subsequent visits in that setting are being reported.

Nursing Facility Services

In the past, nursing facilities (NFs) were divided into skilled nursing facilities (SNFs), intermediate care facilities (ICFs), and long-term care facilities (LTCFs). CPT codes describing nursing facility services also are used to report E/M services provided to a patient in a psychiatric residential treatment facility or a distinct part of a facility utilized for psychiatric care that provides a 24-hour group living arrangement. These services are reported for new or established patients. Services provided in any of these facilities are reported with the following series of CPT codes:

- Initial Nursing Facility Care (99304–99306)
- Subsequent Nursing Facility Care (99307–99310)
- Nursing Facility Discharge Services (99315–99316)
- Other Nursing Facility Services (99318)

Initial Nursing Facility Care CPT codes describing initial nursing facility care are used to report E/M services provided on the day of admission to the facility. If the physician provides services in other settings on that same date prior to admission to the nursing facility, those services are considered part of the initial nursing facility care. Components must meet or exceed three out of three requirements listed in the code descriptor. When time is considered a factor in code selection, the time is the total time spent on the unit or floor. Initial nursing facility care is reported with the codes shown in Table 9.13.

Subsequent Nursing Facility Care Subsequent nursing facility care includes reviewing the medical record, results of diagnostic tests, and changes in the patient's condition since the last visit. Components must meet or exceed two out of three requirements listed in the code descriptor. Table 9.14 describes the requirements for reporting subsequent nursing facility care with an E/M code.

When time is considered a factor in selecting a code for nursing facility care, the time is the total time that a physician spends on the unit or floor.

TABLE 9.13 E/M Codes for Initial Nursing Facility Care

Code	History	Examination	Decision Making	Presenting Problem	Typical Time (minutes)
99304	Detailed or comprehensive	Detailed or comprehensive	Straightforward or low complexity	Low severity	25
99305	Comprehensive	Comprehensive	Moderate complexity	Moderate severity	35
99306	Comprehensive	Comprehensive	High complexity	High severity	45

TABLE 9.14 Requirements for E/M Codes for Subsequent Nursing Facility Care

Code	History	Examination	Decision Making	Patient Condition	Typical Time (minutes)
99307	Problem focused	Problem focused	Straightforward	Stable, recovering, or improving	10
99308	Expanded	Expanded	Low complexity	Responding inadequately or minor complication	15
99309	Detailed	Detailed	Moderate complexity	Significant complication or significant new problem	25
99310	Comprehensive	Comprehensive	High complexity	Unstable or requiring immediate physician attention	35

CODING EXAMPLE

After hip replacement surgery, the patient is admitted to a skilled nursing facility for additional observation and care to allow her to learn to use her new hip. On the initial visit, the physician performs a detailed history, comprehensive exam, and medical decision making of low complexity. On each of the next two subsequent days, he performs a problem-focused history and exam and medical decision making of moderate complexity.

The codes for these visits and exams are 99304, 99307, and 99307.

Nursing Facility Discharge Services Codes 99315 and 99316 are used to report services provided on the final discharge day, including final examination, discussion of the nursing facility stay, instructions for caregivers, and preparation of discharge records, prescriptions, and referral forms. The time the physician spends with the patient need not be continuous time.

- 99315 (Nursing facility discharge day management; 30 minutes or less)
- 99316 (Nursing facility discharge day management; more than 30 minutes)

Other Nursing Facility Services The annual assessment of nursing facility patients is reported with code 99318, the requirements for which are shown in Table 9.15.

TABLE 9.15 Requirements of Code 99318

Code	History	Examination	Decision Making	Patient Condition	Typical Time (minutes)
99318	Detailed	Comprehensive	Low to moderate complexity	Stable, recovering, or improving	30

Patient Type	Code	History	Examination	Decision Making	Presenting Problem	Typical Time (minutes)
New	99324	Problem focused	Problem focused	Straightforward	Low severity	20
	99325	Expanded problem focused	Expanded problem focused	Low complexity	Moderate severity	30
	99326	Detailed	Detailed	Moderate complexity	Moderate to high severity	45
	99327	Comprehensive	Comprehensive	Moderate complexity	High severity	60
	99328	Comprehensive	Comprehensive	High complexity	Patient is unstable or has a significant new problem	75
Established	99334	Problem focused	Problem focused	Straightforward	Self-limited or minor	15
	99335	Expanded problem focused	Expanded problem focused	Low complexity	Low to moderate severity	25
	99336	Detailed	Detailed	Moderate complexity	Moderate to high severity	40
	99337	Comprehensive	Comprehensive	Moderate to high complexity	Patient is unstable or has a significant new problem	60

Domiciliary, Rest Home (e.g., Boarding Home), or Custodial Care Services

These codes are used to report E/M services provided to patients in facilities that provide room, board, and personal assistance services. These codes also are used to report E/M services in an assisted living facility. These facilities do not provide medical services.

E/M services provided to new patients require that all three key components meet the level in the code descriptor. For established patients, two of the three key components must meet the code descriptor level. These requirements are described in Table 9.16.

CODING EXAMPLE

The physician sees a patient for the first time in the rest home. The patient is an 82-year-old female who slipped and fell when getting out of the shower. The physician performs a comprehensive history, a detailed exam, and medical decision making of moderate complexity. When seeing the patient the following week, he performs a comprehensive exam, problem-focused history, and medical decision making of low complexity. What codes describe the services on these two visits?

This patient is considered a new patient the first time the physician sees her and an established patient on the subsequent visit. The components must meet or exceed three out of three requirements on the first visit and two out of three requirements on the subsequent visit. The codes that meet these requirements are 99326 and 99335.

TABLE 9.17 Requirements for New Patient Home Services E/M Codes

Code	History	Examination	Decision Making	Presenting Problem	Typical Time (minutes)
99341	Problem focused	Problem focused	Straightforward	Low severity	20
99342	Expanded problem focused	Expanded problem focused	Low complexity	Moderate severity	30
99343	Detailed	Detailed	Moderate complexity	Moderate severity	45
99344	Comprehensive	Comprehensive	Moderate complexity	High severity	60
99345	Comprehensive	Comprehensive	High complexity	Patient is unstable or has a significant new problem	75

Home Services

A separate set of CPT codes is used to report E/M services provided in a patient's home. Like office E/M codes, these are divided into "new patient" and "established patient" code sets. New patient codes are divided into five levels of services, and each requires that all three key elements must meet the level described in the code descriptor. Established patient codes only require that two out of three key components meet the level described in the code descriptor. However, unlike office-based E/M codes, only four distinct levels of E/M home services are described for established patients.

New Patient The following codes describe E/M services provided to new patients in their homes. Each code requires that all three key components meet the level described in the code descriptor. Table 9.17 describes the requirements for these codes.

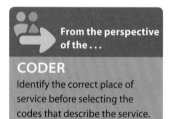

From the perspective of the . . .

CODER

Identify the correct place of service before selecting the codes that describe the service.

Established Patient The following codes describe E/M services provided to established patients in their homes. Each code requires that two out of three key components meet the level described in the code descriptor. Table 9.18 shows the requirements for these codes.

CODING EXAMPLE

A patient is not ambulatory and is unable to go to her doctor's office. The doctor agrees to see this established patient in her home. When he arrives, the physician performs a detailed history and exam with medical decision making of low complexity. What code describes this visit?

Because this is an established patient, only two out of three components must meet or exceed the requirements listed in the code descriptor. In this case, the components meet two of three requirements listed for code 99349.

CODER'S TIP

When a patient is considered a new patient, all three key components must meet or exceed the requirements in the code descriptor.

TABLE 9.18 Requirements for Established Patient Home Services E/M Codes

Code	History	Examination	Decision Making	Presenting Problem	Typical Time (minutes)
99347	Problem focused	Problem focused	Straightforward	Self-limited to mild	15
99348	Expanded problem focused	Expanded problem focused	Low complexity	Low to moderate severity	25
99349	Detailed	Detailed	Moderate complexity	Moderate to high severity	40
99350	Comprehensive	Comprehensive	Moderate to high complexity	Moderate to high severity	60

EXERCISE 9.6

Also available in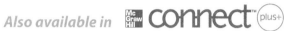

Use the CPT manual to answer the following questions.

1. What code appropriately reports the discharge in less than 30 minutes of a patient from a skilled nursing facility? _____

2. The physician in a nursing facility performs an annual nursing facility assessment with a detailed history, a comprehensive exam, and medical decision making of moderate complexity. What code describes this service?_____

3. The physician goes to the rest home to see a patient for a follow-up visit. He performs a comprehensive exam, problem-focused history, and medical decision making of straightforward complexity. What code describes this visit? _____

4. The physician is seeing a patient in the boarding home for the fourth time. The patient had sustained injuries that required additional nursing services. The physician performs an expanded problem-focused exam and history with medical decision making of low complexity. What code describes these services?
_____

5. The physician is going to see a new patient at the patient's home. The patient has just had his leg amputated below the knee. The physician performs a comprehensive history and exam with medical decision making of high complexity. What code is used to report this service? _____

9.7 Prolonged Services and the Time Factor (99354–99360)

Prolonged Physician Service with Direct Patient Contact

CPT codes 99354–99357 are add-on codes that are used in addition to any other E/M code when a physician provides **prolonged services** that are beyond the usual time for the underlying E/M services in the outpatient or inpatient settings. These codes describe prolonged services involving direct contact with the patient. The prolonged services codes may be reported with any level of E/M code and with CPT codes describing any other services provided during the same session as the underlying E/M service, provided that the E/M code has a typical time designated with that code in the CPT manual.

Similar to the time element of other outpatient E/M services, prolonged services in the outpatient setting are measured in terms of face-to-face time. In contrast, prolonged services in the inpatient setting are measured in terms of unit time. Prolonged

prolonged services
Services that are beyond the usual time for the underlying E/M services in the outpatient or inpatient settings.

services of less than 30 minutes beyond the typical time included in the underlying code descriptor are not separately reported, as that amount of time is considered to be within the appropriate range of time for each E/M code.

CPT code 99354 reports prolonged services of 30–60 minutes provided in the outpatient setting, as measured by face-to-face time with the patient. It is reported in addition to the code that describes the underlying E/M services provided. CPT code 99355 is reported for each additional 15–30 minutes of prolonged services in the outpatient setting beyond the first hour. However, this code is not reported if the prolonged services extend beyond the first hour or any additional 30-minute interval by less than 15 minutes. While there is no maximum number of times that CPT code 99355 may be reported to describe additional 30-minute intervals, the last interval must be 15 minutes or more in length.

CPT code 99356 describes prolonged services of 30–60 minutes provided in an inpatient setting, as measured by the time the physician spends on the unit. This add-on code is reported in addition to the code that describes the underlying inpatient E/M services provided. CPT code 99357 is reported for each additional 30 minutes of unit time provided beyond the first hour. As with the outpatient prolonged services codes, this add-on code may only be used if the prolonged services extend for 15 or more minutes beyond the end of the first hour or any additional 30-minute period.

CODING EXAMPLE

What codes would be used to report 80 minutes of prolonged services involving face-to-face time in the outpatient setting? How would 110 minutes of unit time be reported in the inpatient setting?

In the outpatient setting, the first 60 minutes is reported with add-on code 99354 and the next 20 minutes is reported with add-on code 99355. In the inpatient setting, the prolonged time would be reported with codes 99356 and 99357 X 2.

Prolonged Physician Service without Direct Patient Contact

CPT codes 99358 and 99359 are used to report prolonged services that do not involve direct contact with the patient (face-to-face time for outpatient services or unit time for inpatient services). Prolonged services without direct patient contact must be related to other E/M services provided to the patient, but that E/M service need not occur on the same day as the prolonged services. For example, a physician may review extensive medical records pertaining to a complex condition in a patient whom she has either recently seen or will see in the near future. This review might occur within several days before or after the patient visit.

CPT codes are used to report the total time prolonged services without direct patient contact were provided on each day, but the time need not be continuous. Unlike codes describing prolonged services with direct patient contact, the underlying E/M code need not include a typical time element as part of the information provided in the CPT manual.

CPT code 99358 describes prolonged services of 30–60 minutes without direct patient contact. Prolonged services of less than 30 minutes are not separately reported. CPT code 99359 describes each additional 15–30 minutes of prolonged services beyond the first hour or additional 30-minute periods of prolonged services. Prolonged services less than 15 minutes beyond the first hour or beyond additional 30-minute periods are not reported.

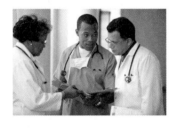

Prolonged service codes are used when a physician provides services that are beyond the usual time for the underlying E/M services in the outpatient or inpatient settings.

CODER'S TIP

When determining whether time spent with a patient meets the requirements to use add-on codes to report the time, it is necessary to understand what time can be counted for that purpose. For outpatient services, only face-to-face time can be counted for prolonged service time. For inpatient services, unit time is counted toward prolonged service time. Unit time need not be face-to-face time with the patient, but may include chart reviews, talking to family, etc.

Physician Standby Services

Sometimes a physician may request that another physician stand by in case his or her services are needed. Physicians who provide the standby service may report this with code 99360 for each 30 minutes of standby time. Physicians can only report this code for each complete 30-minute period. An initial standby period of less than 30 minutes cannot be reported. Subsequent time periods of less than 30 minutes of additional standby time cannot be reported. Physicians reporting standby services for one patient cannot provide services to any other patient during the standby period.

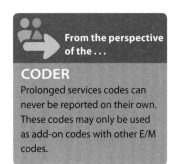

From the perspective of the . . .

CODER

Prolonged services codes can never be reported on their own. These codes may only be used as add-on codes with other E/M codes.

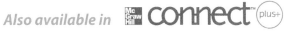

EXERCISE 9.7

Also available in **connect**™ (plus+)

Use the CPT manual to answer the following questions.

1. When selecting a code from the prolonged services category, the coder must know three factors about the time spent providing the service. What are these factors? _____

2. What codes would be reported for 101 minutes of prolonged, direct face-to-face contact with the patient? _____

3. To appropriately code for physician standby services, the services must have been _____.

9.8 Case Management and Care Plan Oversight Services (99363–99364, 99366–99368)

Case Management Services

Case management occurs when a provider provides direct care to a patient and, in addition, coordinates, initiates, supervises, or manages access to other health services the patient requires.

Anticoagulant Management These codes describe the outpatient management of warfarin therapy over ninety days of therapy, including ordering and interpreting international normalized ratio (INR) tests, providing patient instructions, and adjusting the patient's dosage, if necessary. If these codes are reported, these services cannot be the basis for other E/M or care plan oversight services during the 90-day period. If telephone or online services are utilized for anticoagulant management, the telephone and/or online services CPT codes may not be reported either.

Code 99363 describes the initial 90-day therapy period and must include at least eight INR measurements during that period. Code 99364 is used to report each additional 90 days of therapy, with at least three INR measurements during each subsequent 90-day period.

These are outpatient services only. If anticoagulation is initiated or continued during an inpatient stay, a new time period begins after discharge and is reported with CPT code 99364. These codes are not reported if anticoagulation services are provided for less than 60 continuous outpatient days. If fewer than the specified number of INR measurements are performed during the time period, do not report CPT code 99363 or 99364.

CODING EXAMPLE

A physician provides anticoagulation management over a nine-month period. During the first three months, the services include 10 INR measurements, the next three months include 5 INR measurements, and the last three months include 2 INR measurements. How would the physician report these services?

The first three-month period is reported with code 99363. The second three-month period is reported with 99364. The third three-month period cannot be reported because the required number of INR measurements was not provided.

Medical Team Conferences A medical team conference involves face-to-face participation by three or more healthcare professionals from different specialties, each of whom is providing direct care to the patient. It is not necessary for the patient, family member, caregivers, or decision makers to be present during this conference. Each conference participant must have performed a face-to-face evaluation or treatment of the patient within 60 days prior to the conference.

Nonphysician providers report medical team conference services with two CPT codes. Code 99366 is used to report medical team conferences of 30 minutes or more with the patient or family member(s) present during some or all of the conference. Code 99367 describes medical team conferences of 30 minutes or more without the patient or family member(s) present during any part of the conference. Medical team conferences lasting less than 30 minutes are not reported.

Physicians do not use these codes to report medical team conference services with the patient and/or family present during all or part of the conference. If patients and/or family members are present during the medical team conference, physicians report their services using the appropriate E/M service. Physicians report medical team conference services lasting 30 minutes or more without the patient or family present during any part of the conference with CPT code 99368. Similar to nonphysician providers, physicians cannot report medical team conferences lasting less than 30 minutes.

Care Plan Oversight Services

Physicians may report care plan oversight services in addition to other E/M services provided in the office or outpatient setting, hospital, home, nursing facility, or domiciliary setting. These codes describe care plan oversight services provided during a 30-day period, and only one physician may report these services during that period. These codes should not be reported for supervision of patients unless the patient requires recurrent supervision of therapy provided in the various settings.

Care plan oversight services do not include face-to-face time with the patient. Services provided during a face-to-face encounter with the patient are reported with the E/M codes describing services in the location in which the patient was seen.

Specific Code Sets CPT codes 99374 and 99375 describe physician supervision of a patient under the care of a home health agency. Patients may live in their own home, a domiciliary, or other equivalent location. Code 99374 is reported for 15–29 minutes of care plan oversight activities within a calendar month. Code 99375 describes care plan oversight extending for 30 minutes or more during the month.

CPT codes 99377 and 99378 describe physician oversight of a hospice patient. Code 99377 describes 15–29 minutes of care plan oversight during the calendar

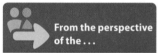

From the perspective of the . . .

CODER

Case management services occur when a physician provides direct care to a patient as well as coordinates, initiates, supervises, or manages access to other health services the patient requires.

month, and code 99378 describes services lasting more than 30 minutes during the month.

CPT codes 99379 and 99380 describe physician supervision of a nursing facility patient provided during the calendar month, with 99379 describing 15–29 minutes of supervision and 99380 describing supervision that lasts for more than 30 minutes during the month.

Two other codes describe care plan oversight services in another section of E/M codes. CPT code 99339 describes physician supervision of a patient at home, in a domiciliary, rest home, assisted living facility, or similar location requiring 15–29 minutes during the calendar month. CPT code 99340 describes similar services requiring 30 minutes or more during the calendar month.

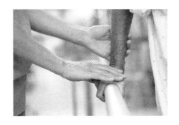

Certain E/M codes describe care plan oversight services. These services do not include supervising the patient unless the patient requires recurrent supervision of therapy.

CODER'S TIP

Ascertain the setting in which the care plan oversight services occurred. The codes used to report these services vary by location.

EXERCISE 9.8

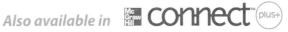

Also available in **Mc Graw Hill connect** plus+

Use the CPT manual to answer the following questions.

1. What time period is associated with anticoagulant management services? _____

2. What code describes a medical team conference of 90 minutes with direct fact-to-face contact by nonphysicians? _____

3. What code describes a medical team conference of 75 minutes by nonphysician providers without the patient present? _____

9.9 Preventive Medicine Services (99381–99387, 99391–99397, 99401–99412)

Preventive medicine services vary depending on the age and sex of the patient. These services include an age-appropriate history and physical exam of the patient, which is often referred to as a comprehensive service. The term *comprehensive* when used in connection with preventive medicine services does not have the same meaning as when it is used in connection with E/M codes in the 99201–99350 range. When used to describe preventive medicine services, comprehensive is used to mean the combination of an age-appropriate history and physical exam.

Preventive medicine services include counseling, anticipatory guidance, and risk factor reduction provided during the time of the preventive medicine visit. If these services are provided at a distinct time other than during the preventive medicine visit, they may be reported separately.

Insignificant or minor problems discovered while performing the periodic preventive medicine examination that do not require additional work or the performance of the key components of a problem-oriented E/M service are not reported separately.

If a significant abnormality is discovered or a preexisting problem is addressed during a periodic preventive medicine examination that requires additional work to perform the key components of a problem-oriented E/M service, then the appropriate office/outpatient E/M code (99201–99215) is reported *in addition to* the preventive medicine service code. Modifier 25 is added to the E/M code to designate that this is a significant, separately identifiable E/M service that is provided by the same physician on the same day as the preventive medicine service.

Other services or products provided during a preventive medicine examination, such as vaccine products; immunization administration; ancillary laboratory or

preventive medicine services
Services that include an age-appropriate history and physical exam of the patient, which is often referred to as a comprehensive service.

TABLE 9.19 Age Requirements for Preventive Medicine Services, New Patient

Code	Age Range
99381	Infant, younger than 1 year of age
99382	Early childhood, age 1–4 years
99383	Late childhood, age 5–11 years
99384	Adolescent, age 12–17 years
99385	18–39 years of age
99386	40–64 years of age
99387	65 years of age and older

radiological studies; vision, hearing, or developmental screening; or other procedures identified with a specific CPT code may be reported separately.

CODER'S TIP

The preventive medicine exam also may be referred to as a well-woman, well-child, or annual exam.

New Patient

The codes listed in Table 9.19 describe the initial comprehensive preventive medicine services for the evaluation and management of a new patient, including an age- and gender-appropriate history, examination, ordering of laboratory procedures, and appropriate anticipatory guidance for patients of various ages.

CODING EXAMPLE

A 16-year-old patient sees a physician for the first time for a comprehensive preventive medicine exam. The physician takes an age-appropriate history, performs an age-appropriate exam, and provides the appropriate anticipatory guidance associated with these services. What code is used to report this service?

Preventive services provided to a new 16-year-old patient are reported with code 99384.

Established Patient

The codes listed in Table 9.20 describe the periodic, comprehensive preventive medicine services for the evaluation and management of an existing patient, including an age- and gender-appropriate history, examination, ordering of laboratory procedures, and appropriate anticipatory guidance for patients of various ages.

CODING EXAMPLE

What code is used to report an annual well-woman exam (preventive services) provided to a 45-year-old woman by her regular gynecologist?

Preventive services provided to an established 45-year-old patient are reported with code 99396.

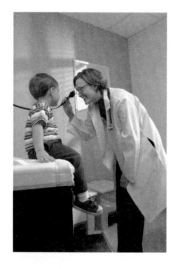

Preventive E/M services are frequently referred to as "well visits."

TABLE 9.20 Age Requirements for Preventive Medicine Services, Established Patient

Code	Age Range
99391	Infant, younger than 1 year of age
99392	Early childhood, age 1–4 years
99393	Late childhood, age 5–11 years
99394	Adolescent, age 12–17 years
99395	18–39 years of age
99396	40–64 years of age
99397	65 years of age and older

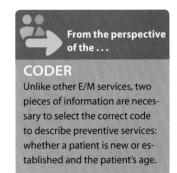

From the perspective of the . . .

CODER

Unlike other E/M services, two pieces of information are necessary to select the correct code to describe preventive services: whether a patient is new or established and the patient's age.

Counseling Risk Factor Reduction and Behavior Change Intervention

Codes 99401–99412 describe services provided directly to patients and/or family to promote health and prevent illness or injury. These may be reported separately from and in addition to other codes describing E/M services provided during the same encounter. However, preventive medicine service codes cannot be reported in combination with these codes. The actual counseling services will vary by age and individual patient circumstances, but unlike the preventive medicine service codes, the individual codes do not vary by age, but by the length of time the services are provided.

These codes are used for both new and established patients and should address issues such as family problems, diet and exercise, substance use and abuse, sexual activity and appropriate precautions, prevention of injury, dental health, and any diagnostic lab/imaging tests available at the time the services are provided. Behavior change interventions are provided to individuals who have a behavior that may be considered an illness in and of itself, such as smoking, drug use and abuse, or obesity.

The following codes describe preventive medicine counseling and risk factor reduction provided to an individual as a separate procedure:

- 99401: Approximately 15 minutes.
- 99402: Approximately 30 minutes.
- 99403: Approximately 45 minutes.
- 99404: Approximately 60 minutes.

There also are specific behavior change interventions that may be provided to individuals, including:

- 99406: Smoking and tobacco use cessation counseling, 3–10 minutes.
- 99407: Smoking and tobacco use cessation counseling, greater than 10 minutes.
- 99408: Alcohol or substance abuse, screening and intervention, 15–30 minutes.
- 99409: Alcohol or substance abuse, screening and intervention, greater than 30 minutes.

Preventive medicine counseling also may be provided as group counseling sessions:

- 99411: Group counseling sessions for approximately 30 minutes.
- 99412: Group counseling sessions for approximately 60 minutes.

Use the CPT manual to answer the following questions.

1. In order to select the appropriate preventive well-visit code, the coder must know two things about the patient. What are these two characteristics? _____

2. A 25-year-old healthy woman presents to her physician's office for her annual checkup as she has each of the past three years. What code would be reported? _____

3. Preventive medicine counseling codes are selected by which measurement? _____

9.10 Special E/M Services (99441–99456)

Certain non–face-to-face physician services may be reported with specific E/M codes, including telephone services and online medical evaluations. Not all telephone services or online medical evaluations may be reported, so coders must understand the circumstances surrounding these services, including other services that may have been provided on other days, to determine whether these services may be reported separately.

Telephone Services

CPT codes 99441–99443 describe non–face-to-face E/M services provided to a patient over the telephone. The codes describe telephone discussions initiated by an established patient. Calls initiated by the physician, such as follow-up calls, are not reported with these codes. The three codes differ only by the amount of time the provider spends providing the medical discussion.

- 99441: Calls of 5–10 minutes.
- 99442: Calls of 11–20 minutes.
- 99443: Calls of 21–30 minutes.

Only physicians who provide telephone services may report these codes. Qualified nonphysicians who provide telephone services report those services with CPT codes 98966–98968.

Not all telephone services can be reported. If the telephone discussion ends with a decision to see the patient within 24 hours, the telephone service cannot be reported separately. The telephone service is considered to be part of the work described by the E/M code used to report the subsequent visit. Also, if the telephone service pertains to an E/M service that occurred within the previous seven days, the telephone service may not be reported separately regardless of whether the telephone service was initiated by the patient or the physician. Similarly, if the telephone call pertains to a prior procedure and occurs within the global period of that procedure, the telephone service may not be reported separately. Those calls are considered to be part of the previous E/M service or procedure.

When reporting codes for E/M services provided over the telephone, pay careful attention to other E/M services documented in the patient's record. If the telephone service is related to another service provided in the past seven days, the telephone service cannot be reported separately.

CODER'S TIP

Parenthetical instructions with the telephone codes instruct coders not to report these codes for telephone services when care plan oversight services are reported with CPT codes 99339–99340 or 99374–99380, as those codes already include telephone services provided as part of the care plan oversight services. Similarly, the telephone services codes cannot be reported for anticoagulant management services reported with CPT codes 99363–99364, as those codes include telephone services provided in conjunction with anticoagulant management.

CODING EXAMPLE

A patient calls her regular physician to discuss a problem that has come up since the last time she saw her doctor six months ago. She asks whether she should be seen immediately or if this can wait. After discussing the problem in detail, the doctor tells her to make an appointment to see him in about a week. The call lasts 15 minutes.

Because this call did not involve an E/M visit that occurred during the previous seven days and did not result in a visit within the next 24 hours, the telephone service is reported with code 99442.

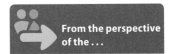

From the perspective of the . . .

CODER

Not all telephone calls can be reported. Only calls that are initiated by the patient or the patient's family qualify. In addition, calls that result in an E/M visit within 24 hours or that occur within seven days of another E/M service cannot be reported.

Online Medical Evaluation

CPT code 99444 describes non–face-to-face E/M services by a physician using the Internet in response to a patient's online request. This service must include the physician's personal timely response to the patient's request, and a permanent record must be maintained of the communication. This code may only be reported once per seven days, regardless of how many individual online communications occur during that time. Multiple physicians may report the code during the same seven-day period, provided each one personally responds to an online request by the patient.

This code cannot be reported if the patient's inquiry is in relation to an E/M service provided during the previous seven days or occurs during the postoperative global period of a previously performed procedure. Those communications are considered to be part of the previously provided E/M service or procedure and are not separately reportable.

Other Special E/M Services

Medical professionals sometimes perform evaluations of individuals prior to the issuance of life or disability insurance policies or examine individuals who claim to be disabled. CPT codes describing these services assume that no active management of medical problems occurred during the encounter. If other E/M services or procedures are provided during the encounter, they should be reported with the appropriate CPT codes.

CPT code 99450 describes a basic life and/or disability examination. CPT code 99455 describes a work or medical disability assessment by the physician who is treating the patient for that problem. CPT code 99456 describes a work or medical disability assessment by a physician other than the one treating the patient for that problem. Each of these codes includes specific elements that must be performed to report these services.

EXERCISE 9.10

Also available in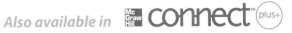

Use the CPT manual to answer the following questions.

1. Can telephone services or online medical evaluation codes be reported for all types of patients? Why or why not? _____

2. Can a physician report two separate online services for the same problem during a five-day period? Why or why not? _____

3. A surgeon receives a request for telephone services from a patient he operated on three weeks earlier. The procedure has a 90-day postoperative global period. He calls the patient and discusses her concerns for approximately 25 minutes. What code would be reported for this telephone service?

9.11 Coding E/M Services for Pediatric Patients (99460–99463)

Newborn Services

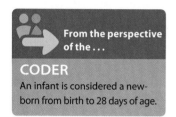

From the perspective of the . . .

CODER

An infant is considered a newborn from birth to 28 days of age.

Newborn services are reported using several groups of CPT codes. A patient is considered a newborn from birth through 28 days of age. These services may be reported in several different settings. E/M services for the newborn include the maternity/fetal history as well as the history of the newborn following birth, physical examination of the newborn, ordering necessary and appropriate diagnostic tests, ordering necessary treatments, meeting with the family, and recording documentation in the medical record.

CPT codes used to report normal newborn services (99460–99463) describe the initial care provided to newborns in the first days after birth before discharge home. If a physician or other provider is in attendance in the delivery room to either stabilize or resuscitate the newborn, CPT codes describing the delivery room attendance or resuscitation (99464–99465) are reported in addition to the codes describing normal newborn services.

When E/M services are provided to infants who are not considered "normal newborns," those services are reported with hospital inpatient E/M service (99221–99233) or neonatal intensive care or critical care codes (99466–99469, 99477–99480). If the physician provides initial services described by the normal newborn service codes and later provides intensive care or critical care on the same day, modifier 25 is added to the intensive care or critical care services code. The normal newborn services are reported without a modifier. Other procedures are not included in the normal newborn service codes and are reported separately if provided.

CODER'S TIP

Coders must know which codes can only be reported once per day.

Normal Newborn Services When reporting normal newborn services, use one of the following codes:

- 99460: Initial care of a newborn in a hospital or birthing center.
- 99461: Initial care of a newborn in settings other than a hospital or birthing center.
- 99462: Subsequent care of a newborn in the hospital.
- 99463: Initial care of a newborn in a hospital or birthing center, when the newborn is admitted and discharged on the same date.

These codes not include any time component and are reported once per day, even if the provider sees the newborn more than once on the same day. At times, one physician may provide the initial care and another provides subsequent care. The second physician would report subsequent day services with code 99462, even if that visit represented the first time that physician treated the newborn.

If the newborn is discharged on the same date as admitted, CPT code 99463 includes all services related to the admission and discharge. If the newborn is discharged subsequent to the initial admission date, the discharge services are described by CPT code 99238 or 99239.

CODING EXAMPLE

What code(s) would be reported for three consecutive days of newborn care of an infant born somewhere other than a hospital and then admitted for an additional two days?

The initial day of care for a newborn provided in a nonhospital setting is reported with code 99461. The subsequent two days of hospital care are reported with code 99462 X 2.

Delivery/Birthing Room Attendance and Resuscitation Services

If the physician delivering a newborn requests another provider to attend the delivery and provide necessary services to the newborn, that second provider may report those services with either CPT code 99464 (if routine stabilization is all that is necessary) or 99465 (if resuscitation is necessary, such as ventilation and/or chest compressions). If other procedures such as intubation or placement of intravascular catheters are necessary as part of the resuscitation efforts, those procedures may be reported separately with the appropriate CPT codes.

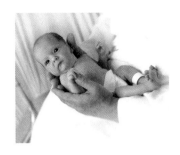

A physician delivering a newborn can request another provider to assist in the delivery. In this case, report the services of the second provider with code 99464 or 99465, depending on the nature of the services.

Inpatient Neonatal Intensive Care and Pediatric/Neonatal Critical Care

Pediatric Critical Care Patient Transport Physicians may provide services during the transportation of a critically ill or critically injured pediatric patient who is 24 months of age or younger. The actual face-to-face time of care provided during the interfacility transport may be reported with these codes. CPT code 99466 describes the first 30–74 minutes of face-to-face transport time. Add-on code 99467 is used to report each additional 30 minutes of face-to-face time. This code is reported in addition to CPT code 99466. Transport services of less than 30 minutes are not reported with these codes. Rather, those services would be reported with E/M codes.

If a physician directs care of a patient during transport through the use of a radio or other two-way communication device, these services are not considered face-to-face care and are not reported with CPT codes 99466 or 99467. Instead, services provided through the use of voice communications are reported with CPT code 99288.

A number of services, if provided during transport, are considered to be included in these transportation codes and are not separately reportable, including: routine monitoring, cardiac output measurements and interpretations, chest x-rays, measurement of pulse oximetry, blood gas interpretation, review and interpretation of information stored in a computer, gastric intubation, temporary pacing, ventilator management, and vascular access procedures. Other procedures not specifically listed in the introductory guidance to this section may be reported separately with the appropriate CPT codes.

Inpatient Neonatal and Pediatric Critical Care These codes describe the initial and subsequent days of critical care services provided to neonates, infants, and children younger than five years of age. The six codes are organized into three pairs (initial and subsequent day), each of which applies to different ages:

- 99468 and 99469: Neonates 28 days of age and younger.
- 99471 and 99472: 29 days through 24 months of age.
- 99475 and 99476: 2 years through 5 years of age.

Critical care services provided to children six years of age or older are reported with CPT codes 99291 and 99292.

The initial day critical care codes (99468, 99471, and 99475) are only reported once per critical care admission. The subsequent day critical care codes (99469, 99472, and 99476) are reported once for each subsequent day of critical care services. These codes are reported only once per day, even if the critical care services are provided over several episodes during that day. Only one physician may report these codes on each day critical care services are provided. Other physicians providing critical care services on those dates may report those services with CPT codes 99291 and 99292.

In those situations where physicians in two different hospitals provide critical care services on the same date of service (e.g., when a critically ill infant or child is transported from one hospital to another), only one physician at the receiving hospital should report services using these codes. All physicians at the initial hospital, as well as additional physicians at the receiving hospital, should report their services with CPT codes 99291 and 99292.

These six E/M codes include many services commonly provided to a critical care patient. All services listed in the guidance associated with CPT codes 99291 and 99292 are also included in these neonatal and pediatric critical care codes. In addition, other services are also considered to be included in these codes, including invasive or noninvasive vital sign monitoring; vascular access procedures; airway and ventilation management; interpretation of blood gases or oxygen saturation; blood transfusions; oral or nasogastric tube placement; bladder catheterization or suprapubic aspiration; and lumbar puncture. Other services not specifically listed in the guidance associated with these codes may be reported separately.

Critical care services provided in an outpatient setting, such as an emergency department or office, are reported with CPT codes 99291 and 99292. Physicians providing critical care services in both outpatient and inpatient settings on the same day should report all services for that day with the neonatal or pediatric critical care codes (99468–99476).

CODER'S TIP

Neonatal and pediatric critical care services include all the services listed in the guidelines for critical care services (99291 and 99292) above. In addition, there is a long list of other services included in neonatal and pediatric critical care beyond those listed for codes 99291 and 99292. These are listed in the guidelines for this section.

Coders must be aware of the services included in the neonatal and pediatric critical care services to avoid reporting those services separately. Because this list may change from year to year, coders should make it a habit to review it when reporting neonatal and pediatric critical care services.

Initial and Continuing Intensive Care Services Neonates 28 days of age or younger may not be critically ill, but may require intensive observation or frequent interventions. CPT code 99477 is reported once to describe the initial day of intensive services for such neonates. CPT codes 99478–99480 describe subsequent days of intensive service, with the choice of code dependent on the patient's weight on that day:

- 99478: Very low birth weight infant (less than 1,500 grams).
- 99479: Low birth weight infants (1,500–2,500 grams).
- 99480: Infants weighing 2,501–5,000 grams.

Subsequent days of intensive care for neonates younger than 28 days of age but weighing more than 5,000 grams are reported with CPT codes 99231–99233.

EXERCISE 9.11

Also available in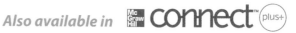

Use the CPT manual to answer the following questions.

1. Newborn care services are categorized by two elements: _____ and _____.

2. Can newborn care codes be reported more than once per day? _____

3. What information must the coder know to select the correct code for neonatal and pediatric critical care services? _____

4. What code(s) would be reported for critical care services for a three-year-old child who fell in her pool in the backyard and has had three days of critical care service by her pediatrician?

_____

5. In addition to the services listed in the CPT guidance, what other services are considered to be included in neonatal critical care? _____

Summary

Learning Outcome	Key Concepts/Examples
9.1 Explain how differences between new and established patients affect E/M code selection in outpatient settings. **Pages 211–213**	A new patient is one who has not been seen by a particular physician or another physician of the same specialty in the same practice during the previous three years. An established patient is one who has been seen by a particular physician or another physician of the same specialty in the same practice during the previous three years. All three key components must meet or exceed the requirements of the code descriptor for new patients, while only two out of three key components must meet or exceed the code descriptor requirements for established patients.
9.2 Differentiate among various categories and subcategories of hospital services. **Pages 213–218**	The categories of hospital E/M services are observation services and inpatient services. Each category is divided into initial day services and subsequent day services. All three key components must meet or exceed the code descriptor requirements for initial day services, while only two out of three key components must meet or exceed those requirements for subsequent day services.
9.3 Describe how consultation codes are different from other E/M services. **Pages 219–221**	Consultation services require a request for the consultation by another provider, recommendations from the consulting physician to the requesting provider, and a report to the referring provider with those recommendations. These services are categorized as either office or inpatient consults. All three key components must meet or exceed the code descriptor requirements.
9.4 Identify factors of E/M codes for emergency services. **Pages 222–223**	Emergency department E/M services are not subdivided by either new vs. established patient or by initial day vs. subsequent days of services. All three key components must meet or exceed the code descriptor requirements for the reported level of E/M code reported.
9.5 Explain how critical care services are reported. **Page 223**	Time is the determining factor used to report critical care services. One code describes the first 30–74 minutes of critical care services while an add-on code describes each additional 30 minutes. The guidance lists services that are included in critical care and may not be reported separately. Other services may be reported separately.
9.6 Describe factors that determine subcategories of E/M services in special settings. **Pages 225–228**	Codes describing E/M services provided in a nursing facility, domiciliary, rest home, or in the patient's home are categorized by whether it is the initial day or subsequent day of service. All three key components must meet or exceed the code descriptor requirements for initial day of service codes, whereas only two out of three key components must meet or exceed the code descriptor requirements for subsequent days.
9.7 Explain how time is calculated and used to report prolonged services. **Pages 229–231**	Prolonged services are reported as add-on codes in addition to the E/M code describing the services. These services are reported on the basis of time when the services require at least 30 minutes additional time over the typical time described in the code descriptor of the designated E/M code. Different codes describe prolonged time in the office and inpatient settings. In each setting, one code describes the first 30–74 minutes of prolonged time, with a second code describing each additional 30 minutes of prolonged services. In the office or other outpatient setting, time is calculated as the total amount of face to face time, while in facilities, time is calculated on the basis of the total time spent on the unit.

(Continued)

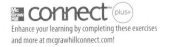
Enhance your learning by completing these exercises and more at mcgrawhillconnect.com!

CHAPTER 9 | EVALUATION AND MANAGEMENT SERVICES, PART II: CODE SELECTION   241

Learning Outcome	Key Concepts/Examples
9.8 Identify the factors that determine which E/M codes are reported for case management and care plan oversight services. **Pages 231–233**	Anticoagulant management and medical team conferences are reported with the case management E/M codes. Care plan oversight E/M services are described by codes based on the place those services are provided, including home, hospice, and nursing facility services.
9.9 Describe preventive medicine services. **Pages 233–235**	Preventive medicine services are divided into two subcategories based on whether the patient is a new patient or an established patient. Within each subcategory, the appropriate code is selected based on the patient's age. Preventive services include age-appropriate history, physical exam, counseling, anticipatory guidance, risk factor reduction, and ordering laboratory and diagnostic tests.
9.10 Identify elements of telephone, online, and special E/M services. **Pages 236–237**	E/M services provided over the telephone may be reported when the patient initiates the call, not the physician. The code is selected on the basis of the total time of the call. These services cannot be reported if the call results in the physician seeing the patient within 24 hours or is related to a visit during the previous seven days. Physicians also may provide E/M services using the Internet in response to a patient's online request. The physician must respond to the request personally to report this service. Physicians may report this service once per seven days, regardless of how many communications occur. This service cannot be reported if it occurs within seven days of a previous E/M visit or during the global period of a previous procedure.
9.11 Contrast E/M coding standards for various newborn services. **Pages 238–240**	Services provided to normal newborns are reported by E/M codes that describe initial day services according to the place those services are delivered and subsequent days of service in any setting. Critical care of a neonate or pediatric patient is reported with E/M codes describing initial and subsequent days of service for various ages of the patient: 28 days or younger; 29 days through 24 months old; and 2 through 5 years of age. Neonatal intensive care services for a patient who is in the NICU but does not require critical care services are reported using codes describing the initial day of service and subsequent days of service based on the infant's current weight.

Using Terminology

Match the key terms with their definitions.

_____ **1.** LO 9.1 Inpatient setting

_____ **2.** LO 9.2 Admit/discharge codes

_____ **3.** LO 9.2 Hospital observation services

_____ **4.** LO 9.7 Prolonged services

_____ **5.** LO 9.9 Preventive medicine services

_____ **6.** LO 9.11 Newborn services

A. Hospital or other facility for an overnight or longer stay

B. A temporary period to determine whether a patient needs to be admitted or can be sent home

C. Set of codes that describe services when a patient is admitted and discharged on the same date

D. E/M services to evaluate baseline health status when no specific disease is treated, such as an annual exam

E. Medical services provided to an infant up to 28 days of age

F. Inpatient or outpatient E/M services involving patient contact that is beyond the usual service

Checking Your Understanding

Each of the following multiple-choice questions includes a clinical vignette. In each case, select the answer with the CPT code(s) that best describe(s) the services provided.

1. LO 9.9 A 33-year-old woman presents to her physician's office for her annual physical exam as she has for each of the past three years. She states she is having trouble sleeping at times, but other than that she feels fine. Her physician performs a detailed history and physical exam; the medical decision making is of low complexity.

   a. 99213
   b. 99203
   c. 99395
   d. 99212

2. LO 9.2 The ENT physician is back to see his patient in the hospital for the third day. The patient is feeling better but is complaining of very sharp pain in her right ear. She also is having drainage of clear fluids from the right ear. The physician performs a problem-focused history and exam; the medical decision making is of moderate complexity.

   a. 99213
   b. 99231
   c. 99323
   d. 99595

3. LO 9.2 A 94-year-old woman presents to her physician's office complaining of cough, shortness of breath, and low-grade fever for the past 48 hours. She also states she has had a sore throat and a cough for the past four days. Her physician performs a detailed history and exam. Her physician orders a chest x-ray to rule out pneumonia. The medical decision making is straightforward.

   a. 99203
   b. 99214
   c. 99204
   d. 99212

4. LO 9.1 A woman is referred to an orthopedic surgeon's office by her primary care physician for evaluation of a fracture of her right humerus. The consulting physician performs a problem-focused history and exam; medical decision making is of low complexity. He also dictates a letter to inform the primary care physician of his findings and treatment plan. What code would report this service?

   a. 99241
   b. 99242
   c. 99204
   d. 99214

5. LO 9.5 A patient is airlifted to the hospital due to traumatic injuries suffered in a fall while hiking a mountain. A bone is protruding through the skin of his arm, and his right leg and ankle appear to be fractured in several places. The patient is unconscious and appears to be suffering from internal injuries. The physician performs critical care services for the next 2 hours and 10 minutes. How would you appropriately report this service?

   a. 99291 X 2
   b. 99291 X 1 and 99292 X 1
   c. 99291 X 1 and 99292 X 2
   d. 99291 X 1 and 99292 X 3

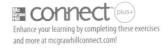
Enhance your learning by completing these exercises
and more at mcgrawhillconnect.com!

CHAPTER 9 | EVALUATION AND MANAGEMENT SERVICES, PART II: CODE SELECTION   243

6. LO 9.2 Over the next several days, the patient in the previous scenario is seen in the hospital by her physician. On day two, the physician performs an expanded problem-focused history and exam with medical decision making of low complexity. On day three, she performs a detailed history and exam with medical decision making of moderate complexity. On day four, she performs a problem-focused history and exam with medical decision making of low complexity. On day five, she takes 25 minutes to discharge the patient to her home, order physical therapy, and arrange a follow-up visit within seven days. What codes would be reported for days 2–5?

   a. 99232, 99233, 99231, 99238
   b. 99233, 99232, 99231, 99239
   c. 99231, 99232, 99232, 99238
   d. 99232, 99233, 99231, 99239

7. LO 9.6 A physician admits his patient to a skilled nursing facility after the patient suffers a fractured femur. He examines her medical chart for her vital signs and stability for hip replacement surgery within the next seven days. He performs a comprehensive history and exam with medical decision making of high complexity. On day two, he performs a problem-focused history and exam with medical decision making of low complexity. On days three and four, he performs a problem-focused history and exam with medical decision making of straightforward complexity. On day five, he discharges the patient from the skilled nursing facility without documenting the time to perform the discharge services. What codes would report the five days of treatment?

   a. 99307, 99306, 99306, 99308, 99316
   b. 99305, 99307, 99307, 99308, 99315
   c. 99306, 99307, 99307, 99307, 99315
   d. 99306, 99307, 99307, 99309, 99316

8. LO 9.11 In a rural part of Northern California, a young couple is trying to comfort their six-day-old infant, who has suddenly developed a fever of 104 degrees. Not knowing what else to do, they call the baby's pediatrician and request that he come to their home to evaluate the infant. After a comprehensive history and exam with medical decision making of high complexity, the physician determines that the baby should be transported to a hospital as soon as possible and requests an air ambulance to the closest hospital. The physician accompanies the infant during the 40-minute transport to the hospital, where another physician admits the infant for critical care. What codes would the pediatrician report for these services?

   a. 99350, 99466
   b. 99350, 99467
   c. 99205, 99285
   d. 99351, 99284

9. LO 9.1 A 52-year-old male presents to the cardiologist's office for an opinion on the advice of a friend after sharing that he had chest pain after walking on the treadmill and has gotten progressively worse each day he uses the treadmill. He tells the cardiologist, "I feel like my chest is pounding so hard it is going to explode." The physician orders an EKG and echo Doppler as soon as possible. He performs a comprehensive history and exam with medical decision making of high complexity. What code describes the cardiologist's services?

   a. 99213
   b. 99245
   c. 99204
   d. 99205

10. L0 9.4 A five-year-old boy presents to the emergency room with his mother. The child has a rusty nail in his foot. The emergency room physician performs an expanded problem-focused history and exam with medical decision making of low complexity. The physician removes the nail and gives the boy a tetanus injection. What code describes this visit?

   a. 99201
   b. 99281
   c. 99291
   d. 99282

11. L0 9.1 A patient goes to his podiatrist's office for the evaluation and management of a hard piece of skin on the bottom of her foot. The doctor has treated this patient for a plantar wart similar to this about two years ago. The physician performs a problem-focused history and exam with medical decision making of straightforward complexity. He also prescribes medications. What code describes this service?

   a. 99212
   b. 99203
   c. 99213
   d. 99241

12. L0 9.9 A 37-year-old woman presents to her physician's office for her annual well-woman exam. She has seen this physician for her exams for six years. What code describes this visit?

   a. 99211
   b. 99291
   c. 99395
   d. 99396

13. L0 9.4 A 21-year-old mother presents to the emergency room with her nine-month-old baby girl who has been up all night crying with a fever of 103 degrees and having difficulty breathing. After the emergency room physician performs a comprehensive exam and history, the physician determines that it is necessary to call the child's pediatrician to have him admit her to the hospital for treatment. He suspects she has respiratory syncytial virus and will be in need of IV antibiotics and breathing treatments. The medical decision making is of high complexity. What code describes this visit?

   a. 99284
   b. 99245
   c. 99285
   d. 99205

14. L0 9.5 In the previous scenario, the child's pediatrician admits her to the hospital and performs 93 minutes of face-to-face critical care services on the baby. He visits and examines the patient daily for the next four days, providing critical care services on each of those days. What code(s) describe(s) the pediatrician's services?

   a. 99471, 99472, 99472, 99472, 99472, or 99471 and 99472 X 4
   b. 99473, 99474, 99474, 99474, 99474, or 99473 and 99474 X 4
   c. 99291, 99292 X 4
   d. 99385 X 4

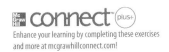
Enhance your learning by completing these exercises
and more at mcgrawhillconnect.com!

15. LO 9.9 A 21-year-old woman goes to her doctor's office for her annual exam. She tells her doctor she feels fine but sometimes during the month she gets sharp pains in her pelvic area. The pain seems to get worse when she is about to start to menstruate. In addition to the annual physical exam, the physician performs a detailed history and exam. What code(s) describe(s) the visit?

    a. 99385-25, 99214
    b. 99395, 99214-25
    c. 99215-25
    d. 99396-25, 99212

16. LO 9.4 A patient presents to the emergency room complaining of chest pain and difficulty breathing. She states that she had gotten into an argument with her boyfriend and was very upset. She is due to get married in three days, and she says the tightness in her chest has been getting worse for the past two days. The physician decides to admit her to observation for additional tests. The physician performs a comprehensive history and exam with medical decision making of low complexity. He determines that the patient has been experiencing anxiety attacks, prescribes some medication, and discharges her four hours later. What code describes the visit?

    a. 99217
    b. 99234
    c. 99218
    d. 99236

17. LO 9.2 A physician is discharging his patient. He spends an hour talking to the patient and his family. He spends an additional 45 minutes completing medical records, referrals, and prescriptions at the nurses' station. He documents the time he started and the time he finished his activities. Which of the following CPT codes describes these services?

    a. 99231
    b. 99238
    c. 99234
    d. 99239

18. LO 9.6 A doctor visits his patient in the rest home. The patient has a history of chronic obstructive pulmonary disease, smoking, shortness of breath, and tightness in his chest. The doctor performs a problem-focused history and exam with medical decision making of moderate complexity. Which of the following CPT codes best describes this physician's services?

    a. 99354
    b. 99334
    c. 99214
    d. 99336

19. LO 9.2 A physician admits his patient to the hospital for treatment of an abscess under the patient's arm. After ordering a CT scan, the physician also requests a consultation by an infectious disease doctor. The consulting physician sees the patient in the hospital, performs a detailed history and exam, and requests that the patient be taken to surgery for incision and drainage of the abscess. The medical decision making is of moderate complexity. What code describes this service?

    a. 99254
    b. 99243
    c. 99253
    d. 99203

20. LO 9.2 A patient is being discharged after being in the hospital for six days. She was admitted after having a cerebrovascular accident (stroke). The physician spends 30 minutes of face-to-face time with the patient to make sure she has an understanding of her treatment plan. The physician also spends 23 minutes documenting in the medical record, writing prescriptions, and discussing the patient's case with the nurse. These services are described by which of the following codes?

a. 99238
b. 99217
c. 99235
d. 99239

21. LO 9.1 A 12-year-old boy presents to his doctor's office with a sore arm after falling on the arm during football practice. The physician performs an expanded problem-focused history and exam, orders an x-ray, and confirms that there is no fracture. The physician determines that the patient sprained his muscles in his wrist, arm, and hand. He orders a bandage and instructs the boy to rest his arm. The medical decision making is of low complexity. What code describes this service?

a. 99203
b. 99214
c. 99213
d. 99202

22. LO 9.4 A patient presents to the emergency department with a laceration to her left eye. She was playing baseball and was attempting to catch the ball when another player collided with her. The other player's elbow broke the patient's glasses and caused a 4-cm laceration to the skin surrounding the eye. The emergency room doctor performs a detailed history and exam, determines that the patient's vision is unaffected, and applies several butterfly bandages. The medical decision making is of moderate complexity. Which of the following codes describes these services?

a. 99282
b. 99202
c. 99284
d. 99214

23. LO 9.2 A pulmonologist is caring for a patient who has severe asthma. The emergency room physician admitted the patient four days ago. The pulmonologist has seen her every day and is ready to discharge her. On day one, he performs a comprehensive history and exam with medical decision making of high complexity. On day two, he sees the patient before and after an inhalation treatment and performs a detailed history and exam with medical decision making of moderate complexity. On day three, he performs a problem-focused history and exam with medical decision making of straightforward complexity. On day four, the patient is ready to be discharged. The physician examines the patient, writes the prescriptions, and completes the medical record. These services are best described by the following CPT codes:

a. 99232, 99221, 99233, 99238
b. 99221, 99233, 99231, 99238
c. 99282, 99223, 99231, 99239
d. 99255, 99233, 99231, 99239

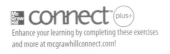

Enhance your learning by completing these exercises
and more at mcgrawhillconnect.com!

24. **L0 9.9** A 49-year-old woman presents to her physician's office for her annual exam. She has been living overseas for approximately four years and now returns to her physician for the exam. The following CPT code describes this visit:

   a. 99386
   b. 99204
   c. 99396
   d. 99214

25. **L0 9.5** An 18-month-old baby is being transported from one hospital to the nearest children's hospital to be treated for internal injuries sustained in an accident. The physician at the treating hospital will be accompanying her on the transport to children's hospital. This trip takes 96 minutes. The physician's services are best described by the following code:

   a. 99471, 99472
   b. 99466, 99467
   c. 99291, 99292
   d. 99466, 99467 X 3

Applying Your Skills

Use the CPT manual to determine the correct code(s) to report the following E/M services, including modifiers where appropriate.

1. **L0 9.1** A 63-year-old female presents to the office for the first time for evaluation and management of chest pain on exertion. The medical assistant aids in obtaining a comprehensive history, and the physician performs a comprehensive exam. The medical decision making is of moderate complexity. _____

2. **L0 9.1** A patient travels out of state and needs a refill of his medication. He calls his usual physician's office to ask that they call in a prescription to a pharmacy near his vacation site. Which code would the physician report? _____

3. **L0 9.1** A 55-year-old male is seen in the medical office for follow-up evaluation and management of his hypertension and fatigue. He is taking a beta-blocker. An expanded problem-focused history and physical exam are performed; medical decision making is of low complexity. _____

4. **L0 9.2** A 72-year-old woman is admitted to the hospital for the examination and treatment of pneumonia. She is given IV antibiotic therapy. A detailed history is obtained. A comprehensive examination is performed, and medical decision making is of low complexity. _____

5. **L0 9.1** A 45-year-old male is following up with his psychiatrist for his 12-year history of bipolar disorder. He is responding well to a combination of pharmacotherapy and psychotherapy. Further psychotherapy and renewal of his prescription are provided. A detailed history of present illness (HPI) and past, family, and social history (PFSH) had already been obtained and documented during a previous office visit. A detailed exam is performed and medical decision making is of moderate complexity. _____

6. **L0 9.2** A 60-year-old male is admitted to the hospital with bronchitis and acute respiratory distress. The patient's condition is of moderate to high severity. A comprehensive history and examination is performed. The social history portion of the PFSH indicates that the patient is a smoker. At least two elements from each of at least nine organ systems or body areas are examined. Medical decision making is of moderate complexity. _____

7. **LO 9.2** A 56-year-old female with type II diabetes mellitus was admitted to the hospital yesterday for regulation of her insulin therapy. The admitting physician performed a problem-focused exam, which includes the performance and documentation of 1–5 elements identified by a bullet in one or more organ systems or body areas. The examination included obtaining the patient's temperature, pulse, respiration, blood pressure, and weight in addition to the following review of systems: cardiovascular, genitourinary, and endocrine. The medical decision making was of low complexity. _____

8. **LO 9.2, LO 9.4** On April 23, John Smith is seen in the emergency room for acute chest pain due to cardiac ischemia and pulmonary embolus. He has a history of myocardial infarction, and changes are seen on his electrocardiogram (EKG). Dr. Koon performs a comprehensive history and exam. The patient is then admitted to the hospital. The admitting physician, Dr. Koon, asks that the attending physician, Dr. Sherman, see the patient for subsequent hospital care. Dr. Sherman performs a level 5 evaluation and management. Which two codes apply in this case? _____

9. **LO 9.4** A 26-year-old female presents to the emergency room for a tetanus toxoid immunization after having cut her leg on metal shelving in a department store. In order to evaluate and manage the patient's care, the physician performs a problem-focused history and exam. The medical decision making is straightforward. The problem-focused history contains the patient's chief complaint and 1–3 elements of the HPI. In this case, location, context, and severity are documented in the patient's medical record. _____

10. **LO 9.5** An 18-year-old is admitted to the hospital after a near-fatal car accident. The patient sustained a traumatic brain injury in addition to a liver laceration after having been struck by an 18-wheeler truck. It takes 4 hours and 15 minutes to evaluate and manage the patient. Assign all codes necessary for this case. _____

11. **LO 9.2, LO 9.7** A 32-year-old female is admitted to the hospital with acute bronchospasm. A comprehensive history and examination is performed, and it is determined that the patient has a history of asthma. The patient's condition worsens. The physician has to spend 1 hour and 30 minutes beyond what is usual for this patient in this setting. Medical decision making is of high complexity. Report all codes that apply in this situation. _____

12. **LO 9.1, LO 9.9** A 45-year-old female was last seen by her physician 90 days ago for the incision and drainage of an abscess. She is now being seen in her doctor's office for an annual physical. A preexisting problem is addressed in the process of evaluating the expanded problem. The problem is significant enough to require additional work. The medical decision making is of low complexity. _____

13. **LO 9.1, LO 9.2** A 39-year-old male is admitted for observation of respiratory distress on April 3rd and discharged the next day, April 4th. A comprehensive history and exam is performed, and medical decision making is of high complexity. The patient is given instructions for continuing his care at home. _____

14. **LO 9.2, LO 9.4** An 87-year-old man arrives at the emergency department on April 3rd with what appear to be psychosis and delirium. An expanded problem-focused history and exam are performed. Medical decision making is of low complexity. The patient is observed for more than 8 hours on April 4th and then discharged on the same day after it is discovered he only has a urinary tract infection (UTI). A more detailed history and exam is obtained on April 4th. He is prescribed an antibiotic. _____

15. **LO 9.2** A 65-year-old female with no insurance is admitted to the hospital for a cerebral vascular accident secondary to an embolism. She has Brocha's aphasia and left sided paralysis. A comprehensive history and exam is performed. Medical decision making is of moderate complexity. The patient's total length of stay is 95 days. On each subsequent day, the healthcare team focuses on the problem as the patient recovers. She has applied for Medicaid and is awaiting approval. _____

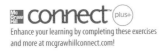

Enhance your learning by completing these exercises
and more at mcgrawhillconnect.com!

16. LO 9.11 An infant born premature at 27 weeks and weighing 1,400 grams suffers from hyaline membrane disease and associated respiratory distress. The infant is admitted to the NICU, intubated, and given surfactant.
_____

17. LO 9.11 In the process of adjudicating a subrogation claim, the law office representing an insurance company wishes to determine if a patient member is eligible for disability due to new-onset epilepsy that is thought to be due to embolic stroke secondary to birth control pill use. Prior to disability insurance certificates being issued, a special evaluation is done by the treating physician that includes completion of a medical history, examination, assessment, and calculation of impairment; development of a medical plan; and completion of necessary documentation for disability certificates. _____

18. LO 9.9 A psychologist who conducts behavioral medicine research and provides ambulatory outpatient therapy for a university sees a patient who is at risk for developing diabetes and heart disease secondary to obesity. The patient is genetically predisposed to both diseases, and her weight is a concern. Baseline data are gathered, and counseling is provided for risk factor reduction. Diet and exercise are the focus of behavioral change for this patient. Barriers to change are identified. In order to test the hypothesis that cognitive behavioral therapy is efficacious in the treatment of eating disorders, psychology students will provide 23 one-hour cognitive behavioral therapy sessions under the auspices of the head psychologist. _____

19. LO 9.10 A violent tornado rips through Tornado Alley, Texas. The high winds down power lines over a 150-mile radius. Two telephone line repairmen are sent out to fix the downed lines, and one worker accidently touches a high-voltage line with his equipment. He dies instantly. As the second repairman tries to save his friend and coworker, he also receives 13,500 volts of electricity, which cause third-degree burns on one forearm and hand. The surviving worker files a medical insurance claim with his employer for worker's compensation of all medical claims resulting from this work-related injury. The patient has authorized a guardian of care to communicate with his provider over the telephone regarding his medical care because the physician will not be seeing the patient within 24 hours or at her next available appointment. The medical discussion takes one hour.
_____

20. LO 9.4 A 36-year-old man met a woman on an online dating site. After two online chats, they decided to meet for a first date. It was love at first sight, and the two began kissing. Prior to meeting, the woman had been eating chocolate-covered peanuts, not realizing that her boyfriend has a food allergy to peanuts. He immediately went into anaphylactic shock, for which emergency medical services was called to transport him to the hospital. The physician directs emergency care in a two-way communication with the ambulance personnel outside the hospital.
_____

21. LO 9.6 An internal medicine physician admits one of his geriatric patients to an assisted living facility, where she can get personal care she could not otherwise provide for herself after having sustained a brain hemorrhage. The physician obtains a detailed history and performs a detailed examination for this newly admitted patient. Medical decision making is of moderate complexity and includes coordination of her care with other healthcare providers and the patient's adult children. _____

22. LO 9.6 A juvenile is mandated by the court to a boarding house for 18 months as an alternative to going to jail as a result of several arrests for aggravated assault and theft. The 16-year-old has dual diagnoses of mental illness and substance abuse. He has been diagnosed with manic depression, generalized anxiety disorder, and obsessive-compulsive disorder. He also displays sociopathy and oppositional defiance. He is undergoing treatment for meth-amphetamine and heroin addiction. The patient also is being treated for hepatitis C resulting from IV drug abuse. A physician provides evaluation and management services for this patient, which includes an expanded problem-focused history and exam. Medical decision making is of low complexity. Medications are checked and prescriptions renewed. _____

23. **LO 9.3** A 40-year-old non-Medicare patient with a history of infectious thyroiditis, hypothyroidism, and parathyroidism sees her primary care physician with a chief complaint of episodic pain radiating through her left side. After baseline radiological evaluation and labs such as C-reactive protein for inflammatory disease are obtained and reviewed, the primary care physician refers the patient to see a rheumatologist to rule out any other autoimmune diseases such as systemic lupus erythematosus. Vitamin and hormone levels are also obtained. Lab results show a severely low vitamin D level. The rheumatologist prescribes 50,000 IU of vitamin D in addition to supplemental calcium to support the parathyroid gland, which pulls calcium and vitamin D from the bones. What code would you report for this consult with medical decision making of moderate complexity?

   _____

24. **LO 9.1** A 56-year-old female with a history of diverticular disease and esophageal esophagitis has spent a significant amount of time in the gastrointestinal unit of the university hospital with a gastrointestinal bleed. As a result of her disease and its complications, she has had poor absorption of nutrients and has often received total parenteral nutrition (TPN). She is now out of the hospital and sees her internal medicine physician for routine follow-up. The physician does not see the patient at this encounter. The medical assistant administers a vitamin B_{12} injection.

   _____

25. **LO 9.2** A patient is driving when she begins to have tunnel vision and shortness of breath. Her heart starts to race and she becomes intensely fearful that she may die. She manages to get herself to the emergency room despite her feelings of impending doom. The patient's blood pressure is abnormally high. Cardiac protocol is followed to ensure the patient is not suffering from cardiac disease. Arterial blood gases (ABGs), chest x-ray (CXR), electrocardiogram (EKG), complete blood count (CBC), complete metabolic profile (CMP), and thyroid levels (T3, T4, and TSH) are normal, so the emergency room physician decides to admit the patient overnight for further observation. The patient is given a beta-blocker to reduce the heart rate and control her anxiety. An endocrinologist is consulted to follow the patient, and he orders a 24-hour urine test to check for catecholamines. The patient does not stay in the hospital more than 24 hours when it is determined that she had a panic attack. A psychiatrist prescribes medications and the patient is discharged. The presenting problem is of high severity, and three out of three key components must be reported for this comprehensive level of care and medical decision making of high complexity. What code(s) would you report for the hospital care? (Each provider will independently bill for his or her respective services.) _____

26. **LO 9.2** A 29-year-old patient with end-stage renal disease is admitted to the transitional care unit. Concurrent care is provided by his primary care physician, his nephrologists, and a pulmonologist. A cardiologist is called on the case later to assess the patient's hypertension secondary to chronic kidney disease. The patient is admitted directly to the hospital after complications in care while undergoing dialysis treatments at an outpatient dialysis facility. He receives a comprehensive examination for his first hospital day and expanded problem focused care on subsequent hospital days. The patient's total length of stay is 30 days. _____

27. **LO 9.6** A 76-year-old female with a 10-year history of transient ischemic attacks sustains a cerebral vascular accident (CVA). After the patient has spent six months in the hospital as an inpatient, the physician makes a decision to discuss nursing home services with the patient and family, because the patient can no longer care for herself. The patient's adult children are not able to be attentive to the care of their mother at home, because they both work full-time and raise small children. After discussions with both the patient and family, a social worker is called to coordinate the patient's transition to the nursing home facility. What code would you report for the admission E/M services involving comprehensive history and physical examination and medical decision making of moderate complexity? _____

connect plus+
Enhance your learning by completing these exercises
and more at mcgrawhillconnect.com!   CHAPTER 9 | EVALUATION AND MANAGEMENT SERVICES, PART II: CODE SELECTION   251

28. LO 9.4 A patient is admitted through the local university's Emergency Psychiatry Department. A multidisciplinary treatment team—consisting of a head psychiatrist, nurse, social worker, medical residents, and psychology students—does an intake and assessment on the patient, who has hallucinations and delusions after sniffing toluene. The patient talks to skeletons coming out of her coffee table while her husband is asleep in the other room. The patient's husband is becoming increasingly concerned, not to mention the disruption it has caused in his sleep due to the loud conversations taking place between the patient and the skeletons. The patient reports that the skeletons are telling her to kill herself. Because of her delusions, the patient poses a significant threat to her own life and physiological functioning. A comprehensive history is obtained by a psychology student. A comprehensive exam is conducted by the medical resident. The medical decision making is discussed by the entire treatment team, and the disposition to admit the patient to a psychiatric care facility is finally determined by the head psychiatrist. What code would you report for the emergency room visit? _____

29. LO 9.8 A 30-year-old health-conscious young mother was at the gym working out on a treadmill when she passed out. Emergency medical services was called, and she was admitted directly to the hospital. The patient's parents and husband arrived promptly to the hospital once they were contacted by the charge nurse on the ventilator care unit. A CT scan of the patient's brain revealed an aneurysm. A neurologist was called on the case to perform an electroencephalogram. After finding two flatline EEGs, an interdisciplinary treatment team of healthcare professionals met face to face with the patient's family to discuss removing life support and do not resuscitate (DNR) orders. The team spent over 30 minutes together in a private waiting room. A transplant doctor was also called to discuss harvesting vital organs. A total of three qualified healthcare professionals from different specialties were involved in the patient's evaluation and management. _____

30. LO 9.8 A 63-year-old male works as a welder at a power plant. During one of his contracted jobs, he steps on a nail that punctures through his boot and into his foot. He has a history of diabetes mellitus. The patient has poor circulation in his extremities due to peripheral neuropathy, a secondary manifestation of the disease. Due to progressive complications in wound healing, the patient requires home health services. Recurrent physician supervision and IV therapy are required to treat progressive local and systemic bacterial infections. Sixty minutes of physician supervision is provided once a month. _____

Thinking It Through

Use your critical-thinking skills to fill in the blanks or provide short answers to the questions below.

1. LO 9.9 Which two factors must be known in order to select the appropriate code for preventive medicine services?

_____

_____

2. LO 9.1 How are evaluation and management codes for office visits categorized?

_____

_____

3. LO 9.1, LO 9.6, LO 9.9 When selecting E/M codes for outpatient services:

   a. How many key components must meet the level defined in the code descriptor for a new patient?

   _____

   b. How many key components must meet the level defined in the code descriptor for an established patient?

   _____

4. LO 9.7 When coding for evaluation and management services for an office visit that lasted longer than expected due to the patient having complications of the underlying disease, is it appropriate to report the prolonged services code alone? Explain the reason for your answer.

_____

_____

5. LO 9.3 A physician refers a Medicare patient to another physician for evaluation and recommendation of further management. Is this service reported with an office consultation code (99241–99245)? Give the main reason for your answer.

_____

_____

6. LO 9.7 How are prolonged services codes for outpatient services reported?

_____

_____

7. LO 9.10 Describe the circumstances in which physicians may report telephone calls.

_____

_____

8. LO 9.2, LO 9.7 What determines the time considered for purposes of selecting E/M codes for hospital inpatient services?

_____

_____

9. LO 9.11 What two factors determine which codes are used to report neonatal and pediatric critical care services?

_____

_____

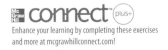

10 ANESTHESIA SERVICES

Learning Outcomes *After completing this chapter, students should be able to:*

10.1 Select anesthesia codes based on surgical procedures.

10.2 Report anesthesia time.

10.3 Use anesthesia modifiers and add-on codes.

10.4 Calculate the total number of anesthesia units for services provided.

10.5 Select anesthesia codes for surgical procedures on specific body parts.

10.6 Choose anesthesia codes for specific procedures.

Key Terms

American Society of Anesthesiologists

Analgesia

Anesthesia assistant

Anesthesiologist

Base unit

Certified registered nurse anesthetist

General anesthesia

Local anesthesia

Monitored anesthesia care

Qualifying circumstances add-on code

Regional anesthesia

Time unit

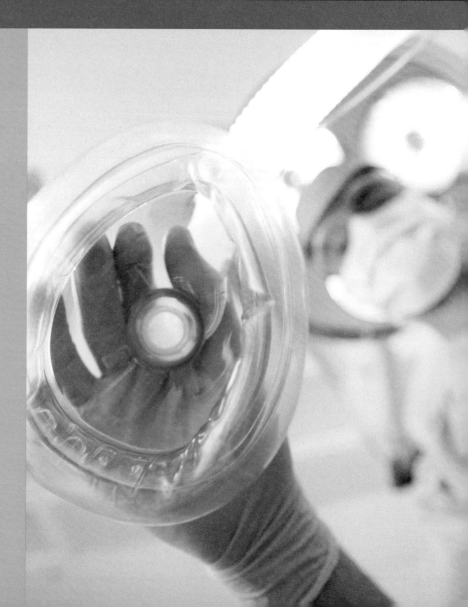

Introduction

Anesthesia involves rendering a patient insensitive to pain by performing procedures and administering medications to patients undergoing surgery or other uncomfortable procedures. Anesthesia services may be administered by several healthcare professionals: **anesthesiologists** (physicians specially trained in anesthesia); **certified registered nurse anesthetists** (CRNAs, specially trained nurses providing anesthesia services, often under the supervision of a physician); or **anesthesia assistants** (AAs, non-nurse professionals trained to provide anesthesia services under the direction of anesthesiologists). In addition to performing procedures and administering medications, anesthesia providers also monitor and manage physiological changes caused by the surgical procedure or by the anesthetic itself.

There are several main types of anesthesia, including general, regional, and local anesthesia. **General anesthesia** involves making the patient unconscious. During this time, it is necessary for the anesthesia provider to carefully monitor the patient's physiological functions, including blood pressure, heart rate, respiration, and oxygen saturation. It is often necessary for the anesthesia provider to either assist the patient's breathing or to take over that function completely by using mechanical ventilators.

Regional anesthesia is the term used when the anesthesia provider performs procedures to make a large portion of the patient's body numb while the patient remains awake. These procedures include spinal or epidural anesthesia that numbs the lower portion of the body or special nerve blocks (injections around large nerves that provide sensation to an entire region of the body) that make an arm or leg numb. **Local anesthesia** is a term used to indicate that the provider makes just the area being operated on numb, usually by injecting local anesthetic agents into the skin and subcutaneous tissues surrounding the operative area. Patients generally remain awake during regional or local anesthesia, although they may be sedated to reduce awareness and anxiety during the procedure.

Monitored anesthesia care (MAC) is another type of anesthesia service. MAC often involves sedating patients through the use of various medications, but not to the extent that they are completely unconscious. During MAC, anesthesia providers monitor the patient's physiological vital signs to detect changes that may pose a threat to the patient's safety, just as they would during other types of anesthesia.

CODER'S TIP

Medicare and some commercial payers will only pay for MAC services when they are medically necessary, based on either the type of surgical procedure the patient is undergoing or the general medical condition of the patient.

10.1 Selecting Anesthesia CPT Codes Based on the Surgical Procedure

Coding for anesthesia services is different than coding for other medical procedures. The codes that describe anesthesia services are not determined by what the anesthesiologist does to or for the patient. Instead, the choice of the CPT code that best describes the anesthesia service is determined by what other providers, such as surgeons, are doing to the patient that makes the anesthesia necessary.

Coders must know the underlying procedures performed on the patient during the anesthetic to select the proper anesthesia code. Except in a very few specific circumstances, CPT codes describing anesthetics do not depend on whether the anesthesia is a general, regional, epidural, spinal, or MAC anesthetic. Also, in most cases the fees for anesthesia services do not depend on the type of anesthetic, thereby eliminating a bias to choose one type over another based on rates.

anesthesiologists
Physicians specially trained in anesthesia.

certified registered nurse anesthetists
Specially trained nurses who provide anesthesia services, often under the supervision of a physician.

anesthesia assistants
Non-nurse professionals trained to provide anesthesia services under the direction of anesthesiologists.

general anesthesia
Involves making the patient unconscious and often requires the anesthesia provider to either assist the patient's breathing or to take over that function completely using mechanical ventilators.

regional anesthesia
The term used when the anesthesia provider performs procedures to make a large portion of the patient's body numb while the patient remains awake or mildly sedated.

local anesthesia
The term used to indicate that the provider makes just the area being operated on numb, usually by injecting local anesthetic agents into the skin and subcutaneous tissues surrounding the operative area.

monitored anesthesia care (MAC)
A type of anesthesia service during which the provider monitors the patient throughout the surgical procedure, often sedating them through the use of various medications, but not necessarily to the extent that they are completely unconscious.

A single anesthesia code may be used to describe anesthesia for a number of different surgical procedures that involve a general area of the body or specific body part. The anesthetics for these surgical procedures may share some common factors, such as patient position, surgical site, access to airway, anticipated blood loss, need for fluid or blood replacement, effects on blood pressure, and other anatomical or physiological factors. Anesthesia codes describing typical anesthesia services for surgery on a particular body part are usually described in general anatomical terms with a "not otherwise specified" notation.

CODER'S TIP

Anesthesia codes are grouped according to the general area of the body that is being operated on by the surgeon. A single anesthesia code may describe anesthesia services for many different surgical procedures. For example, CPT code 00140 (Anesthesia for procedures on the eye; not otherwise specified) may be used to describe anesthesia for more than 150 different surgical procedures on the eye.

More specific codes describe anesthesia for multiple specific surgical procedures, such as CPT code 00142 (Anesthesia for procedures on the eye; iridectomy), which describes anesthesia for about seven specific surgical CPT codes.

Separate anesthesia codes are used to describe anesthetics that are significantly more or less difficult than the typical anesthetic on that particular body part. Specific anesthesia codes are also used to describe procedures that are commonly performed, even if the typical anesthetic for that procedure is similar to anesthetics for other procedures in the "not otherwise specified" group. These specific anesthesia codes may be either stand-alone codes or indented under the "not otherwise specified" code.

The section of CPT codes that describe anesthesia for intracranial procedures consists of one "not otherwise specified" code and eight indented codes:

00210	Anesthesia for intracranial procedures; not otherwise specified
00211	craniotomy or craniectomy for evacuation of hematoma
00212	subdural taps
00214	burr holes, including ventriculography
00215	cranioplasty or elevation of depressed skull fracture, extradural (simple or compound)
00216	vascular procedures
00218	procedures in sitting position
00220	cerebrospinal fluid shunting procedures
00222	electrocoagulation of intracranial nerve

There is no specific code that describes anesthesia for a surgical procedure to remove an intracranial tumor. This is reported with the "not otherwise specified" code 00210. Anesthesia for an intracranial vascular procedure, however, is reported with the specific indented code 00216.

Each indented code (00211–00222) should be read as if it includes the phrase "Anesthesia for intracranial vascular procedures" before the more specific portion of the code descriptor that is printed.

CODER'S TIP

To report anesthesia services, coders should first identify the surgical procedure performed. Next, locate the section of anesthesia CPT codes that would include that procedure. Then determine whether a specific anesthesia CPT code exists to describe

(Continued)

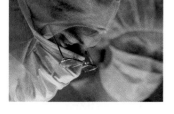

A single anesthesia code may describe anesthesia services for many different surgical procedures.

that anesthetic. If so, that CPT code is used to report the anesthesia procedure. If not, the "not otherwise specified" code describing anesthesia services for surgical procedures in that anatomical region is used to report the anesthetic.

CODING EXAMPLE

An anesthesiologist provides anesthesia for a total knee arthroplasty. To report this anesthetic, the coder would locate the section of anesthesia CPT codes describing anesthesia for procedures on the knee (01320–01444). One indented code, 01402 (total knee arthroplasty) describes this procedure. Because this is an indented code, the full descriptor includes the first part of the descriptor from the nonindented code 01400. Therefore, the full descriptor for code 01402 is "Anesthesia for open or surgical arthroscopic procedures on knee joint; total knee arthroplasty." The coder would report this anesthetic with CPT code 01402.

To report anesthesia for surgery to repair a fracture of the lower femur involving the knee joint, the coder would review the same section of anesthesia CPT codes. In this case, however, there is no specific code to describe that surgical procedure, so the coder would report the anesthesia with the nonspecific code, 01400 (Anesthesia for open or surgical arthroscopic procedures on knee joint; not otherwise specified).

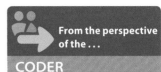

From the perspective of the . . .

CODER
Identify the surgical location and specific surgical procedure to select the correct anesthesia code. The surgical location is usually enough to choose the range of anesthesia codes, but the specific surgical procedure is usually necessary to select the correct anesthesia code.

Each anesthesia CPT code is assigned a number of **base units** that represents the relative value of that anesthetic compared to other anesthetics based on expected or potential difficulties. Base units are whole numbers that range between 3 units (anesthesia for surgical procedures that generally pose little risk to patients) and 30 units (anesthesia for a liver transplant). The number of anesthesia base units is one factor used to calculate payment for anesthesia services.

base unit
Whole number that represents the relative value of one anesthetic compared to other anesthetics based on expected or potential difficulties.

CODER'S TIP

At times, a surgeon may perform more than one surgical procedure during a single operative session. The surgeon will report all those procedures. Anesthesia providers, however, only report one anesthesia code but report time units describing the total time for all the procedures performed during that anesthetic. The anesthesia code used to report the anesthesia services is usually the one that has the highest number of base units. If several anesthesia codes have the same number of base units, the code that represents the major procedure should be reported.

EXERCISE 10.1

Also available in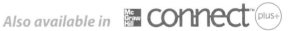

Select the letter that best completes the statement or answers the question.

1. Types of anesthesia include all of the following *except:*
   a. Regional anesthesia
   b. Cerebral anesthesia
   c. MAC
   d. Spinal anesthesia

(Continued)

2. A single anesthesia code is always used to describe anesthesia for the following:

   a. A single surgical procedure.

   b. A group of closely related surgical procedures on a single anatomical area.

   c. One or more surgical procedures.

   d. A single type of surgery performed on multiple anatomical areas.

Insert the word(s) to complete the sentence.

3. The code that describes the anesthesia services provided depends on _____.

10.2 Anesthesia Time Units

Another difference between coding for anesthesia services and coding for other medical services is that anesthesia services are the only procedures that are reported with a CPT code describing the anesthesia service provided plus a separate report of the time that the services were provided. Other medical services outside the anesthesia code range may include a time element as part of the code descriptor, but that is not the same. Unlike E/M codes, anesthesia CPT code descriptors do not include a time element. Instead time is reported separately in addition to the CPT code that describes the anesthesia service.

From the perspective of the . . .

CODER

Anesthesia time begins when the provider begins preparing the patient for the anesthetic and ends when the patient is safely placed under post-anesthesia care. This is likely to be different than the beginning and ending times of the surgical procedure.

CODER'S TIP

It is important to understand the differences between codes that include time as part of their code descriptor and anesthesia codes, which have time reported as a separate element. Codes describing psychotherapy include time elements as part of their code descriptors. See as an example code 90804 (Individual psychotherapy, insight oriented, behavior modifying, and/or supportive, in an office or outpatient facility, approximately 20 to 30 minutes face to face with the patient). In contrast to 90804, anesthesia codes do not contain time elements in their descriptors. Rather, anesthesia time is reported separately from and in addition to the CPT code that describes the anesthetic.

time unit
A specific number of minutes used to measure blocks of anesthesia time.

Anesthesia time begins when the anesthesia provider begins to prepare the patient for anesthesia and ends when the patient is safely placed under postanesthesia supervision. Anesthesia time may be reported in minutes (the total number of minutes anesthesia services were provided) or in **time units** (by converting the minutes into discrete units). Time units are defined as a specific number of minutes. Most payers recognize 15-minute units, with varying rules regarding when the time "clicks over" to the next unit. Some payers recognize 10- or 12-minute units. Medicare also uses 15 minutes per anesthesia time unit but converts the time into tenths of a unit. Medicare assigns one time unit for each full 15-minute interval plus 0.1 units for each additional 1.5 minutes.

Because there is variation among payers regarding time units, coders should assume that time units are calculated on the basis of 15-minute intervals, and any portion of the next time unit is counted as a whole unit.

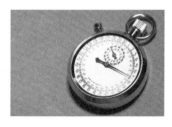

Anesthesia codes differ from other CPT codes in that they consist of a code for the anesthesia service plus a time unit. Other services, including E/M services, incorporate time into their codes but do not contain a separate code to report time spent.

CODING EXAMPLES

An anesthesiologist provides anesthesia for an arthroscopic procedure on the hip joint. Anesthesia begins at 11:15 a.m. and ends at 12:10 p.m. The coder would report this procedure with CPT code 01202 (Anesthesia for arthroscopic procedures of hip

(Continued)

joint) plus time. The time may either be reported as 55 minutes or as four time units (three time units for the first 45 minutes of anesthesia time plus one additional unit for the remaining 10 minutes of time).

CODER'S TIP

Beginning in 2013, the new standards for electronic transmission of claim information will only allow anesthesia time to be reported in minutes, not units. Each payer to which claims are submitted will convert anesthesia time into units for payment purposes based on its individual policies. It is possible that future standards will again allow time to be reported in units, so coders should understand the basics of anesthesia time reporting.

EXERCISE 10.2

Also available in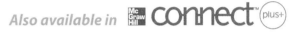

Answer the following questions.

1. Assuming that time is measured in 15-minute time units, how many units would be reported for an anesthetic that was a total of 3 hours and 10 minutes? _____

2. If time is reported in actual minutes, how many units would be reported for anesthesia services lasting from 8:27 a.m. until 10:35 a.m.? _____

3. How are time units reported? _____

10.3 Secondary Aspects of Anesthesia Coding

Selecting the appropriate anesthesia CPT code and calculating anesthesia time are the primary coding activities necessary for reporting anesthesia services. There are several secondary aspects that also must be included to report anesthesia services completely.

Accurately coding anesthesia services includes the use of unique anesthesia modifiers that describe the physical status of the patient, the professional credentials of the individual providing the anesthetic, and reasons for MAC anesthesia. Add-on codes describe qualifying circumstances that make anesthesia more difficult or a greater risk for the patient.

Physical Status Modifiers

Modifiers P1–P6 describe the physical status of the patient to whom an anesthetic is administered. Physical status modifiers describe the underlying health status of the patient in increasing severity:

P1   A normal healthy patient.
P2   A patient with mild systemic disease.
P3   A patient with severe systemic disease.
P4   A patient with severe systemic disease that is a constant threat to life.
P5   A moribund patient who is not expected to survive without the operation.
P6   A brain-dead patient whose organs are being removed for donor purposes.

Some payers allow anesthesia providers to add extra units for procedures provided to patients with physical status described by P3–P5. Medicare does not allow these extra units. Payers that do allow extra units usually allow one extra anesthesia unit for P3, two extra units for P4, and three extra units for P5. P1, P2, and P6 typically do not have any additional unit values associated with those modifiers. Patients with physical status P1 or P2 do not require significant additional anesthesia to justify additional payments. P6 is used to identify a brain-dead patient undergoing organ donation procedures. The physical status of this patient is included in the base unit value of CPT code 01990 (Physiological support for harvesting of organ(s) from brain-dead patient).

CODER'S TIP

Although not every payer recognizes P modifiers for payment purposes, coders should attach a P modifier to each anesthesia CPT code to appropriately report the patient's physical status when reporting anesthesia services. Some coders omit these modifiers when reporting anesthesia services to payers that do not recognize these modifiers for payment purposes, but this may result in lost payments.

The anesthesia provider should determine the appropriate P modifier. Coders usually do not have the necessary clinical information to determine the physical status of the patient. This is primarily a clinical assessment.

Modifiers Identifying Professional Credentials of Anesthesia Providers

Several HCPCS modifiers identify the training and credentials of the individual providing the anesthetic. An anesthesiologist is a physician (MD or DO) with the training and expertise to administer an anesthetic. Other providers, including certified registered nurse anesthetists (CRNA) or resident physicians in training, also may administer anesthetics. Various complex federal rules and state laws determine whether the CRNA or resident must be supervised and how that supervision is structured. HCPCS modifiers may be used to identify those supervisory relationships. The HCPCS modifiers used to identify anesthesia providers are:

AA   Anesthesia services performed personally by an anesthesiologist.
AD   Medical supervision by a physician; more than four concurrent anesthesia procedures.
GC   Anesthesia services provided by a resident physician under the direction of a teaching anesthesiologist.
QK   Medical direction of two, three, or four concurrent anesthesia procedures involving qualified individuals.
QX   CRNA service with medical direction by a physician.
QY   Medical direction of one CRNA by an anesthesiologist.
QZ   CRNA service without medical direction by a physician.

Modifiers Describing Reasons for Monitored Anesthesia Care (MAC)

MAC anesthesia is a specific anesthesia service. MAC usually includes varying levels of sedation and **analgesia**. Anesthesia providers monitor a patient under MAC anesthesia as they would a patient under a general or regional anesthetic. At times, an anesthesia provider may have to convert a MAC anesthesia procedure to a general anesthetic and should be qualified to do so.

Some payers, including Medicare, only pay for MAC anesthesia under specific circumstances. Several HCPCS modifiers are used to describe these, including:

QS   Monitored anesthesia care service.
G8   Monitored anesthesia care for a deep, complex, complicated, or markedly invasive surgical procedure.
G9   Monitored anesthesia care for a patient who has a history of severe cardiopulmonary condition.

analgesia
Lack of the sensation of pain without the loss of consciousness.

Qualifying Circumstances Add-on Codes

Some anesthetics are provided under circumstances that are significantly more difficult than usual or involve additional anesthetic techniques not usually employed during a typical anesthetic. These situations or additional techniques are identified through the use of one or more **qualifying circumstances add-on codes** in addition to the appropriate anesthesia CPT code:

- +99100 Anesthesia for a patient of extreme age, younger than 1 year and older than 70
- +99116 Anesthesia complicated by utilization of total body hypothermia
- +99135 Anesthesia complicated by utilization of controlled hypotension
- +99140 Anesthesia complicated by emergency conditions

Extreme age (younger than 1 year or older than 70 years of age) often makes the administration of anesthesia more difficult even in the absence of other underlying health problems. Total body hypothermia is achieved by cooling the patient's body to a very low temperature. This can cause physiological changes far beyond those usually seen during surgery or anesthesia. Controlled hypotension is achieved by adjusting very powerful medications that decrease blood pressure to levels that potentially can cause complications, such as injuries to the brain, heart, or other organs. Patients undergoing emergency surgery are at increased risk of anesthesia complications.

Some payers recognize qualifying circumstances add-on codes as additional units for payment purposes, typically allowing one additional anesthesia unit for code 99100, five additional anesthesia units for code 99116, five additional anesthesia units for code 99135, and two additional anesthesia units for code 22140.

> **qualifying circumstances add-on code**
> Code used to identify situations that are significantly more difficult than usual or involve additional anesthetic techniques not usually employed during a typical anesthetic.

CODER'S TIP

Add-on codes are never reported alone. They are only reported with other codes that describe primary services. Some add-on codes can only be reported with a specific primary code. Other add-on codes may be reported with a large number of primary codes. The four add-on codes that describe qualifying circumstances may be reported with any anesthesia code. More than one of these add-on codes may be reported.

> **From the perspective of the . . .**
>
> **CODER**
> The codes describing qualifying circumstances are not in the Anesthesia section, but instead are listed in the Medicine section of the CPT manual, which includes the 90000 series of codes.

EXERCISE 10.3

Also available in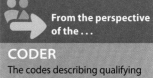

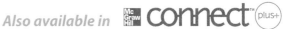

Use the CPT manual to answer the following questions.

1. What is the provider reporting if modifier QZ is added to an anesthesia CPT code?

   _____

2. Which modifier identifies when an anesthesia service is performed on a seven-month-old baby?

   _____

3. What does it mean when the modifier QS is submitted along with the anesthesia CPT code?

   _____

4. Can CPT code 99140 (Anesthesia complicated by emergency conditions) be reported on its own without a CPT code from the anesthesia range? _____

5. When is modifier G8 used? _____

10.4 Calculating Total Anesthesia Units

Anesthesia services are valued in anesthesia units. The total value is the sum of the base units for the particular anesthesia code, time units, physical status modifier units, and qualifying circumstances add-on code units. The basic formula is:

$$\text{Base units} + \text{Time units} + \text{Physical status modifier units} + \text{Qualifying circumstances add-on code units} = \text{Total anesthesia units}$$

Many payers, including Medicare, only recognize the first two elements in this equation. Those payers allow payment for the anesthesia base units plus time units. Coders should still report physical status modifiers and qualifying circumstances add-on codes. This information may be useful to anesthesia providers and payers interested in determining the general health of patients undergoing surgical procedures.

The base units for each anesthesia code are not listed in the CPT manual. The units may be found in other sources, including the *Relative Value Guide* published by the **American Society of Anesthesiologists** or in the Medicare fee schedules published by CMS.

American Society of Anesthesiologists
A professional society representing anesthesiologists.

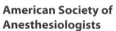
From the perspective of the . . .

CODER

The base units for each anesthesia code are not listed in the CPT manual. The units may be found in other sources, including the *Relative Value Guide* published by the American Society of Anesthesiologists or in the Medicare fee schedules published by CMS.

CODING EXAMPLE

A 72-year-old patient undergoes a total hip arthroplasty. The anesthesiologist assesses the patient before surgery and determines that the patient has severe systemic diseases, including diabetes, hypertension, and coronary artery disease. The patient is taken to the operating room for the procedure, which is accomplished without complications. The patient is taken to the postanesthesia care unit, and care is transferred to the nursing staff. The total anesthesia time is 2 hours and 23 minutes.

The coder is preparing to report the anesthesia services. The anesthesiologist reports time in 15-minute units. The CPT code that describes anesthesia for a total hip arthroplasty is 01214, which has a value of 8 base units. The total time equates to 10 time units. The patient's physical status is reported with modifier P3, which carries a value of 1 unit, and the patient's age is reported with the qualifying circumstances add-on code 99100, which has a value of 1 unit.

The total units reported for this anesthesia service are:

8 (base units) + 10 (time units) + 1 (P3 modifier) +
(extreme age qualifying circumstance) = 20 units

CODER'S TIP

Be aware of all possible modifiers and add-on codes that may be used with anesthesia codes. Even if payers do not recognize the use of these codes for payment purposes, the information obtained through the use of these codes may be important for assessing the overall health of patients undergoing anesthesia.

EXERCISE 10.4

Also available in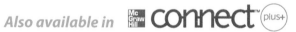

Use your CPT manual to answer the following questions.

1. An anesthesiologist performs an anesthetic with a base value of 5 units. The total anesthesia time is one hour. The physical status is listed as P2, and no qualifying circumstances exist. How many total anesthesia units are reported? _____

2. A CRNA provides anesthesia services with a base value of 7 units. Total time for the anesthesia is 2 hours and 10 minutes. The physical status is reported as P3, and the patient is over 70 years of age. How many total anesthesia units are reported? _____

10.5 Selecting Anatomy-Based Anesthesia CPT Codes (00100–01999)

Anesthesia services are described by CPT codes 00100–01999. Most of these codes are divided into sections by anatomical location. Some anesthesia codes are categorized based on the procedures for which the anesthesia is provided. The anatomical code categories include:

- Head
- Neck
- Thorax (Chest Wall and Shoulder Girdle)
- Intrathoracic
- Spine and Spinal Cord
- Upper Abdomen
- Lower Abdomen
- Perineum
- Pelvis (Except Hip)
- Upper Leg (Except Knee)
- Knee and Popliteal Area
- Lower Leg (Below Knee, Includes Ankle and Foot)
- Shoulder and Axilla
- Upper Arm and Elbow
- Forearm, Wrist, and Hand

Head

The head includes the skull and facial bones (Figure 10.1), cranial cavity, brain, cranial nerves, sinuses, eyes, ears, nose, and structures in the oral cavity. CPT codes used to report "not otherwise specified" procedures on the head include:

- 00120 (Anesthesia for procedures on external, middle, and inner ear including biopsy; not otherwise specified)
- 00140 (Anesthesia for procedures on eye; not otherwise specified)
- 00160 (Anesthesia for procedures on nose and accessory sinuses; not otherwise specified)
- 00170 (Anesthesia for intraoral procedures, including biopsy; not otherwise specified)
- 00190 (Anesthesia for procedures on facial bones or skull; not otherwise specified)
- 00210 (Anesthesia for intracranial procedures; not otherwise specified)

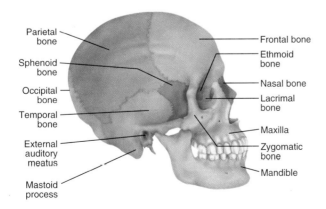

FIGURE 10.1 Skull: Right Lateral View

Therefore, to report a tympanoplasty, use code 00120. A revision or removal of intracranial neurostimulator electrodes would be assigned the code 00210.

Commonly used CPT codes for specific surgical procedures include:

- 00103 (Anesthesia for reconstructive procedures of eyelid [e.g., blepharoplasty, ptosis surgery])
- 00142 (Anesthesia for procedures on eye; lens surgery)
- 00172 (Anesthesia for intraoral procedures; repair of cleft palate)
- 00211 (Anesthesia for intracranial procedures; craniotomy or craniectomy for evacuation of hematoma)
- 00218 (Anesthesia for intracranial procedures; procedures in sitting position)

As an example, a corneal transplant would be coded as 00144.

The above codes include portions of indented codes that only appear in the main code before the semicolon. These parts of the code descriptors are implied as part of the full code descriptor when the indented code only includes the portion of the descriptor that follows the semicolon.

CODER'S TIP

CPT code 00218 is an indented code under 00210. Therefore, it is only used to report intracranial procedures performed in the sitting position. This code is not used to report other procedures performed in the sitting position.

Neck

This section includes anesthesia for procedures on all soft-tissue structures in the neck, including muscles, nerves, esophagus, larynx, trachea, thyroid gland, parathyroid glands, and vascular structures. This section does not include anesthesia for procedures on the cervical spine or spinal cord.

Several codes are used to identify anesthesia for procedures in the neck, including:

- 00300 (Anesthesia for all procedures on the integumentary system, muscles and nerves of the head, neck, and posterior trunk, not otherwise specified)
- 00320 (Anesthesia for all procedures on esophagus, thyroid, larynx, trachea, and lymphatic system of the neck; not otherwise specified, age 1 year or older)
- 00350 (Anesthesia for procedures on major vessels of neck; not otherwise specified)

CODER'S TIP

CPT code 00300 describes anesthesia for procedures on the integumentary system on the head, neck, and posterior trunk. Skin procedures on these areas that are not otherwise described by other codes are reported with this anesthesia CPT code.

Some examples of specific codes describing anesthetics for procedures on the neck are:

- Exploration of a carotid artery wound (00350)
- Esophagoplasty (00320)
- Incision of an infected graft, neck (00350)

Thorax (Chest Wall and Shoulder Girdle)

The chest wall and shoulder girdle area includes structures that are external to the rib cage and do not extend into the thoracic cavity. This includes skin, subcutaneous structures, the breasts, the clavicle, and the scapula. This area does not include the shoulder joint, sternoclavicular joint, or acromioclavicular joint (these are described by CPT code 01630).

Commonly used anesthesia CPT codes include:

- 00400 (Anesthesia for procedures on the integumentary system on the extremities, anterior trunk and perineum; not otherwise specified)
- 00450 (Anesthesia for procedures on clavicle and scapula; not otherwise specified)

Anesthesia for a simple mastectomy is reported with CPT code 00400. More complex breast procedures are reported with CPT codes 00402–00406.

Examples of increasing anesthesia complexity identified through indented codes include the codes indented under CPT code 00400 (Anesthesia for procedures on the integumentary system on the extremities, anterior trunk and perineum; not otherwise specified):

- 00402   (reconstructive procedures on breast [e.g., reduction or augmentation mammoplasty, muscle flap])
- 00404   (radical or modified radical procedures on breast)
- 00406   (radical or modified radical procedures on breast with internal mammary node dissection)

The following are examples of codes describing anesthetics for procedures on the thorax:

- Breast reconstruction (00402)
- Biopsy of the clavicle (00454)
- Repair of clavicle fracture (00450)

Intrathoracic Region

The intrathoracic region includes the heart, lungs, aorta, intrathoracic venous structures, and bronchial structures.

CPT codes describing anesthesia for intrathoracic procedures are organized in groups that designate procedures involving closed-chest procedures (CPT codes 00520–00529), access to the central venous system (CPT codes 00530–00537), procedures on the lungs (CPT codes 00539–00548), and cardiac procedures (CPT codes 00560–00580).

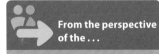

From the perspective of the...

CODER

Make sure you understand the underlying procedure, especially when the differences among those procedures can significantly affect the choice of anesthesia code. If it is unclear what the underlying procedure entailed, ask either the anesthesia provider or the surgeon to clarify these details.

CODER'S TIP

Anesthesia CPT codes are often differentiated by operative differences, the patient's age, or whether the procedure is a new operation or a reoperation. This is especially true for the codes describing anesthesia for cardiac procedures. Carefully review CPT codes 00560–00580 to understand these coding details.

CODING EXAMPLE

A surgeon performs heart surgery on an adult to replace an abnormal aortic valve. This is done using a cardiopulmonary bypass pump. Hypotension and hypothermia are used as part of this procedure. What codes are used to report the anesthesia for this procedure?

The codes describing anesthesia for surgery on the heart, pericardial sac, and great vessels are in the 00560–00580 range. CPT code 00562 further defines this as anesthesia involving a pump oxygenator for patients who are older than one year of age for noncoronary bypass procedures (e.g., valve procedures). Even though this procedure involves the use of hypotension and hypothermia, a parenthetical note in the manual indicates that codes 99116 and 99135 are not reported separately.

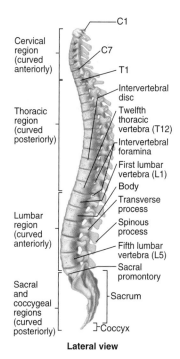

Cervical region (curved anteriorly)

Thoracic region (curved posteriorly)

Lumbar region (curved anteriorly)

Sacral and coccygeal regions (curved posteriorly)

C1
C7
T1
Intervertebral disc
Twelfth thoracic vertebra (T12)
Intervertebral foramina
First lumbar vertebra (L1)
Body
Transverse process
Spinous process
Fifth lumbar vertebra (L5)
Sacral promontory
Sacrum
Coccyx

Lateral view

FIGURE 10.2 Vertebral Column

Spine and Spinal Cord

Codes 00600–00670 are used to report anesthesia for procedures on the bony structures of the cervical, thoracic, lumbar, and sacral spine, as well as procedures on the spinal cord or nerves as they exit the spinal column (Figure 10.2).

The following codes describe common spine procedures:

- 00600 (Anesthesia for procedures on cervical spine and cord; not otherwise specified)
- 00620 (Anesthesia for procedures on thoracic spine and cord; not otherwise specified)
- 00630 (Anesthesia for procedures in lumbar region; not otherwise specified)
- 00670 (Anesthesia for extensive spine and spinal cord procedures [e.g., spinal instrumentation or vascular procedures])

The above codes are only used to describe anesthesia for open procedures on the spine. Anesthesia for closed procedures on the spine is described by CPT code 00640 (Anesthesia for manipulation of the spine or for closed procedures on the cervical, thoracic or lumbar spine). These codes are not used to report anesthesia for diagnostic and therapeutic nerve blocks and injections. Instead, CPT codes 01991 and 01992 are used to report anesthesia for those blocks.

The following are examples of codes describing anesthetics for procedures on the spine:

- Removal of a cervical spine intervertebral disc (00600)
- Lumbar laminectomy (00630)
- Lumbar sympathectomy (00632)

CODER'S TIP

Individual CPT codes describe anesthesia for procedures on the cervical (00600), thoracic (00620), and lumbar (00640) regions of the spinal column. However, CPT code 00670 is the appropriate code to report anesthesia services for procedures on the spine when the surgical procedure is performed on multiple spinal levels, instrumentation is implanted, or add-on codes are attached to the surgical procedure to indicate that the procedure included additional levels regardless of which spinal region is involved.

Upper Abdomen

The upper abdomen includes the upper anterior and posterior abdominal wall (generally above the level of the navel), stomach, duodenum, small intestine, liver, spleen, gallbladder, pancreas, large intestine from the cecum to sigmoid colon, and major abdominal vessels. Even though the appendix is attached to the cecum, it is considered to be in the lower abdomen.

CPT codes describing anesthesia for upper abdominal procedures generally are divided into anesthesia for procedures on the abdominal wall, endoscopic procedures when the endoscope is inserted proximal to the duodenum, hernia repairs, and intraperitoneal procedures. Anesthetics for open and laparoscopic surgical procedures often are described by the same anesthesia CPT code. In the upper abdomen, the most common code describing open or laparoscopic procedures on abdominal organs is code 00790 (Anesthesia for intraperitoneal procedures in upper abdomen including laparoscopy; not otherwise specified).

The following CPT codes are commonly used to describe anesthesia for upper abdominal procedures:

- 00700 (Anesthesia for procedures on upper anterior abdominal wall; not otherwise specified)
- 00730 (Anesthesia for procedures on upper posterior abdominal wall)
- 00740 (Anesthesia for upper gastrointestinal endoscopic procedures, endoscope introduced proximal to duodenum)
- 00790 (Anesthesia for intraperitoneal procedures in upper abdomen including laparoscopy; not otherwise specified)

A surgeon performs a laparoscopic cholecystectomy. What anesthesia code is used to report the anesthesia for this procedure?

The gallbladder is considered part of the upper abdomen. CPT codes describing anesthesia for procedures on the upper abdomen do not include any specific code for anesthesia for cholecystectomy. Therefore, it is necessary to use the "not otherwise specified" code 00790 (Anesthesia for intraperitoneal procedures in upper abdomen including laparoscopy; not otherwise specified) to describe this anesthesia procedure.

CODER'S TIP

Even though procedures on the cecum are considered upper abdominal procedures and the appendix is attached directly to the cecum, procedures on the appendix are considered lower abdominal procedures. CPT code 00840 (Anesthesia for intraperitoneal procedures in lower abdomen including laparoscopy; not otherwise specified) is used to report anesthesia for appendectomies, not CPT code 00790. Coders must be aware of these underlying anesthesia reporting rules.

Lower Abdomen

Anesthesia for procedures in the lower abdomen include those performed on the lower abdominal wall, endoscopic procedures when the endoscope is inserted distal to the duodenum, lower abdominal hernia repairs, intraperitoneal and extraperitoneal procedures in the lower abdomen, appendectomy, procedures on the renal system (including kidneys, ureters, and bladder), and procedures on the major blood vessels of the lower abdomen.

Commonly used CPT codes to describe anesthesia for procedures in the lower abdomen include:

- 00800 (Anesthesia for procedures on lower anterior abdominal wall; not otherwise specified)
- 00810 (Anesthesia for lower intestinal endoscopic procedures, endoscope introduced distal to duodenum)
- 00840 (Anesthesia for intraperitoneal procedures in lower abdomen including laparoscopy; not otherwise specified)
- 00860 (Anesthesia for extraperitoneal procedures in lower abdomen, including urinary tract; not otherwise specified)

The following are examples of codes describing anesthetics for procedures on the lower abdomen:

- Colonoscopy (00810)
- Inguinal hernia repair (00830)
- Kidney transplant (00868)

Perineum

Anesthesia for procedures on the perineum typically includes anesthesia for anorectal surgery and surgery on male and female genitalia. Anesthesia codes for commonly performed perineal procedures include the following:

- 00902 (Anesthesia for; anorectal procedure)
- 00908 (Anesthesia for; perineal prostatectomy)
- 00910 (Anesthesia for transurethral procedures [including urethrocystoscopy]; not otherwise specified)

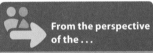

From the perspective of the . . .

CODER

In order to accurately determine which CPT codes describe anesthesia for the hundreds of abdominal surgical codes, it helps to be familiar with abdominal anatomy. Review and understand the use of CPT codes describing anesthesia for specific procedures in the abdomen. Numerous references crosswalk the surgical codes to anesthesia codes, including manuals published by the American Medical Association and the American Society of Anesthesiologists.

- 00914 (Anesthesia for transurethral procedures [including urethrocystoscopy]; transurethral resection of prostate)
- 00920 (Anesthesia for procedures on male genitalia [including open urethral procedures]; not otherwise specified)
- 00921–00938 Specific codes for vasectomy, testicular procedures, radical procedures on the penis, and insertion of penile prostheses.
- 00940 (Anesthesia for vaginal procedures [including biopsy of labia, vagina, cervix, or endometrium]; not otherwise specified)
- 00942–00952 Specific codes for colpotomy, vaginectomy, open urethral procedures, vaginal hysterectomy, and hysterosalpingography.

CODING EXAMPLE

A surgeon performs a transurethral resection of the prostate (TURP) procedure. The coder is reporting the anesthesia services for this surgery. What is the most appropriate code to report this service?

There are several codes that describe anesthesia for transurethral procedures, including 00910 (not otherwise specified), 00912 (transurethral resection of bladder tumors), 00914 (transurethral resection of prostate), 00916 (post-transurethral resection bleeding), and 00918 (removal of ureteral calculus). Because there is a specific code that describes anesthesia for a transurethral resection of the prostate, 00914 is the most appropriate code to report this anesthesia service.

Pelvis (Except Hip)

Codes 01112–01190 describe anesthesia for procedures on the bony pelvis and surrounding structures when part of the procedure on the pelvic bones. Examples of codes describing these procedures include:

- 01112 (Anesthesia for bone marrow aspiration and/or biopsy, anterior or posterior iliac crest)
- 01120 (Anesthesia for procedures on bony pelvis)
- 01170 (Anesthesia for open procedures involving symphysis pubis or sacroiliac joint)
- 01173 (Anesthesia for open repair of fracture disruption of pelvis or column fracture involving acetabulum)

CODER'S TIP

The only surgical procedures described by the anesthesia codes in this section that do not include surgery on the pelvic bones are 01180 (Anesthesia for obturator neurectomy; extrapelvic) and 01190 (Anesthesia for obturator neurectomy; intrapelvic). The obturator nerve is located inside the pelvis and then exits through openings in the pelvic bones. This nerve is occasionally trapped in the pelvis, causing pain. It is sometimes necessary to free the nerve surgically. Depending on the location of the entrapment, the procedure is performed either inside the pelvic bones or external to the pelvis.

The following are examples of codes describing anesthetics for procedures on the pelvis:

- Radical excision of tumor involving pelvis, without amputation (01150)
- Open reduction and internal fixation of acetabular fracture (01173)
- Open reduction and internal fixation of iliac fracture (01120)

Upper Leg (Except Knee)

Codes 01200–01274 describe anesthesia for surgical procedures on the hip joint and upper two-thirds of the femur, including:

- 01210 (Anesthesia for open procedures involving hip joint; not otherwise specified)
- 01214 (Anesthesia for open procedures involving hip joint; total hip arthroplasty)
- 01215 (Anesthesia for open procedures involving hip joint; revision of total hip arthroplasty)
- 01230 (Anesthesia for open procedures involving upper two-thirds of femur; not otherwise specified)
- 01250 (Anesthesia for all procedures on nerves, muscles, tendons, fascia, and bursae of upper leg)

CODER'S TIP

Even though code 01210 describes anesthesia for open procedures involving the hip joint, the most appropriate CPT code to describe anesthesia for a procedure to repair a fracture that involves both the upper femur and the acetabulum would be 01173 (see Pelvis, above).

CODING EXAMPLE

A trauma patient has a subtrochanteric fracture of the upper end of the femur and a supracondylar fracture of the lower end of the femur. The orthopedic surgeon takes the patient to the operating suite, where he performs an open reduction and internal fixation of both fracture sites during one operative session. The total time for both procedures is 3 hours and 15 minutes. The coder is reviewing these procedures to determine how to report the anesthesia services.

The anesthesia services are reported with a single anesthesia code, 01230 (Anesthesia for open procedures involving upper two-thirds of femur; not otherwise specified). The code describing the supracondylar procedure is not reported separately. However, the total time for both procedures is reported. Assuming 15-minute time units, the time would be reported as 16 units.

Knee and Popliteal Area

Codes in the range 01320–01444 describe anesthesia for surgical procedures on the lower one-third of the femur, knee joint (Figure 10.3), popliteal region, and upper ends of the tibia and fibula, including:

- 01320 (Anesthesia for all procedures on nerves, muscles, tendons, fascia, and bursae of knee and/or popliteal area)
- 01360 (Anesthesia for all open procedures on lower one-third of femur)
- 01392 (Anesthesia for all open procedures on upper ends of tibia, fibula, and/or patella)
- 01400 (Anesthesia for open or surgical arthroscopic procedures on knee joint; not otherwise specified)
- 01402 (Anesthesia for open or surgical arthroscopic procedures on knee joint; total knee arthroplasty)

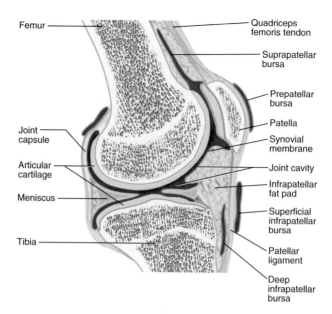

FIGURE 10.3 Section of Knee Joint

Lower Leg (Below Knee, Includes Ankle and Foot)

Codes used to report anesthesia on the lower leg, including ankle and foot, include:

- 01462 (Anesthesia for all closed procedures on lower leg, ankle, and foot)
- 01470 (Anesthesia for procedures on nerves, muscles, tendons, and fascia of lower leg, ankle, and foot; not otherwise specified)
- 01480 (Anesthesia for open procedures on bones of lower leg, ankle, and foot; not otherwise specified)
- 01490 (Anesthesia for lower leg cast application, removal, or repair)

CODER'S TIP

Procedures on the upper end of the tibia and fibula are considered procedures on the knee. Anesthesia for these procedures is reported with codes from the section describing the knee and popliteal area, not the section describing anesthesia for procedures on the lower leg below the knee.

The following are examples of codes describing anesthetics for procedures on the knee, lower leg, ankle, and foot:

- Total knee arthroplasty (01402)
- Arterial repair of popliteal artery (01440)
- Open reduction and internal fixation of tibial shaft fracture (01480)

Shoulder and Axilla

Codes 01610–01682 describe anesthesia for procedures on the shoulder, including procedures involving the humeral head and neck, the shoulder joint (where the humerus meets the scapula), the joints at either end of the clavicle (acromioclavicular joint and sternoclavicular joint), and all the soft tissues surrounding these bony structures. The axilla describes the area commonly referred to as the armpit with all internal soft tissue structures that run through that anatomical structure, such as the brachial plexus, axillary artery, and axillary vein.

Commonly reported anesthesia codes from this section include:

- 01610 (Anesthesia for all procedures on nerves, muscles, tendons, fascia, and bursae of the shoulder and axilla)
- 01630 (Anesthesia for open or surgical arthroscopic procedures on humeral head and neck, sternoclavicular joint, acromioclavicular joint, and shoulder joint; not otherwise specified)
- 01638 (Anesthesia for open or surgical arthroscopic procedures on humeral head and neck, sternoclavicular joint, acromioclavicular joint, and shoulder joint; total shoulder replacement)
- 01650 (Anesthesia for procedures on arteries of the shoulder and axilla; not otherwise specified)
- 01670 (Anesthesia for all procedures on veins of shoulder and axilla)

CODER'S TIP

An interesting coding anomaly is that even though anesthesia for procedures performed at the joints at either end of the clavicle are reported with CPT code 01630 (Anesthesia for open or surgical arthroscopic procedures on humeral head and neck, sternoclavicular joint, acromioclavicular joint, and shoulder joint; not otherwise specified), anesthesia for procedures performed on the clavicle itself are described by CPT code 00450 (Anesthesia for procedures on clavicle and scapula; not otherwise specified) located in the section describing anesthesia for procedures on the thorax.

The following are examples of codes describing anesthetics for procedures on the shoulder and axilla:

- Rotator cuff repair (01610)
- Repair of axillary artery laceration (01650)
- Reduction of shoulder dislocation (01620)

Upper Arm and Elbow

Codes 01710–01782 describe anesthesia for procedures on the bones and soft tissues of the upper arm and elbow. The bones in this region include the humerus below the humeral neck and the upper portion of both the radius (radial head and neck) and ulna (olecranon, the portion of the elbow joint between the lower humerus and ulna). Commonly reported codes include:

- 01710 (Anesthesia for procedures on nerves, muscles, tendons, fascia, and bursae of upper arm and elbow; not otherwise specified)
- 01730 (Anesthesia for all closed procedures on humerus and elbow)
- 01740 (Anesthesia for open or surgical arthroscopic procedures of the elbow; not otherwise specified)
- 01760 (Anesthesia for open or surgical arthroscopic procedures of the elbow; total elbow replacement)

CODER'S TIP

At first glance through the CPT codes describing anesthesia for procedures on the upper arm and elbow, there does not appear to be a code that describes open repair of a humerus fracture. However, by convention, anesthesiologists use CPT code 01744 (Anesthesia for open or surgical arthroscopic procedures of the elbow; repair of nonunion or malunion of humerus) to report open procedures for the repair of humeral shaft fractures.

The following are examples of codes describing anesthetics for procedures on the upper arm and elbow:

- Surgical excision of infected olecranon bursa (01710)
- Open reduction internal fixation of distal humerus fracture (01744)
- Repair brachial artery injury (01770)

Forearm, Wrist, and Hand

Codes 01810–01860 describe anesthesia services for upper extremity procedures beginning below the level of the elbow joint and extending to the fingertips. Commonly reported CPT codes include:

- 01810 (Anesthesia for all procedures on nerves, muscles, tendons, fascia, and bursae of forearm, wrist, and hand)
- 01829 (Anesthesia for diagnostic arthroscopic procedures on the wrist)
- 01830 (Anesthesia for open or surgical arthroscopic/endoscopic procedures on distal radius, distal ulna, wrist, or hand joints; not otherwise specified)
- 01840 (Anesthesia for procedures on arteries of forearm, wrist, and hand; not otherwise specified)

The following are examples of codes describing anesthetics for procedures on the forearm, wrist, and hand:

- Tenolysis, flexor tendon; finger (01810)
- Radical resection of tumor, distal phalanx of finger (01830)
- Closed reduction and casting of distal radius fracture (Colles' fracture) (01820)

EXERCISE 10.5

Also available in **McGraw Hill connect** (plus+)

Use the CPT manual to select the CPT code to describe anesthesia for the following procedures.

1. Procedure performed on the middle ear _____
2. Adenoidectomy _____
3. Partial excision of the thyroid _____
4. Mastopexy _____
5. Incision and drainage of an appendiceal abscess; percutaneous _____
6. Appendectomy _____
7. Aspiration and/or injection of a renal cyst or pelvis by needle, percutaneous _____
8. Excision of a lesion of the pancreas _____
9. Transurethral incision of the prostate _____
10. Excision of a Cowper's gland _____
11. Bone marrow; aspiration only _____
12. Arthroplasty, knee, condyle and plateau; medial compartment _____
13. Osteotomy, distal femur; lengthening _____
14. Arthroscopy, shoulder, surgical biceps tenodesis _____
15. Endoscopic carpal tunnel release _____

10.6 Coding for Specific Procedures

Rather than describing an anatomical region or body part, some anesthesia codes describe the specific procedures that make the anesthetic necessary, including:

1. Radiological procedures.
2. Burn excisions or debridement.
3. Obstetrical anesthesia.
4. Other procedures.

Radiological Procedures

On occasion, it may be necessary to provide anesthesia for a patient undergoing radiological procedures. This is not typically necessary for routine x-rays to visualize a body part, but it may be needed for radiological procedures that result in sufficient discomfort. These CPT codes include:

- 01916 (Anesthesia for diagnostic arteriography/venography)
- 01920 (Anesthesia for cardiac catheterization including coronary angiography and ventriculography [not to include Swan-Ganz catheter])
- 01935 (Anesthesia for percutaneous image-guided procedures on the spine and spinal cord; diagnostic)
- 01936 (Anesthesia for percutaneous image-guided procedures on the spine and spinal cord; therapeutic)

Burn Excisions or Debridement

Anesthetics for patients undergoing surgical treatment of second- and third-degree burns are not reported using the codes that describe procedures on the skin in particular anatomical regions. Instead, there are three separate codes that describe anesthesia for the treatment of burns, two base codes and one add-on code:

- 01951 (Anesthesia for second- and third-degree burn excision or debridement with or without skin grafting, any site, for total body surface (TBSA) treated during anesthesia and surgery; less than 4 percent total body surface area)
- 01952 (between 4 percent and 9 percent total body surface area)
- +01953 (each additional 9 percent total body surface area or part thereof [List separately in addition to code for primary procedure])

Each area of the body is assigned a percentage value. The TBSA is calculated by adding those percentages for the areas treated during the procedure. The assigned percentages for each specific body part include:

- Head, 9 percent (4.5 percent for face, 4.5 percent for back of head)
- Arms, 9 percent each (4.5 percent for front of each arm, 4.5 percent for back of each arm)
- Chest, 9 percent
- Abdomen, 9 percent
- Upper back, 9 percent
- Lower back, 9 percent
- Legs, 18 percent each (9 percent for front of each leg, 9 percent for back of each leg)
- Genitalia, 1 percent

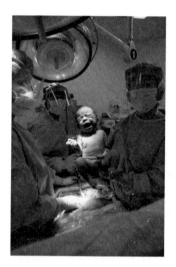

The most common form of obstetrical analgesia is an epidural block, which reduces the pain of labor while allowing the woman to actively push to deliver her child.

Obstetrical Anesthesia

Anesthesia providers perform procedures to produce anesthesia/analgesia for women in labor. This is one of the few services that a single anesthesia provider can perform on multiple patients at the same time. The most common form of labor analgesia is an epidural block that reduces the painful sensations of labor but still allows the woman to actively participate in the delivery by pushing during childbirth.

Most often, the anesthesiologist or CRNA places an epidural catheter and gives a bolus of an anesthetic agent to produce the desired level of analgesia. The anesthesia provider can either periodically inject more anesthetic agent through the catheter or run a continuous infusion through the catheter to maintain the analgesia.

Similar to other anesthesia procedures, anesthesia for labor is reported with a procedure code and time units. However, because the provider may be caring for multiple pregnant patients with catheters in place at the same time, payers have different conventions and requirements for reporting the time units. Common conventions include one time unit per hour, one time unit per 30 minutes, or other periods. Coders must be aware of how each payer wants time units reported.

Another difference that coders must understand about reporting anesthesia for obstetrical services is that, in the event that labor is not allowed to proceed, but instead a cesarean section is performed after a trial of labor, the additional procedure is reported using the base code to describe the labor analgesia and an add-on code to report the cesarean section. If a cesarean section is the only procedure performed, only the code that describes anesthesia for cesarean section is reported. Obstetrical codes include:

- 01960 (Anesthesia for vaginal delivery only) (This code is *not* used to report analgesia for labor, but rather an anesthetic for the delivery.)
- 01961 (Anesthesia for cesarean section only)

The above codes are not used when a labor anesthesia/analgesia has been provided as part of the anesthesia care. The following codes are used to report labor anesthesia/analgesia procedures:

- 01967 (Neuraxial labor analgesia/anesthesia for planned vaginal delivery [this includes any repeat subarachnoid needle placement and drug injection and/or any necessary replacement of an epidural catheter during labor])
- +01968 (Anesthesia for cesarean delivery following neuraxial labor analgesia/anesthesia [List separately in addition to code for primary procedure performed])

Other Procedures

The last few CPT anesthesia codes (01990–01999) are miscellaneous codes reporting anesthesia services that are not otherwise classified, including:

- 01990 (Physiological support for harvesting of organ(s) from brain-dead patient)
- 01991 (Anesthesia for diagnostic or therapeutic nerve blocks and injections [when block or injection is performed by a different provider]; other than the prone position)
- 01992 (Anesthesia for diagnostic or therapeutic nerve blocks and injections [when block or injection is performed by a different provider]; prone position)
- 01996 (Daily hospital management of epidural or subarachnoid continuous drug administration)

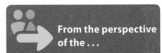

From the perspective of the . . .

CODER

Differentiate between various combinations of obstetrical procedures, such as labor resulting in vaginal delivery, labor converted to cesarean section, and trial of vaginal birth after cesarean (VBAC) procedures, which may be successful or not. Without this knowledge, it is difficult to select the correct combination of codes to report the anesthesia services.

CODER'S TIP

CPT Code 01996 (Daily hospital management of epidural or subarachnoid continuous drug administration) is the only primary anesthesia code in the Anesthesia section that is not reported with time. This code is reported once per day, even if the anesthesia provider makes more than one adjustment to the continuous infusion during a single day.

EXERCISE 10.6

Also available in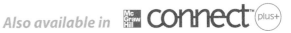

Use the CPT manual to select the CPT code to describe anesthesia for the following procedures.

1. Catheterization of intracerebral aneurysm with placement of therapeutic coil _____
2. Percutaneous placement of artificial disc under radiological image guidance at T11–T12 _____
3. Debridement of burns with split-thickness skin grafting with a TBSA of 36 percent _____
4. Dilation and curettage (D&C) for incomplete spontaneous abortion _____
5. Management of continuous epidural infusion with three separate visits during one day _____

Summary

Learning Outcome	Key Concepts/Examples
10.1 Select anesthesia codes based on surgical procedures. **Pages 255–257**	Coding for anesthesia services is different than coding for any other professional services for two reasons: 1. The choice of code does not depend on what the anesthesia provider did for the patient. Rather, it depends on what the surgeon or other provider is doing that makes the anesthetic necessary. 2. The total time the anesthesia services are provided is reported as a separately identifiable service. A single anesthesia code can describe anesthetics for a large number of surgical procedures. The appropriate anesthesia code can be identified from the code descriptors or from publications that crosswalk surgical codes to the appropriate anesthesia codes. Each anesthesia code is assigned a base unit value that is used by payers to calculate payment for anesthesia services. When selecting anesthesia codes, it is important to review all codes describing anesthesia for specific procedures before selecting the "not otherwise specified" code.
10.2 Report anesthesia time. **Pages 258–259**	Time is a factor that must be reported with each anesthesia code. Time is calculated in different ways, depending on the payer. The two most common methods are either one time unit for each 15 minutes of anesthesia time or the number of minutes. Coders must know how each payer wants time reported.
10.3 Use anesthesia modifiers and add-on codes. **Pages 259–261**	Secondary aspects of anesthesia services are reported with modifiers and add-on codes. Modifiers are added to the anesthesia procedure codes to provide information regarding the physical status of the patient, information regarding who delivered the anesthetic, and the justification for MAC anesthesia. Add-on codes are used to report certain qualifying circumstances, including extremes of age (older than 70 or under one year of age), use of hypotension and/or hypothermia techniques, and whether the case is an emergency procedure. These modifiers and add-on codes may have effects on payment for the anesthesia services, but this varies from payer to payer.
10.4 Calculate the total number of anesthesia units for services provided. **Page 262**	Payment for anesthesia services is based on the total number of anesthesia units that particular case is valued at based on a set formula. The basic formula is: Base units + Time units + Physical status modifier units + Qualifying circumstances add-on code units = Total anesthesia units Not all payers recognize units for physical status modifiers or qualifying circumstances.

CPT only © 2010 American Medical Association. All rights reserved.

Learning Outcome	Key Concepts/Examples
10.5 Select anesthesia codes for surgical procedures on specific body parts. **Pages 263–272**	Most anesthesia codes are classified according to the anatomical location of the underlying surgical procedure. This defines the range of anesthesia codes that may be used to describe the anesthesia services provided. The anatomical divisions include: • Head • Neck • Thorax (Chest Wall and Shoulder Girdle) • Intrathoracic • Spine and Spinal Cord • Upper Abdomen • Lower Abdomen • Perineum • Pelvis (Except Hip) • Upper Leg (Except Knee) • Knee and Popliteal Area • Lower Leg (Below Knee, Includes Ankle and Foot) • Shoulder and Axilla • Upper Arm and Elbow • Forearm, Wrist, and Hand
10.6 Choose anesthesia codes for specific procedures. **Pages 273–275**	Some anesthesia services are classified by the type of procedure that makes the anesthesia necessary. These include anesthesia for: • Radiological procedures. • Burn excision and debridement. • Obstetrical procedures. • Other procedures.

Using Terminology

Match the key terms with their definitions.

_____ **1.** L010.1 Anesthesiologist

_____ **2.** L010.1 Certified registered nurse anesthetist

_____ **3.** L010.1 Anesthesia assistant

_____ **4.** L010.1 General anesthesia

_____ **5.** L010.1 Regional anesthesia

_____ **6.** L010.1 Local anesthesia

_____ **7.** L010.1 Monitored anesthesia care

_____ **8.** L010.2 American Society of Anesthesiologists

_____ **9.** L010.1 Analgesia

_____ **10.** L010.3 Qualifying circumstances add-on codes

A. Involves making the patient unconscious

B. Used when anesthesia is more difficult than usual or involves additional techniques

C. Sedating patients without making them completely unconscious

D. Specially trained nurses who provide anesthesia services

E. Alleviation of pain

F. Physicians specially trained in anesthesia

G. Making a large portion of the patient's body numb

H. A publisher of crosswalks between surgical and anesthesia codes

I. Numbing just the area being operated on

J. Non-nurse professionals trained to provide anesthesia services

Mc Graw Hill **connect** plus+

Enhance your learning by completing these exercises
and more at mcgrawhillconnect.com!

CHAPTER 10 | ANESTHESIA SERVICES   277

Checking Your Understanding

Select the letter that best completes the statement or answers the question.

1. L010.2 Anesthesia time units are determined from the:
   a. Time the patient is put to sleep until the time the patient wakes up.
   b. Time the patient enters the operating room (OR) until the time the patient leaves the OR.
   c. Time the patient first receives medication until the anesthesiologist leaves.
   d. Time the patient is prepared for anesthesia until the time the patient is placed in postanesthesia care.

2. L010.1 Which of the following forms of anesthesia renders the patient unconscious?
   a. Regional
   b. MAC (monitored anesthesia care)
   c. General
   d. Local

3. L010.1 Which characteristics determine the groupings of CPT anesthesia codes?
   a. The type of anesthesia performed (e.g, general, MAC, local, or regional)
   b. The general area of the body that is being operated on by the surgeon
   c. The degree of invasiveness of the surgery
   d. The duration of the anesthesia rounded up to the nearest 15-minute interval

4. L010.2 Anesthesia CPT codes require a separate report defining units of:
   a. Medication used for anesthesia.
   b. Time in the operating room.
   c. Time of anesthesia care services.
   d. Comorbid conditions or diseases affecting anesthesia care.

5. L010.5 A patient is hospitalized for multiple burns, upper leg fractures, and head injury after a motor vehicle collision and is sent for an MRI of her head to check for brain injury. The patient requires general anesthesia to allow her to hold completely still during the MRI. The anesthesia CPT code from which of the following categories should be used for this anesthesia care?
   a. 01951–01953
   b. 01916–01936
   c. 01200–01274
   d. 00100–00218

6. L010.6 Anesthesia CPT codes for burn excision and debridement are determined by:
   a. The degree of the burn (first, second, third).
   b. The location of the burn on the patient.
   c. The percentage of total body surface area that is burned.
   d. The percentage of total body surface area that is excised or debrided.

7. L010.6 A pregnant patient receives anesthesia during labor for a planned vaginal delivery but ultimately requires a cesarean section due to fetal distress. Which pair of codes describes the anesthesia services performed?

   a. 01967, 01968
   b. 01961, 01968
   c. 01960, 01961
   d. 01968, 01960

8. L010.5 Which of the following primary anesthesia codes are not reported with time units?

   a. 01967 (epidural anesthesia for planned vaginal delivery)
   b. 01996 (maintenance of epidural or subarachnoid continuous medication administration)
   c. 01935 (anesthesia for percutaneous image-guided procedures on spine and spinal cord)
   d. 01992 (anesthesia for diagnostic or therapeutic nerve blocks and injections, prone position)

9. L010.3 Which of the following modifiers identifying professional credentials of anesthesia providers is incorrect?

   a. AA—Anesthesia services personally performed by an anesthesiologist
   b. QX—CRNA service with medical direction by a physician
   c. QZ—CRNA service without medical direction by a physician
   d. AD—Anesthesia services provided by the surgeon

10. L010.5 Which anesthesia add-on code would be used for services provided to a patient who was taken to the OR emergently for laparotomy after a motor vehicle collision?

    a. 99100
    b. 99116
    c. 99135
    d. 99140

11. L010.2 Which of the following is never added to base units when calculating total anesthesia units?

    a. Time units
    b. Physical status modifier units
    c. Anesthesia gas units
    d. Qualifying circumstances add-on codes

12. L010.5 For an esophagoduodenoscopy, a patient is placed supine, anesthetized, and an endoscope is placed into the mouth, through the esophagus, and into the duodenum for a biopsy. Which anatomical body part would be used to index the correct anesthesia code?

    a. Head
    b. Neck
    c. Thorax
    d. Upper abdomen

13. L010.6 An adult patient receives anesthesia care for debridement of third-degree burns involving all of his right leg and lower back. Which combination of anesthesia codes is correct for this service?

    a. 01952, 01953
    b. 01952, 01953, 01953
    c. 01951, 01953
    d. 01951, 01953, 01953

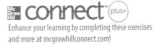

14. L010.3 Which physical status modifier would be most appropriate to use when coding for anesthesia services provided for a patient with hypertension, hypothyroidism, and congestive heart failure?

 a. P3
 b. P2
 c. P3 and P2
 d. Whichever is documented by the anesthesia provider

15. L010.3 Which of the following modifiers does not indicate a MAC anesthesia service?

 a. QS
 b. Q8
 c. G8
 d. G9

16. L010.6 Which of the following codes would be used for anesthesia services provided for a patient undergoing a diagnostic heart catheterization?

 a. 00410
 b. 00532
 c. 01920
 d. 00560

17. L010.1 Which method of anesthesia commands the highest fee for a given surgical procedure?

 a. General
 b. Regional
 c. Epidural
 d. None of these

18. L010.2 An anesthesiologist evaluates a patient at 12:00 and puts the patient on cardiopulmonary monitoring. At 12:23, a sedative is given. At 12:32, the patient is taken to the OR suite. The patient is put under general anesthesia at 12:45 and awakened at 1:19. The patient is transferred to postanesthesia care at 1:39. Using a time unit of 15 minutes, how many time units would be calculated for this case?

 a. 5
 b. 6
 c. 7
 d. 8

19. L010.6 Which code or codes would be used for epidural anesthesia during labor and vaginal delivery of twins?

 a. 01967
 b. 01967, 01967
 c. 01967, 01968
 d. 01960

20. L010.3 Which of the following scenarios justifies the use of the add-on code 99135?

 a. A patient with essential hypertension
 b. A patient who becomes profoundly hypotensive during surgery
 c. A patient with hypotension intentionally induced for surgery
 d. A patient with hypothermia intentionally induced for surgery

Applying Your Skills

Use the CPT manual to determine the correct code to report anesthesia associated with the following procedures.

1. L010.5 Cesarean delivery only

_____

2. L010.5 Rhinoplasty, primary; including major septal repair

_____

3. L010.5 Injection procedure for temporomandibular joint arthrography

_____

4. L010.5 Decompression of orbit only, transcranial approach

_____

5. L010.5 Craniectomy

_____

6. L010.5 Excision of a pilonidal cyst or sinus; complicated

_____

7. L010.5 Mastectomy for gynecomastia

_____

8. L010.5 Intranasal biopsy

_____

9. L010.5 Pancreatic islet cell transplantation through portal vein, open

_____

10. L010.5 Transcatheter biopsy

_____

11. L010.5 Interstitial radiation source application; complex

_____

12. L010.5 Closed treatment of a radial shaft fracture; without manipulation

_____

13. L010.5 Incision and drainage, forearm and/or wrist; deep abscess or hematoma

_____

14. L010.5 Arthroplasty, radial head

_____

15. L010.5 Arthroscopy, shoulder, surgical; with rotator cuff repair

_____

Enhance your learning by completing these exercises
and more at mcgrawhillconnect.com!

CHAPTER 10 | ANESTHESIA SERVICES   281

16. L010.5 Tenotomy, shoulder area; single tendon

_____

17. L010.5 Radical resection of tumor; tibia

_____

18. L010.5 Biopsy of lower leg muscle; superficial

_____

19. L010.5 Excision; ischial bursa

_____

20. L010.5 Vaginal repair that is not part of an obstetrical delivery

_____

21. L010.5 Amputation of penis; partial

_____

22. L010.5 Vulvectomy, radical, complete

_____

23. L010.5 Laparoscopy, surgical; ureterolithotomy of upper ureter

_____

24. L010.5 Nephrolithotomy; removal of calculus

_____

25. L010.5 Pancreatectomy, total

_____

26. L010.5 Amniocentesis

_____

27. L010.5 Culdoscopy

_____

28. L010.5 Total elbow replacement

_____

29. L010.6 Urgent hysterectomy following delivery (childbirth)

_____

30. L010.6 D&C for missed abortion

_____

Thinking It Through

Use your critical-thinking skills to answer the questions below.

1. L010.1 What are the four main categories of anesthesia?

   _____

   _____

2. L010.2 For the purpose of calculating anesthesia care time units, how is the total duration of anesthesia service determined?

   _____

   _____

3. L010.3 What is the significance of including physical status modifiers (P1–P6) with the anesthesia CPT codes?

   _____

   _____

4. L010.3 How should a coder indicate that an anesthesia service was provided under circumstances that are significantly more difficult than usual or involve additional anesthetic techniques?

   _____

   _____

5. L010.2, 10.3 Identify the four components that comprise the total anesthesia units and indicate which components are always recognized and which ones are only recognized by some payers.

   _____

   _____

6. L010.6 What two variables must a coder know about an obstetrical case in order to accurately choose a CPT code for anesthesia services during childbirth?

   _____

   _____

connect plus+

Enhance your learning by completing these exercises and more at mcgrawhillconnect.com!

CHAPTER 10 | ANESTHESIA SERVICES   283

11 RADIOLOGY SERVICES

Learning Outcomes *After completing this chapter, students should be able to:*

11.1 Define positions, projections, and planes in terms of radiology services.

11.2 Explain the process for reporting radiology services.

11.3 Use modifiers with radiology CPT codes.

11.4 Discuss parameters surrounding CPT coding for various radiology services.

Key Terms

Anteroposterior (AP)

Computed tomography (CT)

Contrast material

Coronal plane

Decubitus

Digital x-ray system

Fluoroscopy

Left lateral decubitus

Magnetic resonance imaging (MRI)

Mammography

Modifier 26

Modifier TC

Nuclear medicine

Oblique

Posteroanterior (PA)

Prone

Radiological supervision and interpretation

Right lateral decubitus

Sagittal plane

Standing

Supine

Tomogram

Transverse plane

Ultrasound

X-ray film

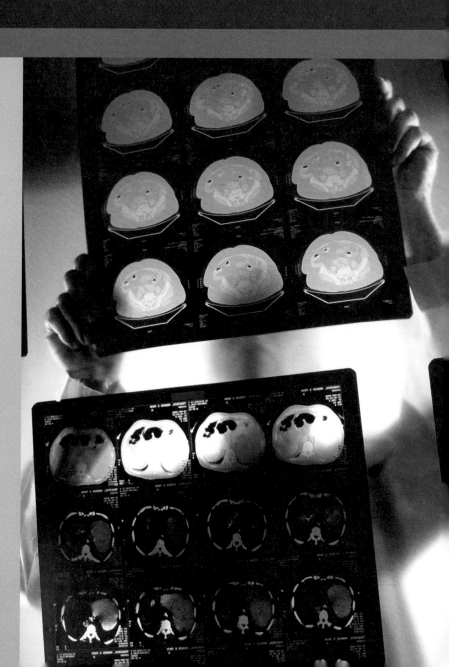

Introduction

Radiology is the branch of medicine that utilizes various imaging techniques to diagnose and treat diseases. Imaging techniques include **x-ray films, digital x-ray systems, computed tomography (CT), magnetic resonance imaging (MRI), positron emission tomography (PET), ultrasound, nuclear medicine**, and **fluoroscopy**. Diagnostic radiology uses these imaging techniques to identify disease processes, whereas interventional radiology uses imaging to assist physicians in performing minimally invasive procedures. Radiation oncology, or radiation therapy, is another branch of radiology, in which high doses of radiation are used to treat patients with some cancers.

11.1 Positions, Projections, and Planes

X-rays or other images are often described by noting the anatomical parts imaged, the position the patient was in when the image was created, and the direction of the x-ray beam or the body plane shown by the image. When imaging techniques are performed, the most common patient positions are **standing, supine** (back side down), **prone** (stomach side down), or **decubitus** (one side down). In some cases, the patient may be positioned somewhere between these standard positions, which are often described as **oblique** positions.

Projection describes the direction of the x-ray beam used to create the image. The beam begins in an x-ray source, passes through the patient's body, and then lands on a film or other x-ray detector to form an image. Projections are identified by describing the direction of the beam, beginning where it enters the body and ending with the part of the body closest to the film. For example, the **anteroposterior (AP)** projection describes a beam that enters at the front of the body (anterior) and exits at the back (posterior). A common AP film is a chest x-ray, where the beam is aimed at the patient's chest and the film is placed along the patient's back.

The **posteroanterior (PA)** projection is where the beam is aimed at the patient's back (posterior) and the film is placed along the front side of the patient (anterior). The **right lateral decubitus** and **left lateral decubitus** positions are used to describe situations where the beam enters one side of the body and exits the other. The "left" or "right" designations signify the side of the body closest to the x-ray film, which is almost always the side of the body that is lying against the table or bed.

Some imaging techniques, such as CT or MRI, utilize a computer to combine thousands of individual images into a composite view of the body in a particular plane. A **tomogram** is a two-dimensional image of a section of a three-dimensional object. A tomogram represents a plane or slice through the body. The most common anatomical planes are **transverse** (a view of a horizontal cross section), **sagittal** (a view of a front-to-back cross section), and **coronal** or frontal (a view of a side-to-side cross section).

---

x-ray film
An x-ray detector upon which the x-ray beam is cast to form an image of the body plane being examined.

digital x-ray system
A system that uses computerized data for radiological imaging instead of conventional x-ray film.

computed tomography (CT)
The use of multiple x-rays to produce cross-sectional images.

magnetic resonance imaging (MRI)
The use of a powerful magnetic field and special injectable materials to produce images.

positron emission tomography (PET)
A radiographic imaging technique that measures functional activity in specific organs and body tissues by injecting radionuclides into the venous system and measuring activity in various anatomic structures.

ultrasound
A procedure that uses sound waves to create permanent images and measurements of body parts or as guidance during other procedures.

nuclear medicine
Involves placing radioactive materials within the body and then monitoring the radioactive emissions from those elements; provided for either diagnostic or therapeutic purposes.

CODER'S TIP

The three standard anatomical planes commonly used in imaging studies are:

- Coronal or frontal plane: A vertical plane that divides the body into front and back (anterior and posterior) portions.
- Sagittal: A vertical plane that divides the body into right and left portions.
- Transverse: A horizontal plane that divides the body into upper (superior) and lower (inferior) portions.

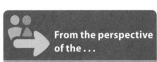

From the perspective of the . . .

CODER

Understanding the different imaging techniques is essential to correctly selecting the appropriate codes to report those services. Notations identifying position and projections provide information regarding the number of services provided.

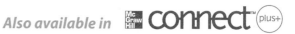
Fill in the blanks to complete each statement below.

1. If the medical record indicates that an x-ray was taken in the left lateral decubitus position, how do you describe this position in general terms? _____

2. A computer-generated image is displayed showing a cross-sectional, front-to-back slice of the body that demonstrates the internal structures as if viewed from the side. This is known as the _____ plane.

3. A patient has a chest x-ray taken in which he is standing up with his chest against the film and the x-ray beam passes through him from back to front before striking the film. This is known as the _____ projection.

---

fluoroscopy
A technique used to produce real-time images of the body by using an x-ray source and a viewing screen.

standing
One position in which an imaging may be performed.

supine
A common position for imaging procedures in which the patient is lying back side down.

prone
A common position for imaging procedures in which the patient is lying stomach side down.

decubitus
A common position for imaging procedures in which the patient is lying one side down.

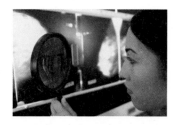

Sometimes one physician performs a surgical procedure, while another physician, a radiologist, performs an associated radiological service or interprets the results of a radiological service. In these cases, each physician reports the services that he or she performed.

11.2 Reporting Radiology Services

Some of the terms included in the CPT codes that describe radiology services can be confusing. For example, many radiology CPT codes include the term "separate procedure" within the code descriptor. These procedures are often performed as part of other procedures. When a radiological procedure is performed as part of another procedure, those codes should *not* be listed in addition to the codes that describe those other procedures.

There are times, however, in which procedures that include "separate procedure" in their code descriptors are either performed alone or with other procedures to which they are not related. In such instances, the radiology service that includes "separate procedure" in its descriptor may be reported with modifier 59 to indicate that the procedure is not a part of another procedure. This may be appropriate when the "separate procedure" service is performed during a different session, with a different surgical procedure, or on a different body part.

Another source of potential confusion is the use of the term **radiological supervision and interpretation** in the code descriptor. These codes often describe radiological services performed in combination with other services described by CPT codes in the surgical or other sections of the CPT manual. Sometimes one physician performs the procedure, while a radiologist performs the radiological service. In those instances, each provider reports the services he or she performed. If a single physician performed both the procedure and the radiological service, that provider reports both the radiological CPT code and the procedure code from outside the 70000 series. This is known as *component coding* or *combination coding*. Examples of these combination procedures include placing stents, guide wires, or catheters. Sometimes it is necessary to inject **contrast material** during procedures. When the radiologist injects contrast material, a procedure code from the surgical section is used to indicate the injection procedure.

CODER'S TIP

Most radiological codes have an inherent supervision and interpretation component, but only some codes include this term in their descriptors. Radiologists report routine diagnostic radiological services by adding modifier 26 to the code describing the exam. The codes that include the term "radiological supervision and interpretation" are those that describe radiological services commonly used by nonradiologists when performing other procedures. These codes describe services that are professional services only, so modifier 26 is not added.

Unlisted Codes

If the particular radiology service provided is not described by a specific CPT code, the coder should use one of the "unlisted" radiology CPT codes at the beginning of the Radiology section in the CPT manual. Unlisted codes describe many specific types of radiology services, including fluoroscopic, CT, MRI, radiological, ultrasound, therapeutic radiology treatment planning, therapeutic radiology treatment management, clinical brachytherapy, and diagnostic nuclear medicine procedures.

When an unlisted code is used to report a service, the provider should document the specifics of that service. This should include a description of the service; the need for the procedure; and the time, effort, and equipment necessary to perform the service.

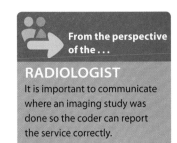

EXERCISE 11.2

Also available in McGraw Hill **connect** (plus+)

Provide brief definitions of the following terms.

1. Separate procedure _____

2. Radiological supervision and interpretation _____

3. Unlisted code _____

11.3 Modifiers

The most common modifiers used to report radiology procedures are **modifier 26** and **modifier TC**. Radiology services utilize complex and expensive equipment to create the desired images. In many cases, the professionals who interpret the images do not own the equipment used to create them. For example, radiologists may review x-rays taken in a hospital and issue official interpretations of their findings. Those professionals would report their services with the CPT codes that describe the specific x-rays, along with modifier 26 to indicate they are reporting the professional services.

CODER'S TIP

When reporting professional services for the radiologist's interpretation of a study, it is almost always necessary to add modifier 26 to the code that identifies the imaging study.

Entities that own or lease x-ray equipment add modifier TC to the appropriate CPT codes to report the technical component of the imaging procedure. In some cases, a single entity owns the equipment used to create images and employs the professionals who interpret those images. In those cases, the single entity reports the code describing the particular radiology service without attaching either the 26 or TC modifier. This is referred to as the global code. It is incorrect to report a code with both modifiers.

In addition to the professional and technical component modifiers, other modifiers may be used to describe radiology services. Anatomical modifiers, such as RT and LT, are often used to differentiate particular locations. If an x-ray of a particular finger or toe is used, the appropriate anatomical modifiers may be added to the claim. Modifier 50 is used to indicate that bilateral images were created and interpreted. This is only used when the exact same image is created on both sides of the body.

Other modifiers may be used to describe unusual circumstances. Modifiers discussed in Chapter 7 may be attached to radiology CPT codes when it is appropriate to

oblique
A position for imaging procedures in which the patient is lying between standard positions.

anteroposterior (AP)
An x-ray projection in which a beam enters at the front of the patient's body (anterior) and exits at the patient's back (posterior).

posteroanterior (PA)
An x-ray projection in which the beam is aimed at the patient's back (posterior) and the film is placed along the front side of the patient (anterior).

right lateral decubitus
Position used to describe situations where the beam enters the left side of the body and exits the right side, with the right side closest to the x-ray film.

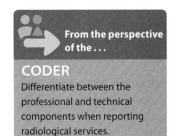

left lateral decubitus
Position used to describe situations where the beam enters the right side of the body and exits the left side, with the left side closest to the x-ray film.

tomogram
A two-dimensional image of a section of a three-dimensional object, which represents a plane or slice through the body.

transverse plane
A common anatomical plane that is a view of a horizontal cross section of the body.

do so. Such circumstances might include situations when services that are not usually reported together should be considered as separate services (modifier 59) and when it is necessary to repeat a procedure (modifier 76 or 77).

CODING EXAMPLE

An MRI without contrast material is performed on a patient's head, followed by a second scan with contrast material. The radiologist interprets these images. How would the hospital and radiologist report their services?

Both the hospital and radiologist use the same code to report the scans: 70546 (Magnetic resonance angiography, head; without contrast material[s], followed by contrast material[s] and further sequences). The hospital reports this code with the TC modifier: 70546-TC. The radiologist reports this code with modifier 26: 70546-26.

EXERCISE 11.3.1

Also available in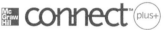

Using the CPT manual, assign the correct modifier to each of the following parts of an encounter involving radiology services.

1. To report the physician's interpretation of a film taken at the hospital. _____

2. An x-ray is taken in the physician's office, and the physician interprets the film at the time of service. _____

3. To report the use of the x-ray equipment only. _____

EXERCISE 11.3.2

Also available in Mc Graw Hill **connect**™ (plus+)

Using your critical-thinking skills, answer the following questions.

1. Is it necessary to append modifier 26 to report an x-ray when the supervision and interpretation are part of the code descriptor? Why or why not? _____

2. List two circumstances when modifier 59 can be used to report two codes that are not usually reported together. _____

sagittal plane
View of a front-to-back cross section of the body.

coronal plane
View of a side-to-side cross section of the body.

radiological supervision and interpretation
Professional services often reported by nonradiologists as part of other procedures.

11.4 Radiology CPT Coding (70010–79999)

The Radiology section of the CPT manual is divided into the following sections:

- Diagnostic Radiology (Diagnostic Imaging)
- Diagnostic Ultrasound
- Radiologic Guidance
- Breast, Mammography
- Bone/Joint Studies
- Radiation Oncology
- Nuclear Medicine

Each of these sections may be further divided by anatomical region or type of service.

Diagnostic Radiology (Diagnostic Imaging)

The Diagnostic Radiology section (70010–76499) is divided first by anatomical region and then by type of service. The major anatomical regions listed in this section include:

- Head and Neck
- Chest
- Spine and Pelvis
- Upper Extremities
- Lower Extremities
- Abdomen
- Gastrointestinal Tract
- Urinary Tract
- Gynecological and Obstetrical
- Heart
- Vascular Procedures
- Other Procedures

Within each of these sections, procedures describing particular imaging techniques, such as radiological exams, CT or MRI studies, or other techniques are often grouped together. Students should become familiar with the structure of the coding sections to correctly identify the code that most appropriately describes the service provided.

Coders must use the index to identify the CPT code that best describes the radiological procedure. The index categorizes procedures by type under headings such as CT Scan, Fluoroscopy (Figure 11.1), Magnetic Resonance Angiography, Magnetic Resonance Imaging (Figure 11.2), Positron Emission Tomography (Figure 11.3), Ultrasound, and X-rays (Figure 11.4). Within each of these index headings, specific procedures are listed with a cross-reference to the associated CPT code.

In addition to listing radiological procedures, the index lists anatomical locations and body parts. Under each of these subheadings is a list of procedures performed on those structures, including radiological procedures, along with their associated CPT codes. With proper use of the index, coders should be able to identify the appropriate CPT code that describes the particular radiological procedure provided to the patient.

The use of contrast material as part of the radiological imaging exam often distinguishes one CPT code from another. Terms used include *without contrast, with contrast,* or *without contrast followed by contrast.* Coders must pay attention to the type of exam performed and the code descriptors to correctly report radiological services involving contrast material.

Examples of diagnostic radiological procedures include barium enemas, PET scans, and MRIs.

contrast material
Material used to enhance viewing of anatomical structures during radiological procedures.

modifier 26
When reporting professional services for the radiologist's interpretation of a study, a common modifier added to the code that identifies the imaging study.

modifier TC
A common modifier added to report the technical component of the imaging procedure by entities that own x-ray equipment.

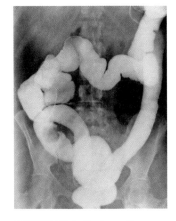

FIGURE 11.1 Barium Enema Showing Cancer of the Colon (orange area)

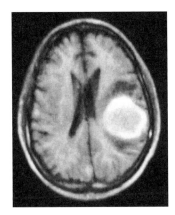

FIGURE 11.2 MRI of the Brain Showing Metastatic Tumor

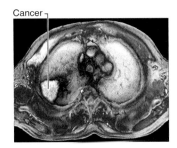

Cancer

FIGURE 11.3 PET Scan Showing Cancer in the Right Lung

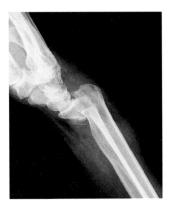

FIGURE 11.4 X-ray of Colles' Fracture with Radius and Ulna Involved

At times, a patient has CT scans of both the abdomen and the pelvis. Until the 2011 edition of the CPT manual, these procedures were reported as separate procedures with CPT codes 74150–74170, which described three types of CT scans of the abdomen (without contrast, with contrast, and without contrast followed by contrast material and further scans), and CPT codes 74192–74194, which described the same three CT scans of the pelvis.

Beginning with the 2011 CPT manual, when a CT scan of the abdomen is combined with a CT scan of the pelvis, a single code is used to report both procedures. These three new codes are 74176 (without contrast), 74177 (with contrast), and 74178 (without contrast followed by contrast material and further sections in one or both body parts). Magnetic Resonance Angiography of the abdomen and pelvis with contrast is reported with CPT code 74174.

The CPT manual includes a grid to show coders how to report these combinations of procedures. If both the abdomen and pelvis are scanned without contrast, code 74176 is reported. If both regions are scanned with contrast material, code 74177 is reported. If either or both regions are scanned without contrast material followed by the use of contrast material and further scans, code 74178 is reported. If one region is scanned without contrast and the other is scanned with contrast material, code 74178 is reported.

CODER'S TIP

Medicare and some other payers may allow contrast material to be reported separately by the facility performing the exam. If allowed, the contrast material is usually reported with HCPCS A-codes and Q-codes. Coders should understand how to report contrast material used during a radiological exam.

CODER'S TIP

Physicians reporting professional services only cannot report contrast material. Facilities performing the exams may report these codes. When physicians own the equipment and report services using the global codes, they may report contrast material.

CODING EXAMPLE

A bilateral x-ray of the ribs with three views was performed. What would be the correct code for this service?

Because this was a radiological examination of the ribs, bilateral, and contained three views, the correct code is 71110.

Is a modifier necessary to report that the service was done bilaterally? If so, what modifier?

Because the description of code 71110 states that the service is bilateral, no modifier should be used to report the laterality of the procedure.

Diagnostic Ultrasound

To report diagnostic ultrasound exams as separate procedures (using codes 76506–76999), it is necessary to record permanent images, including measurements when clinically indicated. When the sole purpose of the ultrasound exam is to obtain a biometric measurement, it is not necessary to retain permanent recorded images because the measurements themselves document the exam. In addition to the permanent images, a final written report should be included in the medical record.

The CPT codes describing diagnostic ultrasound procedures are divided into anatomical subsections, including:

- Head and Neck
- Chest
- Abdomen and Retroperitoneum
- Spinal Canal
- Pelvis (further divided into Obstetrical and Nonobstetrical subsections)
- Genitalia
- Extremities

CPT codes describe complete ultrasound exams and limited ultrasound exams. If the CPT code describing a complete exam is reported, each element required for the complete exam should be included in the written report or, if not visualized as part of the exam, the reason it could not be visualized. The required elements for each complete exam are listed in the particular anatomical subsection. If all of the elements of a complete exam are not included in the exam, the code for the limited exam should be reported. It is improper coding to report both a complete and limited exam on the same anatomical region during the same session.

Ultrasound also may be used as guidance during other procedures. CPT codes describing ultrasonic guidance procedures are listed in the last subsection of the Ultrasound Guidance Procedures section. Ultrasound guidance procedures also require permanent recorded images and documentation of the localization process. This documentation may be written as a separate report or included in the written report of the underlying procedure for which the guidance is used.

Several different types of ultrasound exams may be performed:

- A-mode: A one-dimensional ultrasonic measurement.
- M-mode: A one-dimensional ultrasonic measurement with movement of the trace to show the amplitude and velocity of the moving structures.
- B-scan: A two-dimensional ultrasonic scan with a two-dimensional display.
- Real-time scan: A two-dimensional ultrasonic scan with a two-dimensional display of structure and movement with time.

Most codes in the Diagnostic Ultrasound section identify the type of scan or combination of scans performed for that procedure.

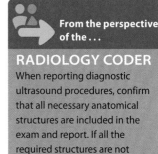

From the perspective of the . . .

RADIOLOGY CODER

When reporting diagnostic ultrasound procedures, confirm that all necessary anatomical structures are included in the exam and report. If all the required structures are not included, the code for the complete study should not be reported. In such circumstances, only the limited exam should be reported. If there is no report or permanent copy of the ultrasound, the diagnostic ultrasound codes should not be reported.

CODER'S TIP

Performing an ultrasound examination without evaluating the anatomical region and organs, documenting the images, and preparing a final written report is not a separately reportable service. If the images are documented and a report is prepared, but all required organs are not identified in the ultrasound exam, the limited exam code must be reported, not the complete exam code.

Radiologic Guidance

Various imaging techniques may be used as guidance when performing other procedures. This section (77001–77032) is divided into subsections based on the type of imaging technique utilized for guidance, including fluoroscopic, computed tomography, magnetic resonance, and other radiological guidance techniques.

Each of these subsections includes CPT codes that describe the purpose of the underlying procedure that requires the guidance. For example, the three fluoroscopic guidance codes describe use of the guidance for vascular procedures; needle placement for biopsy, aspiration, injection, or localization; and spine or paraspinous diagnostic or therapeutic injection procedures. The use of radiological guidance codes in combination with the procedure codes describing the underlying procedures is another example of component or combination coding.

mammography
An x-ray of the breast used in the screening for breast cancer.

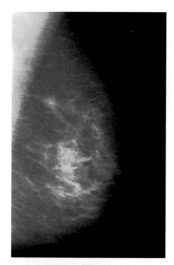

(a)

Breast, Mammography

Codes 77051–77059 describe various **mammography** exams, including screening and diagnostic studies (Figure 11.5). Some codes differentiate between bilateral and unilateral exams. This section also includes add-on codes that are reported when computer-aided detection is used to analyze digital images to identify potential lesions. Separate codes are used to report magnetic resonance imaging of the breast.

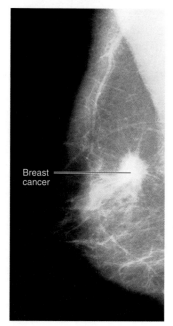

Breast cancer

(b)

FIGURE 11.5 Mammograms Showing (a) Fibrocystic Disease of the Breast (b) Breast Cancer

Bone/Joint Studies

Specific radiological studies of the bones and joints are listed in this section (77071–77084). These do not include diagnostic x-rays, CTs, MRIs, or other imaging studies of bony structures performed as part of routine diagnostic radiological exams. This section includes CPT codes describing bone age studies, bone density studies, osseous surveys for metastases, and MRI studies of the blood supply to the bone marrow.

Radiation Oncology

CPT codes in the Radiation Oncology section (77261–77799) describe the professional and technical components of the radiation services used to treat certain cancers. A radiation oncologist may see a patient in consultation prior to beginning treatment. That service would be reported with the appropriate evaluation and management code. Radiation therapy treatments may be complex and involve several stages, including:

- Clinical treatment planning: Involves tumor localization, determining the dose and timing of treatments, choice of modalities, number and shape/size of ports, and other factors unique to the treatment plan. There are three levels of planning.
- Treatment simulation: Involves evaluating the treatment areas and ports to ensure proper aim and disbursement of the radiation. There are four levels of simulation described by these codes.

- Medical radiation physics, dosimetry, treatment devices, and special services: Involves the choice of treatment modality, dose, and treatment device. Dosimetry is the calculation of the radiation dose and how it is placed to treat the individual tumor.
- Radiation treatment delivery: These codes are used to report the technical component only. The choice of code depends on the total amount of radiation delivered to the patient and the number of areas treated and ports and blocks used.
- Radiation treatment management: These codes are used to report the professional component. Physicians may report radiation treatment management services in addition to the actual radiation treatment procedures. Radiation treatment management is reported in units of five fractions or treatment sessions. These services need not be delivered on consecutive days. CPT code 77427 (Radiation treatment management, 5 treatments) is reported once for every five treatments provided. This code also may be reported if three or four treatments are provided beyond a multiple of five treatments. It is not reported if only one or two treatments are provided beyond a multiple of five treatments. CPT code 77431 may be used once to report a course of treatment that consists of only one or two treatments in total.

  Radiation treatment management includes multiple services, such as record review, dose delivery, dosimetry, patient treatment setup, port films, and treatment parameters.
- Proton beam treatment delivery: Utilizes particles that are positively charged with electricity. The choice of codes in this section is determined by whether it is a simple, intermediate, or complex delivery.
- Hyperthermia: Increases body temperature in the region of the cancer. Heat may be generated through the use of ultrasound, microwaves, or by other means. The heat source may be external, interstitial, or intracavitary.
- Clinical brachytherapy: Involves placing radioactive material directly into a tumor or in the tissues surrounding the tumor. The radioactive material may be placed in the interstitial tissues or within a body cavity.

CODING EXAMPLE

How should radiation treatment management be reported if the treatment consists of 14 treatments? Seven treatments? Two treatments?

These services are reported with CPT code 77427 (Radiation treatment management, 5 treatments). This code is reported once for every five treatments. It also may be reported if three or four treatments are provided beyond a multiple of five treatments. It is not reported if only one or two units are provided beyond a multiple of five treatments. If treatment consists of only one or two fractions, they may be reported with CPT code 77431.

In the case of 14 treatments, this treatment management would be reported with code 77427 X 3. In the case of seven treatments, this treatment management would be reported with code 77427 X 1. In the case of two treatments, this treatment management would be reported with code 77431.

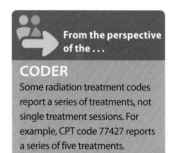

From the perspective of the . . .

CODER

Some radiation treatment codes report a series of treatments, not single treatment sessions. For example, CPT code 77427 reports a series of five treatments.

Nuclear Medicine

Nuclear medicine involves placing radioactive material within the body and then monitoring the radioactive emissions from those elements. Nuclear medicine services may be provided for either diagnostic or therapeutic purposes. CPT codes describing diagnostic nuclear medicine procedures (78000–79999) are selected based on the anatomical or physiological system tested and the type of nuclear medicine test utilized. The CPT codes describing diagnostic tests do not include the radiopharmaceutical or drug used for the test. These are reported separately.

Therapeutic nuclear medicine procedures are reported using a small set of codes (79005–79999). If the radiopharmaceutical agent is administered either orally or intravenously, the CPT code includes administration. For intra-arterial, intracavitary, or intra-articular administration of therapeutic nuclear medicine agents, the appropriate injection or procedure code is reported in addition to the nuclear medicine administration code. This is another example of component or combination coding.

EXERCISE 11.4.1   *Also available in* Mc Graw Hill **connect** (plus+)

Use the CPT manual, including the Radiology section guidelines, to answer the following questions:

1. What code describes an MRI scan of the brain without contrast material, followed by a second scan with contrast material? _____

2. What code is used to report a unilateral x-ray of the temporomandibular joint (TMJ) with open and closed views? _____

3. In the TMJ scenario above, what additional information must be reported with that code? _____

4. If an ultrasound of the abdomen is performed but there is no permanent image or report in the medical record, should the coder report the ultrasound? _____

5. When reporting CPT code 77750, is it also appropriate to report E/M codes describing hospital admission and daily visits? _____

EXERCISE 11.4.2   *Also available in* Mc Graw Hill **connect** (plus+)

Using your CPT manual, assign the correct code(s) for each radiology scenario below.

1. Magnetic resonance guidance for the monitoring of parenchymal tissue ablation _____

2. Mammographic guidance for needle placement of a breast lesion _____

3. Unilateral mammography _____

4. Bilateral two-view screening mammography _____

5. Medicare beneficiary who has a bilateral diagnostic digital image mammogram _____

6. Bone age study _____

7. Osseous survey of an infant _____

8. Dual-energy x-ray absorptiometry (DXA) body composition study _____

9. What code describes each of the following nuclear medicine studies?

    a. Thyroid, imaging only _____

    b. Liver and spleen imaging; static only _____

    c. Bone and/or joint imaging; three-phase study _____

    d. Platelet survival study _____

    e. Brain imaging less than four static views; with vascular flow _____

Summary

Learning Outcome	Key Concepts/Examples
11.1 Define positions, projections, and planes in terms of radiology services. **Page 285**	Radiology services are described according to the position the patient is in during the imaging procedure and the direction of the x-ray beam used to create the image, known as the projection. Positions include standing, supine, prone, decubitus, and oblique. Projections include anteroposterior and posteroanterior. Information from imaging procedures, such as CT or MRI scans, may be organized into two-dimensional images representing a cross-sectional image through several planes, including the transverse, sagittal, or coronal planes.
11.2 Explain the process for reporting radiology services. **Pages 286–287**	Some radiological codes include the term "separate procedure" in their descriptors. This designation means that the procedure may be reported separately if it is performed as the only procedure. If the service is performed as part of another procedure, the code is not reported separately. The term "radiological supervision and interpretation" designates radiological services performed as part of other services described by codes in the surgical or other sections of the CPT manual. These codes describe professional services only, and the use of modifier 26 is not necessary. These radiology codes are often used by nonradiologists to report their use of radiology imaging during other procedures. The Radiology section of the CPT manual includes a number of "unlisted" codes. Many types of radiology services include unlisted codes to report those types of services when no specific code describes the particular service.
11.3 Use modifiers with radiology CPT codes. **Pages 287–288**	Modifiers are used to provide more specific information about the radiological services provided. The most commonly used are modifiers 26 and TC. Modifier 26 indicates that the provider reporting the service only performed the professional services to indicate what the image shows. Modifier TC is reported by the entity that owns the imaging equipment and is only reporting the technical component, not the professional services of interpreting the image.
11.4 Discuss parameters surrounding CPT coding for various radiology services. **Pages 288–294**	Radiology codes are divided into sections by the type of imaging or other radiology services. These sections include: • Diagnostic Radiology (Diagnostic Imaging) • Diagnostic Ultrasound • Radiologic Guidance • Breast, Mammography • Bone/Joint Studies • Radiation Oncology • Nuclear Medicine Some of the sections, such as Diagnostic Radiology and Diagnostic Ultrasound, are further divided by anatomical location or types of procedures (e.g., x-ray, CT, MRI, etc.). Mammography codes include screening and diagnostic exams. The bone and joint studies do not include diagnostic x-rays or other imaging studies used as part of diagnostic radiological exams. This section includes bone age studies, bone density studies, bone surveys for metastatic diseases, and bone marrow blood supply studies. Radiation oncology codes describe services included in these treatments, such as planning, simulation, delivery, and radiation treatment management. Nuclear medicine involves the placement of radioactive materials within the body as diagnostic procedures or to treat tumors. CPT codes describing diagnostic procedures are selected based on the anatomical or physiological system tested. Therapeutic procedures are reported by codes describing the route of administration or location.

Using Terminology

Match each term with its definition.

_____ **1.** L011.4 Computed tomography (CT)
_____ **2.** L011.2 Contrast material
_____ **3.** L011.1 Coronal plane
_____ **4.** L011.1 Fluoroscopy
_____ **5.** L011.4 Mammography
_____ **6.** L011.2 Magnetic resonance imaging (MRI)
_____ **7.** L011.4 Nuclear medicine
_____ **8.** L011.1 Oblique
_____ **9.** L011.2 Radiological supervision and interpretation
_____ **10.** L011.1 Supine
_____ **11.** L011.1 Sagittal plane
_____ **12.** L011.1 Tomogram
_____ **13.** L011.1 Transverse plane
_____ **14.** L011.4 Ultrasound
_____ **15.** L011.1 X-ray film

A. The use of radioactive elements and radiation beams to treat illnesses
B. An x-ray detector upon which the x-ray beam is cast to form an image of the body plane being examined
C. A substance used to highlight specific structures in the body
D. View of a front-to-back cross section of the body
E. A technique used to view real-time images of the body by using an x-ray source and a fluoroscope
F. View of a horizontal cross section of the body
G. The use of a powerful magnetic field and special injectable materials to produce an image
H. A position in which the patient is lying between standard positions
I. Two-dimensional image of a section of a three-dimensional object
J. An x-ray of the breast, used in the screening for breast cancer
K. When a radiologist performs the supervision and provides a report of his or her findings
L. View of a side-to-side cross section of the body
M. A procedure that uses sound waves to create permanent images and measurements of body parts or as guidance during other procedures
N. The use of multiple x-rays to produce cross-sectional images
O. A position in which the patient is lying back-side down

Checking Your Understanding

Select the letter that best completes the statement or answers the question.

1. L011.1 Which of the following is a plane of view used when performing radiology procedures?

   a. Anteroposterior projection
   b. Prone
   c. Frontal
   d. Posteroanterior projection

2. L011.1 Which of the following is not the correct positioning for radiographic procedures?

   a. Anteroposterior projection
   b. Oblique projection
   c. Lateral projection
   d. Midsagittal projection

3. L011.1 Which of the following is true regarding the coronal plane?

    a. It vertically divides the body through the midline into two equal left and right halves.

    b. It horizontally divides the body into superior and inferior portions.

    c. It divides the body into anterior and posterior or ventral and dorsal portions at a right angle to the sagittal plane, separating the body into front and back.

    d. The patient is positioned at a right angle so that the body is divided into unequal left and right portions.

4. L011.1 In which type of projection is the patient positioned with his or her back parallel to the film and the x-ray beam travels from front to back, or anterior to posterior?

    a. Oblique projection

    b. Transverse projection

    c. Anteroposterior projection

    d. Posteroanterior projection

5. L011.4 Which of the following is a radiological procedure?

    a. Injection for catheter

    b. PET scan

    c. Ablation

    d. CABG

6. L011.4 Which of the following produces high-frequency sound waves that bounce off internal organs and create echoes?

    a. Venography

    b. Ultrasonography

    c. Nuclear imaging

    d. Fluoroscopy

7. L011.4 Which of the following takes x-rays of different angles to create cross-sectional images of organs, bones, and tissues to visualize blood flow in arterial and venous vessels throughout the body?

    a. MRI

    b. Single-photon emission computerized tomography (SPECT)

    c. Angiography

    d. Computed tomography angiogram (CTA)

8. L011.4 Which code would be reported for a computed tomographic angiogram, abdominal aorta and bilateral iliofemoral lower extremity runoff with contrast material and image processing?

    a. 75635

    b. 75658

    c. 75671

    d. 75736

9. L011.3 Which of the following describes supervision of the performance of the diagnostic imaging procedure and the provision of an interpretation of the images?

    a. Global service

    b. TC modifier

    c. Imaging supervision and interpretation

    d. Modifier 26

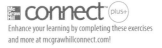

10. L011.2, L011.4 Which three things are not considered when coding for radiology procedures?

    a. The way the patient is positioned, the amount of equipment and supplies used, special reports

    b. Performance, supervision, and interpretation

    c. Type of service, use of contrast material, anatomical site

    d. Age, date of birth, and occupation of the patient

11. L011.1 Several radiology codes within the CPT manual contain the words *separate procedure*. What do the words *separate procedure* instruct the coder to report?

    a. Code the separate procedure in addition to another procedure.

    b. Provide only the code for the separate procedure.

    c. The separate procedure may be an integral part of a major procedure and should always be coded separately.

    d. The separate procedure may be an integral part of a major procedure and may not be coded.

12. L011.3 Which modifiers are often used to report radiology services?

    a. 25, 51, 50, TC, 22, 24, 54, 59

    b. 25, 26, and TC, 79, 91, GG

    c. 26, 50, 76, 77, and TC

    d. R0076, R0076, 26, 25, 50, 76, 77, and TC

13. L011.3 Which code would be used to report radiological supervision and interpretation for bilateral venography?

    a. 78522

    b. 75822

    c. 75833

    d. 75860

14. L011.4 Which code would be used to report transvaginal ultrasound of a pregnant uterus, real time with documentation of image?

    a. 76801

    b. 76813

    c. 76817

    d. 76645

15. L011.2 Which code would be used to report an x-ray of the knee, anteroposterior, both knees standing?

    a. 73564

    b. 73560

    c. 73719

    d. 73565

16. L011.4 Which of the following is not considered when reporting diagnostic ultrasound procedures?

    a. Is the diagnostic ultrasound a limited or complete exam?

    b. Are all of the required elements of a complete examination documented?

    c. Should both a limited and complete ultrasound examination be reported for procedures performed during the same session?

    d. Is there a thorough evaluation of organ(s) or anatomical region, image documentation, and a final written report?

17. L011.2, L011.4 A certified medical coder is reporting professional services for a radiologist who provided services at the hospital that day. She is reviewing a medical record when she notices a diagnostic mammogram was ordered for which there are no signs, symptoms, or evidence of breast cancer. She is unsure why a diagnostic mammogram was ordered rather than a screening mammogram. What should the coder do in this case?

  a. Make an inquiry to the physician to see if there is additional information before coding.
  b. Report a screening code.
  c. List the first-listed diagnosis.
  d. Report a diagnostic mammogram.

18. L011.2, L011.3 Medical tests are performed and the results are back. The radiology report has not yet been reviewed in order to make a definitive diagnosis. With no physician interpretation, which of the following would the correct method of coding?

  a. Make a diagnosis based on your experience.
  b. Do not code the case until the physician interprets the findings and provides a definitive diagnosis.
  c. Code only the admitting diagnosis.
  d. Code symptoms or diagnoses provided by the referring provider.

19. L011.3 Assume it is medically necessary to perform several chest x-rays on the same day for a patient with respiratory distress. How would the radiologist interpreting all these x-rays report the multiple tests?

  a. Report only one x-ray for the day.
  b. Add modifier 76 to the code for all the chest x-rays.
  c. Report three tests on the first day and the remainder on subsequent days.
  d. Report the chest x-ray code with modifier 26 for the first x-ray, and report subsequent x-rays with modifiers 26 and 76.

20. Assume it is medically necessary to perform several chest x-rays on the same day for a patient with respiratory distress. What code(s) would be reported if another radiologist read any of the subsequent x-rays?

  a. Report the chest x-ray code with modifier 26 for the first x-ray, and report subsequent x-rays with modifiers 26 and 76.
  b. Modifier 26 for professional services for all tests
  c. X-ray code with modifiers 26 and 77 for repeat procedure or service provided by another physician
  d. TC modifier for radiological supervision and interpretation

Applying Your Skills

Each of the following scenarios involves radiological procedures. Many include other services, but for purposes of these exercises, pay attention to the radiological services only. Use the CPT manual to determine the correct code to report the radiological services associated with each of the following procedures.

  1. L011.4 A patient has neoplastic tumors of the liver that are not amenable to surgical resection. The physician performs a minimally invasive surgical laparoscopy for radiofrequency ablation. What code describes ultrasonic imaging to visualize the tumors? _____

  2. L011.4 A physician performs a needle biopsy to determine whether a tumor on the patient's prostate is cancerous. A needle is inserted into the prostate under ultrasonic visualization, and a tissue sample is obtained. Which code describes the ultrasonic guidance? _____

  3. L011.3 Radiological supervision and interpretation is required to catheterize a patient to introduce contrast material for saline infusion sonohysterography (SIS). Which codes describe the radiological portions of the catheterization and ultrasound sonohysterography? _____

Mc Graw Hill **connect**™ (plus+)
Enhance your learning by completing these exercises and more at mcgrawhillconnect.com!

CHAPTER 11 | **RADIOLOGY SERVICES**   299

4. L011.3 A patient is diagnosed with cervical cancer and requires clinical brachytherapy by insertion of Heyman capsules. An intracavitary insertion of eight radioactive elements near the target tissue is done using radiological guidance. What code describes the radiological supervision and guidance required? _____

5. L011.3 A surgeon performs an endovascular repair of an infrarenal abdominal aortic aneurysm. What code would be reported for the imaging performed with this procedure?_____

6. L011.4 A 45-year-old woman presents to her gynecologist's office for her annual physical exam. The physician performs a Pap smear and breast exam. The breast exam reveals lumps that require further investigation. The physician orders a bilateral diagnostic mammography that will be performed by the radiological technologist that same day within the medical office. Which codes would be reported for the mammography? _____

7. L011.4 A patient has not been able to metabolize lipids appropriately, causing gastrointestinal complications. Because bile from the gallbladder is responsible for metabolizing fats, the physician obtains real-time images of the soft tissue of the gallbladder using high-frequency sound waves. Coding from the doctor's order, which code would you report for the diagnostic ultrasound? _____

8. L011.4 A 55-year-old male patient is evaluated for poor blood flow to his kidneys. The patient's past family and social history reveals that vascular disease runs in his family, he is a smoker, and he eats a high-fat diet. After further workup, the patient is scheduled for a percutaneous transluminal balloon angioplasty of both renal arteries with radiological supervision and interpretation. Which codes would you report for the imaging?

_____

9. L011.2 A line worker at an automotive manufacturing plant has been putting in a lot of mandatory overtime and is having difficulty performing his job of manually installing parts on a new line of vehicles. His primary care physician orders a two-view x-ray of his wrists. Which codes would you report for this radiology procedure?

_____

10. L011.3 In order to determine if a patient's cancer has spread, a physician performs an MRI of the pelvis. This staging procedure will use high resolution to provide the physician with images from multiple planes. What code is used to report the interpretation of the MRI? _____

11. L011.3, L011.4 A patient presents to the emergency room with shortness of breath, tachycardia, anxiety, and hyper-ventilation. Psychiatric disorders are ruled out. The physician suspects the patient has a pulmonary embolism and orders a computed tomographic angiogram with contrast to obtain images of the pulmonary arteries. Which code describes the radiologist's interpretation of the CT scan? _____

12. L011.3, L011.4 A medical assistant student is preparing to do her externship and must obtain a tuberculosis (TB) skin test before she can begin clinical rotations. The TB skin test reveals a hard wheal indicating a positive result. The student has a two-view chest x-ray as follow-up for the positive skin test. Which code describes the interpretation of these x-rays? _____

13. L011.3, L011.4 A 35-year-old woman on a family vacation at an amusement park experienced neck pain while riding a roller coaster. When she got home, she discovered she could not sleep at night because the pain was getting worse. Her primary care doctor suspected whiplash and wrote an order for her to have an x-ray of the soft tissue in her neck. Which code would you report for the interpretation of these x-rays? _____

14. L011.3, L011.4 A woman was driving to work in New York City one morning when she was broadsided by a truck driver who was running late for his delivery. She sustained a traumatic brain injury. Her physician ordered an MRI of the brain, including the brain stem, with contrast material. Which code would you report for the MRI of the brain? _____

15. L011.3, L011.4 A patient is diagnosed with diabetes mellitus after her hemoglobin A1C comes back abnormal. The physician suspects the patient has lost physiological functioning of the beta cells of her islets of Langerhans within the pancreas. The patient has had poor insulin hormone production and utilization, as evidenced by her lab results and the physician's inability to stabilize her blood sugars. The physician orders a percutaneous needle biopsy of the pancreas with fluoroscopic guidance to determine what, if any, disease may be present in the pancreas. Which code describes the radiological imaging, supervision, and interpretation? _____

16. L011.3, L011.4 A patient sees her primary care physician for back pain, abdominal pain, fever, and malaise. Labs and a radiological examination of her gastrointestinal tract with an x-ray of her kidneys, ureters, and bladder (KUB) are ordered and performed. The results reveal that she has some bacterial infection secondary to the diverticular disease in her intestines. The disease has progressed to the point of developing a retroperitoneal abscess that may need to be drained percutaneously if it does not respond to antibiotics. What code describes the test that has already been performed, documented, and signed? _____

17. L011.3, L011.4 A 70-year-old woman with a history of morbid obesity has been having some complications with her weight-bearing joints. In addition to being placed on a protein-sparing modified fast, prescribed potassium supplementation, and instructed to walk daily, her physician orders a three view radiological examination of her knees. Which code would you report for this radiological procedure? _____

18. L011.3, L011.4 A 56-year-old woman sees her primary care physician with the complaint of pain radiating into her thigh. After a complete medical evaluation, the physician orders a computed tomography of the abdomen without contrast followed by contrast and further sections. The results show that the patient has a rare sarcoma. The signed radiology report is in the chart. What code identifies the radiological services? _____

19. L011.4 A patient has neoplastic disease of the chest, which will require a targeted approach of delivering radiation therapy to avoid damage to surrounding tissue. Stereoscopic x-ray guidance for localization of target volume for the delivery of radiation therapy is performed in a freestanding imaging center. What code describes this service? _____

20. L011.3, L011.4 A radiation oncologist develops a patient's treatment plan to deliver 15 MeV of radiation to a single area of the cervix in order to kill the cancer found there. It is thought that this procedure will prevent any recurrence of the disease. Which code describes this radiation treatment? _____

21. L011.4 In the course of providing treatment for a patient with neoplastic disease, a nurse practitioner examines the patient. A radiation oncologist reviews the dictation, greets the patient, and verifies that everything is set up in the treatment room for radiation treatment management. The patient is to receive five radiation treatments. What code is used to report this procedure? _____

22. L011.4 A patient presents to the emergency room with visible signs of diaphoresis, forceful tachycardia, and extreme hypertension. She is extremely anxious and fearful. The emergency room physician suspects the patient may have a pheochromocytoma, which is a rare tumor of the adrenal gland. To rule out this tumor, the physician orders nuclear imaging of the adrenal cortex. Which code describes imaging of the adrenal cortex? _____

23. L011.3, L011.4 A 35-year-old woman is seen by her primary care provider for her annual physical. Baseline laboratory tests are acquired. The complete blood count comes back abnormal. The patient has extremely low monocyte and lymphocyte counts. Upon further inquiry and study, the physician documents a diagnosis of aplastic anemia. Because blood is manufactured in the bone marrow, the physician orders a three-phase nuclear imaging study of the bones. It has not been determined whether the patient will need a bone marrow transplant. Which code describes this bone imaging technique? _____

connect plus+

Enhance your learning by completing these exercises and more at mcgrawhillconnect.com!   CHAPTER 11 | RADIOLOGY SERVICES   301

24. LO11.3, LO 11.4 A 50-year-old male has been complaining of feelings of impending doom, chest pain, jaw pain, and erratic-feeling heartbeats in his chest when he lies down to go to sleep at night. The patient has a history of hypokalemia and has an abnormal EKG. The patient's cardiologist performs an echocardiogram and cardiac stress test, as well as myocardial perfusion imaging including quantitative wall motion, with multiple studies at rest and during stress due to pharmacological agents. What code describes the myocardial perfusion imaging?

_____

25. LO11.3, LO 11.4 A 76-year-old woman with a history of chronic cigarette smoking, hypertension, and transient ischemic attacks sustained a cerebral vascular accident (CVA) within the past six months. She has right-sided paralysis and is unable to speak. To assess the risks for further damage, the patient's physician orders radiological imaging of the brain for vascular flow. What code describes radiological imaging of the brain for vascular flow?

_____

26. LO11.4 A 68-year-old male has a history of significant heart disease including coronary atherosclerosis, congestive heart failure, and cardiomegaly. The patient's cardiologist wishes to assess the patient's right ventricular ejection fraction by first-pass technique. The radiological study involves cardiac blood pool imaging and gated equilibrium. A single study at rest is performed. What code(s) would you report for this radiological imaging?

_____

27. LO11.3, LO11.4 An Olympic ice skater falls on the ice and sustains an ankle injury. Her manager will not allow her to go back to skating until her ankle has healed. She sees her physician, who orders a radiological exam of the ankle with three views. Which code describes the interpretation of these x-rays? _____

28. LO11.3, LO11.4 A 21-year-old male and his friend went to their usual stop on Friday night during happy hour— Eat at Joe's Sports Bar and Grill. In between hot-and-spicy buffalo wings and pitchers of beer, the man was enjoying one of his other favorite pastimes—bungee jumping and rock climbing—when he landed on the ground and dislocated his shoulder. What code describes the interpretation of a single-view diagnostic x-ray of the shoulder? _____

29. LO11.3, LO 11.4 A 45-year-old female went to see her gastroenterologist due to complaints of diarrhea, constipation, and rectal pain. After a physical exam, the physician determined that the patient had irritable bowel syndrome and prescribed a motility agent in addition to scheduling a radiological exam of the colon with barium contrast material, including a KUB. Which code would you report for the radiologist's interpretation of this exam of the colon? _____

30. LO11.4 A 50-year-old man is involved in an automobile accident. He is brought to the emergency department, where he is examined. He complains of diffuse abdominal pain over most of the middle and lower abdominal regions. The ED physician orders a CT scan of the abdomen and pelvis, with and without contrast. Which code describes the professional services associated with this exam? _____

Thinking It Through

Use your critical-thinking skills to answer the questions below.

1. L011.3 Radiology procedures involve two separate components that are commonly described by the use of modifiers added to the code. What are these two components?

   _____

   _____

2. L011.3 The professional component of a diagnostic procedure includes interpretation of the study and a written report. How do radiologists report these services?

   _____

   _____

3. L011.3 If a provider owns or leases the equipment used to perform the radiological exam and provides the interpretation, along with documentation of that interpretation in the medical record, what modifier is added to the radiology code?

   _____

   _____

4. L011.3 An imaging center owns complex imaging equipment but does not employ the radiologists who interpret the imaging studies performed there. How would the imaging center report the imaging studies?

   _____

   _____

5. L011.3 Many procedures require radiological guidance to be performed. Describe how these procedures are reported in each of the following circumstances.

   a. The physician performs the procedure and provides the radiological guidance.

   _____

   _____

   b. One physician performs the procedure and another physician provides the radiological guidance.

   _____

   _____

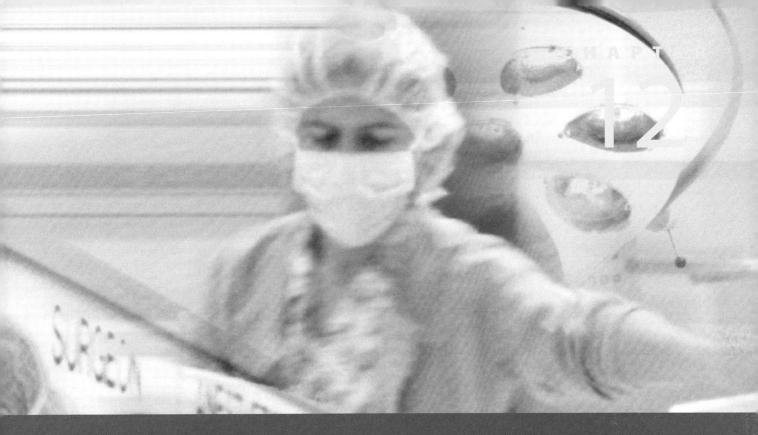

SURGERY CODES
Coding for Surgical Procedures
on Specific Organ Systems

Module 12.1
General and Integumentary System

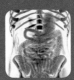

Module 12.4
Digestive System

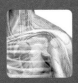

Module 12.2
Musculoskeletal System

Module 12.5
Urinary System, Male and Female Genital Systems, and Maternity Care and Delivery

Module 12.3
Respiratory, Cardiovascular, Hemic, and Lymphatic Systems, Mediastinum, and Diaphragm

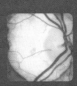

Module 12.6
Endocrine, Nervous, Ocular, and Auditory Systems

Introduction

The term *surgical procedure* encompasses thousands of different services, ranging from the simplest excision of a skin tag to the most complex procedures deep inside the brain. Most of these procedures are described by CPT codes in the range of 10021–69990. In some instances, a single code describes a distinct surgical procedure, while in other situations a family of codes is used to describe slight variations among closely related procedures. Sometimes one code describes the basic procedure and add-on codes are used to indicate additional components of the procedure, either in terms of the number of services provided or the extent of the procedure.

Surgical procedure codes include a number of services beyond the surgical procedure itself. Services considered to be included in the surgical procedure described by a CPT code include the following:

- One E/M service, including a history and physical exam, on the day of or the day before the surgical procedure.
- Infiltration of local anesthesia, application of topical anesthesia, or provision of a digital block anesthetic of one or more fingers or toes.
- The surgical procedure itself.
- Postoperative care in the postanesthesia recovery area.
- Writing postoperative orders, dictating operative notes, and talking with the patient's family and other physicians caring for the patient.
- Routine postoperative follow-up care.

Follow-up Care

The extent of follow-up care that is considered to be included in the surgical procedure is limited to the care that is related to the procedure itself. Postoperative care after therapeutic surgical procedures includes the care that is typically necessary following that particular surgery. The treatment of complications, recurrences of the underlying disease, exacerbations, or the occurrence of other conditions may be separately reported in addition to reporting the surgical procedure. For diagnostic procedures such as arthroscopies, endoscopies, or injections for diagnostic radiographic procedures, the postoperative care included in the procedure is only the care related to recovery from the diagnostic procedure. Care provided after the diagnostic procedure that is related to the underlying condition for which the diagnostic test was performed or for other medical conditions requiring treatment is not included under the diagnostic procedure CPT code and may be reported separately.

Many surgical procedures have a global period associated with them. A significant number of procedures do not have an associated global period. Medicare, for example, assigns either a 10- or 90-day global period to many surgical procedures, but it does not assign a global period to many other codes. In general, all follow-up care provided during the global period that is related to the procedure, including E/M services, wound checks, dressing changes, and other routine postoperative care, is included in the payment for the surgical procedure. While payment methodologies are beyond the scope of basic coding courses, it is important for coders to understand that how the services are reported affects payments.

Multiple Procedures and "Separate Procedures"

When more than one procedure is performed on the same date of service, it is necessary to add one or more modifiers to the CPT codes describing the additional services. Modifiers should not be used to report services typically included in the surgical package unless documentation shows that the procedure is not part of the surgical package in that particular case.

Many CPT codes that describe procedures routinely performed as part of other surgical procedures include the term "separate procedure" as part of their descriptors. This does not mean that these codes are reported separately when the services described by those codes are performed as part of another service. The "separate procedure" designation means that if the procedure is performed as a stand-alone service, not related to another, larger procedure, then it is reported with that CPT code.

When a provider performs a service described by a CPT code with the "separate procedure" designation, and that service is not part of other services provided on that date of service, the CPT code describing that separate service should be listed with modifier 59 added. The most common situations for adding modifier 59 are when the service is performed on a different body part, through a separate incision, to treat a separate injury, or at a different time on the same date of service.

Structure of the Surgical Section of the CPT Manual

Surgical CPT codes are divided into numerical sections, each of which may be subdivided into subsections based on anatomy or physiology. This chapter is divided into six modules based on the numerical sections listed in Table 12.1 below. Each module provides instructions regarding the codes in that section, including exercises related to those codes.

Because of the large number of codes included in these sections, coders should become familiar with using the index to identify the individual codes or family of codes that describe particular surgical procedures. Once these codes are identified, it is necessary to review the detailed description of each one to determine the most appropriate code to report the service provided.

TABLE 12.1 Sections of Surgical Section in CPT Manual

Section/Code Series	Subsections
10000	General and Integumentary System
20000	Musculoskeletal System
30000	Respiratory System (30000–32999) Cardiovascular System (33010–37799) Hemic and Lymphatic System (38100–38999) Mediastinum and Diaphragm (39000–39599)
40000	Digestive System
50000	Urinary System (50010–53899) Male Genital System (54000–55899) Female Genital System (56405–58999) Maternity Care and Delivery (59000–59899)
60000	Endocrine System (60000–60699) Nervous System (61000–64999) Eye and Ocular Adnexa (65091–68899) Auditory System (69000–69979) Operating Microscope (69990)

Learning Outcomes   *After completing this module, students should be able to:*

12.1.1 Identify procedures of the skin and subcutaneous tissues.

12.1.2 Determine how to group wounds together according to anatomical location and type of closure for reporting purposes.

12.1.3 Describe the differences between graft, flap, and burn procedures.

12.1.4 Report tissue destruction of benign and malignant tissues by various techniques.

12.1.5 Select the appropriate codes for surgical procedures on the breast.

12.1.6 Code anesthesia services for procedures in the 10000 series.

Key Terms

Abscess

Adjacent tissue transfer

Allograft

Autograft

Complete mastectomy

Complex wound repair

Debridement

Excision

Fine needle aspiration

Hematoma

Hidradenitis

Incision and drainage

Intermediate wound repair

Modified radical mastectomy

Mohs micrographic surgery

Necrotizing infection

Partial mastectomy

Radical mastectomy

Simple wound repair

Tissue flap

Xenograft

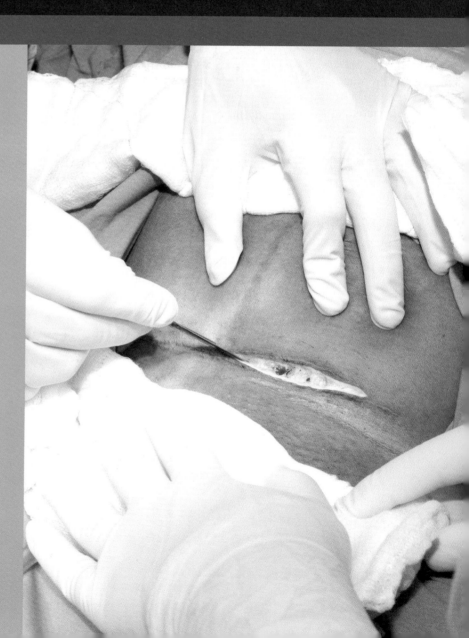

Introduction

The CPT manual divides the 10000 code series into two main sections: General and Integumentary System. The General section consists of only two codes; for convenience, these are discussed with the first series of codes describing procedures of the skin and subcutaneous tissues.

12.1.1 Reporting Procedures of the Skin and Subcutaneous Tissues (10021–11983)

General

This section consists of only two codes, one describing **fine needle aspiration** without imaging guidance (10021) and the other fine needle aspiration with imaging guidance (10022). These codes describe the fine needle aspiration itself, with parenthetical notes identifying codes describing associated services. There also is a parenthetical note identifying codes that describe percutaneous needle biopsies that are not fine needle aspirations.

For example, CPT code 10022 includes a parenthetical remark directing coders to use CPT code 76942 (ultrasound), 77002 (fluoroscopy), 77012 (CT), or 77021 (MRI) for the radiological supervision and interpretation associated with the particular imaging guidance modality used during the procedure.

In the CPT manual, the parenthetical note at the end of this section identifies codes that describe percutaneous needle biopsies other than fine needle aspirations, including:

- 20206 Muscle
- 32400 Pleural
- 32405 Lung or mediastinum
- 42400 Salivary gland
- 47000 and 47001 Liver
- 48102 Pancreas
- 49180 Abdominal or retroperitoneal mass
- 60100 Thyroid
- 62267 Nucleus pulposus, intervertebral disk, or paravertebral tissue
- 62269 Spinal cord

Each of these codes also includes a parenthetical remark directing coders to CPT codes 10021 and 10022 for fine needle aspiration.

Coders must become familiar with using parenthetical notes to identify the most appropriate codes to describe particular services. These notes also provide instructions on whether a particular combination of codes may be reported together. For example, many nerve block codes now include fluoroscopic guidance as an inherent service within the code, whereas other blocks do not. If fluoroscopic guidance is included, the radiology code for that service cannot be reported separately. When not included, an additional code describing the radiology service may be reported separately. The number of codes describing blocks that include image guidance has increased with each new edition of the CPT. This underscores the need for coders to use the most recent edition of the CPT manual to avoid errors.

Superficial Procedures

CPT codes describing integumentary procedures are divided into sections by the type of procedure rather than by location. Some sections include guidance or parenthetical comments instructing coders on specific coding elements unique to codes in that section.

fine needle aspiration
The use of a needle to collect cells for clinical examination.

In some sections, the codes are further subdivided by the size of the involved area, the type of closure performed, or anatomical location.

Incision and Drainage

incision and drainage
A procedure in which the skin is punctured or an incision is made without closing the skin afterwards, allowing for the removal of fluid.

Incision and Drainage **Incision and drainage** procedures (10040–10180) typically involve puncturing the skin or making an incision but not closing the skin at the end of the procedure. Some code descriptors include the reason for performing the procedure, such as to remove a foreign body or to drain an **abscess, hematoma,** or other fluid collection. Parenthetical comments direct coders to use other codes to describe exploration of wounds due to penetrating trauma or open fractures. CPT code 10180 describes incision and drainage of postoperative wound infections.

abscess
Pus collection in an infected site, usually accompanied by inflammation and pain.

hematoma
Collection of blood that has escaped from the blood vessels into tissue.

debridement
The removal of injured or necrotic tissue.

Debridement Two codes describe **debridement** of skin due to eczema or infection. CPT code 11000 is reported to identify the first 10 percent of body surface area, and code 11001 is reported for each additional 10 percent of body area or part of an additional 10 percent.

CODING EXAMPLE

A surgeon performs debridement of 23 percent of the total body surface area. How would a coder report this procedure?

Because of the surface area involved in this procedure, the coder would report 11000 X 1 and 11001 X 2 (once for the additional surface area between 10 and 20 percent and a second time for the additional 3 percent).

necrotizing infection
Severe inflammation that produces tissue death.

Debridement procedures for **necrotizing infections** are described by CPT codes 11004–11006. An add-on code (11008) describes removal of prosthetic material or mesh as part of a debridement procedure. Like all add-on codes, code 11008 is reported in addition to the code that best describes the underlying procedure.

A series of codes (11010–11012) describes debridement procedures related to open fractures. These codes are differentiated from each other by the extent of tissues debrided during the surgical procedure. Another series of codes (11040–11047) describes debridement of tissue during surgical procedures that are not associated with open fractures. A parenthetical comment instructs coders not to report these codes with codes describing active wound management (codes 97597–97602).

Paring or Cutting These codes describe paring or cutting of benign hyperkeratotic lesions, such as corns or calluses. Code 11055 is used for one lesion; 11056 for 2–4 lesions; and 11057 for more than four lesions.

Biopsy Biopsies of skin lesions are not typically reported separately. Skin tissue is most often excised as part of another procedure, in which case the biopsy is part of that other procedure and the biopsy codes are not reported separately. Biopsy codes may be reported separately if the skin biopsy is performed independently rather than as part of another procedure. CPT code 11100 is used to report the first lesion, and add-on code 11101 is used to report each additional separate lesion.

Removal of Skin Tags These codes are used to report the removal of skin tags by any method. Coders should report CPT code 11200 once to describe the removal of 1–15 skin tags, while CPT code 11201 is used to report each additional 10 lesions or portions thereof.

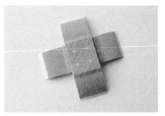

A physician removes 29 separate skin tags from a patient's neck, chest, abdomen, and perineal areas. The coder reports these procedures with CPT codes 11200 X 1 (for the first 15 lesions) and 11201 X 2 (once for lesions 16–25 and again for lesions 26–29).

When coding for procedures of the skin, note the location where the procedure was performed and the amount of skin involved.

Shaving of Epidermal or Dermal Lesions Shaving consists of slicing horizontally through epidermal or dermal layers of skin to remove a lesion without excising the full thickness of skin. Because the deeper layers of skin are intact, no sutures are necessary to close the wound. Cautery may be necessary to stop bleeding if the incision goes into the dermal layers, which include blood vessels that bring oxygen and nutrients to the skin. Cautery is included in these code descriptors. This family of codes (11300–11313) is first divided into three groups by location: (1) trunk, arms, or legs; (2) scalp, neck, hands, feet, or genitalia; and (3) face, ears, eyelids, nose, lips, or mucous membranes. Each group is further divided into four individual CPT codes by lesion size: (1) 0.5 cm or less; (2) 0.6 to 1.0 cm; (3) 1.1 to 2.0 cm; and (4) over 2.0 cm.

Excision of Benign and Malignant Lesions Excision refers to the full-thickness removal of a lesion and surrounding tissues. The excision codes include local anesthesia and simple wound repair of the defect created by the removal of the lesion. A simple wound repair is a single-layer closure of the skin defect. If more extensive wound repairs are necessary, such as intermediate or complex closures, the appropriate wound repair code is reported in addition to the excision code. Wound repair procedures are discussed in detail below. Each benign or malignant lesion excised is reported separately using the CPT code that most accurately describes that excision.

Separate families of codes describe excisions of benign and malignant lesions. Both code families are divided into three groups based on anatomical location, and then each group is subdivided into individual CPT codes by the size of the lesion excised. The anatomical groups include (1) trunk, arms, or legs; (2) scalp, neck, hands, feet, or genitalia; and (3) face, ears, eyelids, nose, lips, or mucous membranes. Each anatomical group is divided into six specific codes by the size of the excised lesion, including margins: (1) less than 0.5 cm; (2) 0.6 to 1.0 cm; (3) 1.1 to 2.0 cm; (4) 2.1 to 3.0 cm; (5) 3.1 to 4.0 cm; and (6) over 4.0 cm. The total size is calculated by adding the largest diameter of the lesion to the smallest necessary margins.

The Excision—Benign Lesions section also includes six codes describing excision of skin and subcutaneous tissue for **hidradenitis,** a chronic condition affecting sweat glands in the axilla, groin, or other regions. These codes (11450–11471) differentiate these excisions by three anatomical regions and whether a simple or complex wound repair is necessary (see wound repair discussion below).

Malignant lesions are often sent to the pathology laboratory to make sure the margins are tumor free. If the margins are not "clean" or tumor free, additional tissue must be excised. If this is performed during the same operative procedure, only the single CPT code that describes the tumor plus the total margin size is reported. On rare occasions, it may be necessary to return to the operating room to excise further tissue during a separate operative session. In those cases, the CPT code that best describes the size of the additional tissue excised is reported for the repeat procedure. Modifier 58 is added to the code if the second procedure is performed during the global period of the first procedure.

Nails; Pilonidal Cyst; Introduction CPT codes 11719–11765 describe various procedures on the nails, including debridement, avulsion, evacuation of hematoma, excision of nail and nail matrix, biopsy, repair, reconstruction, and wedge

excision
Removal of tissues, organs or other anatomical structures.

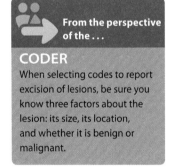

From the perspective of the . . .

CODER

When selecting codes to report excision of lesions, be sure you know three factors about the lesion: its size, its location, and whether it is benign or malignant.

hidradenitis
A chronic condition affecting sweat glands in the axilla, groin or other regions.

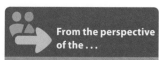

From the perspective of the . . .

PROVIDER

Knowing a lesion's size is crucial to selecting the right code for the lesion's removal. When performing this procedure, record the sizes of lesions removed in the operative notes for use by the coder.

resection for an ingrown toenail. Excision of pilonidal cysts is reported with CPT codes 11770–11772. A parenthetical note with these codes provides the instruction that incisions of pilonidal cysts are reported with codes 10080–10081. The Introduction section includes injections; tattooing; subcutaneous injections of filling material; insertion, removal, and replacement of tissue expanders (other than breast); insertion, removal, and reinsertion of implantable contraceptive capsules; and insertion, removal, and reinsertion of drug delivery implants.

When skin is removed, it is important that coders understand how to calculate the total diameter of the lesion. Lesions are not usually uniformly circular in size. Rather, the size of the lesion depends on which direction is measured. A lesion's size is usually calculated based on the following equation:

Maximum lesion diameter + Narrowest margin on two sides = Total lesion diameter

CODER'S TIP

When lesions are surgically removed, surrounding tissue is often removed in addition to the lesion itself. The amount of surrounding tissue depends on the type of lesion (i.e., benign or malignant). The total diameter of the surgical excision is determined by measuring the *maximum* distance across the lesion plus the *narrowest* margin surrounding the lesion on two sides. The total diameter is one factor that determines the correct CPT code.

CODING EXAMPLE

When determining which CPT code describes the excision of a 2 cm by 1 cm lesion with 0.5 cm margins on all sides, what is the diameter of the lesion? Keep in mind that the lesion's size is equal to its maximum diameter plus its narrowest margin on two sides. The total diameter of this lesion is 2 cm (largest distance across the lesion) plus 0.5 cm margin on one side of the lesion plus 0.5 cm margin on the other side of the lesion. This is a total of 3.0 cm.

EXERCISE 12.1.1

Also available in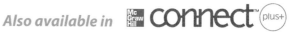

Use the CPT manual to select the code(s) to describe the following services.

1. Procedures on pilonidal cysts

    a. Incision and drainage of a complicated pilonidal cyst _____

    b. Excision of pilonidal cysts _____

2. Incision and drainage of a hematoma on the scalp _____

3. Removal of glass pieces and debridement of an open fracture of the femur _____

4. Debridement of subcutaneous tissue and muscle _____

5. Paring or cutting of five benign hyperkeratotic lesions _____

6. Debridement of nails _____

7. Complicated excision of a 1.3 cm benign lesion on the hand _____

8. Repair of a nail bed _____

9. Excision of a 4.2 cm malignant lesion on the right leg _____

12.1.2 Wound Repair (Closure) (12001–13160)

Wound Repair or Closure

Wound repair involves the placement of sutures, staples, or adhesives to hold the edges of a wound together until healing occurs. When adhesive strips are used as the only method of wound closure, surgical wound repair codes should not be used to describe the service provided. Instead, the procedure is described with the E/M code that best describes the level of services provided during the procedure.

Wound repairs are classified according to the level of difficulty involved:

- **Simple repair:** A one-layer closure of a wound with sutures or a device.
- **Intermediate repair:** A multilayer closure of a wound with one or more layers of subcutaneous tissue closure in addition to the skin closure.
- **Complex repair:** A wound repair requiring more than a multilayer closure, such as debridement, undermining of wound margins, scar revisions, or the use of retention sutures or stents.

A separate family of codes describes each wound repair technique—simple, intermediate, and complex. Each family of codes is divided into groups based on the anatomical location of wounds. These groups are subdivided into individual CPT codes based on wound length.

Simple repairs (12001–12018) are divided into two anatomical groups. The first includes superficial wounds of the scalp, neck, axillae, external genitalia, trunk, and extremities. For simple repairs, the term "extremities" *includes* the hands and feet. The second group includes superficial wounds of the face, ears, eyelids, nose, lips, and mucous membranes. Within each group, individual codes describe simple repairs of wounds of varying lengths ranging from 2.5 cm or less up to over 30.0 cm. Coders must pay particular attention to the sizes of the wounds to correctly identify the correct codes.

The Simple Repair section also includes two codes that describe treatment of superficial wound dehiscence. Code 12020 describes simple closure, while code 12021 describes packing of the wound dehiscence.

Intermediate repairs (12031–12057) are divided into three anatomical groups:

- Scalp, axillae, trunk, and extremities, *excluding* the hands and feet.
- Neck, hands, feet, and external genitalia.
- Face, ears, eyelids, nose, lips, and mucous membranes.

Similar to the simple repair code groups, these groups are subdivided into individual codes based on wound length ranging from 2.5 cm or less up to over 30.0 cm.

Complex repairs (13100–13153) are divided into four anatomical groups:

- Trunk.
- Scalp, arms, or legs.
- Forehead, cheeks, chin, mouth, neck, axillae, genitalia, hands, and feet.
- Eyelids, nose, ears, and lips.

Each of these groups is subdivided based on the length of the wound, but these lengths differ from those described under simple or intermediate repairs. The first code in each group describes complex repairs of wounds of 1.1 to 2.5 cm in length. The second code describes wounds of 2.6 to 7.5 cm. Each group includes an add-on code that describes each additional 5 cm or less of wound length that is listed in addition to the second code in each group to account for the actual wound length.

Code 13160 describes secondary closure of a surgical wound or wound dehiscence.

A parenthetical note with each group instructs coders not to use the complex closure codes for wounds of 1.0 cm or less. These must be reported with the simple or intermediate closure codes. Another parenthetical note at the beginning of this section directs coders to other sections for full-thickness repairs of the lip or eyelid.

simple wound repair
A one-layer closure of a wound with sutures or a device.

intermediate wound repair
A multilayer closure of a wound with one or more layers of subcutaneous tissue closure in addition to the skin closure.

complex wound repair
A wound repair requiring more than a multilayer closure, such as debridement, undermining of wound margins, scar revisions, or use of retention sutures or stents.

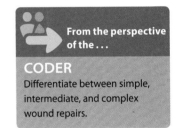

From the perspective of the . . .

CODER
Differentiate between simple, intermediate, and complex wound repairs.

CODER'S TIP

Pay close attention to the locations and lengths of the wounds closed by each repair type. The anatomical grouping of wounds is not the same in the three wound repair sections (simple, intermediate, and complex). Similarly, the wound lengths included in each CPT code within the anatomical groups vary by both closure type and anatomical location.

Coding Wound Repair Services

When reporting wound repair services, use the following guidelines:

1. The length of each wound repair is measured in centimeters (cm).
2. Wounds treated by the same type of repair (simple, intermediate, or complex) are grouped together.
3. The wounds from each group identified above are divided by the anatomical locations included in each subgroup of CPT codes under that repair type.
4. The lengths of multiple wounds treated with the same type of repair and from the same anatomical grouping associated with that repair type are added together.
5. The total length of repairs in each group identifies the specific CPT code used to report the wound repairs included in that group.

CODING EXAMPLE

Determine the CPT codes used to report the repair of the following wounds, all performed as one procedure on one patient:

A. A 2.5 cm wound of the abdomen closed with an intermediate repair
B. A 4.5 cm wound on the forearm closed with a simple repair
C. A 5.0 cm wound of the chest wall closed with a simple repair
D. A 2.0 cm wound of the hand closed with an intermediate repair
E. A 6.5 cm wound of the thigh closed with an intermediate repair

First, group the wounds by repair type. This results in two groups: B and C (simple repairs) and A, D, and E (intermediate repairs). Next, review anatomical groupings in the CPT manual to determine whether the two groups must be further divided. Repairs B and C are considered together, as both of these are included in the same anatomical group of codes. These two wounds add up to 9.5 cm total. The correct CPT code to describe these repairs is 12004.

The remaining three repairs (A, D, and E) must be further divided. Repairs A and E are part of the same anatomical grouping described under the Repair—Intermediate family of repair codes. These two wounds add up to 9.0 cm and are described by CPT code 12034. Unlike simple repairs, intermediate repairs of hand or foot wounds are not in the same group as extremity wounds. Therefore, repair D is part of a different group and is reported with CPT code 12041.

EXERCISE 12.1.2

Also available in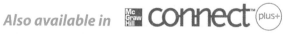

Use the CPT manual to select the code(s) to describe the following services.

1. Repair of a 22.5 cm superficial wound of the left calf _____
2. Simple repair of a 4.3 cm wound of the eyelid _____

3. Intermediate repair of a 7.2 cm scalp wound and a 12.0 cm arm wound _____

4. Complex repairs of a 9.5 cm arm wound and 4.0 cm cheek wound _____

5. Intermediate repairs of a 4.5 cm neck wound and 3.0 cm hand wound plus a 5.0 cm scalp wound _____

12.1.3 Skin Repair Procedures (14000–16036)

Adjacent Tissue Transfer or Rearrangement

Codes 14000–14350 describe excision procedures and/or wound repairs when adjacent tissue is transferred (**adjacent tissue transfer**) or rearranged to cover part of the primary wound. Numerous procedures are used to transfer adjacent tissues to cover a primary wound, including Z-plasty, W-plasty, rotation flaps, island flaps, and advancement flaps.

adjacent tissue transfer
A skin repair procedure in which adjacent tissue is transferred or rearranged to cover part of the primary wound.

The primary defect is the initial wound or excision area. Transferring or rearranging tissues often creates a secondary defect. The sizes of the primary and secondary defects are added together to determine which code is selected to describe the procedure.

The codes are divided into groups based on anatomical locations:

- Trunk.
- Scalp, arms, or legs.
- Forehead, cheeks, chin, mouth, neck, axillae, genitalia, hands, or feet.
- Eyelids, nose, ears, or lips.

Each group consists of two codes describing the total size of the defect as less than 10.0 sq cm or 10.1 to 30.0 sq cm. Two additional codes are used to report tissue transfers involving larger defects. Code 14301 describes tissue transfers for defects of 30.1 to 60.0 sq cm, and add-on code 14302 is used for each additional 30.0 sq cm or part thereof.

Skin Replacement Surgery and Skin Substitutes

CPT codes 15002–15005 are used to report the preparation of the recipient area to which skin replacement materials will be applied. CPT codes 15002 and 15004 describe preparation of the first 100 sq cm of the defect area in adults and children over 10 years of age. They are also used to describe the first 1 percent of body surface area in infants and children under 10 years of age. These two codes differ according to the anatomical location of the recipient area. CPT codes 15003 and 15005 are add-on codes that describe each additional 100 sq cm or 1 percent of body surface area, or any part thereof.

autografts
Tissues transferred from one part of a patient's body to another part.

CPT codes 15100–15261 describe various split-thickness and full-thickness **autografts** (tissues transferred from one part of a patient's body to another part), including tissues cultured for tissue autografts. As with many other sections of codes describing procedures involving the integumentary system, the codes are divided into groups by anatomical location. Each anatomical group has a primary code describing the initial area (100 sq cm or 1 percent of body surface area in infants and children) and an add-on code for reporting any additional surface area.

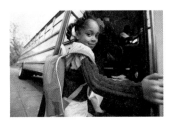

CODING EXAMPLE

A surgeon performs split-thickness skin grafts to burned areas of a patient's lower legs. The skin is harvested from the patient's abdomen and upper thighs (a total of 225 sq cm). The coder reports these procedures with 15100 X 1 for the first 100 sq cm and add-on code 15101 X 2 for the next 125 sq cm.

When coding skin repair procedures, verify the patient's age. Requirements for some codes differ depending on whether the patient is younger or older than 10 years of age.

allografts
Human tissue or organ transplant grafts from another person.

xenografts
Nonhuman tissue grafts.

CPT codes 15271–15278 describe applications of skin substitutes, including **allografts** (human skin grafts from another person), **xenografts** (non-human skin substitute grafts), and biological products that form scaffolding for skin growth. These codes are not reported for application of non-graft wound dressings (e.g., gel, ointment, foam, or liquid) or injected skin substitutes. These codes are divided by anatomic location. Each anatomic group is further divided by total size of the graft applied. The two anatomic groups are: 1) trunk, arms, legs (includes wrists and ankles), and 2) face, scalp, eyelids, mouth, neck, ears, orbits, genitalia, hands, feet, and/or digits.

Codes in each anatomic group are divided by size of the defect—up to 100 sq cm and 100 sq cm or more. One code in each anatomic group describes the first 25 sq cm with an add-on code describing each additional 25 sq cm or part thereof, for wounds up to 100 sq cm. Another code describes the first 100 sq cm with an add-on code describing each additional 100 sq cm or part thereof for wounds equal to or greater than 100 sq cm.

CODER'S TIP

When reporting skin grafts, coders must differentiate the graft type (autograft, allograft, or xenograft), the anatomical location of the graft, and the total graft area in square centimeters.

Flaps; Other Procedures; Excision of Pressure Ulcers

tissue flap
A transfer of tissue to a site that is more distant from the donor site than an adjacent tissue transfer.

A **tissue flap** is a transfer of tissue to a site that is more distant from the donor site than an adjacent tissue transfer. These may be performed in a single procedure or in stages. Anatomical regions included in CPT code descriptors refer to the recipient area when the graft is attached to its final site at the time of the procedure. Anatomical regions in CPT code descriptors refer to the donor site when the tissue is arranged into a graft tube for later transfer to its final site. Codes 15570–15777 describe various types of flaps, including skin and subcutaneous flaps, myocutaneous flaps (which include muscle and skin tissues), and pedicle flaps (which include vascular and/or neural tissues).

CPT codes 15780–15999 describe various other procedures, including dermabrasion, chemical peels, blepharoplasties, excision of excess skin, and the treatment of decubitus ulcers with excisions and flaps.

Burns

Code range 16000–16036 includes codes that describe debridement and dressings for partial-thickness burns affecting varying body surface areas. These codes are selected based on the size of the area treated, described as the percentage of total body surface area (TBSA). Code 16020 describes dressing or partial debridement of partial-thickness burns that are less than 5 percent of TBSA. Code 16025 describes treatment of burns that are 5 to 10 percent of TBSA, and code 16030 describes treatment of burns that are greater than 10 percent of TBSA.

Total body surface area is usually estimated using the rule of nines, which assigns different areas of the body a percentage value. The rule of nines is illustrated in Figure 12.1.1.

Escharotomy is a procedure to release the pressure caused by swelling that is secondary to burns, especially on the extremities. This pressure can cut off blood flow to the more distal portions of the extremities. Escharotomies are reported with two codes: CPT code 16035 describes the first incision, while add-on code 16036 describes each additional incision.

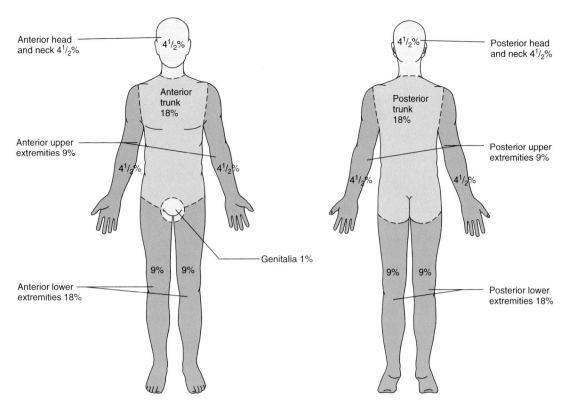

FIGURE 12.1.1
Rule of Nines

Anterior head and neck 4$^1/_2$%

Anterior trunk 18%

Anterior upper extremities 9%

4$^1/_2$% 4$^1/_2$%

Genitalia 1%

9% 9%

Anterior lower extremities 18%

Posterior head and neck 4$^1/_2$%

Posterior trunk 18%

Posterior upper extremities 9%

4$^1/_2$% 4$^1/_2$%

9% 9%

Posterior lower extremities 18%

CODER'S TIP

To calculate the total body surface area of a burn, use the rule of nines.

EXERCISE 12.1.3

Also available in **connect** plus+

Use the CPT manual to select the code(s) to describe the following services.

1. Surgical preparation of a 320 sq cm recipient site by excision of an open wound of the right arm _____

2. A 210 sq cm skin autograft of the left leg _____

3. Xenograft skin for temporary wound closure of the hands, 97 sq cm _____

4. Free fascial flap with microvascular anastomosis _____

5. Escharotomy involving three incisions _____

6. Adjacent tissue transfer of 51.5 sq cm to the cheek and chin _____

12.1.4 Destruction of Lesions (17000–17999)

Destruction of Benign or Premalignant Lesions

Code range 17000–17250 describes destruction of benign or premalignant tissues by any method. "Any method" includes electrosurgery, cryosurgery, laser treatment, and chemical treatments. These procedures include any required local anesthesia but do not usually require skin closure. CPT codes 17000–17004 describe destruction of premalignant lesions. CPT code 17000 refers to the destruction of the first lesion, with add-on code 17003 for each additional lesion between 2 and 14 lesions. CPT code 17004 describes the destruction of 15 or more lesions.

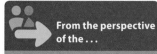

From the perspective of the...

CODER

When reporting destruction of benign or premalignant lesions, verify how many lesions were treated.

CPT codes 17106–17108 describe destruction of cutaneous vascular lesions. Code 17106 describes destruction of lesions of less than 10 sq cm. Code 17107 is used to report destruction of lesions that are 10.0 to 50.0 sq cm, and code 17108 is used for lesions over 50.0 cm. CPT codes 17110 and 17111 describe destruction of benign lesions other than skin tags or vascular lesions. Code 17110 describes destruction of up to 14 lesions, and code 17111 describes destruction of 15 or more lesions.

Destruction of Malignant Lesions

Destruction of malignant lesions is described by CPT codes 17260–17286. These codes are divided into three groups based on the anatomical location of the lesion. Each group is divided into individual codes based on the size of the lesion. The anatomical regions include: (1) trunk, arms, or legs (17260–17266); (2) scalp, neck, hands, feet, and genitalia (17270–17276); and (3) face, ears, eyelids, nose, lips, and mucous membranes (17280–17286). Within each group, six individual codes describe lesions of varying diameter: less than 0.5 cm, 0.6 to 1.0 cm, 1.1 to 2.0 cm, 2.1 to 3.0 cm, 3.1 to 4.0 cm, and over 4.0 cm.

Mohs Micrographic Surgery

Mohs micrographic surgery
A technique for removal of malignant skin lesions and examination of removed tissue by the same practitioner.

Mohs micrographic surgery (or Mohs surgery) is a technique for removal of malignant skin lesions and pathological examination of all tissue margins by a single provider acting as both surgeon and pathologist. Codes 17311–17315 describe Mohs surgery.

CODER'S TIP

Codes 17311–17315 are only used if one physician acts as both surgeon and pathologist. They are not used if one physician performs the surgical excision and a second provider performs the pathological examination of the tissues.

The provider excises the tumor and embeds the tissues into a tissue mounting block for microscopic pathological examination. The choice of the initial code (either CPT code 17311 or 17313) depends on the anatomical location from which the tissue is excised. The initial code describes the first stage of the excision process and includes up to five tissue blocks. If it is necessary to excise additional tissue after the microscopic exam, these additional stages are reported with add-on codes specific for each initial code (CPT code 17312 or 17314). If more than five tissue blocks are prepared during any excision stage, each additional block is reported with add-on code 17315.

CODING EXAMPLE

A physician performs Mohs microsurgery for excision of multiple malignant skin cancers involving the nose and cheeks of a patient. During the initial excision, the provider prepares eight tissue blocks for microscopic tissue examination. After examining all tissues, the provider determines that she needs to remove additional tissues from several sites and prepare six more tissue blocks. After examining those tissue samples, the provider determines that sufficient tissue has been removed and the margins are free of residual tumor.

When reporting these procedures, the initial excision is reported with one unit of CPT code 17311 (based on the anatomical location of the lesions) and three units of add-on code 17315 to describe the three additional tissue blocks beyond the first five. The additional stage is reported with one unit of add-on code 17312 for the excision and first five tissue blocks and one unit of add-on code 17315 for the sixth tissue block prepared during the second stage.

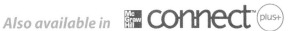

EXERCISE 12.1.4

Also available in McGraw Hill connect™ plus+

Use the CPT manual to select the code(s) to describe the following services.

1. Destruction by cryosurgery of 12 lesions _____

2. Destruction of a 3.3 cm malignant lesion on the left arm by electrosurgery _____

3. First stage of Mohs micrographic surgical removal of a tumor of the right leg with associated services, including obtaining specimens, mapping, color coding of specimens, and microscopic exam of three tissue blocks by the surgeon _____

4. Cryosurgery of a 2.5 cm malignant lesion on the scalp _____

5. Laser procedure of a cutaneous vascular lesion of the face measuring 17 sq cm _____

12.1.5 Procedures on the Breast (19000–19499)

The section of the CPT manual that describes procedures on the breast is divided into subsections describing incision, excision, introduction, mastectomy, and repair and/or reconstruction procedures of the breast.

Incisions

The procedures described by codes 19000–19030 include aspiration of cysts, drainage of abscesses, and injections for mammary ductograms. CPT code 19000 describes aspiration of a single breast cyst. Code 19001 is an add-on code describing aspiration of each additional cyst.

Excisions

Codes 19100–19272 describe some types of biopsies, removal of benign or malignant breast lesions, and the surgical removal of malignant tumors arising from the chest wall. Biopsies include percutaneous and open procedures and the excision of masses identified with radiological markers. Codes in this section are used to report the excision of chest wall malignancies arising from soft tissues or the ribs, but not from the lungs or pleura.

CODER'S TIP

When reporting breast biopsy procedures, verify how the specimen was obtained. Was it an open or percutaneous procedure?

Introduction

Code range 19290–19298 describes preoperative placement of needle localization wires and percutaneous placement of localization clips under image guidance. This section also includes codes that describe the placement of expandable catheters into the breast for radiation therapy, but not the introduction of tissue expanders for breast reconstruction.

Mastectomy Procedures

Codes 19300–19307 describe **partial mastectomy** and **complete mastectomy** procedures, including **radical mastectomies** and **modified radical mastectomies**. Partial mastectomies are reported when less than the entire breast is removed (e.g., a lumpectomy). A complete mastectomy includes excision of the entire breast. A radical mastectomy includes removal of the entire breast, axillary lymph nodes, and both the

partial mastectomy
Removal of part of the breast.

complete mastectomy
Removal of the entire breast.

radical mastectomy
Removal of the entire breast, axillary lymph nodes, and both the pectoralis major and pectoralis minor muscles.

modified radical mastectomy
Removal of the entire breast and axillary lymph nodes, with or without removal of the pectoralis minor muscle.

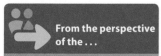
pectoralis major and pectoralis minor muscles. A modified radical mastectomy does not include removal of the pectoralis major muscle. The pectoralis minor muscle may or may not be removed in a modified radical mastectomy.

Parenthetical comments following these codes provide instructions regarding the insertion of an implant following mastectomy. CPT code 19340 describes the immediate insertion of an implant following mastectomy. CPT code 19342 describes the delayed insertion of an implant following mastectomy.

Repair and/or Reconstruction

Codes 19316–19396 are used to report numerous types of repair and reconstruction procedures, including:

- Mastopexy (19316)
- Reduction mammaplasty (19318)
- Augmentation mammaplasty, without or with a prosthetic implant (19324, 19325)
- Removal of implants (19328, 19330)
- Immediate or delayed insertion of tissue expanders following mastectomy (10340, 19342)
- Nipple and/or areola reconstruction (19350, 19355)
- Breast reconstruction using muscle or other tissue flaps (19357–19369)
- Periprosthetic capsulotomy or capsulectomy (19370, 19371)
- Revision of previous breast reconstruction procedure (19380)

CODING EXAMPLE

A patient has a modified radical mastectomy on one breast and a subcutaneous mastectomy on the other breast, followed by the immediate insertion of breast implants on both sides.

The coder reports these procedures with the following codes:

- 19307 (Mastectomy, modified radical, including axillary lymph nodes, with or without pectoralis minor muscle, but excluding pectoralis major muscle)
- 19304 (Mastectomy, subcutaneous)
- 19340-50 (Immediate insertion of breast prosthesis following mastopexy, mastectomy or in reconstruction)

A parenthetical note at the beginning of the Repair and/or Reconstruction section directs coders to use modifier 50 to report bilateral procedures.

Also available in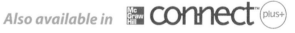

EXERCISE 12.1.5

Use the CPT manual to select the code(s) to describe the following services.

1. Breast augmentation with a prosthetic implant _____
2. Excision of a chest wall tumor including ribs _____
3. Cryosurgical ablation of three fibroadenomas with ultrasound guidance _____
4. Modified radical mastectomy with immediate insertion of a prosthesis _____
5. Placement of a tissue expander for reconstruction at the site of a previous mastectomy _____

12.1.6 Anesthesia Associated with Procedures on the Integumentary System

Anesthetics provided for most procedures on the integumentary system are reported with CPT codes 00300 (Anesthesia for all procedures on the integumentary system, muscles and nerves of the head, neck, and posterior trunk, not otherwise specified) or 00400 (Anesthesia for procedures on the integumentary system on the extremities, anterior trunk and perineum; not otherwise specified).

Exceptions to this general rule include anesthesia for procedures that include debridement of subcutaneous tissues or open fractures. Anesthetics for those procedures are usually reported with anesthesia codes for procedures on deep tissues such as 00700, 00800, 00820, 00904, 01250, 01320, 01470, 01610, 01710, and 01810. Anesthesia codes for debridement of wounds due to open fractures include 00190, 00450, 01120, 01210, 01360, 01392, 01480, 01630, 01740, and 01830. CPT codes 00402, 00404, and 00406 are used to report anesthesia for procedures on the breast.

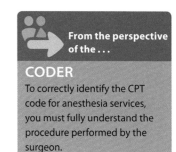

From the perspective of the . . .

CODER
To correctly identify the CPT code for anesthesia services, you must fully understand the procedure performed by the surgeon.

CODER'S TIP

When selecting the code to describe anesthesia for procedures described by CPT codes in the 10000 range, coders should determine whether the underlying procedure involved skin and subcutaneous tissues only or deeper structures, such as muscles or bones. The choice of the correct anesthesia code depends on the structures involved in the procedure.

CODING EXAMPLE

A patient is admitted to the emergency department with an open fracture of the tibia. The orthopedic surgeon takes the patient to the operating room for debridement of the skin, subcutaneous tissue, and muscle. He decides not to repair the fracture at this time because of the degree of contamination of the fracture site.

The coder is reporting both the surgical and anesthesia codes. CPT code 11011 (Debridement including removal of foreign material at the site of an open fracture and/or an open dislocation [e.g., excisional debridement]; skin, subcutaneous tissue, muscle fascia, and muscle) describes the surgical procedure. The choice of this code depends on the types of tissues removed during the debridement procedure, not the site of the fracture. CPT code 01470 describes the anesthesia. The choice of this code depends on the site of the fracture, not the particular tissues removed during the procedure.

EXERCISE 12.1.6

Also available in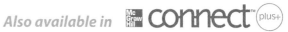

Use the CPT manual to select the code(s) to describe the anesthesia for the following procedures.

1. Debridement of skin, subcutaneous tissue, and muscle of the lower abdominal wall _____

2. Excision of a 1.5 cm malignant lesion of the face _____

3. Wound repair with adjacent tissue transfer of 22 sq cm on the chest _____

4. Incision and drainage of an abscess on the back of the neck _____

5. Debridement and dressing of a burn between 5 and 10 percent of TBSA _____

MODULE **12.1** REVIEW

Summary

Learning Outcome	Key Concepts/Examples
12.1.1 Identify procedures of the skin and subcutaneous tissues. **Pages 309–312**	Superficial procedures on the integumentary system include incision and drainage, debridement, biopsies, removal of skin tags, shaving of skin lesions, and excision of benign and malignant lesions. Selecting the correct code to describe some of these procedures may require the coder to determine the total number of lesions involved, the anatomical location and size of the lesion, and whether the lesion is benign or malignant.
12.1.2 Determine how to group wounds together according to anatomical location and type of closure for reporting purposes. **Pages 313–314**	Wound repairs are differentiated from one another depending on a number of factors. Selecting the correct code to describe these repairs depends on the type of closure necessary to close the wounds (simple, intermediate, or complex), the anatomical location of the wounds, and the total length of the wounds repaired by each closure type and anatomical group.
12.1.3 Describe the differences between graft, flap, and burn procedures. **Pages 315–317**	Large skin defects may be covered using a variety of surgical techniques, including skin advancement, skin grafts with a number of different materials, and various procedures involving flaps. Treatment of burns and pressure ulcers are also described by codes in this section.
12.1.4 Report tissue destruction of benign and malignant tissues by various techniques. **Pages 317–318**	A series of codes describes the destruction of benign and malignant lesions. Selecting the correct code involves determining whether the lesion is benign, premalignant, or malignant; the anatomical location of the lesion; and either the total number of lesions destroyed (for benign or premalignant lesions) or the total size of the lesion destroyed (for malignant lesions).
12.1.5 Select the appropriate codes for surgical procedures on the breast. **Pages 319–320**	Procedures on the breast include incision, excision, introduction, mastectomy, and reconstruction. Parenthetical notes associated with these codes include essential information for correctly reporting these procedures.
12.1.6 Code anesthesia services for procedures in the 10000 series. **Page 321**	Anesthesia for most of the surgical procedures described by codes in the 10000 series of CPT codes is described by CPT codes 00300 or 00400 if the procedure involves only skin structures. Some surgical procedures in this range describe procedures on tissues below the skin. Anesthesia for those procedures is reported by CPT codes that depend on the anatomical location of the surgical procedure.

Using Terminology

Match each term with its definition.

_____ **1.** [LO 12.1.1] Abscess
_____ **2.** [LO 12.1.3] Allograft
_____ **3.** [LO 12.1.3] Autograft
_____ **4.** [LO 12.1.2] Complex repair
_____ **5.** [LO 12.1.1] Debridement
_____ **6.** [LO 12.1.1] Excision
_____ **7.** [LO 12.1.1] Fine needle aspiration
_____ **8.** [LO 12.1.1] Hematoma
_____ **9.** [LO 12.1.1] Incision and drainage
_____ **10.** [LO 12.1.2] Intermediate repair
_____ **11.** [LO 12.1.4] Mohs micrographic surgery
_____ **12.** [LO 12.1.2] Simple repair
_____ **13.** [LO 12.1.3] Xenograft

A. Repair of wounds that requires more than layered closure of the epidermis, dermis or subcutaneous tissue

B. A diagnostic procedure utilizing a very thin needle to aspirate tissue samples for examination by a pathologist

C. Moving or transplanting the patient's own tissue from one area to another

D. Surgical removal by the cutting away of tissue

E. A technique that removes complex or ill-defined skin cancer and enables the surgeon to perform a histological examination of all of the surgical margins of the tumor specimen

F. Application of a non-human skin graft or wound dressing

G. Blood that has been trapped in the skin or inside an organ if the blood then clots, hardens and causes pain to the patient

H. Suture repair of a wound that requires a layered closure of one or more deeper layers of subcutaneous tissue and the closure of the epidermal and dermal layers of the skin

I. Application of a human skin graft from a donor to the patient

J. Suture repair of a wound that is only superficial and requires a one-layer closure of the epidermis or dermis layer of the skin

K. A surgical cut into an organ or space within the body with subsequent removal of fluids from the body cavity

L. A localized infection that may cause a cavity to be filled with pus and surrounded by inflamed tissue

M. The removal of damaged tissue, foreign objects, or dirt from a wound

Checking Your Understanding

Select the letter that best completes the statement or answers the question.

1. LO12.1.3 The physician used a porcine graft in a procedure. What type of graft is this and what range of codes would be used?

   a. Allograft, 15271–15278
   b. Autograft, 15100–15261
   c. Xenograft, 15271–15278
   d. Adjacent tissue, 14000–14350

2. LO12.1.5 The radiologist performed preoperative placement of a needle localization wire for a single lesion of the breast. What would be the appropriate code(s) to report for this procedure?

   a. 19290, 19125   **c.** 19290
   b. 19125   **d.** 19295

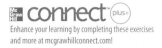

Enhance your learning by completing these exercises
and more at mcgrawhillconnect.com!

3. L012.1.2 A patient in the emergency room has lacerations on the left arm. There are two lacerations: the first is 7 cm, and the second is 9 cm. They are closed with layered sutures. Which code(s) would be assigned?

 a. 12045   c. 12002, 12004
 b. 12035   d. 12004

4. L012.1.3 Which code would be assigned for an initial, local treatment of a first-degree burn?

 a. 16000   c. 16030
 b. 16035   d. None of these

5. L012.1.3 The patient receives a rotation flap after excision of a malignant lesion of the neck, 2 cm by 4 cm. How would this be coded?

 a. 14040, 11624   c. 14040
 b. 14041, 11623   d. 14041

6. L012.1.1 Thirty skin tags (benign lesions) were removed from a patient's neck. How would this procedure be coded?

 a. 11400   c. 11200, 11201 X 2
 b. 11200   d. 11201

7. L012.1.1 Incision and drainage of an infected pilonidal cyst would be coded as _____.

 a. 10040   c. 10080
 b. 10060   d. 10081

8. L012.1.1 A 2.5 cm lesion with a 0.5 cm margin on each side of the lesion was removed from the patient's right arm. The pathology report stated that the lesion was a squamous cell carcinoma. This procedure would be coded as _____.

 a. 11404
 b. 11424
 c. 11604
 d. 11624

9. L012.1.4 What CPT code would be used to report the destruction of a malignant lesion by cryosurgery? The lesion was located on the trunk and measured 3.6 cm.

 a. 17264
 b. 17363
 c. 11404
 d. 11604

10. L012.1.4 A physician performed Mohs surgery on a patient's leg. The physician was both the surgeon and the pathologist. The procedure was performed in two stages with a total of five blocks in each stage. Which codes would be assigned for this procedure?

 a. 17311, 17312, 88314
 b. 17313, 17314
 c. 17311, 17312, 17315
 d. 17313, 17314, 17315

Applying Your Skills

Use the CPT manual to determine the correct code to report the following procedures.

1. L012.1.1 Incision and drainage of a deep abscess located on the patient's gluteus maximus _____

2. L012.1.1 Repair of a nail bed _____

3. L012.2.2 A multilayer intermediate closure of a 16 cm wound in the axilla _____

4. L012.2.2 Burrow's operation involving a 55 sq cm adjacent tissue transfer of the abdomen _____

5. L012.1.3 An island pedicle flap _____

6. L012.1.3 The excision of a 3.4 cm benign lesion on the lip and a 1.4 cm benign lesion on the neck

   _____

7. L012.1.2 Adjacent tissue transfer, 42.3 cm _____

8. L012.1.1 Puncture aspiration of an abscess, hematoma, bulla, or cyst _____

9. L012.1.1 Debridement of skin, subcutaneous tissue, muscle, and fascia for necrotizing soft tissue infection; external genitalia, perineum, and abdominal wall with fascial closure _____

10. L012.1.1 Paring of more than four benign hyperkeratotic lesions (e.g., corns or calluses) _____

11. L012.1.1 Biopsy of four lesions involving skin, subcutaneous tissue, and/or mucous membrane _____

12. L012.1.1 Shaving of a 1.7 cm dermal lesion on the face and a 2.3 cm dermal lesion on the nose _____

13. L012.1.1 Excision of a 2.6 cm benign lesion on the leg _____

14. L012.1.1 Wedge excision of the nail fold (e.g., for ingrown toenail) _____

15. L012.1.1, 17 intralesion injections _____

Thinking It Through

Use your critical-thinking skills to answer the questions below.

1. L012.1.1 Explain the different criteria that must be considered before determining the correct code for repairs.

   _____

   _____

2. L012.1.1 Explain the criteria that must be considered before determining the correct code for excisions.

   _____

   _____

3. L012.1.2 Give examples of simple, intermediate, and complex repairs.

   _____

   _____

Key Terms

Anterior vertebral structure
Arthrodesis
Arthroscopy
Cast
Cervical spine
Closed fracture
Closed treatment
Comminuted fracture
Fascia
External fixation
Internal fixation
Lumbar spine
Manipulation
Open or compound fracture
Open treatment
Osteotomy
Penetrating wound
Percutaneous skeletal fixation
Posterior vertebral structure
Spinal instrumentation
Splint
Strapping
Subcutaneous
Thoracic spine
Traction

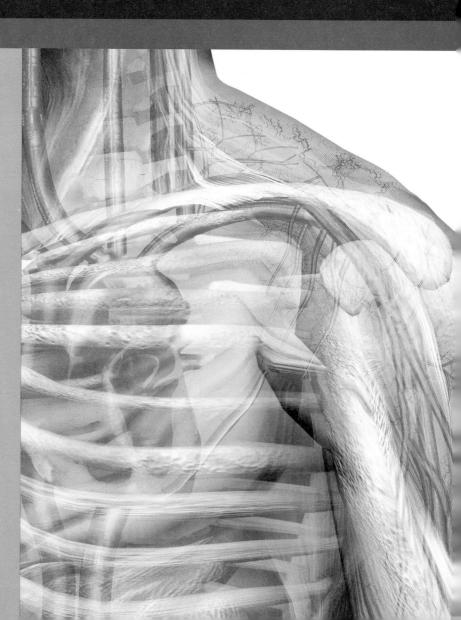

Introduction

The CPT codes in the 20000 series describe procedures on the musculoskeletal system. This series is divided into subsections based on anatomical location and includes more codes than any other section of the CPT.

The anatomical subsections include:

- Head
- Neck (Soft Tissue) and Thorax
- Back and Flank
- Spine (Vertebral Column)
- Abdomen
- Shoulder
- Humerus (Upper Arm) and Elbow
- Forearm and Wrist
- Hand and Fingers
- Pelvis and Hip Joint
- Femur (Thigh Region) and Knee Joint
- Leg (Tibia and Fibula) and Ankle Joint
- Foot and Toes
- Application of Casts and Strapping
- Endoscopy/Arthroscopy

Each of these anatomical subsections is further divided by procedure type. Most of the anatomical sections include common procedures. Some sections include additional procedures that are unique to those sections. The procedures included in most anatomical sections are incision; excision; introduction or removal; repair, revision, and/or reconstruction; fracture and/or dislocation; arthrodesis; and amputation.

12.2.1 Musculoskeletal System Treatments

The codes in the 20000 series describe numerous procedures on the bones and soft tissues of the musculoskeletal system. Many codes include terms commonly used to describe the treatment of soft tissue and bone abnormalities that coders should understand. Coders should be familiar with the terms described below, which are used in CPT code descriptors to denote the type of treatment.

In **closed treatment**, the fracture site is not surgically opened during treatment of the fracture. There are three types of closed treatments:

- Without manipulation
- With manipulation
- With or without traction

In **open treatment**, the fracture is surgically exposed as part of the treatment. In most cases, this is done through an excision that exposes the ends of the fracture, allowing the surgeon to manipulate the bones into proper position. The bones may be held in place with **internal fixation** (Figure 12.2.1), such as plates and screws to allow healing to occur in correct alignment. In some cases, the actual fracture is not exposed, but the broken bone is exposed above or below the fracture site and a device known as an intramedullary nail is inserted down the middle of the bone to keep both ends in alignment during healing.

Percutaneous skeletal fixation is performed when the fracture is not surgically exposed but pins or other devices are placed through the skin to hold the ends of the fracture in place.

closed treatment
A treatment for a fracture during which the fracture site is not surgically opened.

open treatment
A treatment for a fracture during which the fracture is surgically exposed as part of the treatment.

internal fixation
A fracture treatment using devices such as plates and screws to maintain bone alignment.

percutaneous skeletal fixation
A treatment for a fracture during which the fracture is not surgically exposed but pins or other devices are placed through the skin to hold the ends of the fracture in place.

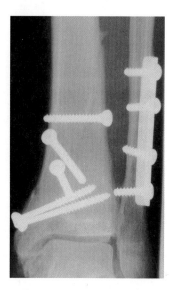

FIGURE 12.2.1 Internal Fixation of a Fracture with Screws and a Plate

traction
The application of force to a limb through pins or wires attached to bones or through strapping applied directly to the skin to align bones to their original length and/or position.

external fixation
A fracture treatment using casts, splints, traction, and/or external fixators to maintain bone alignment.

manipulation
Manually applying external forces to align bones or joints to their normal anatomical position.

subcutaneous
Below the skin.

Traction refers to the application of force to a limb through pins or wires attached to bones or through strapping applied directly to the skin to align bones to their original length and/or position. **External fixation** involves the use of pins through the bones plus an external mechanism to hold the bones in position to treat bony deformities.

Manipulation refers to the manual application of external forces to align bones or joints to their normal anatomical position.

To report excision of soft tissue and bone tumors, coders must differentiate between excision of **subcutaneous** soft tissue tumors and tumors that extend deeper into the **fascia** or muscle. Some procedures for tumor excision are described as "radical resections" to denote that not only is the tumor removed, but a wide margin of normal tissue is also surgically removed. This is usually done for malignant or very aggressive benign tumors. Radical resections may involve only soft tissue or include resection of bone.

Fractures fall into three types:

- **Closed fracture:** A fracture in which the skin overlying the fracture site is not compromised and the fracture is not exposed to the external environment.

- **Open or compound fracture:** A fracture in which the skin is open and the fracture is exposed to external elements.

- **Comminuted fracture:** A fracture in which the bone is broken into more than two pieces. Comminuted fractures may be either closed or open.

CPT code descriptors refer to the type of fixation used to treat the fracture. These terms are similar to the descriptions of closed, open, and comminuted fractures, but coders should not confuse them. One set describes the fracture, while the other describes the method of treatment. Some code descriptors refer to the type of fracture treated as well as the treatment utilized.

In spite of the similarity of the terms, the type of fracture (closed, open, or compound) does not correlate to the type of treatment (closed, open, or percutaneous). Fracture treatment codes describe the treatment of fractures and joint injuries by the type of manipulation and stabilization. These codes may be used with either open or closed fractures.

CODER'S TIP

Fractures are often described as closed, open/compound, or comminuted. When coding, differentiate between the type of fracture and the type of fixation used to treat the fracture.

EXERCISE 12.2.1

Also available in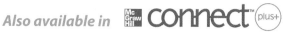

Using your knowledge of treatments of the musculoskeletal system, answer the questions below.

1. Closed treatments can be classified into three types. What are these types? _____

_____

2. Identify two types of open fracture treatment. _____

_____

3. Describe the difference between open and closed fractures. _____

_____

12.2.2 General Codes and Codes Describing Procedures on the Head, Neck (Soft Tissues), and Thorax (20005–21899)

General

The anatomical subsections are preceded by an introductory General section of codes that describe some procedures that are essentially the same regardless of the area of the body on which the services are performed. For example, incision of a subfascial soft tissue abscess is described by CPT code 20005, regardless of where the abscess is located. A parenthetical note provides guidance that incision and drainage of cutaneous or subcutaneous abscesses are reported with CPT codes 10060 and 10061.

Similarly, the exploration of a **penetrating wound,** such as a stab wound or gunshot wound, is described by CPT codes 20100–20103. These codes refer to penetrating wounds that do not extend into the thorax or abdomen. If a wound exploration requires a thoracotomy or laparotomy, then other, more specific codes are used to describe the procedures.

Codes in the General section also describe certain injections (e.g., sinus tract, tendon sheath, trigger point, joint, or bursa); excision of foreign bodies; application of halo (circular) and external fixation devices; replantation of completely severed body parts; and certain types of grafts. Coders should be familiar with the codes in this section.

fascia
Sheet of fibrous connective tissue usually over muscle tissue.

closed fracture
A fracture in which the overlying skin is not compromised and the fracture is not exposed to the external environment.

open or compound fracture
A fracture in which the skin is open and the fracture is exposed to external elements.

comminuted fracture
A fracture in which the bone is broken into more than two pieces. Comminuted fractures may be either closed or open fractures.

penetrating wound
A wound that penetrates the skin, such as a stab wound or gunshot.

CODER'S TIP

Aspirations of joints are described by a series of codes that differ from one another by the size of the joint on which the aspiration is performed. CPT code 20600 describes aspiration of small joints (e.g., fingers or toes). Code 20605 is used to describe aspiration of intermediate joints, such as the temporomandibular joint, acromioclavicular joint, wrist, elbow, or ankle. Code 20610 describes aspiration of major joints, including the shoulder, hip, and knee.

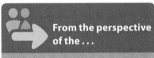

From the perspective of the . . .

CODER
In order to select the correct code to describe wound exploration procedures, the coder must know the anatomical location of the wound.

CPT codes describing bone and tissue grafts (20900–20938) are included in the General section of codes. If the graft material is harvested from a surgical site that is separate from the location to which it is grafted (i.e., through a separate incision), the harvesting should be reported separately. Some codes used to report graft procedures will have a descriptor that states that the procedure includes obtaining the graft material, in which case a separate code is not used to report obtaining the graft.

A series of add-on codes (20936–20938) describes the use of bone grafts in conjunction with surgery procedures on the spine. These descriptors specifically state that the procedure includes harvesting the graft.

CODING EXAMPLE

A surgeon performs a spinal fusion on the T10–T12 levels using morselized bone graft obtained from the patient's iliac crest through a separate incision. The coder reports these procedures as follows: 22610 (arthrodesis of the thoracic spine, first level), add-on code 22614 (additional level), and add-on code 20937 (morselized autograft through a separate incision).

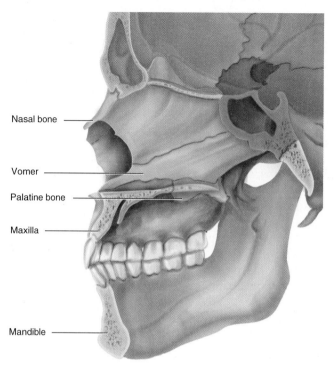

Nasal bone

Vomer

Palatine bone

Maxilla

Mandible

FIGURE 12.2.2 Facial Bones

Head

Codes 21010–21499 describe procedures on the skull, facial bones (Figure 12.2.2), and temporomandibular joint (TMJ). The only incision code in this section is 21010, which describes arthrotomy of the TMJ. A number of codes are used to describe excision of different benign and malignant tumors of the face or scalp. The specific code selected depends on the location and size of the tumor excised, the method of excision, and whether an osteotomy is performed as part of the procedure.

CODING EXAMPLE

Mandibular fracture treatments are described by a series of CPT codes (21450–21470) that differ from each other by whether the treatment is open or closed and whether the treatment includes interdental fixation.

A surgeon performs an open treatment of a mandibular fracture with interdental fixation. The coder reports this procedure with CPT code 21462 (Open treatment of mandibular fracture; with interdental fixation).

If interdental fixation is performed for any condition other than a fracture, it is reported with CPT code 21497.

Codes in this section describe prostheses used to treat deficiencies of the face, eyes, ears, or oral cavity when the physician prepares the prosthesis. An outside laboratory does not use these codes to report services. Numerous codes describe repairs, reconstructions, and treatment of fractures of the facial bones and mandible. A parenthetical note instructs coders to use CPT codes 62000–62010 to report operative repairs of skull fractures.

Neck (Soft Tissue) and Thorax

Most of the codes in code range 21501–21899 describe soft tissue procedures on the neck and thorax, including excision of tumors. Excision procedures (21550–21632) are differentiated by the size of the soft tissue tumors excised and which bones, if any, are included in the procedure. The only fracture repair and reconstruction procedures described by these codes are those involving the ribs or sternum, not spinal structures. Codes describing reconstruction procedures for pectus excavatum or pectus carinatum (21740–21743) are divided based on whether it is an open procedure, a minimally invasive procedure without thoracoscopy, or an invasive procedure with thoracoscopy.

Use the CPT manual to select the appropriate codes for the following procedures.

1. Exploration of a penetrating wound to the chest _____
2. Halo application for thin skull osteology _____
3. Removal of an external fixation device under anesthesia _____
4. Excision of a malignant tumor of the mandible _____
5. Closed treatment of a nasal bone fracture without stabilization _____
6. Excision of facial bones for osteomyelitis _____
7. Biopsy of soft tissue of the neck _____
8. Open treatment of a sternum fracture with skeletal fixation _____
9. Partial excision of a rib _____
10. Radical resection of the sternum with mediastinal lymphadenectomy _____

12.2.3 Codes Describing Procedures on the Back and Flank, Spinal Column, and Abdomen (21920–22999)

Back and Flank

Most of the codes in the Back and Flank section (21920–21936) describe soft tissue excisions of tumors. The appropriate code to describe the excision of subcutaneous tumors depends on whether the tumor is less than 3 cm (21930) or equal to or greater than 3 cm (21931). The choice of codes describing subfascial tumors, however, depends on whether the tumor is less than 5 cm (21932) or equal to or greater than 5 cm. Similarly, the choice of codes describing radical resection of tumors also depends on whether the tumor is less than 5 cm (21935) or equal to or greater than 5 cm.

Spine (Vertebral Column)

Code range 22010–22899 describes procedures on the **cervical, thoracic,** and **lumbar spine.** In many cases, the initial code in a series describes a procedure followed by a description of a particular portion of the spine. The initial code is typically followed by indented codes denoting the same procedure on other portions of the spine.

Excision codes in this subsection describe resection of bony structures, not soft tissues of the back. These codes are divided into two groups. The first group (22100–22103) describes excisions of **posterior vertebral structures** (spinous process, lamina, and facet joint), whereas the second group (22110–22116) describes the **anterior vertebral structure** or vertebral body. Each group has four codes, three of which describe the procedure on a single segment in each portion of the spine. These are followed by a single add-on code that is used to report procedures on each additional segment. Excision codes are followed by numerous parenthetical comments directing coders to use specific codes or to use specific combinations of codes for certain procedures.

cervical spine
The seven vertebrae of the neck.

thoracic spine
The twelve vertebrae of the thoracic region that adjoin to the ribs.

lumbar spine
The five vertebrae lying between the thoracic vertebrae and the sacrum.

posterior vertebral structure
Spinous process, lamina, and facet joint.

anterior vertebral structure
Vertebral body.

A surgeon performs a three-level lumbar laminectomy to relieve pressure on the spinal cord. The coder is reporting this procedure. She selects CPT code 22102 to describe the first level and add-on code 22103 X 2 to describe the additional two levels.

spinal instrumentation
The use of surgically implanted devices to immobilize the spine for correct healing.

Treatment of spinal diseases often requires several procedures to correct the underlying abnormality. For example, several vertebral bodies may be fused together (arthrodesis) using bone graft material to facilitate bone healing and **spinal instrumentation** to hold the vertebral bodies in correct alignment. Each of these procedures is reported with separate CPT codes. Coders should understand how these procedures relate to one another. For example, bone grafting and instrumentation are never performed without arthrodesis. Other procedures, such as a laminectomy, may be performed alone or in combination with arthrodesis. When arthrodesis is performed in addition to another procedure (e.g., laminectomy or fracture repair), the arthrodesis is reported with modifier 51 (multiple procedures).

CODER'S TIP

On occasion, two surgeons work together as co-surgeons to perform complex spine procedures such as those performed on the anterior portion of the spinal column. The anterior spine is usually approached through the thorax or abdomen, depending on the level of the procedure. In those cases, a general surgeon or cardiothoracic surgeon often works with the spinal surgeon as a co-surgeon. Each surgeon reports the same CPT code for the underlying procedure, but both surgeons attach modifier 62 to the code to indicate that they performed as co-surgeons, not as one surgeon and an assistant surgeon.

osteotomy
A surgical procedure in which a bone is cut to shorten, lengthen or change its alignment.

arthrodesis
The fusion of two bones.

A series of codes (22206–22226) describe **osteotomies** (cutting the bone to change its alignment during deformity-correcting procedures). These procedures are often performed with other spinal procedures, including arthrodesis and spinal instrumentation.

The term **arthrodesis** refers to the fusion of two bones. Spinal fusions may be performed anteriorly on the vertebral bodies or on the posterior spinal structures (spinous process, lamina, and facet joints). The spinal structures operated on during these procedures may be reached by several different approaches, including lateral; anterior or anterolateral; transoral (used for skull to C2 procedures only); and posterior or posterolateral approaches. For each approach, an individual code describes the initial procedure on the first interspace in each portion of the spine. A single add-on code is used to describe additional interspaces at any level.

A separate group of codes (22800–22819) is used to describe arthrodesis procedures for the correction of spinal deformities such as scoliosis or kyphosis. These are divided into posterior and anterior procedures, and then further divided into specific codes depending on how many spinal segments are involved. These codes only describe the arthrodesis. Bone grafts and/or spinal instrumentation procedures are reported using the appropriate codes and modifier 51.

When two surgeons work together as co-surgeons to perform an arthrodesis through an abdominal or thoracic approach, they should each report the appropriate procedure code with modifier 62 added. Other procedures performed in addition to the arthrodesis, such as bone grafts and/or spinal instrumentation, are not reported with modifier 62. If the second surgeon continues to assist the primary surgeon performing the bone grafting or instrumentation procedures, the second

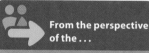

From the perspective of the . . .

CODER

It is much easier to code spinal procedures when you have a detailed understanding of spinal anatomy and terminology. Coders must understand spinal segments (e.g., cervical, thoracic, and lumbar) as well as the anterior and posterior spinal structures.

surgeon would add modifier 80 (assistant surgeon) to the codes describing the additional procedures.

Spinal instrumentation is used to hold spinal segments in alignment. Segmental instrumentation refers to devices that are attached to the spine at each end and at least one additional point between the two ends. Nonsegmental instrumentation is attached to the spine only at the two ends and may span a number of segments without attaching to any of them. Codes describing the insertion of spinal instrumentation (22840–22848, 22851) are add-on codes and must be reported in addition to codes describing the primary procedure. Codes describing instrumentation procedures that are not performed at the same time as the primary procedure, such as removal of instrumentation devices, are stand-alone codes.

Abdomen

The only codes describing abdominal procedures in the 20000 series are those that describe excision or radical resection of tumors from the soft tissues of the abdominal wall (22900–22905). The excision codes are first divided by tumor location (subcutaneous or intramuscular) and then by tumor size. Codes describing the excision of subcutaneous tumors are differentiated by whether the tumor is less than 3 cm (22902) or equal to or greater than 3 cm (22903). Codes describing excision of subfascial tumors are divided by whether the tumor is less than 5 cm (22900) or equal to or greater than 5 cm (22901). Similarly, codes describing the radical resection of tumors from the abdominal wall are differentiated from one another by whether the tumor is less than 5 cm (22904) or equal to or greater than 5 cm (22905).

EXERCISE 12.2.3

Also available in **McGraw Hill connect™** (plus+)

Use the CPT manual to select the appropriate codes for the following procedures.

1. Exploration of spinal fusion _____

2. Single-level arthrodesis of the thoracic spine, posterior technique _____

3. Removal of anterior spinal instrumentation _____

4. Excision of a 2.5 cm subcutaneous tumor of the back or flank _____

5. Radical resection of a 7.5 cm tumor from the abdominal wall _____

12.2.4 Codes Describing Procedures on the Extremities and Joints (23000–28899)

Shoulder

The shoulder (Figure 12.2.3) includes two bones (scapula and clavicle), part of a third bone (head and neck of the humerus), and three joints (glenohumeral, sternoclavicular, and acromioclavicular). Incision procedures (23000–23044) include drainage of abscesses, shoulder capsule release, and simple arthrotomy of any of the three joints.

Excision procedures (23065–23220) describe excisions and radical resections of soft tissue tumors, arthrotomies with biopsy or joint exploration, removal of bone cyst or infected bone, resection of the humeral head, and radical resections of bone tumors. The Introduction or Removal section (23330–23350) includes codes describing removal of foreign bodies and injections for arthrography. Multiple parenthetical comments following these codes direct coders to the correct combination of codes to report radiographic procedures involving injections of the shoulder.

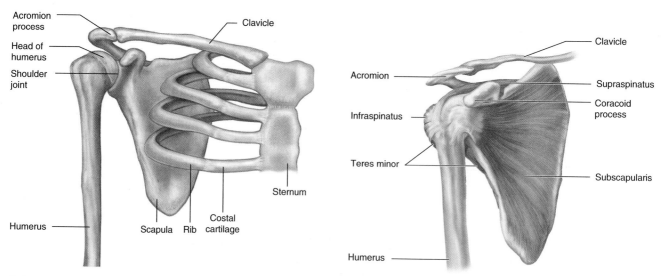

FIGURE 12.2.3 Anatomy of the Shoulder Joint

FIGURE 12.2.4 Rotator Cuff Muscles

Repair, revision, and reconstruction codes (23395–23491) include muscle and tendon repairs, ligament reconstruction and releases, rotator cuff repairs (Figure 12.2.4), and both hemiarthroplasties and total shoulder arthroplasties. The remainder of the codes in the Shoulder section describe repair, reconstruction, treatment of fractures and dislocations, arthrodesis, and amputation of shoulder structures (23500–23921).

CODER'S TIP

Each anatomical section includes families of codes describing treatment of fractures and dislocations. These are grouped according to the type of reduction and fixation utilized during the procedure. The codes may be used to describe treatments of either open or closed fractures.

Humerus (Upper Arm) and Elbow; Forearm and Wrist; Hand and Fingers

The humerus and elbow codes (23930–25999, 26010–26989) describe procedures on the upper arm below the level of the humeral neck extending across the elbow, including the olecranon and the radial head and neck. The forearm and wrist codes describe procedures on the radius, ulna, carpal bones, and wrist joint. The hand and fingers codes describe procedures on the metacarpals and phalanges (finger bones), joints between these bones, and soft tissue structures.

Each of these subsections includes codes describing incisions, excisions, introduction and removal, repair and reconstruction, treatment of fractures/dislocations, arthrodesis, and amputations. The procedures described by the codes within these subsections differ from one another by the specific details contained within the code descriptors. For example, the appropriate excision code is selected based on the specific tissue excised and the location of that tissue. Reconstruction codes are selected based on the anatomical structure, and fracture treatment codes are selected based on the treatment type and specific bone. Some codes describe procedures on one bone (e.g., "radius OR ulna"), whereas others describe the same procedure on multiple bones (e.g., "radius AND ulna"). Codes in the Hand section may describe specific structures, the number of digits, or the particular type of fracture treatment. Coders must pay particular attention to specific wording in code descriptors to determine the correct code.

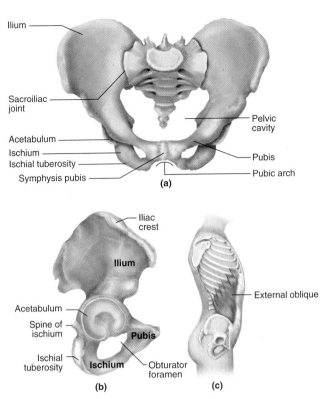

FIGURE 12.2.5 Anatomy of the Pelvis. (a) Front view; (b) Side view; (c) Abdominal muscles supporting the pelvic girdle

Pelvis and Hip Joint

Code range 26990–27299 describes procedures on the bony pelvis (Figure 12.2.5) and hip joint, including the femoral head and neck. These codes include procedures on the muscles overlying the pelvis. Incision codes describe tenotomy (incision of a tendon to release muscles and reduce contractures across the joint) and arthrotomy of the hip joint. Parenthetical comments instruct coders to add modifier 50 to some tenotomy codes when the procedure is performed bilaterally.

Excision codes include biopsy of soft tissues, excision and radical resections of tumors, arthrotomy with excision of joint tissue, excision of bone cysts and bursa, and coccygectomy (removal of the coccyx). The Introduction or Removal section includes codes that describe sacroiliac joint injections and removal of previously implanted hip prostheses. Parenthetical comments instruct coders regarding the use of radiology codes to describe supervision and interpretation for hip and sacroiliac joint arthrography.

The repair and reconstruction codes include those describing hemiarthroplasty and total hip replacement procedures (27125–27138). However, coders are instructed to use a different code (27236) if a prosthesis is used to treat a hip fracture.

CODING EXAMPLE

A surgeon performs an elective hip hemiarthroplasty using a femoral stem prosthesis. The coder reports this procedure with CPT code 27125.

The same surgeon treats a femoral neck fracture by using the same femoral stem prosthesis. This procedure, however, is reported with CPT code 27236.

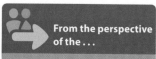

From the perspective of the . . .

CODER

It is important to understand skeletal anatomy to report procedures on the musculoskeletal system. Medical records may only briefly refer to the anatomical location by referring to a specific bone or group of bones. Without understanding skeletal anatomy, it is almost impossible to select the correct code.

Fracture treatment is described with a series of codes describing a variety of procedures, including closed reduction, percutaneous pinning, open fracture repair with plates and screws, and the replacement of the femoral head and neck with a prosthesis.

Femur (Thigh Region) and Knee Joint; Leg (Tibia and Fibula) and Ankle Joint; Foot and Toes

Codes 27301–28899 follow the same general structure as others in the 20000 series. The only special instruction in these sections is that the knee joint includes the tibial plateau. These sections include specific parenthetical instructions related to proper reporting of certain procedures.

EXERCISE 12.2.4

 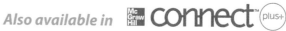

Use the CPT manual to select the appropriate codes for the following procedures.

1. Closed treatment of a scapular fracture with manipulation _____
2. Muscle transfer of the shoulder _____
3. Radical resection of a 6 cm tumor of the upper arm _____
4. Arthroplasty of the wrist _____
5. Closed treatment of a radial shaft fracture _____
6. Bilateral open tenotomy of the hip adductors _____
7. Open treatment of a femoral neck fracture with prosthetic replacement _____

12.2.5 Casting, Strapping, Endoscopy, and Arthroscopy (29000–29999)

Application of Casts and Strapping

cast
A molded circumferential immobilization device applied to a body part to allow healing of a fracture or other injury.

splint
A non-circumferential device used to prevent motion of a joint or broken bone.

strapping
The use of adhesive tape to hold a body part in place for correct healing.

arthroscopy
Visual examination of the interior of a joint using an endoscope.

Codes 29000–29750 describe the application of **casts**, **splints**, and the use of **strapping** as either definitive treatment for an injury or as replacement for an initial cast applied at the time of another treatment. Treatment of fractures, dislocations, or other injuries includes the initial cast application, so these codes cannot be used in addition to the codes describing those treatments.

If one physician applies an initial cast or splint and another performs other restorative or fracture treatment procedures, both may report their services with the appropriate CPT codes. A separate E/M service is not reported when a replacement cast or splint is applied unless significant separately identifiable services are provided. However, if a cast or splint is intended to be the definitive treatment of a fracture, an E/M service may be reported at the time of the initial treatment in addition to the appropriate casting code.

Endoscopy/Arthroscopy

Code range 29800–29999 describes **arthroscopy** procedures. According to instructions at the beginning of this section of codes, a surgical arthroscopic procedure always includes a diagnostic arthroscopic procedure on the same joint if one is performed.

If two or more arthroscopic procedures are performed during the same setting, the additional procedures are reported with modifier 51. If both an arthroscopy and arthrotomy are performed, the arthroscopy is reported with modifier 51.

From the perspective of the . . .

PHYSICIAN

Initial cast applications are not reported separately. When the physician treats a fracture, dislocation, or other injury, the treatment code includes any necessary cast application.

CODER'S TIP

Even if the medical records state that a diagnostic arthroscopy and surgical arthroscopy were performed on the same joint, only the surgical arthroscopy procedure is reported. If a diagnostic arthroscopy is performed on one joint and a surgical arthroscopy is performed on the same joint on the opposite side, both may be reported. In that case, it is very important to identify the joints with the RT and LT anatomical modifiers to make it clear that these procedures involved different anatomical sites.

CODING EXAMPLE

A surgeon performs a diagnostic arthroscopy of the knee. Based on his findings, he decides he cannot perform the necessary surgical procedure through the arthroscope. He proceeds to perform an open osteochondral autograft.

The coder reviews the medical records and reports these procedures with CPT codes 29870 (diagnostic arthroscopy) and 27416 (open osteochondral autograft of the knee). A parenthetical note states that this code includes the harvesting of the autograft, so no additional code is reported.

EXERCISE 12.2.5

Also available in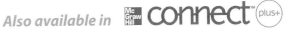

Use the CPT manual to select the appropriate codes for the following procedures.

1. Application of a patellar tendon bearing cast, not associated with initial treatment _____

2. Diagnostic arthroscopy of the knee followed by arthrotomy with medial and lateral meniscectomy _____
_____

3. Application of a long arm cast (shoulder to hand) _____

4. Application of a short leg splint (calf to foot) _____

5. Wedging of a clubfoot cast _____

12.2.6 Anesthesia Associated with Procedures on the Musculoskeletal System

Numerous CPT codes describe anesthesia for procedures on the musculoskeletal system. The anatomical regions of the musculoskeletal system and the anatomical divisions of the anesthesia codes are somewhat similar, but they are not necessarily in perfect alignment. This does make selecting anesthesia codes for surgical procedures on the musculoskeletal system easier than for some other surgical sections.

Some examples of these codes are listed in Table 12.2.1. However, this is not meant to be a complete list of codes describing anesthesia services. For clarity, the anesthesia codes are listed according to the anatomical region of the musculoskeletal system to which they apply, which does lead to some repetition of anesthesia codes.

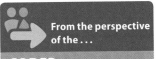

From the perspective of the . . .

CODER

Be sure to compare the surgical procedure code and the anesthesia code to ensure that both describe the same anatomical area.

TABLE 12.2.1 Anesthesia Codes by Anatomical Region

Anatomical Region	Anesthesia Codes
Head and facial bones	00100–00210, 00300, 00400
Neck and thorax	00300, 00320, 00400, 00470, 0472, 00474, 00520, 00550
Back and flank	00300, 00400
Spinal column	00600–00670, 01996
Abdominal wall	00700, 00730, 00800, 00820
Shoulder and upper extremity	00450, 01610–01860
Pelvis, hip, and lower extremity	01112–01490
Arthroscopy (procedure)	00190, 01202, 01400, 01464, 01622, 01630, 01732, 01740, 01829, 01830

CODER'S TIP

It is typically easier to identify the appropriate anesthesia code for procedures on the musculoskeletal system than for other anatomical systems. This is because both the procedure codes and anesthesia codes are organized by anatomical location.

CODING EXAMPLE

A surgeon performs a surgical arthroscopy of the wrist joint with synovectomy (29845). The coder reviews options to report the anesthesia for this procedure. She selects code 01830 (Anesthesia for open or surgical arthroscopic/endoscopic procedures on distal radius, distal ulna, wrist, or hand joints; not otherwise specified). This code descriptor matches the surgical procedure code descriptor with respect to the anatomical location (wrist) and procedure (surgical arthroscopy).

EXERCISE 12.2.6

Also available in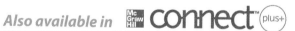

Use the CPT manual to select the anesthesia code for the following surgical procedures.

1. Open treatment of an orbital floor blowout fracture; periorbital approach _____

2. Open treatment of a vertebral fracture, posterior approach, cervical spine performed in the sitting position _____

3. Arthrodesis, lateral approach, lumbar spine _____

4. Resection of the humeral head _____

5. Total hip replacement _____

6. Hemiarthroplasty of the hip _____

7. Arthrotomy of the knee with medial meniscectomy _____

8. Open treatment of a medial malleolus fracture _____

9. Open rotator cuff repair for chronic injury _____

10. Closed treatment of a Colles' fracture with manipulation _____

Summary

Learning Outcome	Key Concepts/Examples
12.2.1 Differentiate among musculoskeletal treatment modalities. **Pages 327–328**	Treatment options for musculoskeletal injuries include closed treatment, open treatment, percutaneous skeletal fixations, traction, and manipulation. Soft tissue procedures include incision and excision.
12.2.2 Identify CPT codes that describe general procedures on the musculoskeletal system and procedures on the head, neck, and thorax. **Pages 329–331**	Codes in the General section of the musculoskeletal system codes describe procedures that are performed on many parts of the musculoskeletal system, such as incision of an abscess, exploration of a penetrating wound, and injections into tendon sheaths or joints. Procedures on the head described by codes in this section include excision of tumors, repairs of facial fractures, and operative procedures on the mandible. Repairs of skull fractures are not described by codes in this section. A parenthetical note provides instructions to code skull fractures with codes from 62000 to 62010. Most procedure codes for the neck and thorax describe excision of tumors from these areas. The only fractures described by codes in these sections are fractures of the ribs and sternum.
12.2.3 Describe procedures on the back and flank, spine, and abdomen. **Pages 331–333**	Procedures on the back, flank, and abdomen include excision of soft tissue tumors. Procedures on the spine (vertebral column) are more extensive, including incision and excision procedures as well as numerous procedures on the vertebral bones of the spine and the intervertebral spaces, such as fracture repair, arthrodesis or fusion, correction of spinal deformities, and placement of instrumentation to maintain spinal alignment.
12.2.4 Determine codes describing procedures on the upper and lower extremities. **Pages 333–336**	Procedures on the extremities include incision, excision, repair or reconstruction of soft tissue injuries, fracture treatment, arthrodesis, and amputation. These are divided by anatomical regions, including: • Shoulder • Humerus and elbow • Forearm, wrist, hand, and fingers • Pelvis and hip • Femur and knee • Leg, ankle, foot, and toes
12.2.5 Identify codes that describe the application of casts, strapping, and arthroscopy procedures. **Pages 336–337**	Several series of codes describe casting, splinting, and strapping procedures. A separate series of codes describes diagnostic and surgical arthroscopy procedures on the joints of the extremities.
12.2.6 Code anesthesia services for procedures of the musculoskeletal system. **Pages 337–338**	There is a wide range of codes that describe anesthesia for surgical procedures on the musculoskeletal system reported with codes from the 20000 series. The anesthesia codes are organized by anatomical region as well as by the type of surgical procedure for which the anesthetic is given.

Using Terminology

Match each term with its definition.

_____ **1.** L012.2.1 Open treatment
_____ **2.** L012.2.1 Closed treatment
_____ **3.** L012.2.1 Internal fixation
_____ **4.** L012.2.1 External fixation
_____ **5.** L012.2.1 Traction
_____ **6.** L012.2.5 Casting
_____ **7.** L012.2.5 Strapping
_____ **8.** L012.2.5 Splinting
_____ **9.** L012.2.3 Arthrodesis
_____ **10.** L012.2.1 Subcutaneous
_____ **11.** L012.2.5 Arthroscopy
_____ **12.** L012.2.3 Osteotomy
_____ **13.** L012.2.3 Spinal instrumentation
_____ **14.** L012.2.1 Manipulation

A. Fusion of two or more bones

B. Fracture site is not surgically opened during treatment of the fracture

C. Under the skin

D. Manually applying external forces to align bones or joints to their normal anatomical position

E. Fracture site is surgically exposed as part of treatment

F. Visual examination of the interior of a joint

G. Immobilization of a limb or other body part with circumferential rigid materials, such as plaster or fiberglass

H. Fracture immobilization via surgical approach

I. The use of metal devices to immobilize the spine

J. Application of a pulling force to treat muscle and skeletal disorders

K. Fracture immobilization through the use of devices attached without surgical approach to the fracture

L. Removal of a portion of the vertebra to realign the spine

M. Immobilization of a limb with noncircumferential rigid materials to prevent motion of a joint of the ends of a fractured bone

N. Immobilization of a limb or other body part with soft materials only, such as compression bandages

Checking Your Understanding

Select the letter that best completes the statement or answers the question.

1. L012.2.2 Exploration of a penetrating wound (e.g., stab wound or gunshot) has a range of codes (20100–20103). These codes do not include penetrating wounds that require the following:

   a. Thoracotomy.
   b. Laparotomy.
   c. Thoracotomy and laparotomy.
   d. Either thoracotomy or laparotomy.

2. L012.2.4 A patient has a fracture of the ulna that is not exposed to the environment. In order to treat the fracture, the surgeon makes an incision to expose the ends of the fracture and then manipulates the bones into the proper position. Which types of fracture and treatment are described by this scenario?

   a. Open fracture, open treatment
   b. Open fracture, closed treatment
   c. Closed fracture, open treatment
   d. Closed fracture, closed treatment

3. L012.2.3 When arthrodesis is performed in addition to another procedure (unless the code includes the arthrodesis, such as bone grafting or instrumentation), the arthrodesis is also reported with which modifier?

a. Modifier 51
b. Modifier 59
c. Modifier 22
d. None of these; it does not require a modifier

4. L012.2.3 When two surgeons work together to perform separate parts of a procedure, which modifier is used to show they performed as co-surgeons and not as assistant surgeons?

a. Modifier 81
b. Modifier 62
c. Modifier 80
d. Modifier 51

5. L012.2.3 In order to select the appropriate code to describe excision of benign and malignant tumors of the musculoskeletal system, a coder must know the following:

a. The location and size of the tumor excised.
b. Whether it was a simple excision or a radical resection.
c. Whether an osteotomy was performed as part of the procedure.
d. All of these.

6. L012.2.2, L012.2.3 The surgeon performed a posterior arthrodesis of L5–S1 for degenerative joint disease using mor-selized autograft iliac bone graft harvested through a separate fascial incision. The appropriate code(s) would be:

a. 22612
b. 22612, 20937
c. 22610, 20937
d. 22612, 22614, 20937

7. L012.2.4 The surgeon performed a radical resection of a tumor, shaft or distal humerus. The appropriate code would be:

a. 24151
b. 24150
c. 24152
d. 24149

8. L012.2.5 A diagnostic arthroscopic exam of the meniscus was performed and a tear was confirmed. A surgical repair of the tear was performed arthroscopically. Which of the following statements is correct?

a. Only the surgical arthroscopy would be coded.
b. Both the diagnostic arthroscopy and the surgical arthroscopy would be coded.
c. Both procedures would be coded with a modifier 51 attached to the diagnostic arthroscopy.
d. Only the diagnostic arthroscopy would be coded.

9. L012.2.5 Casting and strapping codes apply when:

a. The cast application or strapping is a replacement procedure used during or after the period of follow-up care.
b. The cast application or strapping is an initial service performed without a restorative treatment or procedure to stabilize or protect a fracture, injury, or dislocation and/or to afford comfort to the patient.
c. The physician who applies the initial cast, strap, or splint also assumes all of the subsequent fracture, dislocation, or injury care.
d. The cast application or strapping is both a replacement procedure and an initial service.

10. L012.2.4 An injection procedure for enhanced CT arthrography of the shoulder with contrast using fluoroscopic guidance is performed. The appropriate code(s) would be:

a. 23350
b. 23350, 77002, 73202
c. 23350, 77002, 73201
d. 23350, 73040

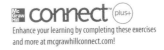

Applying Your Skills

Use the CPT manual to determine the correct code to report the following procedures.

1. L012.2.2 Excision of a cyst on the cheekbone _____
2. L012.2.2 Reconstruction of mandibular rami with internal rigid fixation _____
3. L012.2.4 Deep excision of a tumor on the hand _____
4. L012.2.4 Closed treatment of a tibia shaft fracture with manipulation _____
5. L012.2.4 Implant removal from the elbow joint _____
6. L012.2.5 Diagnostic arthroscopy of the elbow without synovial biopsy _____
7. L012.2.4 Amputation of the arm through the humerus with primary closure _____
8. L012.2.2 Exploration of a gunshot wound through the patient's arm _____
9. L012.2.4 Deep excision biopsy of the thigh area _____
10. L012.2.5 Endoscopic plantar fasciotomy _____
11. L012.2.5 Surgical arthroscopy of the subtalar joint, with removal of foreign body _____
12. L012.2.4 Osteochrondral autografts of the knee _____
13. L012.2.4 Conversion of a previous hip surgery to a total hip arthroplasty _____
14. L012.2.5 Repair of a spica jacket _____
15. L012.2.2 Closed treatment of a mandibular fracture with manipulation _____

Thinking It Through

Use your critical-thinking skills to answer the questions below.

1. L012.2.1 Describe the format of the Musculoskeletal System section in the CPT manual.

_____

_____

2. L012.2.3 Give an example of when modifier 62 would be used in the musculoskeletal section.

_____

_____

3. L012.2.5 A patient is seen by Dr. Michaels, who applies the initial cast for a tibia fracture. Dr. Johnson then performs other restorative fracture treatment. Explain how each physician may code these procedures. How would a coder know that this is the accurate way to code this scenario?

_____

_____

Respiratory, Cardiovascular, Hemic, and Lymphatic Systems; Mediastinum and Diaphragm

Learning Outcomes
After completing this module, students should be able to:

12.3.1 Differentiate among the surgical procedures performed on the respiratory system.

12.3.2 Describe the various types of procedures performed on the cardiac system, including coronary artery bypass grafts, repairs of cardiac abnormalities, and procedures on the great vessels.

12.3.3 Identify CPT codes to report open and endovascular arterial repairs, bypass procedures, angioplasties, shunts, and vascular access procedures.

12.3.4 Describe procedures on the hemic and lymphatic systems, mediastinum, and diaphragm.

12.3.5 Code anesthesia services for procedures in the 30000 series of CPT codes.

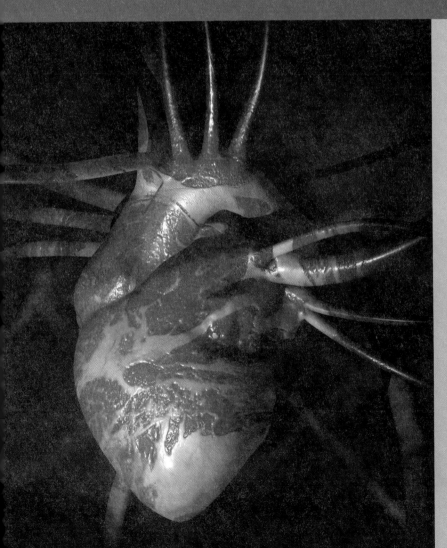

Key Terms

Aneurysm

Angioplasty

Bronchi

Bronchoscopy

Cardiopulmonary bypass

Cardiotomy

Central venous access device

Diagnostic thoracoscopy

Embolectomy

Endoscopy

Ethmoid sinus

Extracorporeal membrane oxygenation

Frontal sinus

Hemodialysis

Maxillary sinus

Mediastinum

Pericardium

Pleura

Shunt

Sinusotomy

Sphenoid sinus

Surgical thoracoscopy

Thrombectomy

Trachea

Turbinate

Introduction

Procedures described by the 30000 series of CPT codes include those performed on the respiratory, cardiovascular, hemic, and lymphatic systems. Procedures of the mediastinum and diaphragm are also included in the 30000 series.

The respiratory system includes the nose, sinuses, larynx, trachea, bronchi, lungs, and pleura. The cardiovascular system is divided into the heart and great vessels, arteries, and veins. The hemic and lymphatic systems include the spleen, bone marrow, lymph nodes, and lymphatic channels. The **mediastinum** is the area between the lungs. It includes the structures in the chest that lie between the right and left lungs, including the esophagus, trachea, main bronchi, heart, pericardium, and great vessels.

12.3.1 Procedures on the Respiratory System (30000–32999)

Procedures on the respiratory system are divided into the following anatomical sections:

- Nose (30000–30999)
- Accessory Sinuses (31000–31299)
- Larynx (31300–31599)
- Trachea and Bronchi (31600–31899)
- Lungs and Pleura (32035–32999)

Each of these sections includes subsections of codes describing some or all of the following types of procedures:

- Incision
- Excision
- Introduction
- Repair
- Destruction
- Endoscopy

Some of these anatomical sections include codes that describe procedures specific to that particular anatomical structure, such as lung transplantation.

Nose

Procedures on the nose are described by codes 30000–30999. Incision codes describe drainage of abscesses and hematomas of the nose by internal approaches and nasal septum. Incisions involving an external approach are reported with codes from the 10000 series (10060–10180). Excision codes describe the removal of various tissues, including lesions, cysts, inferior **turbinates,** and bony nasal structures. Other procedures described by codes in this section include rhinoplasty procedures, repair of nasal vestibular stenosis, septoplasty procedures, and control of nasal hemorrhage.

Accessory Sinuses

Codes 31000–31299 describe procedures on any of the four sinuses (**frontal, ethmoid, sphenoid,** and **maxillary**). Incision procedures include **sinusotomy** and obliterative procedures. Most of the remaining codes in this section describe sinus **endoscopy** procedures.

Surgical endoscopy procedures include diagnostic endoscopy and sinusotomy procedures, if performed. Unless otherwise specified in the code descriptor, these codes describe unilateral procedures. If performed bilaterally, modifier 50 is added to the code. Some codes, such as 31231 (Nasal endoscopy, diagnostic, unilateral or bilateral [separate

---

mediastinum
Area between the lungs that contains the heart, great vessels, trachea, main bronchi, and esophagus.

turbinate
One of the spongy, scroll-shaped bones in the nasal passages.

frontal sinus
Either of the two air filled cavities within the frontal bone.

ethmoid sinus
Air-filled cavity located at the top of the nasal cavities between the eyes.

sphenoid sinus
One of two cavities in the sphenoid bone that communicate with the nasal cavities.

maxillary sinus
One of a pair of air cavities in the maxilla (upper jaw) that connect with the nose.

sinusotomy
Incision into a sinus.

endoscopy
The visual inspection of a body cavity or canal with an endoscope.

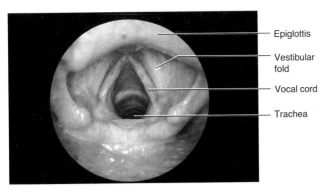

FIGURE 12.3.1 View of the Larynx Using a Laryngoscope

procedure]), specify that even when performed bilaterally, modifier 50 is not added to the code. This code descriptor also identifies this as a "separate procedure." This means that this code is reported when this is the only procedure performed. But, as noted above, diagnostic endoscopy is included as part of surgical endoscopy procedures.

Larynx

Excision codes describe laryngotomy and laryngectomy procedures, or procedures performed on the larynx (Figure 12.3.1). The numerous codes in the Endoscopy subsection (31505–31579) describe laryngoscopy with associated procedures. Some codes include the use of an operating microscope or telescope as part of the code descriptor. Following each of these codes is a parenthetical remark instructing the coder not to report code 69990. Codes describing reconstruction with graft material often note that the procedure includes obtaining the graft material. Parenthetical remarks following such codes include instructions not to report those codes with other codes that describe obtaining the grafts.

Trachea and Bronchi

Code range 31600–31899 describes procedures on the **trachea** and **bronchi**. Most of the codes in this section describe tracheostomy and endoscopy procedures. The endoscopy code group includes various combinations of **bronchoscopy** with other procedures. Many of these combinations are indented under a primary procedure code. A significant number of codes include a symbol that indicates that conscious sedation is inherent in the procedure and cannot be reported separately. These codes are also listed in Appendix G.

Several code descriptors indicate that the code is reported for a single lobe. Add-on codes are used to report the same procedure in additional lobes.

trachea
Air tube from the larynx to the bronchi.

bronchi
Subdivisions of the trachea to each lung and individual lobes of the lungs.

bronchoscopy
Examination of the interior of the tracheobronchial tree with an endoscope.

CODING EXAMPLE

A pulmonologist performs four biopsies in the right upper lobe and two biopsies in the right lower lobe through a bronchoscope while providing conscious sedation to his patient. The coder reviews coding guidelines to report these procedures and reports them with CPT code 31628 and add-on code 31632, listing each code only once. The physician questions her, stating that the codes should be reported with the number of units corresponding to the number of biopsies. When she disagrees, the physician asks her to show him instructions to support a single use of each code. He also wants her to report the conscious sedation as a separate service.

(Continued)

Reviewing the guidelines in the Endoscopy section, the coder shows the physician that CPT code 31628 includes a parenthetical instruction that the code is only reported once regardless of how many biopsies are performed in a lobe. She also points out the parenthetical note associated with this code instructs coders to use add-on code 31632 to report biopsies in a second lobe. Turning to that code, the parenthetical note states that this code is only reported once regardless of how many biopsies are taken in the additional lobe. She then shows the pulmonologist that CPT code 31628 is marked with the bull's-eye sign, indicating conscious sedation cannot be reported separately. Add-on codes do not independently determine whether conscious sedation can be reported separately. Rather, they follow the rules for the parent code.

pleura
Membrane covering the lungs and lining the ribs in the thoracic cavity.

diagnostic thoracoscopy
Examination of the thoracic cavity with an endoscope.

surgical thoracoscopy
Surgical endoscopy done as part of a thoracic procedure.

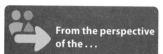

From the perspective of the . . .

CODER

Most endoscopic procedures are unilateral unless the code descriptor specifically states that it is a bilateral procedure. If the surgeon performs bilateral endoscopies, these should be reported independently with either modifier 50 to indicate that the same procedure was performed bilaterally or anatomical modifiers to differentiate the two procedures.

Excision and repair codes describe procedures such as tracheoplasty (31750), carinal reconstruction (31766), bronchoplasty (31770), tracheal stenosis excision repair (31780), surgical closure of tracheostomy (31820), and revision of tracheostomy scar (31830).

Lungs and Pleura

Codes describing procedures on the lungs and **pleura** (32035–32999) are divided into the usual incision, excision, removal, and endoscopy codes. The Endoscopy section includes two main codes: **diagnostic thoracoscopy** and **surgical thoracoscopy**. Each of these two codes has numerous associated indented codes describing additional procedures performed with the thoracoscopy. Surgical thoracoscopy always includes a diagnostic thoracoscopy.

This section includes codes describing procedures associated with lung transplants, including harvesting organs from the cadaver donor, backbench work to prepare the donor organ, and four codes to describe transplant procedures—single and double lung transplants with and without cardiopulmonary bypass.

CODER'S TIP

Surgical thoracoscopy procedures are described with a family of 16 separate codes. Each of these includes a specific surgical procedure performed with the thoracoscopy. None of these codes describe nonspecific procedures or not otherwise specified procedures.

EXERCISE 12.3.1

Also available in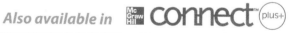

Use the CPT manual to select the best code to describe the following procedures.

1. Unilateral repair of nasal vestibular stenosis _____

2. Diagnostic nasal endoscopy _____

3. Emergency endotracheal intubation _____

4. Bronchoscopy, flexible diagnostic with placement of multiple fiducial markers _____

5. Lobectomy, single lobe _____

12.3.2 Procedures on the Heart and Pericardium (33010–33999)

The cardiovascular system is complex, ranging from the heart and great vessels in the chest to the smallest arteries and veins of the fingers and toes. Numerous types of procedures may be performed on these structures. Coders must understand the anatomy of the cardiovascular system as well as the structure of the code sections to select the correct code to report procedures on these structures.

Codes in the Heart and Pericardium section of the CPT manual describe procedures on the heart and great vessels (aorta, pulmonary artery, and large veins entering the left and right atria). Some procedures involve structures on the surface of the heart, while others involve opening the heart and repairing or replacing anatomical structures within the heart itself, such as the valves.

Codes describing these procedures are grouped together based on anatomical location, type of procedure, or both. Some sections have specific instructions associated with them, and those instructions will be discussed with those codes. Understanding the anatomical structures and their relationships to each other is critical to selecting the right code for procedures on the heart and pericardium.

Pericardium; Cardiac Tumor; Transmyocardial Revascularization

The **pericardium** is the sac that surrounds the heart. Fluid may collect inside the pericardium but outside the heart. If a significant amount of fluid collects in this space, it may decrease the ability of the heart to pump blood. Most procedures performed on the pericardium are designed to remove such fluid or prevent it from occurring.

pericardium
The sac that surrounds the heart.

Pericardiocentesis (33010 and 33011) is a procedure by which fluid is withdrawn from the pericardial sac, usually through the use of a needle (or catheter) and a syringe. If fluid continues to collect within the pericardium, a window or opening in the pericardium can be created surgically to allow the fluid to drain out of the pericardium (33025). In severe cases, most or all of the pericardium may be surgically removed (33030–33031). On occasion, a cyst or tumor may form in the pericardium that requires excision (33050).

Heart tumors may form either inside the heart (intracardiac) or on the outside of the heart (external tumor). Excision of these tumors is reported with CPT code 33120 or 33130.

Transmyocardial revascularization is a procedure in which a laser is used to create holes in the heart muscle (myocardium) as a treatment for myocardial ischemia. This promotes the flow of blood into the myocardium and the formation of new blood vessels. When this procedure is performed as the only procedure on the heart, it is reported with CPT code 33140. If it is performed with other cardiac procedures, use CPT code 33141.

Pacemaker or Pacing Cardioverter-Defibrillator

Pacemakers or pacing cardioverter-defibrillators include one or more leads, an electronic pulse generator, and a battery. The leads are threaded into the heart through one of the veins leading back to the heart or attached to the outside of the heart (epicardium). The pulse generator/battery usually is implanted subcutaneously below the clavicle or under the abdominal muscles.

Pacemakers may be either single chamber (sending an electrical signal through one lead to either the right atrium or right ventricle) or dual chamber (sending electrical signals through two electrodes to both the right atrium and right ventricle). CPT codes 33202–33223 describe various combinations of these procedures, including insertion

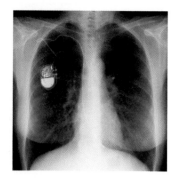

Pacemakers send electrical signals to the heart. The type of pacemaker determines how it is coded.

of temporary pacemakers, insertion of a permanent pacemaker generator with one, two, or multiple leads, and insertion or replacement of only the generator or only the leads when necessary to repair or replace one part of the system.

In some cases, it is necessary to provide biventricular pacing (sending electrical signals through two leads to the right and left ventricles). To do this, a separate lead must be placed into the coronary sinus that leads into the veins of the left ventricle. CPT code 33224 is used to report this procedure if the lead is placed and attached to a previously installed generator. If the left ventricle lead is placed through the coronary sinus at the same time that the generator is initially implanted, the generator placement code is reported with the add-on code 33225 to report placement of the left ventricular lead. CPT codes 33226–33249 (with several out of sequence codes) describe various procedures for repositioning, removing, and replacing pacemaker or cardioverter-defibrillator components. The CPT manual now includes a table to guide coders in selecting the correct codes for these procedures.

Electrophysiologic Operative Procedures; Patient-Activated Event Recorder

It is sometimes necessary to surgically excise or ablate tissues that cause supraventricular dysrhythmias. These may be performed as primary procedures (33250–33256) or in addition to other procedures (add-on codes 33257–33259). To determine the correct code, coders must pay particular attention to whether these procedures are performed with or without cardiopulmonary bypass. When these procedures are performed via endoscopy, CPT codes 33265–33266 are used to report the procedure with or without cardiopulmonary bypass.

In some instances, it is necessary to implant devices that record cardiac events and later remove these devices. These procedures are reported with CPT codes 33282–33284.

Wounds of the Heart and Great Vessels

Even minor wounds involving the heart or great vessels (aorta, pulmonary artery, pulmonary vein, and vena cava) may be life threatening and require surgical exploration and/or repair. Cardiac wound repairs are reported with CPT code 33300 or 33305, depending on whether it is necessary to utilize cardiopulmonary bypass during the repair.

Cardiotomy (opening the heart to explore the interior chambers) is reported with CPT codes 33310 and 33315. These procedures include removing any foreign body from the heart, including a thrombus (blood clot). When blood clots are removed as part of other cardiac procedures, these codes are not reported separately unless a separate incision is made in the heart that would not typically be necessary as part of the other procedure. In that case, CPT code 33310 or 33315 may be reported with modifier 59 to indicate that it is a separate procedure.

Suture repairs and insertions of graft into the great vessels may require the use of **cardiopulmonary bypass** or a **shunt** (insertion of a tube that temporarily allows blood to bypass the area of the vessel being repaired). Codes identifying these procedures differentiate whether cardiopulmonary bypass, shunt bypass, or neither is used during the repair/graft procedure (33320–33322; 33330–33332).

Cardiac Valves

The heart contains four valves. The mitral valve separates the left atrium and ventricle. The aortic valve separates the left ventricle and aorta. On the right side of the heart, the tricuspid valve separates the right atrium and ventricle, while the pulmonary valve separates the right ventricle from the pulmonary artery. At times, it is necessary to repair or replace one or more of these valves. The CPT has separate codes for procedures on each of these valves.

The range of procedures varies by valve. That is, not all procedures that are performed on the aortic valve have corresponding procedures on the other valves. Coders must know what procedure was performed and on which valve. If the surgeon operates

cardiotomy
Opening the heart to explore the interior chambers.

cardiopulmonary bypass
A surgical procedure to divert blood around the heart and lungs, most often during surgical procedures on the heart or great vessels.

shunt
Insertion of a tube that temporarily allows blood to bypass the area of the vessel being repaired.

on more than one valve during the same surgical procedure, each procedure is reported separately. Modifier 51 is added to the secondary valve procedure(s).

Coronary Artery Anomalies

Codes 33500–33507 describe various procedures performed to repair anomalies of the coronary arteries. When the surgeon also performs an **angioplasty** or endarterectomy, those procedures are included in the basic codes for the coronary artery repair.

angioplasty
Recanalization of a blood vessel by surgery or with a balloon tip catheter.

Coronary Artery Bypass Graft (CABG) Procedures

Coronary artery bypass graft (CABG, pronounced "cabbage") procedures restore blood circulation to the myocardium when the patient's own arteries are too narrow to allow sufficient blood flow to supply oxygen to the heart muscle. Depending on the underlying circulatory abnormality, the surgeon may perform as few as one bypass graft or as many as six or more grafts.

The grafts may be venous grafts, arterial grafts, or a mixture of the two. The saphenous vein is often used for venous grafts. In some instances, other veins are harvested and used for the graft. The internal mammary artery is the artery used most often as an arterial graft. In some cases, a combination of internal mammary artery graft and saphenous vein graft is used. Other veins and/or arteries may be used as part of the bypass procedure. Reporting these procedures correctly depends on what types of grafts are used (venous, arterial, or both) and where the grafts were harvested.

Venous Grafting Only for Coronary Artery Bypass When only venous grafts are used, coders should report the procedures with CPT codes 33510–33516. These codes are not reported if an arterial graft is performed in combination with the venous graft procedure. The only difference between these codes is the number of venous grafts used in the procedure. These procedures include harvesting of the saphenous vein, so the harvesting procedure is not reported separately. If a surgical assistant performs only the saphenous vein harvesting, the assistant adds modifier 80 to CPT codes 33510–33516 to report his or her services. This code and modifier are also used if the assistant surgeon assists with other parts of the procedure.

If other veins are harvested from either the upper or lower extremities, then add-on codes 35500 (Harvest of upper extremity vein, 1 segment, for lower extremity or coronary artery bypass procedure [List separately in addition to code for primary procedure]) or 35572 (Harvest of femoropopliteal vein, 1 segment, for vascular reconstruction procedure [e.g., aortic, vena caval, coronary, peripheral artery] [List separately in addition to code for primary procedure]).

Combined Arterial-Venous Grafting for Coronary Bypass A bypass procedure with both arterial and venous grafts is reported with a combination of two codes, one to report the appropriate arterial graft procedure (33533–33536, see below) and the appropriate add-on code describing the venous graft portion of the procedure (33517–33523). These codes describe the number of venous grafts utilized. Add-on codes 33517–33523 are never reported alone.

As with the codes describing venous-grafting-only procedures, obtaining the saphenous vein graft is included in these add-on codes and is not reported separately. If other veins are harvested from the upper or lower extremities, add-on codes 33500 or 33572 are reported to describe the harvesting procedure. Harvesting the arterial graft is included in the arterial graft bypass procedure codes and is not reported separately unless an arterial graft is obtained from the upper extremity, with the exception of a radial artery graft (see below). If an upper extremity artery is harvested, that procedure is reported with add-on code 33600 in addition to the bypass procedure codes. Modifier 80 is added to the CPT code that describes the bypass procedure (33517–33523 or 33533–33536) if a surgical assistant performs the artery or vein harvesting procedure.

Arterial Grafting for Coronary Artery Bypass CPT codes 33533–33536 are used to report arterial grafting for CABG procedures when performed alone or in combination with venous grafting. Arterial graft procedures may include use of the internal mammary, gastroepiploic, epigastric, radial, and other arteries. The four codes differ from one another by the number of arterial grafts performed. These codes include harvesting the arteries used in the graft procedure with the exception of a graft harvested from the upper extremity, in which case add-on code 33600 is reported in addition to the arterial coronary grafting code. As discussed above, if the surgeon performs a combined arterial-venous graft procedure, both the arterial graft code and the venous graft add-on code are reported together.

Repair of Cardiac and Great Vessel Anomalies/Defects

CPT codes describing repairs of cardiac anomalies and defects are grouped together by the location of the anomaly or type of repair. The CPT includes the following groups:

- Single Ventricle and Other Complex Cardiac Anomalies (33600–33619)
- Septal Defect (33641–33697)
- Sinus of Valsalva (33702–33722)
- Venous Anomalies (33724–33732)
- Shunting Procedures (33735–33768)
- Transposition of the Great Vessels (33770–33783)
- Truncus Arteriosus (33786–33788)
- Aortic Anomalies (33800–33853)
- Thoracic Aortic Aneurysm (33860–33877)
- Endovascular Repair of Descending Thoracic Aorta (33880–33891)
- Pulmonary Artery (33910–33926)

Within each subsection, the type of defect and the particular surgical repair differentiate one code from another. Coders must be familiar with the descriptions of these procedures. Many cardiac anomalies are congenital abnormalities that require surgical repair shortly after birth. Codes describing procedures commonly performed on infants include parenthetical notes directing coders not to add modifier 63 (procedure performed on infants weighing less than 4 kg) to that particular code. Coders also must pay attention to the numerous parenthetical notes providing directions regarding which codes can or cannot be reported with other codes.

CODING TIP

Many, but not all, of the codes that describe cardiac and great vessel repair procedures cannot be reported with modifier 63, which identifies procedures on infants weighing less than 4 kg. The code descriptors do not usually identify these procedures as only for infants, but they are very often performed on very young and small infants.

CODING EXAMPLE

A surgeon performs a repair of an atrial septal defect (33647) on an infant weighing 3.2 kg. Although this would typically be reported with modifier 63, a parenthetical note below this code provides the instruction, "Do not report modifier 63 in conjunction with 33647." This code is also listed in Appendix F, which identifies all codes that are modifier-63 exempt.

The only codes listed above with specific guidance are those in the family of codes describing endovascular repairs of the descending thoracic aorta. Codes describing endovascular repairs include introduction, manipulation, positioning, placement, and deployment of the device. Any associated angioplasties or stent placements in the region treated by the endovascular device are not reported separately. However, associated arteriotomies, guide wire and catheter insertions, and extensive repairs or replacements of the artery are separately reported. If the patient undergoes one or more surgical procedures in association with the endovascular repair, these additional procedures should be reported separately.

The two main codes describing endovascular repairs of the descending thoracic aorta (33880 and 33881) differ from one another depending on whether the device covers the beginning of the left subclavian artery where it comes off the aorta. These two codes include additional distal segments added to the original endovascular device. Proximal segments, however, are reported separately with CPT code 33883 for the first proximal extension and add-on code 33884 for each additional proximal extension in addition to the main code.

Fluoroscopic guidance associated with endovascular repair of the descending aorta is reported with CPT codes 75956–75959. CPT codes 75956 and 75957 are reported with 33880 and 33881, respectively. Fluoroscopic guidance associated with placement of proximal extensions is reported with CPT code 75958. CPT code 75959 is used to report fluoroscopic guidance for the placement of distal extensions.

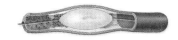

Angioplasty involves the insertion and inflation of a balloon to clear a circulatory pathway. If associated with an endovascular repair, angioplasty is not reported separately from that procedure.

CODER'S TIP

Endovascular repairs of the descending aorta require fluoroscopic guidance. Both the surgical codes (33880–33886) and the fluoroscopic guidance codes (75956–75959) are reported to fully describe these procedures.

Heart and Heart/Lung Transplantation

Organ transplants include three main components: (a) cadaver donor organ resection; (b) backbench work to prepare the donor organ for implantation; and (c) recipient organ transplantation. CPT codes 33930, 33933, and 33935 describe these three components for heart-lung transplant procedures. CPT codes 33940, 33944, and 33945 describe the same three components for heart transplants.

Cardiac Assist

A variety of devices may be used to provide circulatory assistance. Extracorporeal circulation devices are external devices that provide mechanical assistance to pump blood throughout the body when the heart is incapable of doing so on its own. Extracorporeal circulation is described by CPT code 33960 for the first 24 hours and add-on code 33961 for each additional 24 hours. The use of intra-aortic balloon assist devices is described with CPT codes 33967–33974. These codes describe percutaneous and open procedures to insert and remove balloon assist devices. CPT codes 33975–33979 are used to report the insertion and removal of ventricular assist devices.

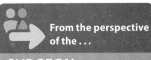

From the perspective of the . . .

SURGEON

It is important to communicate the specific details regarding all three components of heart or heart-lung transplants to the professional coder reporting these services. The three components include: (a) cadaver donor resection; (b) backbench work to prepare the organ; and (c) the transplant procedure in the recipient.

EXERCISE 12.3.2

Also available in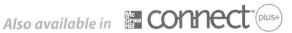

Use the CPT manual to select the best code to describe the following procedures.

1. Replacement of an electrode for a temporary dual-chamber pacemaker _____
2. Subsequent pericardiocentesis _____

(Continued)

3. Surgical endoscopic limited tissue ablation of the atria _____

4. Closed heart valvotomy, pulmonary valve; transventricular _____

5. Mitral valve valvuloplasty, with cardiopulmonary bypass _____

6. Suture repair of aorta without shunt or cardiopulmonary bypass _____

7. Embolectomy, pulmonary artery; with cardiopulmonary bypass _____

8. Reimplantation of an anomalous pulmonary artery _____

9. Subclavian to pulmonary artery shunt _____

10. Percutaneous insertion of an intra-aortic balloon assist device (balloon pump) _____

12.3.3 Procedures on the Arteries and Veins (34001–37799)

Codes 34001–37799 describe procedures on both the arterial and venous systems. Most but not all of these procedures are intended to establish or reestablish blood flow. Vascular procedures intended to establish blood flow include all elements necessary to establish blood inflow and outflow as part of the procedure. Some procedures, such as arterial or venous ligation, do not contemplate establishing blood flow.

When a surgeon performs intraoperative arteriograms as part of the procedure, those are also included in the primary procedure code and are not reported separately. Procedures that require fluoroscopic or other guidance as part of the procedure include parenthetical notes identifying the correct radiology code to describe imaging for the particular procedure.

embolectomy
Surgical removal of an embolus.

thrombectomy
Surgical removal of a blood clot.

aneurysm
A weak area of an artery that can rupture, causing extreme blood loss, damage, and possible death.

Embolectomy/Thrombectomy; Venous Reconstruction

The codes describing arterial **embolectomy** or **thrombectomy** procedures (34001–34203) and venous thrombectomy procedures (34401–34490) are divided into groups by whether they are arterial or venous procedures. The codes are furthered divided by the anatomical location and particular artery or vein on which the procedure is performed. Some venous reconstruction procedure codes (34501–34530) describe procedures to repair specific veins.

Endovascular Repair of Abdominal Aortic Aneurysm; Endovascular Repair of Iliac Aneurysm

An **aneurysm** is a weak area of an artery that can, without treatment, suddenly rupture causing extreme blood loss, damage to surrounding anatomical structures, and possible death. Endovascular repair of an aortic aneurysm involves insertion of an endovascular device into the femoral or iliac artery, maneuvering the device into correct position in the aorta, opening the device to provide a reinforced conduit for blood flow within the vessel, and repairing the artery through which the device was inserted. This relieves pressure on the aneurysm to prevent the rupture of the weakened artery.

A family of codes describes endovascular repairs of aortic aneurysms with various types of endovascular grafts (e.g., a simple tube in the aorta alone, a bifurcated graft with one limb extending into one iliac artery, or a bifurcated graft with two limbs extending into both iliac arteries). The codes also describe whether an open procedure is performed to place the endovascular device in the femoral or iliac

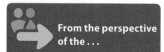

From the perspective of the . . .

CODER

According to the guidelines associated with endovascular repair of abdominal aortic aneurysms, additional interventional procedures performed at the same time are reported separately. These might include procedures on the renal arteries, intravascular ultrasound, balloon angioplasty, or placement of stents.

arteries. A single procedure code (34900) is used to report endovascular repair of iliac aneurysms.

Balloon angioplasties and the placement of stents in the same vessel as the endovascular grafts are included in the procedure and are not separately reported. Other procedures, such as placement of guide wires or extensive repair of one of the arteries, are reported separately in addition to the underlying code. Fluoroscopic guidance is reported with CPT code 75952, 75953, or 75954, depending on whether it is part of a primary aortic aneurysm endovascular graft, an extension of the primary graft, or an iliac artery graft.

Direct Repair of Aneurysm or Excision and Graft Insertion

The codes in this section describe direct (open) procedures for aneurysm repair or excision of aneurysm with placement of an arterial graft. Most of these procedures are described by a pair of codes—the first describing procedures to treat an aneurysm prior to rupture, the second to treat an aneurysm after it has ruptured. These codes are only used when the artery has an aneurysm with or without occlusive disease associated with the aneurysm. If the graft procedure is performed because of occlusive disease only, those procedures are reported with CPT codes (35201–35286).

Repair Arteriovenous Fistula

Arteriovenous fistulas (abnormal direct connections between an artery and vein) are divided into those that are congenital and those that are acquired or secondary to trauma. Each of these fistula types is further divided by anatomical location of the fistula: (a) head and neck; (b) thorax and abdomen; and (c) extremities. Codes 35180–35190 describe the repair of arteriovenous fistulas.

Repair Blood Vessel Other Than for Fistula

Code range 35201–35286 describes repairs of arteries and veins. The codes are first divided by the type of repair (direct, vein graft, or graft other than a vein) and then further divided by anatomical location (e.g., neck, upper extremity, intrathoracic [with and without bypass], intra-abdominal, or lower extremity).

Thromboendarterectomy

Thromboendarterectomies involve opening an artery, removing a blood clot or plaque, and then closing the vessel. This series of codes describe procedures on various vessels and includes one add-on code. CPT code 35305 describes the procedure on the initial tibial or peroneal artery, while CPT code 35306 describes procedures on each additional tibial or peroneal artery. These codes include harvesting an upper extremity or saphenous vein graft if used to repair the artery.

Transluminal Angioplasty; Transluminal Atherectomy

Each of these families of codes is divided into open and percutaneous procedures. Each group is further subdivided into separate codes for each vessel. Parenthetical notes direct coders to the associated radiological supervision and interpretation codes reported with these codes. If these procedures are performed as part of another procedure, they should be reported with modifier 51 (multiple procedures) or 52 (reduced services).

CODER'S TIP

Transluminal angioplasties are described with two families of codes (35450–35460 and 35471–35476). One family describes open procedures and the other describes percutaneous procedures. Each family includes four codes to describe procedures on renal or other visceral arteries, aorta, brachiocephalic vessels, and veins.

An open transluminal angioplasty of the aorta is reported with code 35452, whereas a percutaneous transluminal angioplasty of the aorta is reported with code 35472.

CODER'S TIP

The importance of always using the most up-to-date CPT manual can be illustrated by comparing the 2010 edition to the 2011 edition. Transluminal atherectomy procedures were reported with codes 35480–35495 in 2010. This entire family of codes was deleted in 2011. Some procedures are now reported with new codes in the 37220–37235 range of codes. Others were deleted and converted to Category III codes. Any coder using the 2010 edition would report these procedures incorrectly.

Bypass Graft

Veins are often used as graft material when a bypass graft is performed to surgically treat arterial insufficiency. In most cases, the saphenous vein or other veins are harvested and moved to the arterial site. Both ends of the harvested vein are then attached to the artery to allow blood to flow through the vein from the proximal anastomosis (attachment of the vein to the artery) to the distal anastomosis. CPT codes 35501–35671 describe specific bypass grafts procedures, each of which is differentiated from the others by the location of the proximal and distal anastomoses.

Harvesting the saphenous vein is included in the descriptors of CPT codes 35501–35587, and no other code is used to report that service. If it is necessary to harvest other vein grafts, those services are reported separately with CPT add-on codes 35500 (Harvest of upper extremity vein, 1 segment, for lower extremity or coronary artery bypass procedure) or 35572 (Harvest of femoropopliteal vein, 1 segment, for vascular reconstruction procedure [e.g., aortic, vena caval, coronary, peripheral artery]). Each of these codes includes parenthetical remarks listing the CPT codes for bypass procedures that may be reported with these add-on codes.

In some cases, bypass grafts may be performed with a combination of synthetic grafts and harvested vein grafts or with veins harvested from multiple locations. Those procedures are reported with add-on codes 35681 (Bypass graft; composite, prosthetic and vein); 35682 (Bypass graft; autogenous composite, 2 segments of veins from 2 locations); or 35683 (Bypass graft; autogenous composite, 3 or more segments of vein from 2 or more locations). Only one of these add-on codes may be reported with a primary code describing the primary bypass procedure.

Excision, Exploration, Repair, Revision

Code series 35700–35907 describes various procedures to explore vascular structures (35701–35860), repair previous grafts (35870–35876), revise grafts (35879–35884), or excise (remove) infected grafts (35901–35907). Guidance and parenthetical remarks direct coders to the use of specific codes for each type of procedure.

Vascular Injection Procedures

central venous access device
A catheter inserted into the heart or venous trunk through a large vein of the arm, leg, neck, or shoulder.

Code range 36000–36598 describes placement of catheters in specific vascular structures for diagnostic or therapeutic procedures (36000–36522) and **central venous access** procedures (36555–36598). In most cases, a catheter is introduced into either the vena cava or aorta through a percutaneous insertion of the catheter.

Coders often find coding vascular catheterization procedures confusing. To fully understand the coding of these procedures, it is necessary to understand the anatomy of the vascular system and how the various arteries are designated for coding purposes. As explained in more detail below, coding catheterization procedures depends on where within the vascular anatomy the catheter is positioned for the procedure. Refer to Appendix L while studying this section. An abbreviated version of the information in Appendix L appears at the end of this module.

Although the CPT manual lists venous procedures first, followed by arterial procedures, this section will address these in reverse order. The aorta is the major artery leading from the heart to the rest of the body. Each main vessel branching off the aorta is referred to as a first-order vessel. The first-order vessels have several vessels branching off of them, each of which is designated as a second-order vessel. Similarly, most second-order vessels have other vessels branching from them, each of which is designated as a third-order vessel. Even though the arterial system continues branching into many smaller vessels beyond those designated as third-order vessels, for coding purposes it is sufficient to understand the anatomy to this level.

Catheterization procedures are reported with codes that indicate the most distal (farthest) vessel into which the catheter is placed. For arterial catheterization, the procedures typically begin with the placement of a catheter in the aorta. If the catheter is not positioned into any vessels beyond the aorta, the procedure is reported with CPT code 36200 (Introduction of catheter, aorta). If the catheter is positioned into any vessels beyond the aorta, code 36200 is not reported.

If the catheter tip is placed into any first-order vessel, but not beyond, the procedure is reported with one of two codes that describe the first-order vessel: code 36215 (Selective catheter placement, arterial system; each first order thoracic or brachiocephalic branch, within a vascular family) or 36245 (Selective catheter placement, arterial system; each first order abdominal, pelvic, or lower extremity artery branch, within a vascular family). These two codes essentially divide the arterial system into two parts—one providing blood to the head, thorax, and upper extremities; the other to the abdomen, pelvis, and legs. The code descriptors for these two codes specify they are reported for each first-order vessel. If the catheter tip is placed in two or more first-order vessels, but no further, these codes are reported with the number of units that correspond to the number of first-order vessels catheterized.

If the catheter is advanced from the first-order vessel into a second-order vessel, but no further, the code describing first-order vessel catheterization is not reported. Instead, either indented code 36216 (initial second order thoracic or brachiocephalic branch, within a vascular family) or indented code 36246 (initial second order abdominal, pelvic, or lower extremity artery branch, within a vascular family) is reported for the second-order vessel catheterization, depending on the anatomical location of the second-order vessel.

Similarly, if the catheter is advanced into a third-order vessel or beyond, the code describing catheterization of the second-order vessel is not reported. Instead, either code 36217 (initial third order or more selective thoracic or brachiocephalic branch, within a vascular family) or code 36247 (initial third order abdominal, pelvic, or lower extremity artery branch, within a vascular family) is reported, depending on the anatomical location of the third-order vessel.

Two add-on codes, one for each anatomical group of arteries, report additional third-order vessels catheterized from a second-order vessel or additional second-order vessels catheterized from a first-order vessel. The two add-on codes are 36218 (additional second order, third order, and beyond, thoracic or brachiocephalic branch, within a vascular family [List in addition to code for initial second or third order vessel as appropriate]) and 36248 (additional second order, third order, and beyond,

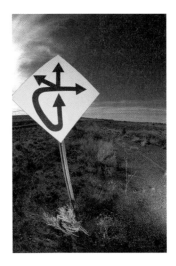

Coding for vascular catheterization procedures can be complex. As a first step, determine where the procedure was conducted using the clinical documentation and your own knowledge of anatomy.

abdominal, pelvic, or lower extremity artery branch, within a vascular family [List in addition to code for initial second or third order vessel as appropriate]).

As explained above, additional first-order vessels are reported with additional units of the codes describing first-order vessel catheterization, not with the add-on codes. However, if those additional first-order vessel catheterizations also involve second- or third-order catheterizations, then the reporting system begins again with an initial second- or third-order vessel catheterization code, because this is the initial second- or third-order vessel in a new vascular family. If additional second- or third-order vessels are catheterized, the appropriate add-on codes are used to report those additional catheterizations.

A third set of codes (36251–36254) describes first- and second-order catheter placement in renal arteries. First-order procedures include selective catheterization of the renal artery and any accessory renal arteries. Second-order procedures include superselective (second-order or higher) catheterization of renal artery branches. Separate codes describe unilateral and bilateral procedures.

CODING EXAMPLE

A patient has a procedure in which the following vessels are selectively catheterized: right internal carotid, right external carotid, left internal carotid, left external carotid, and the right and left common iliac arteries. How is this coded?

The initial step is to identify the number of first-order vessels catheterized without further placement of the catheter. There are two first-order vessels, the right and left common iliac vessels, catheterized without further catheter placement. These are reported with CPT code 36245 X 2 (once for each first-order vessel with no further catheterization in that vascular family).

Next, identify second-order vessels catheterized without further catheterization of third-order vessels in that family. The left internal carotid and left external carotid arteries are second-order vessels without further catheterization. The first second-order vessel is reported with CPT code 36216. The other second-order vessel is part of the same vascular family, so it is reported with add-on code 36218.

The right internal carotid and right external carotid arteries are third-order vessels that are part of the same vascular family (i.e., they are branches of the same second-order vessel, the right common carotid artery). These two vessels are reported with 36217 and add-on code 36218.

The entire procedure is reported as 36245 X 2, 36216, 36217, and 36218 X 2.

The above coding system applies to the catheterization of systemic arterial vessels only. Catheterization of the coronary circulation, including coronary arteries, venous coronary artery bypass grafts, or arterial conduits performed in conjunction with a concomitant cardiac catheterization, is reported with codes from the 90000 series (see Chapter 14).

Procedures on the venous system are reported in a similar fashion. CPT code 36010 (Introduction of catheter, superior or inferior vena cava) describes placement of a catheter in either the superior or inferior vena cava. CPT code 36011 (Selective catheter placement, venous system; first order branch [e.g., renal vein, jugular vein]) describes placement in a first-order branch, and code 36012 (Selective catheter placement, venous system; second order or more selective, branch [e.g., left adrenal vein, petrosal sinus]) describes placement in a second-order or higher branch. CPT codes 36013–36015 describe placement of a catheter into the right heart or main pulmonary artery, left or right pulmonary artery, or selective segmental pulmonary arteries.

Procedures on the venous system, including venipuncture procedures that require a physician's skill, transfusions, injections of sclerosing agents, ablation of incompetent veins, and various therapeutic apheresis procedures are reported with CPT codes 36400–36522.

Central venous access procedures, including the placement of percutaneous catheters or implanted subcutaneous ports, are described by CPT codes 36555–36598. Arterial puncture or catheter placement is described by CPT codes 36600–36660.

Hemodialysis Access, Intervascular Cannulation for Extracorporeal Circulation, or Shunt Insertion

Hemodialysis, extracorporeal membrane oxygenation (ECMO), and other procedures that process blood externally require fistulas, grafts, or cannulas to take blood from the patient's circulatory system and return it after processing. Placement of fistulas, grafts, or cannulas is described by CPT codes 36800–36870.

Portal Decompression Procedures; Transcatheter Procedures; Endovascular Revascularization; Intravascular Ultrasound; Endoscopy; Ligation; Other Procedures

Portal hypertension (elevated pressure in the portal vein of the liver) is a serious condition that often requires surgical treatment to relieve the pressure. Surgeons will often connect one abdominal vein to a second vein in the abdomen. The most common procedure is a portacaval shunt in which the portal vein is connected to the inferior vena cava. CPT code 37140 describes this venous anastomosis. CPT codes 37145–37183 describe similar procedures.

CPT codes 37184–37216 describe transcatheter procedures that are performed through a catheter placed within either the arterial or venous systems. These procedures include mechanical thrombectomies, thrombolysis, occlusion or embolization, and placement of noncoronary stents.

Endovascular revascularization procedures of the lower extremities are now described by a series of codes that were introduced in the CPT in 2011. These codes are reported for both open and percutaneous procedures. For purposes of reporting these procedures, the lower extremity is divided into three arterial vascular territories. The iliac vascular territory includes three vessels—the common iliac, internal iliac, and external iliac arteries. The femoral/popliteal vascular territory is considered a single vessel for purposes of reporting these procedures on the femoral or popliteal arteries. The tibial/peroneal vascular territory includes three vessels—the anterior tibial, posterior tibial, and peroneal arteries.

Procedures on the iliac arteries are reported with a single primary code (37220 or 37221) for procedures on the first vessel and either one or two add-on codes (37222 or 37223) for the other vessels, if treated. Add-on codes are not used to report treatment of additional lesions in the same vessel.

Procedures on the femoral/popliteal artery are reported with a single code (37224–37227). Because this is considered one vessel for purposes of describing these procedures, no add-on codes are used. If several procedures are performed on this vessel territory, the code describing the most complex procedure is reported. The codes are numbered according to increasing complexity.

Procedures on the tibial/peroneal territory are reported with a primary code (37228–37231) for the first vessel and add-on codes (37232–37235) for each additional vessel. Only two additional vessels may be reported, because the territory consists of a total of three vessels. Add-on codes are only used to report procedures on additional vessels, not for the treatment of additional lesions in the same vessel.

Ligation is a procedure in which an artery or vein is tied off to disrupt blood flow through that vessel. This might be necessary because of a malformation, tumor, aneurysm, trauma, varicose veins, or other abnormal conditions. CPT codes 37565–37785 describe these procedures. The code descriptors vary by the specific vessel that is ligated.

Penile revascularization procedures (37788 and 37790) are included in the Other Procedures section, along with the unlisted vascular surgery procedure code (37799).

hemodialysis
Artificial filtration to remove excess waste materials and fluid directly from the blood.

extracorporeal membrane oxygenation
Technique that externally provides respiratory and cardiac functions to assist a patient whose lungs and heart cannot function on their own.

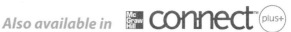

Use the CPT manual to select the best code to describe the following procedures.

1. Open transluminal balloon angioplasty of the brachiocephalic trunk and branches _____

2. Direct repair of a ruptured popliteal artery aneurysm _____

3. Endovascular repair of an abdominal aortic aneurysm with a modular bifurcated prosthesis with two docking limbs _____

4. Introduction of an intravenous catheter into a vein _____

5. Collection of blood by venipuncture _____

6. Open caval-mesenteric venous anastomosis _____

12.3.4 Procedures on the Hemic and Lymphatic Systems, Mediastinum, and Diaphragm (38100–39599)

Hemic and Lymphatic Systems

The Hemic and Lymphatic Systems section describes procedures involving the spleen, lymph nodes, bone marrow, and stem cells. Procedures on the spleen (CPT codes 38100–38200) include excision (removing the spleen), repair, and laparoscopic splenectomy. Bone marrow aspiration and transplant procedures are described by CPT codes 38207–38242.

CODING EXAMPLE

Bone marrow transplants involve donor cells from the recipient (autologous transplant) or from another donor (allogeneic). These transplants are reported with separate CPT codes: code 38240 for allogeneic donor cells and code 38241 for autologous donor cells. CPT code 38230 describes harvesting of bone marrow cells regardless of whether they will be used for an autologous or allogeneic transplant procedure.

CODER'S TIP

CPT codes 38207–38215 describe procedures to prepare bone marrow or stem cells for the transplant procedure. These are reported only once per day, regardless of the amount of bone marrow or stem cells prepared.

Procedures on the lymphatic system can range from a simple biopsy on a superficial lymph node to extensive procedures to remove all lymph nodes from within the thorax or abdominal cavities. Lymphadenectomy procedures may be limited (removing the lymph nodes only) or radical (extensive tissue removal for the treatment of malignancies). CPT codes 38300–38999 describe these procedures.

Mediastinum and Diaphragm

CPT codes 39000–39599 describe procedures on the mediastinum and diaphragm, including mediastinotomies, mediastinoscopies, and surgical repairs on the diaphragm.

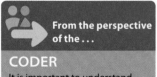

From the perspective of the . . .

CODER

It is important to understand the anatomy of the mediastinum and the structures associated with this space.

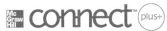
Also available in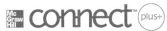

EXERCISE 12.3.4

Use the CPT manual to select the best code to describe the following procedures.

1. Total splenectomy _____
2. Bone marrow harvesting for transplant _____
3. Open excision biopsy of the deep cervical lymph nodes _____
4. Mediastinoscopy with biopsies _____
5. Repair of a chronic diaphragmatic hernia in an adult _____

12.3.5 Anesthesia for Procedures in the 30000 Code Series

Determining which code to use to report anesthesia for procedures in the 30000 code series is one of the most challenging aspects of anesthesia coding. Not only are the anesthesia codes located in numerous anatomical sections of the anesthesia codes, but there also are a number of different anesthesia codes within each section. At times, relatively minor differences in the surgical procedure change the choice of anesthesia code. Some of the factors that should be considered when selecting anesthesia codes are outlined below.

Anesthesia for procedures on the respiratory tract depends on location. Anesthesia for procedures on the nose and sinuses is described by code 00160. Anesthesia for procedures on the larynx and the portion of the trachea within the neck is described by code 00320. Anesthesia codes in the 00520–00529 or 00539–00548 ranges describe anesthesia for procedures on the portions of the respiratory system within the thorax.

Different CPT codes describe anesthesia for transvenous insertion of a permanent pacemaker (00530) and transvenous insertion of a pacing cardioverter-defibrillator (00534). Codes describing anesthesia for procedures on the lungs depend on whether both lungs are ventilated throughout the procedure (00540) or one-lung ventilation (mechanically inflating only one lung during the surgical procedure) is utilized for part of the procedure (00541).

The choice of anesthesia code for cardiac procedures can be confusing. CPT code 00560 describes anesthesia for procedures on the heart, pericardial sac, and great vessels of the chest, without a pump oxygenator (cardiopulmonary bypass pump), for patients of any age. In contrast, CPT code 00561 describes anesthesia for similar procedures with a pump oxygenator for patients who are younger than one year of age. For patients who are older than 1 year of age and undergoing cardiac procedures with a pump oxygenator, the code that describes anesthesia depends on the procedure. Code 00562 describes anesthesia for all non–coronary bypass procedures, such as a valve replacement (Figure 12.3.2), or for reoperations for coronary bypass procedures that occur more than one month after the original bypass graft. Codes describing anesthesia for coronary artery bypass graft procedures depend on whether the procedure is performed without a pump oxygenator (00566) or with a pump oxygenator (00567). As mentioned above, if the procedure is a reoperation more than one month after the original bypass graft procedure, it is reported with code 00562 if the procedure involves the use of a pump oxygenator.

Anesthesia codes for vascular procedures depend on the location of the vessel on which the surgery is performed. Most anatomical code selections are fairly obvious, but anesthesia for vascular procedures on abdominal vessels depends on whether the vessel is in the upper abdomen (00770) or lower abdomen (00880).

Examples of common anesthesia codes used with procedures from the 30000 series are shown in Table 12.3.1.

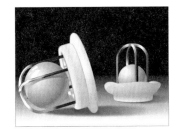

FIGURE 12.3.2 Artificial Heart Valve

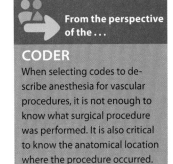

From the perspective of the . . .

CODER

When selecting codes to describe anesthesia for vascular procedures, it is not enough to know what surgical procedure was performed. It is also critical to know the anatomical location where the procedure occurred.

TABLE 12.3.1 Common Anesthesia Codes for Procedures in the 30000 Series

Code Range	Procedures Reported
00160	Procedures on the nose and accessory sinuses
00320	Procedures on the esophagus, thyroid, larynx, trachea, and lymphatic system of the neck
00350	Procedures on the major vessels of the neck
00500–00580	Intrathoracic procedures
00770	Procedures on major abdominal blood vessels
00880	Procedures on major lower abdominal blood vessels
01260–01274	Vascular procedures of the upper leg
01430–01444	Vascular procedures of the knee and popliteal area
01500–01522	Vascular procedures of the lower leg
01650–01670	Vascular procedures of the shoulder and axilla
01770–01782	Vascular procedures of the upper arm and elbow
01840–01852	Vascular procedures of the forearm, wrist, and hand

CODER'S TIP

Each anesthesia code describes anesthesia for many surgical procedures. Even so, small differences in those surgical procedures can mean that a different anesthesia code would be reported.

CODING EXAMPLE

A 65-year-old man has a coronary artery bypass graft (CABG) procedure with a pump oxygenator approximately eight years after his first CABG operation. How would the coder report the anesthesia for this procedure?

The coder would report this with code 00562. The procedure was performed with a pump oxygenator; the patient is older than one year of age; the surgical procedure is a repeat CABG; and the original CABG procedure occurred more than one month prior to this procedure.

To select the correct code to report anesthesia for open heart procedures, coders must consider the following:

1. *Whether the procedure was done with or without cardiopulmonary bypass.* If done without bypass, only codes 00560 or 00566 should be considered as possible codes. If done with bypass, only codes 00561, 00562, 00563, or 00567 are possible anesthesia codes.

2. *Whether the procedure was a coronary artery bypass graft or other procedure.* If the procedure is a new CABG procedure, only codes 00566 or 00567 should be considered as appropriate anesthesia codes. If not a CABG, do not consider these codes. Anesthesia for a reoperation for a CABG procedure originally performed more than one month previously is reported with code 00562.

3. *Patient age.* Procedures on children less than one year of age that involve the use of cardiopulmonary bypass are reported with code 00561.

CODING EXAMPLE

A six-month-old infant undergoes cardiac surgery to correct a congenital anomaly of the great vessels. The procedure is performed with a pump oxygenator and hypothermia. How would the coder report this anesthetic?

The anesthetic is reported with code 00561 (Anesthesia for procedures on heart, pericardial sac, and great vessels of chest; with pump oxygenator, younger than 1 year of age).

EXERCISE 12.3.5

Also available in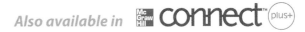

Use the CPT manual to select the best code to describe anesthesia for the following procedures.

1. Radical sinusotomy (Caldwell-Luc) _____

2. Total laryngectomy with radical neck dissection _____

3. Bronchoscopy of both lungs with biopsies _____

4. Left lower lobectomy with single lung ventilation _____

5. Insertion of pacemaker via subclavian vein _____

6. Mitral valve replacement with cardiopulmonary bypass _____

7. Coronary artery bypass graft (CABG) without cardiopulmonary bypass _____

8. Repair of ventricular septal defect with cardiopulmonary bypass in three-week-old infant _____

9. Iliofemoral bypass graft _____

10. Splenectomy _____

Summary

Learning Outcome	Key Concepts/Examples
12.3.1 Differentiate between the surgical procedures performed on the respiratory system. **Pages 344–346**	Procedures on the respiratory system include procedures on the nose, sinuses, larynx, trachea, bronchi, lungs, and pleura. These procedures include incisions, excisions, removal, repair, destruction, endoscopy, and transplants. Coders must understand the differences between these procedures to select the correct codes to report them.
12.3.2 Describe the various types of procedures performed on the cardiac system, including coronary artery bypass grafts, repairs of cardiac abnormalities, and procedures on the great vessels. **Pages 347–351**	Procedures on the heart range from those that do not involve exposing the heart, such as pericardiocentesis or placement of cardiac pacemakers, to coronary artery bypass grafts (CABGs) that are performed on the surface of the heart, to valve replacements and corrections of cardiac abnormalities that involve operating on interior structures of the heart. The great vessels include the aorta, the pulmonary artery, the pulmonary vein returning from the lungs to the left atrium, and the two vena cava vessels returning from the body to the right atrium. Coders must be able to identify the type of procedure and the anatomical structures involved to correctly report these procedures.
12.3.3 Identify CPT codes to report open and endovascular arterial repairs, bypass procedures, angioplasties, shunts, and vascular access procedures. **Pages 352–357**	Procedures on the arterial and venous systems include endovascular and open repairs, bypass procedures, angioplasties, shunts, and vascular access procedures. It is important to understand the anatomy and the surgical procedure to determine the correct code to describe these procedures.
12.3.4 Describe procedures on the hemic and lymphatic systems, mediastinum, and diaphragm. **Page 358**	The hemic and lymphatic systems include the spleen, bone marrow, lymph nodes, and lymph channels. These procedures include open and laparoscopic procedures. Selecting the correct codes requires coders to identify the particular anatomical structures involved in the surgical procedure, the specific surgical procedure performed, and whether the procedure is open or laparoscopic. The mediastinum is the space between the lungs, including the anatomical structures within that space, such as the trachea, esophagus, heart, and the great vessels. The diaphragm lies between the thorax and the abdomen.
12.3.5 Code anesthesia services for procedures in the 30000 series of CPT codes. **Pages 359–361**	CPT codes describing anesthesia for procedures in the 30000 series come from a large number of anesthesia code sections. This is not surprising, considering the wide range of anatomical structures described by procedures in the 30000 series.

Using Terminology

Match each term with its definition.

_____ **1.** L012.3.1 Sinusotomy
_____ **2.** L012.3.1 Turbinate
_____ **3.** L012.3.1 Maxillary sinus
_____ **4.** L012.3.1 Bronchoscopy
_____ **5.** L012.3.1 Endoscopy
_____ **6.** L012.3.2 Central venous access device
_____ **7.** L012.3.2 Angioplasty
_____ **8.** L012.3.2 Cardiopulmonary bypass
_____ **9.** L012.3.2 Pericardium
_____ **10.** L012.3.2 Mediastinum
_____ **11.** L012.3.3 Thrombectomy
_____ **12.** L012.3.3 Aneurysm
_____ **13.** L012.3.3 Shunt
_____ **14.** L012.3.3 Extracorporeal membrane oxygenation

A. Ridge-shaped cartilage inside the nose
B. Recanalization of a blood vessel by surgery
C. Procedure involving a scope inserted into the trachea and bronchial structures
D. A surgical procedure to divert blood around the heart and lungs
E. Incision into the sinus cavity
F. The sac that surrounds the heart
G. Area between the lungs
H. Weak area of an artery that can, without treatment, suddenly rupture
I. Related to one of the spongy, scroll-shaped bones of the nasal passages
J. A device inserted through the venous system into the superior or inferior vena cava or the right side of the heart
K. Surgical removal of a blood clot
L. Visual inspection of a body cavity or canal with an endoscope
M. Insertion of a tube that temporarily allows blood to bypass the area of the vessel being repaired
N. Technique that externally provides respiratory and cardiac aid to a patient whose lungs and heart cannot function on their own

Checking Your Understanding

Select the letter that best completes the statement or answers the question.

1. L012.3.4 Procedures performed on the mediastinum and diaphragm are coded from which range of codes in the CPT manual?

a. 30000
b. 40000
c. 20000
d. None of these

2. L012.3.1 If performed bilaterally, code 31231 (Nasal endoscopy, diagnostic, unilateral or bilateral) requires which of the following?

a. Modifier 50
b. Modifier 51
c. No modifier
d. LT and RT modifiers

3. L012.3.1 Procedures described by codes 31505–31579 describe laryngoscopy with associated procedures. Parenthetical remarks following those codes instruct the coder:

a. Not to use 69990 (operating microscope), as this is part of the code description.
b. Not to report codes associated with obtaining the graft material for reconstruction.
c. To use 31599 (unlisted procedure) for reconstruction of a vocal cord with allograft.
d. All of these.

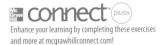

Enhance your learning by completing these exercises
and more at mcgrawhillconnect.com!

4. L012.3.1 A flexible bronchoscopy with two transbronchial lung biopsies of the left lower lobe would be coded with which of the following code(s)?

    a. 31625, 31625
    b. 31628, 31632
    c. 31628
    d. 31628, 31628

5. L012.2.2 The sac surrounding the heart is called the _____.

    a. Myocardium
    b. Pericardium
    c. Epicardium
    d. Endocardium

6. L012.2.2 A permanent pacemaker generator was inserted with the leads (electrodes) placed in the atrium and the ventricle. Which code(s) would be used to report this procedure?

    a. 33208
    b. 33249
    c. 33208, 33217
    d. 33207

7. L012.2.2 Which valve separates the left ventricle and aorta?

    a. Mitral valve
    b. Pulmonary valve
    c. Aortic valve
    d. Tricuspid valve

8. L012.2.2 Organ transplants include which of the following components?

    a. Recipient organ transplantation
    b. Backbench work to prepare the donor organ for implantation
    c. Cadaver donor organ resection
    d. All of these

9. L012.3.4 Codes 38207–38215 describe procedures to prepare bone marrow or stem cells for the transplant procedure. The guidelines above these codes tell the coder that this range of codes may be used:

    a. As often as needed for the amount of bone marrow/stem cells required.
    b. Once per day regardless of the quantity of bone marrow/stem cells required.
    c. Only one time.
    d. None of these.

10. L012.3.3 Arteriovenous fistulas (abnormal direct connections between an artery and vein) are divided into which of the following categories in order to determine the appropriate CPT code?

    a. Congenital
    b. Acquired or secondary to trauma
    c. Anatomical location of the fistula
    d. All of these

Applying Your Skills

Use the CPT manual to determine the correct code to report the following procedures.

1. L012.3.1 Simple excision of a dermoid cyst of the nose _____
2. L012.3.3 Interruption of the femoral vein _____
3. L012.3.1 Open pleural biopsy; percutaneous needle _____
4. L012.2.2 Repair of a pulmonary valve _____
5. L012.2.2 Removal of a pacemaker from the heart _____
6. L012.3.4 Exploration of lymph nodes of the neck _____
7. L012.3.3 Exploration of a blood vessel in the abdomen _____
8. L012.2.2 Implantation of a cardiac event recorder _____
9. L012.2.2 Allograft preparation of the heart _____
10. L012.2.1 Transtracheal injection for bronchography _____
11. L012.3.1 Single lung transplant without cardiopulmonary bypass _____
12. L012.3.1 Bilateral diagnostic nasal endoscopy _____
13. L012.3.3 Reconstruction of a vena cava with resection _____
14. L012.3.4 Bone marrow needle biopsy _____
15. L012.3.4 Unlisted procedure of the hemic system _____

Thinking It Through

Use your critical-thinking skills to answer the questions below.

1. L012.3.2 Identify the four heart valves, their anatomical locations, and their functions.

   _____

   _____

2. L012.3.2 What information must a coder have to correctly report a pacemaker or implantable cardiac defibrillator procedure?

   _____

   _____

3. L012.3.2 Explain when harvesting of vein and artery grafts for a CABG may be reported.

   _____

   _____

12.4 Digestive System

Learning Outcomes

After completing this module, students should be able to:

12.4.1 Identify procedures on the digestive system from the lips to the throat.

12.4.2 Describe procedures on the digestive tract from the esophagus to the anus.

12.4.3 Identify procedures on organ systems attached to the gastrointestinal tract.

12.4.4 Code anesthesia services for procedures in the 40000 series.

Key Terms

Appendix
Backbench work
Colonoscopy
Endoscopic retrograde cholangiopancreatography (ERCP)
Fistula
Gastrointestinal
Intestines
Laparoscopy
Proctectomy

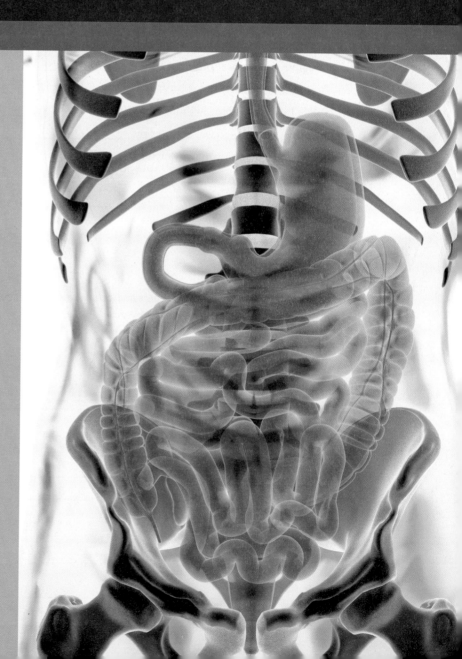

Introduction

The entire 40000 series of CPT codes describes procedures on the digestive system. The digestive system includes the **gastrointestinal** tract, which begins at the lips and continues uninterrupted through irregular tubular structures to the anus. The digestive system also includes additional organ systems and structures attached to these tubular structures.

The CPT codes that describe procedures on the digestive system are divided according the anatomical structures involved. CPT codes within each anatomical division are subdivided according to the type of procedure (e.g., incision, excision, repair, **endoscopy**, and **laparoscopy**).

The anatomical divisions include:

- Lips (40490–40799)
- Vestibule of Mouth (40800–40899)
- Tongue and Floor of Mouth (41000–41599)
- Dentoalveolar Structures (41800–41899)
- Palate and Uvula (42000–42299)
- Salivary Gland and Ducts (42300–42699)
- Pharynx, Adenoids, and Tonsils (42700–42999)
- Esophagus (43020–43499)
- Stomach (43500–43999)
- Intestines (Except Rectum) (44005–44799)
- Meckel's Diverticulum and the Mesentery (44800–44899)
- Appendix (44900–44979)
- Rectum (45000–45999)
- Anus (46020–46999)
- Liver (47000–47399)
- Biliary Tract (47400–47999)
- Pancreas (48000–48999)
- Abdomen, Peritoneum, and Omentum (49000–49999)

12.4.1 Procedures on the Mouth and Throat (40490–42999)

Lips

CPT codes 40490–40799 describe excisions and repairs of the lips. CPT codes in the 40000 series do not describe procedures performed on the skin surrounding the lips. (Those procedures are described by codes in the 10000 series.)

Full-thickness repairs of the lip are described by CPT codes 40650–40654, depending on the extent of the injury or abnormality (vermilion only, less than half the vertical height of the lip, or more than half the vertical height of the lip). Repairs of cleft lip and nasal deformities are described by CPT codes 40700–40761.

> ### CODER'S TIP
>
> CPT codes in this section do not describe reconstruction procedures of the lips except for cleft lip repairs. Other reconstruction procedures are described by CPT codes in the Integumentary section (see the parenthetical notes following CPT codes 40530 and 40761).

Vestibule of Mouth

The vestibule includes the mucosal tissues of the lips and cheeks (i.e., the tissues inside the mouth but outside the teeth and gums). Procedures on these structures include

---

gastrointestinal
The irregular tubular structures beginning at the lips and ending at the anus, including the mouth, pharynx, esophagus, stomach, small intestines and large intestines.

endoscopy
Examination of the interior of an organ or body cavity using an endoscope.

laparoscopy
Examination of the contents of the abdomen using a laparoscope or endoscope.

incisions to drain abscesses or remove foreign bodies; excisions to biopsy suspicious tissues or remove a lesion; and repairs of lacerations within these structures. Instructions following CPT code 40845 direct coders to use other codes (e.g., 15002) to describe skin graft procedures on vestibular structures.

Tongue and Floor of Mouth

Codes 41000–41599 describe procedures on the tongue and tissues behind the dental structures. The incision codes describe both intraoral and extraoral approaches used to drain abscesses, cysts, or hematomas from the tongue or floor of the mouth. Procedures on the tongue, such as excision of lesions or repairs, are differentiated by whether the procedure is performed on the anterior two-thirds or posterior one-third of the tongue. The choice of codes describing resection of the tongue (glossectomy) depends on what part of the tongue is removed and whether other procedures are performed in combination with the glossectomy.

Dentoalveolar Structures

Codes 41800–41899 describe procedures on the tissues surrounding the teeth, including the gums and bony structures in which the teeth are embedded. CPT codes do not describe procedures on the teeth. Procedures on the teeth are described by dental codes instead of the CPT code set. CPT codes 41800–41850 describe incision (drainage or removal of foreign bodies) and excision of soft tissue and surrounding bony structures.

CPT codes 41870–41874 describe other procedures on the dentoalveolar structures, including periodontal mucosal grafting, gingivoplasty, and alveoloplasty. Coders should note that the gingivoplasty and alveoloplasty code descriptors include a designation of "each quadrant" that allows the code to be reported with up to four units if all four quadrants are operated on at the same time. It is more likely, however, that these procedures would involve only one or two quadrants during a single operation.

Palate and Uvula

The palate, or roof of the mouth, extends from behind the front upper teeth backwards to the pharynx. The uvula marks the posterior extension of the palate. Code range 42000–42299 includes a number of codes that describe palatoplasty procedures (cleft palate repair). The correct code to report these procedures depends on the extent of the repair and the specific oral structures involved.

CODER'S TIP

Repair codes in this and several other sections describe lacerations that are over a certain size or that are complex. Simple repairs must be over the size specified to report that code. A complex repair of a laceration of *any* size, however, is described by that CPT code.

Salivary Gland and Ducts

The salivary glands include the parotid, submandibular, and sublingual glands. Some codes in the 42300–42699 range describe procedures performed on any of these glands, whereas others differentiate between procedures on the parotid gland and similar procedures on the other glands. Procedures involving excision of the parotid gland are further defined as to whether the facial nerve, which runs within the parotid gland tissue, is dissected and preserved or is sacrificed with the parotid gland.

Pharynx, Adenoids, and Tonsils

The pharynx is the area of the throat beyond the posterior tongue and palate that extends to the larynx and esophagus. The pharynx connects the mouth and nose to the respiratory tract and alimentary canal. It can be further divided into the oropharynx and the nasopharynx.

The tonsils and adenoids are lymphoid tissues. Tonsils are located at the lateral periphery of the oropharynx. The adenoids are located at the back end of the nasal passages where they join the nasopharynx.

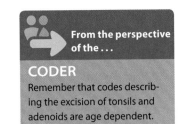

From the perspective of the . . .

CODER
Remember that codes describing the excision of tonsils and adenoids are age dependent.

CODING EXAMPLE

A physician performs a tonsillectomy and adenoidectomy on a five-year-old and forwards the information to his coder. The coder looks up *tonsils* in the index and finds that excision with adenoids is reported with codes 42820–42821. Turning to those codes, he finds that code 42820 describes a tonsillectomy and adenoidectomy in a patient younger than 12 years of age. Code 42821 describes the same procedure in patients 12 years of age or older. The coder reports code 41820.

Several CPT codes describe biopsies of pharyngeal structures, depending on the area of the pharynx from which the biopsy is taken. Tonsillectomy and adenoidectomy procedures are described by codes that describe a tonsillectomy alone, adenoidectomy alone, or a combined procedure where both the tonsils and adenoids are excised. Each of these procedures is further divided depending on the age of the patient (younger than 12 years of age versus age 12 or older).

EXERCISE 12.4.1

Also available in **McGraw Hill connect** plus+

Use the CPT manual and index to select the best code for the following procedures.

1. V-excision of the lip with primary direct linear closure _____
2. Complicated removal of a foreign body embedded in the vestibule of the mouth _____
3. Repair of the tongue over 2.6 cm _____
4. Complex repair of a 1.5 cm laceration of the palate _____
5. Excision of the entire parotid gland with preservation of the facial nerve _____
6. Radical resection of the tonsil and related structures without closure _____

12.4.2 Procedures on the Gastrointestinal Tract from the Esophagus to the Anus (43020–46999)

Esophagus

Codes 43020–43499 describe multiple types of procedures on the esophagus, including incision, excision, endoscopy, and laparoscopy.

Incisions and Excisions Two incision codes describe esophagotomy procedures to remove a foreign body, one designating a cervical and the other a thoracic approach.

The Excision section includes numerous codes describing partial or total esophagec-tomies. The choice of the correct code depends on whether the procedure is performed with a cervical approach or through a thoracotomy and whether a portion of the colon is interspersed between the upper and lower ends of the resected tissue as a replacement for the esophagus. For example, CPT code 43116 (Partial esophagectomy, cervical, with free intestinal graft, including microvascular anastomosis, obtaining the graft and intesti-nal reconstruction) describes an intestinal graft that is not only attached to the proximal and distal ends of the remaining esophagus but also includes microvascular connections of blood vessels. Coders must note the parenthetical remarks following this code.

The first parenthetical note instructs coders not to report add-on code 69990 (Microsurgical techniques, requiring use of operating microscope [List separately in addition to code for primary procedure]) with this code. Add-on code 69990 is not reported with procedures designated as microsurgical in their descriptors. The second parenthetical note instructs coders to add modifier 52 to the code if another surgeon performs the free intestinal or free jejunal graft with microvascular anastomosis. The third parenthetical note directs coders to use CPT code 43496 to report a free jejunal graft with microvascular anastomosis performed by another physician.

CODER'S TIP

It is important for coders to not only review the CPT code descriptors, but also to review all associated guidance and parenthetical notes. These instructions provide essential information regarding when codes can or cannot be reported and what conditions require that modifiers be attached to a code.

Endoscopy The Endoscopy subsection includes several large families of codes. One describes endoscopy procedures of the esophagus (esophagoscopy). A second family of codes describes upper gastrointestinal endoscopy, which includes the stom-ach, duodenum, and/or jejunum in addition to the esophagus.

The first code in each family (43200 and 43235) describes diagnostic endoscopy alone. These are followed by a number of codes describing different surgical endos-copy procedures. Coders should report the CPT code that most closely describes the surgical procedure performed. When a surgical endoscopy code is reported, the diag-nostic endoscopy is included and therefore is not reported separately.

A third family of codes describes diagnostic and surgical **endoscopic retrograde cholangiopancreatography (ERCP)** procedures. A diagnostic ERCP (CPT code 43260) involves the insertion of a catheter through the ampulla of Vater to inject con-trast material for x-ray or other imaging examination of the hepatobiliary system, in-cluding the pancreatic ducts, hepatic ducts, common bile duct, and gallbladder (if not previously removed). This code is followed by a number of surgical procedures on these structures. The surgical ERCP procedures include diagnostic ERCP. One add-on code (43273) is reported when an endoscope, rather than a catheter, is passed through the ampulla of Vater to allow direct visualization of hepatobiliary structures.

Laparoscopy Unlike the endoscopy codes, this group of codes only describes surgi-cal laparoscopic procedures on the esophagus and the top of the stomach (fundus) where the esophagus attaches. Surgical laparoscopy always includes diagnostic laparoscopy. Diagnostic laparoscopy is reported with CPT code 49320 (Laparoscopy, abdomen, perito-neum, and omentum, diagnostic, with or without collection of specimen[s] by brushing or washing) according to the instructional notes at the beginning of this section.

Repair This series of codes describes esophageal repair procedures, including esophagoplasty, esophagogastrostomy, esophagogastric fundoplasty, and esophagotomies combined with other surgical procedures. To choose the correct code to describe a procedure, coders must understand the structures involved.

endoscopic retrograde cholangiopancreatography (ERCP)
A procedure that uses a combi-nation of x-rays and an endo-scope to diagnose disorders of the liver, gallbladder, bile ducts, and pancreas; also used to sur-gically correct such disorders.

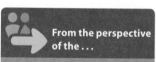

From the perspective of the . . .

CODER

Every code within the endos-copy range is designated with the bull's-eye sign and listed in Appendix G, which indicates that conscious sedation is an inherent part of these procedures and is not reported separately when provided by the same physician who is performing the endoscopic procedure. If another provider administers sedation during the procedure, that provider may report the service.

Stomach

Codes 43500–43999 describe various procedures on the stomach.

Incision and Excision The incision codes (43500–43520) describe several procedures performed through a gastrostomy incision, including removal of foreign bodies, repair of bleeding ulcers, or repair of a preexisting esophagogastric laceration, also known as a Mallory-Weiss tear.

Excision codes (43605–43641) describe open and closed biopsy procedures, excision of ulcers or benign lesions, and total and partial gastrectomy procedures with various methods of reconnecting the remaining portions of the digestive tract.

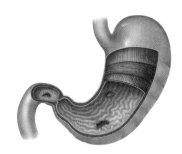

Repairs of bleeding stomach ulcers are included in the procedures reported by codes 43500–43520.

Laparoscopy Laparoscopic procedures (43644–43659) on the stomach include bypass procedures, implantation of gastric neurostimulator electrodes, transection of the vagus nerves for the treatment of ulcers, and bariatric procedures to treat morbid obesity.

Introduction This section of codes (43752–43761) describes procedures that involve gastric or duodenal intubation, which generally must be done by a skilled physician. Code selection depends on where the tube is placed and how it is used.

Bariatric Surgery A variety of bariatric procedures may be performed as open procedures or through a laparoscope. Band devices may be implanted and adjusted to control the size of the stomach. Alternatively, the stomach can be permanently stapled to reduce the amount of food it can hold. Some procedures involve permanent anatomical bypasses of the intestines. Coders must be aware of the specific procedure to report the correct code.

Intestines (Except Rectum)

Codes 44005–44799 describe procedures on the **intestines.** This includes the small intestine, which begins at the duodenum and extends through the jejunum and ileum, ending at the ileocecal junction. The large intestine includes the ascending colon, transverse colon, descending colon, sigmoid colon, and rectum, ending at the anus. Procedures on the rectum and anus are included in separate sections of codes.

intestines
The digestive tubes from the stomach to the anus.

Incision and Excision The incision codes (44005–44055) include codes describing the exploration of each separate anatomical division of the small and large intestines. These procedures are commonly used for biopsies or removal of foreign bodies from inside the intestines. CPT code 44005 (Enterolysis [freeing of intestinal adhesion]) does not involve opening the intestines; rather, it involves incising adhesions attached to the outside surface of the intestines. A parenthetical comment directs the use of code 44180 if enterolysis is performed through a laparoscopic approach.

The excision codes (44100–44160) describe a number of procedures on the intestines, including biopsies; resection of a portion of the intestine with anastomosis of remaining structures; resection of the intestines with the formation of an ileostomy, cecostomy, or colostomy; and transplanting intestines from either a cadaver or living donor.

CODER'S TIP

Some procedures described by the codes in this section may include the rectum, but these codes do not describe procedures performed primarily on the rectum. For example, CPT code 44155 (Colectomy, total, abdominal, with proctectomy; with ileostomy) describes a procedure involving multiple structures, including the rectum. Procedures performed primarily on the rectum are included in a separate section of codes.

Laparoscopy This family of codes (44180–44238) describes a variety of procedures performed through a laparoscope. CPT code 44180 (Laparoscopy, surgical, enterolysis [freeing of intestinal adhesion]) is the companion code to CPT code 44005, which describes open surgical enterolysis. Several codes describe the creation of an enterostomy, where the intestinal structures remain continuous but an opening is created through the skin for feeding, decompression, or evacuation.

Codes in this section also describe partial and total enterectomies/colectomies performed through a laparoscope. Some of these codes describe resections of part of the intestines with an anastomosis, while others describe resections with the formation of an enterostomy or colostomy. The selection of the proper code to describe these procedures depends on the details of the actual surgical procedure.

Enterostomy—External Fistulization of Intestines These codes describe open procedures to create enterostomies, including ileostomies, cecostomies, and colostomies. Coders must pay particular attention to the parenthetical remarks that give instructions regarding codes that cannot be reported with the codes in this section.

Endoscopy, Small Intestine and Stomal These codes describe diagnostic and surgical endoscopy of the small intestine. Surgical endoscopy always includes diagnostic endoscopy. These codes are organized into several groups of codes describing similar procedures. One group (44360–44373) describes endoscopy beyond the second portion of the duodenum but not including the ileum. Another group (44376–44379) describes endoscopic procedures that include the ileum.

A third group of codes (44380–44397) describes diagnostic and surgical ileoscopy and **colonoscopy** procedures through an existing stoma (an opening through the skin into the intestine). These codes are not used to report colonoscopies performed through the rectum. A separate group of codes describes those procedures.

Repair Codes in this section (44602–44680) describe repairs of intestinal structures that are performed to correct a perforation, including those caused by an ulcer, diverticulum, wound, or rupture of the intestine. Separate codes describe repairs of the small and large intestine.

These codes also describe closures of enterostomies, intestinal cutaneous **fistulas**, enteroenteric or enterocolic fistulas, and enterovesical fistulas. Several parenthetical remarks follow the codes describing closure of different types of fistulas direct coders to other sections to report closures of renocolic, gastrocolic, and rectovesical fistulas. As always, coders must review the entire code range to be sure there are no parenthetical remarks that are relevant to the procedure they are reporting.

Meckel's Diverticulum and the Mesentery; Appendix

A relatively small number of codes describe excision of a Meckel's diverticulum and other mesentery lesions.

Abscesses of the **appendix** may be drained through open or percutaneous procedures. Open drainage is reported with CPT code 44900 (Incision and drainage of appendiceal abscess; open), whereas percutaneous drainage is reported with CPT code 44901 (Incision and drainage of appendiceal abscess; percutaneous). According to the parenthetical remark that follows the percutaneous code, providers also may report CPT code 75989 for radiological supervision and interpretation when the physician performing the percutaneous procedure uses radiological guidance such as fluoroscopy, ultrasound, or CT as part of the percutaneous drainage procedure.

CPT code 44950 (Appendectomy) describes an open procedure, while CPT code 44970 (Laparoscopy, surgical, appendectomy) is used to report a laparoscopic appendectomy.

A surgeon is performing an excision of the descending and sigmoid colon. He inspects the entire small and large intestine during the procedure, notices that the appendix is slightly inflamed and swollen, and performs an appendectomy due to early appendicitis. How should the coder report this appendectomy procedure?

The coder looks up *appendix* in the index, where she finds excision codes listed in the 44950–44960 range. She then turns to these codes to determine which is the most appropriate for this situation. Code 44950 (Appendectomy) describes an open procedure. Add-on code 44955 describes an appendectomy done for an indicated purpose at the time of another major procedure. Because the surgeon performed the appendectomy while excising a major part of the colon, the coder reports add-on code 44955 to describe the appendectomy.

Rectum

Procedures on the rectum are described by codes 45000–45999.

Incision, Excision, and Destruction Three codes (45000–45020) describe the incision and drainage of rectal abscesses or pelvic abscesses through the rectum, depending on the location of the abscess. Excision codes (45100–45172) describe **proctectomy** procedures with and without an anastomosis, excision of rectal tumors, pelvic exenteration for colorectal tumors, and excision of rectal strictures. Several codes differ from one another based on the approach to the rectal tumor, including transsacral, transcoccygeal, or transanal. CPT code 45190 describes destruction of rectal tumors by a number of techniques through an anal approach.

proctectomy
Surgical resection of the rectum.

Endoscopy Endoscopic procedures of the large intestine are divided into three broad categories. Proctosigmoidoscopy includes endoscopic examination of the rectum and sigmoid colon. Sigmoidoscopy includes the rectum and entire sigmoid colon and may include a portion of the descending colon. Colonoscopy includes the entire colon from the rectum to the cecum and may include a portion of the distal ileum.

Each of the three families of endoscopy codes begins with a code describing diagnostic endoscopy (CPT codes 45300, 45330, and 45378) followed by a number of surgical endoscopy procedures. Each of the endoscopy codes includes conscious sedation when provided by the same practitioner performing the underlying endoscopy service.

Laparoscopy Several procedures may be performed on the rectum through a laparoscope. CPT codes 45395 and 45397 describe laparoscopic proctectomy with colostomy or anastomosis, respectively. CPT codes 45400 and 45402 describe proctopexies for rectal prolapse, either without or with sigmoid resection.

Repair Rectal repair codes describe proctoplasties, proctoplexies through several different approaches, and rectocele repairs. These codes also describe procedures to close several specific fistulas, including rectovesical and rectourethral fistulas.

Anus

Guidance at the beginning of code range 46020–46999 instructs coders on which codes to use for certain procedures, including incision of thrombosed external hemorrhoids, ligation of internal hemorrhoids, excision of internal or external hemorrhoids, and other specific methods used to treat hemorrhoids.

Incision codes (46020–46083) describe various abscess drainage procedures. These codes also describe the placement and removal of a seton, a special suture used to close anal fistulas. Excision codes (46200–46288) describe various hemorrhoidectomy procedures. These codes differ from one another by treatment method and the number of hemorrhoid groups treated. It is important for coders to note that several of these codes are out of numerical order so that codes describing similar procedures can be grouped together in the CPT manual. The excision codes also describe the treatment of anal fissures and fistulas.

The endoscopy codes (46600–46615) describe diagnostic and surgical anoscopy procedures. Surgical anoscopy includes biopsies, removal of foreign bodies, removal of tumors by various techniques, and control of bleeding. Surgical anoscopy procedures always include diagnostic anoscopy.

The repair codes (46700–46947) describe anoplasty procedures; repair of anal fistulas, imperforate anus, and cloacal anomalies; and sphincteroplasties for incontinence. The destruction codes (46900–46942) also describe methods to destroy anal lesions, including electrodessication, cryosurgery, laser surgery, and surgical excision.

CODER'S TIP

Several codes describing anal repair procedures include parenthetical comments stating that these codes are not reported with modifier 63, which identifies procedures performed on infants weighing less than 4 kg. These procedures are most commonly performed on infants, and no special identification of this is necessary.

A complete list of procedures that should not be reported with modifier 63 can be found in Appendix F of the CPT manual.

EXERCISE 12.4.2

Also available in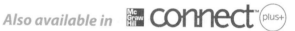

Use the CPT manual and index to select the best code for the following procedures.

1. Diagnostic upper gastrointestinal endoscopy including collection of specimens _____

2. ERCP _____

3. Gastric bypass for morbid obesity _____

4. Open partial colectomy _____

5. Laparoscopic appendectomy _____

6. Partial-thickness excision of a rectal tumor using a transanal approach _____

12.4.3 Procedures on Organs Connected to the Digestive Tract (47000–49999)

Liver

The incision codes (47000–47015) describe percutaneous needle biopsy procedures and drainage of hepatic abscesses by open or percutaneous approaches. Excision codes (47100–47130) describe wedge biopsy procedures and various liver resections.

Liver transplantation codes (47133–47147) describe harvesting donor organs from cadaveric and living donors. Because living donors only have a portion of their livers removed for transplant, several different codes describe the portion of the liver removed, including whether the right or left lobe was donated.

Repair codes (47300–47362) describe management of hepatic wounds and bleeding. The laparoscopic codes describe surgical ablation of hepatic tumors by radiofrequency and cryosurgery. Other codes describe open ablation of hepatic tumors by radiofrequency and cryosurgery.

Codes in the Laparoscopy section (47370–47379) describe laparoscopic ablation of hepatic lesions. Codes in the Other Procedures section (47380–47399) describe open ablation procedures of hepatic tumors.

Biliary Tract

The biliary tract includes the gallbladder, cystic duct, common bile duct, and extrahepatic portion of the hepatic duct. Abdominal surgical procedures commonly involve these structures.

Incision procedures (47400–47480) involve opening one or more of the biliary tract structures for drainage or to remove calculi (stones) from within the biliary tract. Introduction procedures (47490–47530) include placement of a needle, catheter, or tube into the biliary tract for drainage or to inject contrast material for cholangiography.

Endoscopy codes (47550–47556) in this section describe intraoperative endoscopy or percutaneous endoscopy through a tube or other tract into the biliary structures. Endoscopy procedures or ERCPs performed through an endoscope inserted through the esophagus are reported with the endoscopy codes from the Esophagus section of codes. Several codes (47560–47579) describe laparoscopy procedures, including cholecystectomy and commonly associated procedures such as cholangiography or exploration of the common bile duct.

The excision codes (47600–47715) describe open procedures on the biliary tract, including cholecystectomy with or without associated procedures such as cholangiography or exploration of the common bile duct; removal of stones from the biliary tract; and excision of cysts or biliary tumors. Repair codes (47720–47900) describe reconstructive procedures of the biliary ducts and anastomoses involving the biliary and hepatic ducts and the gastrointestinal tract.

Pancreas

Pancreatic procedures described by the incision codes (48000–48020) are usually performed to drain abscesses or remove stones from the pancreas. Excision procedure codes (48100–48160) describe biopsies, debridement of pancreatic tissues, excision of pancreatic cysts, and partial and total pancreatectomies with various anastomoses to reconnect the remaining structures. Repair codes (48500–48548) describe procedures designed to reconnect pancreatic structures to various gastrointestinal structures.

The pancreatic transplant codes (48550–48556) describe three distinct phases of transplants: harvesting of the donor organ, **backbench work** to prepare the donor organ, and implantation of the organ into the recipient.

backbench work
Work done to prepare a donor organ for transplantation.

Abdomen, Peritoneum, and Omentum

Code range 49000–49999 describes procedures within the abdominal cavity, including the peritoneum and omentum. Coders should review the anatomy of the abdomen. It is important to understand which organs are within the peritoneum (intraperitoneal) and which are outside the peritoneum (extraperitoneal or retroperitoneal).

Incision procedures (49000–49084) include exploratory laparotomy (exploration of intraperitoneal organs and structures), exploration of retroperitoneal structures, and drainage of intraperitoneal and retroperitoneal abscesses. These abdominal exploratory procedures include biopsies of structures within these areas.

Several codes (49203–49205) describe the excision or destruction of one or more intra-abdominal tumors, cysts, or endometrial masses. The size of the largest tumor determines which code is selected to describe the procedure. A separate code describes a staging laparotomy for Hodgkin's disease or lymphoma (49220). This staging

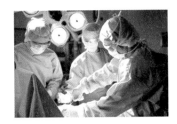

Pancreatic transplant codes differentiate between the three phases of transplants: organ harvesting, organ preparation, and organ implantation.

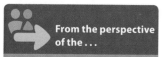

From the perspective of the . . .

CODER

When multiple intra-abdominal tumors, cysts, or endometrial masses are excised or destroyed, the size of the largest tumor determines which code is reported. Code 49203 is used when the largest tumor is 5 cm or less in diameter, code 49204 is reported when the largest tumor is 5.1 to 10.0 cm in diameter, and code 49204 is reported when the largest tumor is greater than 10.0 cm.

procedure includes a splenectomy and biopsies of both lobes of the liver. This procedure may include biopsies or excisions of one or more abdominal lymph nodes, bone marrow biopsy, and possibly repositioning the ovaries in women undergoing the procedure. Code 49255 describes excision of the omentum.

The laparoscopy codes describing abdominal procedures are located within two separate code sections. CPT codes 49320–49329 describe intra-abdominal diagnostic or surgical laparoscopies such as aspiration of cysts, biopsies, or placement of intra-peritoneal catheters. CPT codes 49650–49659 describe laparoscopic procedures on the abdominal wall to repair various hernias.

CPT codes 49400–49465 describe placement of various cannulas, tubes, shunts, or devices for radiation therapy. These codes also describe the percutaneous placement or replacement of tubes in the stomach, small intestine, or large intestine. CPT code 49446 describes the percutaneous conversion of a gastrostomy tube to a gastrojejunostomy tube. If this conversion is performed at the time of the initial gastrostomy tube placement, coders should report both 49446 and 49440.

CODER'S TIP

Guidance in the CPT manual instructs coders that if one tube is removed and another tube is placed through a separate incision, this is not coded as a replacement but as the placement of a new tube. Percutaneous placement and replacement procedures include fluoroscopic guidance, the injection of contrast material, and a report of the imaging procedure. No separate code is reported for the imaging procedure.

Hernia repairs are described by CPT codes 49491–49659. These codes differ from one another by the type of hernia (inguinal, femoral, incisional, or ventral); age of the patient; whether the hernia is reducible or incarcerated; whether it is a primary hernia repair or a recurrent hernia repair; and whether the hernia repair is an open or laparoscopic procedure. Coders must determine which CPT code best describes the procedure by considering all of these factors.

CODING EXAMPLE

A surgeon repairs an initial inguinal hernia that is reducible in a four-year-old child. The coder reviews the codes that describe inguinal hernia repairs and finds two codes that describe this procedure in a patient this age. Code 49500 describes the repair of an initial inguinal hernia that is reducible in patients from six months to five years of age. Code 49501 describes the same procedure when the hernia is incarcerated. The coder reports this procedure with CPT code 49501.

EXERCISE 12.4.3

Also available in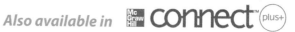

Use the CPT manual and index to select the best code for the following procedures.

1. Wedge biopsy of the liver _____

2. Open cholecystectomy _____

3. Excision of pancreatic lesions _____

4. Exploration of the retroperitoneal area with biopsies _____

5. Laparoscopic insertion of a tunneled intraperitoneal dialysis catheter _____

6. Repair of a reducible inguinal hernia in a four-year-old boy _____

12.4.4 Anesthesia for Procedures Included in the 40000 Series of CPT Codes

Anesthesia codes for procedures on the gastrointestinal (GI) tract and associated organs are categorized according to the anatomical location of the portion of the GI tract on which the procedure is performed. The GI tract extends from the head, through the neck and thorax, and into the abdominal cavity before ending at the anus.

Codes for anesthesia for these procedures are listed in several anatomical locations, including the head, neck, intrathorax, upper abdomen, lower abdomen, and perineum. The most commonly reported CPT codes to report anesthesia for procedures located in the 40000 series of codes are shown in Table 12.4.1.

CODING EXAMPLE

An anesthesiologist performs a general anesthetic for a laparoscopic cholecystectomy. The coder reviews the anesthesia codes to determine which code describes this anesthesia procedure. CPT code 00790 (Anesthesia for intraperitoneal procedures in upper abdomen including laparoscopy; not otherwise specified) is the most appropriate code to report this anesthesia service.

CODER'S TIP

The descriptor for CPT code 00500 (Anesthesia for all procedures on the esophagus) may be confusing. This code is in the Intrathoracic section of anesthesia codes. It is used to describe anesthesia for all open procedures on the portion of the esophagus within the thoracic cavity. This code does not describe anesthesia for open procedures on the portions of the esophagus outside the thorax. Instead, CPT code 00320 (Anesthesia for procedures on the esophagus, thyroid, larynx, trachea and lymphatic system of the neck) is used to describe open procedures on the portion of the esophagus in the neck. CPT code 00790 (Anesthesia for intraperitoneal procedures in upper abdomen including laparoscopy; not otherwise specified) describes anesthesia for surgical procedures on the portion of the esophagus within the abdominal cavity between the diaphragm and the stomach. CPT code 00320 describes anesthesia for all closed procedures on the esophagus.

EXERCISE 12.4.4

Also available in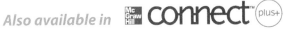

Use the CPT manual and index to select the code that describes anesthesia for each of the following procedures.

1. Tonsillectomy and adenoidectomy, younger than 12 years of age _____
2. Esophagotomy, cervical approach, with removal of foreign body _____
3. Esophagotomy, thoracic approach, with removal of foreign body _____
4. Cholecystectomy _____
5. Laparoscopy with aspiration of an ovarian cyst _____
6. Hepatectomy, partial lobectomy _____

TABLE 12.4.1 Anesthesia for Common Procedures on the Digestive System

Code	Related Procedures
00100	Anesthesia for procedures on salivary glands
00102	Anesthesia for procedures involving plastic repair of cleft lip
00170	Anesthesia for intraoral procedures
00172	Anesthesia for repair of cleft palate
00174	Anesthesia for excision of retropharyngeal tumor
00176	Anesthesia for intraoral radical surgery
00300	Anesthesia for procedures on the integumentary system of the head
00320	Anesthesia for procedures on the esophagus
00500	Anesthesia for open procedures of the esophagus
00700–00797	Anesthesia for procedures of the upper abdomen
00800–00848	Anesthesia for procedures of the lower abdomen
00902	Anesthesia for anorectal procedures
00904	Anesthesia for radical perineal procedures

Summary

Learning Outcome	Key Concepts/Examples
12.4.1 Identify procedures on the digestive system from the lips to the throat. **Pages 367–369**	The initial portion of the gastrointestinal tract is contained primarily within the head. It consists of the lips, vestibule of the mouth, tongue, floor of the mouth, dentoalveolar structures, palate, uvula, salivary glands and ducts, pharynx, adenoids, and tonsils. Procedures on these structures include incisions, excisions, and repairs.
12.4.2 Describe procedures on the digestive tract from the esophagus to the anus. **Pages 369–374**	The remainder of the gastrointestinal tract runs through the interior of the neck, thorax, and abdomen before ending at the anus. The anatomical structures consist of the esophagus, stomach, intestines, rectum, and anus. The intestines include the three portions of the small intestines (duodenum, jejunum, ileum) and the large intestines (cecum, appendix, ascending colon, transverse colon, descending colon, and rectum). Procedures on these anatomical structures include incision, excision, endoscopy, laparoscopy, repair, destruction, and transplantation for several organs.
12.4.3 Identify procedures on organ systems attached to the gastrointestinal tract. **Pages 374–376**	The organ systems that connect with the gastrointestinal tract include the liver, biliary tract, and pancreas. Procedures on each of these structures include some but not necessarily all of the following: incision, excision, endoscopy, laparoscopy, repair, and transplantation. In addition, the abdomen contains the peritoneum and omentum. Procedures on these structures include incision, excision, laparoscopy, and repair, including hernia repairs.
12.4.4 Code anesthesia services for procedures in the 40000 series. **Pages 376–378**	Codes describing anesthesia services for procedures on the digestive system come from several sections of anesthesia codes. The choice of the correct anesthesia code depends on the anatomical structure on which surgery is performed and, in some situations, the specific surgical procedure.

Using Terminology

Match the key terms with their definitions.

_____ **1.** LO12.4.2 Laparoscopy

_____ **2.** LO12.4.3 Backbench work

_____ **3.** LO12.4.2 Colonoscopy

_____ **4.** LO12.4.2 Endoscopic retrograde cholangiopancreatography (ERCP)

_____ **5.** LO12.4.2 Gastrointestinal

_____ **6.** LO12.4.2 Fistula

_____ **7.** LO12.4.2 Intestines

_____ **8.** LO12.4.2 Appendix

_____ **9.** LO12.4.2 Proctectomy

A. Visualization of the colon through a scope

B. Work done to prepare the donor organ for transplantation

C. Surgical resection of the rectum

D. Duodenum, jejunum, ileum, and all segments of the colon

E. Visualization of the abdominal cavity through a scope

F. A procedure that uses a combination of x-rays and an endoscope to diagnose disorders of the liver, gallbladder, bile ducts, and pancreas

G. Narrow, tubelike appendage of the colon

H. An abnormal opening between an organ and the body surface or another organ

I. Relating to the stomach and intestines

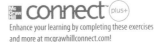

Enhance your learning by completing these exercises and more at mcgrawhillconnect.com!

MODULE 12.4 | **DIGESTIVE SYSTEM**   379

Checking Your Understanding

Select the letter that best completes the statement or answers the question.

1. L012.4.1 CPT codes in the 40490-40799 series describe excisions and repairs of the lip tissue. Procedures performed on the skin surrounding the lips are described in what series of codes?

   a. 30000   **c.** 20000
   b. 10000   **d.** 40000

2. L012.4.1 A repair of a 1.5 cm laceration of the posterior one-third of the tongue would be reported with code:

   a. 41250
   b. 41251
   c. 41252
   d. 12011

3. L012.4.1 Code 41010 (frenotomy) describes what type of procedure?

   a. Excision
   b. Suturing
   c. Incision
   d. Repair

4. L012.4.1 Procedures on teeth and not the tissues surrounding the teeth are coded using which coding resource?

   a. CPT
   b. Dental codes instead of CPT codes
   c. ICD-9
   d. CPT and HCPCS Level II D-codes

5. L012.4.1 The salivary glands include the following:

   a. Parotid
   b. Submandibular glands
   c. Sublingual glands
   d. All of the above

6. L012.4.2 Partial esophagectomy, cervical, with free intestinal graft, including microvascular anastomosis, obtaining the graft and intestinal reconstruction using an operating microscope would be coded with which CPT code(s)?

   a. 43116-52
   b. 43116, 69990
   c. 43116
   d. 43116, 43496

7. L012.4.2 Codes 43752–43761 describe procedures involving gastric or duodenal intubation. Which is true about this range of codes?

   a. They generally require the skill of a physician to place the tube.
   b. Code selection can depend on where the tube is placed.
   c. Code selection can depend on how the tube is used.
   d. All of these statements are true.

8. L012.4.2 The large intestine includes the
   a. Duodenum and jejunum.
   b. Ascending colon, transverse colon, descending colon, sigmoid colon, and rectum.
   c. Anus.
   d. Duodenum, jejunum, ileum, and ascending colon.

9. L012.4.2 Percutaneous placement and replacement gastrointestinal tube codes include which of the following procedures that cannot be coded separately?
   a. Fluoroscopic guidance
   b. Injection of contrast material
   c. Report of imaging procedure
   d. All of the above

10. L012.4.3 What would be the appropriate CPT code for an initial open repair of a strangulated ventral hernia in a 35-year-old patient?
    a. 49560
    b. 49561
    c. 49654
    d. 49565

Applying Your Skills

Use the CPT manual to determine the correct code to report the following procedures.

1. L012.4.3 Repair of an abscess of the liver _____

2. L012.4.1 Incision and drainage of an abscess; peritonsillar _____

3. L012.4.2 Incision of the anal sphincter _____

4. L012.4.2 Laparoscopy, surgical, gastric restrictive procedure; with gastric bypass and small intestine reconstruction _____

5. L012.4.2 Destruction of a tumor in the rectum _____

6. L012.4.2 Excision of a tumor in the stomach _____

7. L012.4.1 Laser surgery of a lesion in the mouth _____

8. L012.4.1 A needle biopsy of the salivary gland _____

9. L012.4.1 Placement of an orogastric tube _____

10. L012.4.3 Reconstruction of the anastomosis in the bile duct _____

11. L012.4.2 Stent enteroscopy _____

12. L012.4.2 Incision and removal of a foreign body in the stomach _____

13. L012.4.1 Suture of a throat wound _____

14. L012.4.3 Laparoscopy with drainage of lymphocele to peritoneal cavity _____

15. L012.4.2 Proctectomy, partial, without anastomosis, perineal approach _____

Mc Graw Hill **connect** (plus+)

Enhance your learning by completing these exercises and more at mcgrawhillconnect.com!

MODULE 12.4 | DIGESTIVE SYSTEM   381

Thinking It Through

Use your critical-thinking skills to answer the questions below.

1. L012.4.4 Using the CPT guidelines, explain the information a coder would need to assign the appropriate code(s) for hernia repair.

   _____

   _____

2. L012.4.1 List three of the anatomical structures that make up the digestive system. What are the main functions of these structures? What are some procedures that are performed on these structures?

   _____

   _____

3. LO 12.4.4 Describe the three distinct phases of a liver transplant.

   _____

   _____

Urinary System, Male and Female Genital Systems, and Maternity Care and Delivery

Learning Outcomes

After completing this module, students should be able to:

12.5.1 Report codes for procedures on the urinary system.

12.5.2 Describe codes for procedures on the male genital system.

12.5.3 Describe codes for procedures on the female genital system.

12.5.4 Explain codes used to report maternity care services.

12.5.5 Select anesthesia codes for procedures in the 50000 series.

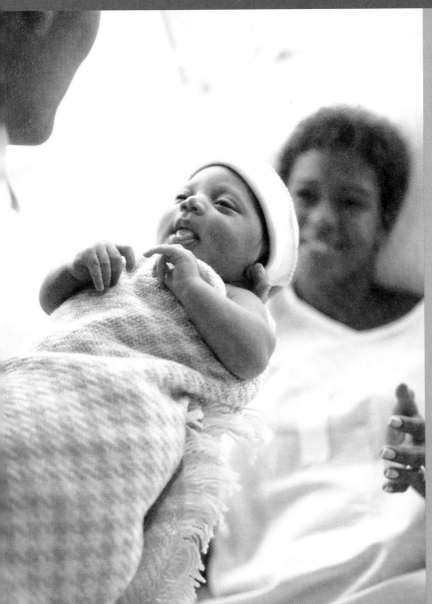

Key Terms

Allotransplantation
Antepartum care
Bartholin's gland
Bladder
Cervix
Cesarean section
Colposcopy
Cystocele
Endometrium
Enterocele
Epididymus
Epispadius
Hypospadius
Kidney
Myometrium
Orchiopexy

Postpartum care
Prostate
Rectocele
Renal calculus
Seminal vesicles
Testis or testicle
Tunica vaginalis
Ureter
Urethra
Vagina
Vaginal delivery
Vas deferens (spermatic cord)
VBAC procedure
Vulva

Introduction

The 50000 code series describes procedures on the urinary system and both male and female genitalia, as well as maternity services. As with other organ systems, it is imperative that coders understand the anatomical structures described by these codes. The urinary system consists of the **kidneys, ureters, bladder,** and **urethra.** With the exception of the urethra and structures surrounding it, the anatomical relationships between these structures are essentially the same in males and females. The major differences in male and female urinary system anatomy involve the urethra and surrounding structures between the outlet of the bladder and the meatus.

12.5.1 Procedures on the Urinary System (50010–53899)

Codes in the 50000 series describing procedures on the urinary system are organized into sections according to the anatomical structures involved—the kidneys, ureters, bladder, and urethra. Each section is divided by the type of procedure, including incisions, excisions, introductions, repairs, laparoscopies, and endoscopies. Guidelines in some sections provide specific instructions regarding how the codes are to be reported.

Kidney

Incision procedures on the kidney (50010–50135) include renal exploration, drainage of a renal abscess, removal of a **renal calculus** (kidney stone), and placement of a nephrostomy tube. Separate codes describe open versus percutaneous procedures. Coders must identify whether the procedure was performed through an open or percutaneous approach to determine the correct code to report the services.

Excision procedures (50200–50290) describe biopsy, partial or total nephrectomy, radical nephrectomy, renal mass ablation, and excision of renal cysts. Several different codes describe nephrectomy procedures. These differ from one another based on whether the surgeon performed other procedures in addition to the nephrectomy.

Codes describing procedures associated with kidney transplants include living or cadaver donor nephrectomy (50300–50320), backbench work on donor organs (50323–50329), and organ transplantation (50360–50380).

> ## CODER'S TIP
>
> A kidney transplant may include nephrectomy of one or both recipient kidneys. An associated nephrectomy is included in the description of CPT code 50365 (Renal **allotransplantation,** implantation of graft; with recipient nephrectomy). The nephrectomy is not reported separately. However, if a nephrectomy is performed at some other time on a transplant recipient, that procedure is described with CPT code 50340 (Recipient nephrectomy [separate procedure]).

The codes included in the Introduction section describe the removal and the removal and replacement of indwelling ureteral stents via percutaneous and transurethral approaches. Other codes describe the removal and the removal and replacement of externally accessible ureteral stents.

> ## CODER'S TIP
>
> Most of the codes in the Introduction section describe removal of an existing ureteral stent. One code in this section (50393) describes the percutaneous placement of a
>
> *(Continued)*

---

kidney
Organ of excretion that produces urine and helps regulate certain chemicals in the blood.

ureter
Tube that connects the kidney to the urinary bladder.

bladder
Hollow sac that holds fluid (e.g., urine or bile).

urethra
Canal leading from the bladder to outside the body.

renal calculus
Kidney stone.

allotransplantation
Implantation of a graft or tissue from one person to another.

CPT codes 50541–50580 describe various laparoscopic and endoscopic procedures on the kidney. Laparoscopy procedures include ablation of renal cysts, partial and total nephrectomies, radical nephrectomies, and donor nephrectomies for transplantation. Endoscopic procedures may be performed through an existing or new opening (nephrostomy or pyelostomy). Separate codes differentiate between these procedures.

Ureter

Incision codes (50600–50630) describe opening the ureter for drainage, placement of ureteral stents, or removal of stones from different sections of the ureter (upper third, middle third, and lower third). Only two excision codes (50650 and 50660) describe the removal of the ureter, but numerous codes (50700–50940) describe repair procedures involving the ureter.

One reason so many codes are necessary to describe ureteral repair procedures is that numerous repair procedures might be performed, depending on the underlying reason for the repair. Ureteral repairs may involve only the ureter itself; reattachment of the ureter to the bladder or other abdominal organs; creation of a replacement bladder when the original bladder is removed (including attaching the ureters to the replacement structure); or bringing the ureter through the skin to drain into an external urinary bag.

Ureteral procedures may be performed with the use of a laparoscope (50945–50949) or an endoscope (50951–50980). Laparoscopic procedures include removal of ureteral stones and placement of ureteral stents. Similar to renal endoscopic procedures, ureteral endoscopic procedures may be performed through an existing or newly established ureterotomy.

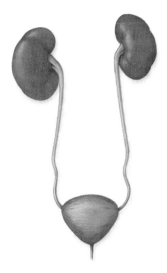

Many different codes are used to report ureteral repair procedures. This is because there are separate underlying causes for each type of repair.

Bladder

Incision codes (51020–51080) describe opening the bladder to destroy tumors, drain bladder contents, remove urinary stones from the bladder, or insert a ureteral stent. Removal codes (51100–51102) describe draining the bladder or placing a suprapubic catheter. Excision codes (51500–51597) describe partial or total removal of the bladder with reattachment or reimplantation of ureters into other structures. Some codes within this range describe these procedures combined with pelvic lymph node dissections. The last code in this section (51597) describes a complete pelvic exenteration for tumors arising from the lower urinary tract, including the bladder, prostate, and urethra.

The codes in the Introduction section (51600–51720) describe injections for cystography or urethrocystography, bladder irrigation, instillation of anticancer agents, straight catheterization for one-time drainage of the bladder, and placement of a temporary indwelling catheter.

CPT codes 51725–51798 describe urodynamic measurement procedures. These procedures may be performed individually or in various combinations. Like radiology codes, these codes include both professional and technical components. To use the global code to report the service, the physician must provide all the equipment necessary to perform the procedure. If the physician only interprets the results of the test, modifier 26 is added to the code to report only the professional services. Examples of these measurements include cystometrograms, voiding pressure studies, uroflowmetry, electromyography (EMG), evoked response measurements, and ultrasonic measurement of postvoiding residual urine and/or bladder volume.

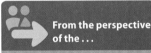

From the perspective of the . . .

CODER

In order to select the correct CPT code to report a procedure, it is sometimes necessary to know the diagnosis or the reason the procedure was done. For example, CPT code 51597 describes pelvic exenteration for urinary tract tumors, but a parenthetical note following this code instructs coders to use code 58240 if the reason for the surgery is a gynecological tumor.

CODER'S TIP

One add-on code (51797) is included in the Urodynamics section. This code is used in combination with CPT codes 51727 and 51728 to identify those instances when the voiding pressure studies described by those codes are performed with intra-abdominal pressure measurements using rectal, gastric, or intraperitoneal pressure devices.

Repair codes (51800–51980) describe various procedures on the bladder, including cystoplasties (repairs of the bladder); cystourethroplasty (repair of the bladder and bladder neck); suspension of the bladder to repair urinary incontinence; and repair of various fistulas, including vesicovaginal and vesicouterine fistulas.

CODER'S TIP

Parenthetical remarks in the Repair section provide instructions that repairs of fistulas between the bladder and intestinal structures (e.g., vesicoenteric and rectovesical fistulas) are reported with codes from the 40000 series. It is important for coders to understand how to use the index to locate the appropriate section of codes to describe these procedures.

CPT codes 51990 and 51992 describe laparoscopic procedures for the treatment of urinary stress incontinence. Cystoscopy and cystourethroscopy are terms used to describe endoscopy procedures of the urinary system. CPT codes 52000–52700 describe various groups of cystourethroscopy procedures. The first group of codes (52000–52010) describes diagnostic cystourethroscopy, irrigation, and placement of ureteral catheters. The next group of codes (52204–52318) describes cystoscopy procedures on the urethra and bladder, including fulguration of bladder tumors, internal urethrotomy, insertion of urethral stents, and removal of urinary stones from the bladder.

CODING EXAMPLE

A surgeon performs a laparoscopic bladder sling operation for urinary incontinence. How should the coder report this procedure?

The coder looks up *laparoscopy* in the index and finds a "Bladder" subheading, which includes an indented listing for sling operation and a reference to code 51992.

CPT codes 52320–52355 describe cystourethroscopy procedures on the ureter and renal pelvis (the portion of the kidney that connects to the ureter). Guidance notes preceding this group of codes provide specific instructions regarding codes that cannot be billed together. Therapeutic procedures include diagnostic procedures described by CPT codes 52000 and 52351. Insertion of a temporary ureteral catheter with subsequent removal (CPT code 52005) is included in any of the procedures described by CPT codes 52320–52355.

CODER'S TIP

The insertion of an indwelling ureteral stent during another procedure is reported separately with CPT code 52332 (Cystourethroscopy, with insertion of indwelling ureteral stent) in addition to other procedures described by CPT codes 52320–52355.

(Continued)

Modifier 51 is added to this code if it is performed in addition to another procedure. CPT code 52332 describes a unilateral procedure. Modifier 50 is added to this code if stents are placed bilaterally. Therefore, coders should report CPT code 52320 with both modifier 50 and modifier 51 if bilateral indwelling ureteral stents are placed in addition to other procedures.

CPT codes 52400–52700 describe therapeutic cystourethroscopy of the bladder neck and prostate. CPT code 52601 describes a transurethral resection of the prostate (TURP) procedure, one of the most common procedures from this group. This procedure is performed through a cystoscope using an electrocautery knife to excise the tissue and cauterize bleeding using the same instrument. Other codes (52647–52649) describe the removal of prostate tissue using a laser device.

Urethra

Code range 53000–53665 reports therapeutic procedures on the meatus and urethra. Incision codes (53000–53085) describe meatotomy procedures and drainage of abscesses. The excision codes (53200–53275) describe biopsy procedures, urethrectomies, and excision of glands located around the urethra.

CPT codes 53400–53520 describe repairs involving the urethra, including urethroplasty, insertion of artificial sphincters, and repair of injuries to the urethra. Urethral dilation and other manipulation procedures are described by CPT codes 53600–53665.

EXERCISE 12.5.1

Also available in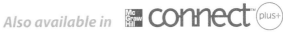

Use the CPT manual and index to select the code for each of the following procedures.

1. Nephrolithotomy and removal of a calculus _____
2. Open donor nephrectomy from a living donor _____
3. Ureteroplasty _____
4. Aspiration of the bladder with insertion of a suprapubic catheter _____
5. Complete transurethral resection of the prostate (TURP) _____
6. Reconstruction of the female urethra (urethroplasty) _____

12.5.2 Procedures on the Male Genital System (54000–55899)

CPT codes describing procedures on the male genital system are divided by the anatomical structures into the following sections:

- Penis (54000–54450)
- Testicles (or Testes) (54500–54699)
- Epididymis (54700–54901)
- Tunica Vaginalis (55000–55060)
- Scrotum (55100–55180)
- Vas Deferens (55200–55450)
- Spermatic Cord (55500–55559)
- Seminal Vesicles (55600–55680)
- Prostate (55700–55899)

Each section of CPT codes describing procedures on the male genital system includes some or all of the following types of procedures: incision, destruction, excision, laparoscopy, introduction, repair, manipulation, and suture. Coders should familiarize themselves with the anatomy of the male genital system and the procedures commonly performed on each of these structures.

Penis

Three CPT codes describe incision procedures on the penis. Two of these (54000 and 54001) describe the same procedure (Slitting of prepuce, dorsal or lateral [separate procedure]). CPT code 54000 describes the procedure on a newborn, whereas code 54001 describes the same procedure when it is not performed on a newborn. The "separate procedure" parenthetical in the code descriptor indicates that this code is used when the incision is the only procedure performed. When incisions are part of other procedures performed on the penis, these codes are not reported separately; rather the incision is considered a part of those other procedures.

Several CPT codes describe destruction of various lesions of the penis. If this is a "simple" procedure, separate codes (54050–54060) describe the procedure based on the method used to destroy the lesion (e.g., chemical, electrical, cryosurgical, laser surgery, or surgical excision). Only one code (54065) describes the destruction of lesions that are considered "extensive," regardless of the method used.

CODING EXAMPLE

A patient undergoes cryosurgical destruction of lesions on his penis. The coder looks in the index under "Lesion" and finds a subheading for "Penis" with several codes listed under "Destruction," including 54056 for cryosurgery. The coder also notes other entries under "Destruction," including codes for electrodesiccation (54055), laser surgery (54057), and surgical excision (54060).

The coder reports CPT code 54056.

Excision procedures include simple biopsies, removal of foreign bodies, amputations, and several circumcision procedures. Coders should note that several codes describe similar procedures that differ only by the age of the patient.

CODER'S TIP

When CPT code descriptors include a reference to neonates, there is often a parenthetical instruction not to add modifier 63 to the code. That modifier is used when a procedure that can be performed on a patient of any age is actually performed on a neonate.

Repair procedure codes (54300–54440) describe a number of surgical procedures to treat **hypospadius, epispadius**, erectile dysfunction, and penile injuries.

Testis

Excision codes (54500–54535) include biopsy, excision of lesions, and orchiectomy procedures. Separate codes describe simple, partial, or radical orchiectomy procedures. CPT codes 54550 and 54560 describe exploration procedures for an undescended **testis.**

hypospadius
A birth defect in which the urethra opens on the underside of the penis.

epispadius
A congenital defect in which the urethra opens on the top side of the penis.

testis or testicle
One of the male reproductive glands.

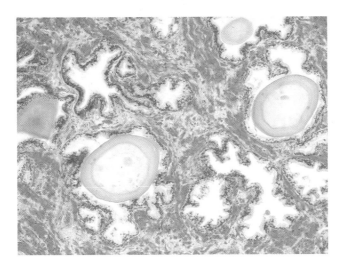

FIGURE 12.5.1 Micrograph of the Prostate Gland and Tubuloalveolar Glands

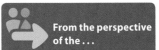

Repair codes (54600–54680) describe reduction of testicular torsion (twisted testicle); **orchiopexy**; repair of testicular injuries; and transplantation of the testicle to the thigh, which may be necessary if the scrotal sac is destroyed. CPT codes 54690 and 54692 describe laparoscopic orchiectomy and orchiopexy. As with all surgical laparoscopic procedures, a diagnostic laparoscopy, if performed, is included in the surgical laparoscopic procedure.

CPT codes describing procedures on the **epididymis, tunica vaginalis,** scrotum, **vas deferens (spermatic cord),** and **seminal vesicles** are organized first by anatomical structure and then by type of procedure. Coders must understand both the anatomy and the procedure to identify the correct codes.

orchiopexy
Surgical fixation of a testis in the scrotum.

epididymus
A coiled structure in the testis for the storage and transport of sperm to the vas deferens.

tunica vaginalis
A layer of tissue surrounding the testicle.

vas deferens (spermatic cord)
Tube that receives sperm from the epididymis.

seminal vesicle
Sac of the vas deferens that produces seminal fluid.

prostate
Organ surrounding the beginning of the urethra in males.

Prostate

Codes 55700–55899 describe procedures on the prostate gland (Figure 12.5.1). CPT codes describing incisions of the **prostate** (55700–55725) include biopsy and drainage of abscess procedures. Excision codes (55801–55865) describe prostatectomy procedures performed through an open approach (i.e., through an excision). Parenthetical notes direct coders to use CPT codes from other sections to describe a transurethral approach for removal or destruction of the prostate. The only laparoscopic procedure described in this section is CPT code 55866, which describes a radical retropubic prostatectomy with nerve sparing.

EXERCISE 12.5.2

Also available in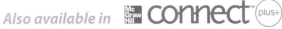

Use the CPT manual and index to select the code for each of the following procedures.

1. Penile plethysmography _____
2. Simple repair of hypospadias complications _____
3. Surgical reduction of torsion of a testis _____
4. Partial orchiectomy _____
5. Repair of a testicular injury _____
6. Perineal radical prostatectomy _____

12.5.3 Procedures on the Female Genital System (56405–58999)

CPT codes describing procedures on the female genital system are divided by anatomical structure and then subdivided by type of surgical procedure. The anatomical structures appear in the following sections:

- Vulva, Perineum, and Introitus (56405–56821)
- Vagina (57000–57426)
- Cervix Uteri (57452–57800)
- Corpus Uteri (58100–58579)
- Oviduct and Ovary (58600–58770)
- Ovary (58800–58960)
- In Vitro Fertilization (58970–58999)

As in the male genital system, each anatomical section includes some, but not necessarily all, of the following procedures: incision, destruction, excision, introduction, repair, manipulation, endoscopy, and laparoscopy. The Female Genital System section has several parenthetical guidance notes at the beginning of the section that direct coders to specific codes for various procedures. Coders should be familiar with these instructions.

Vulva, Perineum, and Introitus

Code range 56405–56821 includes instructions that differentiate between simple, radical, partial, and complete vulvectomy procedures (56620–56640). Incision procedures include drainage of abscesses and cysts of the **vulva**, perineum, and **Bartholin's glands**. Excision codes describe biopsy procedures and various vulvectomy procedures (simple/partial, simple/complete, radical/partial, and radical/complete). Coders must fully understand the surgical procedure to select the correct code.

vulva
Female external genitalia.

Bartholin's gland
Gland located on the labia minora at the side of and below the vaginal opening that secretes a lubricating fluid when stimulated.

CODER'S TIP

A number of codes describe vulvectomy procedures. Four codes differentiate simple from radical procedures and partial from complete procedures:

- 56620 (Vulvectomy, simple; partial)
- 56625 (Vulvectomy, simple; complete)
- 56630 (Vulvectomy, radical; partial)
- 56633 (Vulvectomy, radical; complete)

Several other codes describe the two radical procedures with either unilateral or bilateral inguinofemoral lymphadenectomy (56631, 56632, 56634, and 56637). A single code (56640) describes a radical complete vulvectomy with inguinofemoral, iliac, and pelvic lymphadenectomy. If this procedure is performed bilaterally, it is reported with modifier 50.

CODING EXAMPLE

A gynecologist is examining a woman during her annual pelvic exam. He notices several lesions of the vulva and proceeds to perform biopsies of three of those lesions. How should the coder report these procedures?

Looking up *biopsy* in the index, the coder finds a subheading of "Vulva" with references to codes 56605–56606. Looking up these codes shows that code 56605 describes a biopsy of one lesion of the vulva or perineum, and code 56606 is an add-on code describing a biopsy of each additional lesion. In this case, the coder reports 56605 and 56606 X 2.

Vagina

CPT codes 57000–57023 describe incision and drainage procedures of the **vagina**, including abscess and hematoma drainage. Codes 57061 and 57065 describe simple and extensive destruction of vaginal lesions.

The excision codes (57100–57135) describe various vaginectomy procedures. These include partial and complete procedures that are either simple or radical. As with other procedures, coders must fully understand the procedure to select the correct code.

CPT codes (57200–57335) describe repair procedures based on the underlying defect, including **cystocele, rectocele, enterocele,** and other pelvic floor defects. These codes differentiate between vaginal and abdominal approaches. This section of codes also describes repairs of several different types of vaginal fistulas, including rectovaginal, urethrovaginal, and vesicovaginal fistulas.

The Endoscopy/Laparoscopy section describes endoscopic and/or laparoscopic procedures of the vagina. As with other laparoscopic procedures, any diagnostic procedures are included in the surgical procedure code.

Cervix Uteri

CPT codes in code range 57452–57800 primarily describe endoscopy and excision procedures of the **cervix**. Endoscopy codes (57452–57461) describe **colposcopy** alone and in combination with various biopsy procedures. The excision codes (57500–57558) describe biopsies of the cervix, cervical curettage, conization, and partial and complete excision of the cervix, including radical procedures.

Corpus Uteri

The excision codes in this section (58100–58294) describe biopsy of the **endometrium,** dilation and curettage, excision of fibroids from the uterine **myometrium,** and a number of hysterectomy procedures, including abdominal and vaginal approaches combined with other procedures. The codes also identify the size of the uterus and whether the procedure is a simple or radical hysterectomy. It is important to note that the codes in this subsection do not describe laparoscopic hysterectomy procedures.

Codes in the Introduction section (58300–58356) describe a number of procedures, including insertion or removal of an intrauterine device (IUD), fallopian tube catheterization, endometrial ablation, and insertion of capsules for brachytherapy. The Laparoscopy/Hysteroscopy section (58541–58579) is comprised of a number of procedures, including laparoscopic hysterectomy procedures and vaginal hysterectomies performed with laparoscopy, hysteroscopy procedures, biopsies, lysis of adhesions, and laparoscopic excision of fibroid tissues.

Oviduct/Ovary

Codes 58600–58779 describe open procedures on the fallopian tubes and laparoscopic procedures on both the tubes and ovaries, but they do not describe open procedures on the ovaries. The incision codes (58600–58615) describe tubal ligation and/or transection as a separate procedure, during the postpartum period, or at the time of cesarean section.

The laparoscopic codes (58660–58679) describe a number of surgical procedures or a combination of procedures on adnexal structures (ovary and tube). The excision codes (58700 and 58720) describe salpingectomy (excision of tube) and salpingo-oophorectomy (excision of tube and ovary). The repair codes (58740–58770) describe open procedures such as lysis of adhesions or tubal repairs. Laparoscopic repairs are reported with laparoscopic surgery codes.

vagina
Female genital canal extending from the uterus to the vulva.

cystocele
Hernia of the bladder into the vagina.

rectocele
Hernia of the rectum into the vagina.

enterocele
A hernia sac containing a portion of the small intestine.

cervix
The lower part of the uterus.

colposcopy
Examination of the vagina using a colposcope.

endometrium
Inner lining of the uterus.

myometrium
Muscle wall of the uterus.

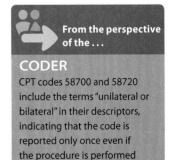

From the perspective of the . . .

CODER
CPT codes 58700 and 58720 include the terms "unilateral or bilateral" in their descriptors, indicating that the code is reported only once even if the procedure is performed on both sides.

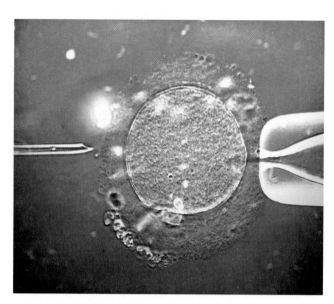

FIGURE 12.5.2 In Vitro Fertilization of a Human Egg

Ovary

Codes 58800–58960 describe open procedures on the ovaries, including incisions for drainage of abscesses, biopsies, excision of ovarian structures as part of radical procedures, tumor resection, and staging procedures.

In Vitro Fertilization

Codes 58970–58976 describe procedures related to in vitro fertilization (Figure 12.5.2), including oocyte (egg) retrieval and embryo intrauterine transfer.

EXERCISE 12.5.3

Also available in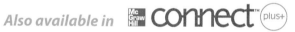

Use the CPT manual and index to select the code for each of the following procedures.

1. Colposcopy and biopsy of the vulva _____
2. Vaginectomy including removal of the vaginal wall _____
3. Cervicectomy _____
4. Total abdominal hysterectomy _____
5. Bilateral complete salpingo-oophorectomy _____
6. Bilateral biopsies of the ovary _____

12.5.4 Maternal Care and Delivery (59000–59899)

antepartum care
Prenatal care.

postpartum care
Care following childbirth.

Maternity services during an uncomplicated delivery include **antepartum care**, delivery, and **postpartum care**. Antepartum (prenatal) care includes an initial history; physical exams; monitoring of weight, blood pressure, fetal heart tones, and urinalysis; and follow-up visits to update these findings. Ideally the pregnant woman is seen at least monthly for the first seven months (28 weeks), every two weeks for the next two months (8 weeks), and then weekly until delivery. Additional visits or services are reported separately.

CODER'S TIP

Maternity care consists of three separate components—prenatal care, delivery, and postpartum care. Combinations of these components are reported with a single code.

Delivery services include the hospital admission history and physical exam, management of labor, and **vaginal delivery** (with or without episiotomy and with or without forceps) or **cesarean section**. Postpartum care includes hospital and office visits following delivery.

Medical problems during the pregnancy that require additional services beyond the usual services provided during uncomplicated pregnancies may be reported using the usual E/M codes. Surgical complications may be reported using the surgical CPT codes. When one physician provides antepartum or postpartum services, but does not perform the delivery, the services provided are reported using CPT code 59425, 59426, or 59430.

The Maternal Care and Delivery section is divided into subsections based on the care provided, including:

- Antepartum and Fetal Invasive Services (59000–59076)
- Excision (59100–59150)
- Repair (59300–59350)
- Vaginal Delivery, Antepartum and Postpartum Care (59400–59430)
- Cesarean Delivery (59510–59525)
- Delivery after Previous Cesarean Delivery (59610–59622)
- Abortion (59812–59847)
- Other Procedures (59866–59899)

Antepartum and Fetal Invasive Services

Code series 59000–59076 describes prenatal testing procedures such as amniocentesis, fetal contraction stress test, fetal nonstress test, fetal scalp blood sample, and fetal monitoring during labor. These codes do not describe antepartum care of the pregnant woman. That care is described by codes in subsequent sections.

Excision

Codes 59100–59150 describe abdominal hysterotomy and various procedures for the treatment of ectopic pregnancies by abdominal, vaginal, or laparoscopic approaches. The approach used to treat an ectopic pregnancy depends on its location (e.g., within a tube, free within the abdomen, or within the uterine wall).

Vaginal Delivery, Antepartum and Postpartum Care

A single code (59400) describes the entire package of services associated with routine vaginal deliveries, including antepartum care; vaginal delivery (with or without episiotomy and with or without forceps); and postpartum care. Separate codes describe the delivery alone (59409), delivery plus postpartum care (59410), antepartum care only (59425 and 59426), and postpartum care only (59430). The difference between the two antepartum codes is that code 59425 describes four to six visits, whereas code 59426 describes seven or more visits. Less than four antepartum visits are reported with the appropriate E/M codes for those visits rather than the bundled antepartum visit codes.

vaginal delivery
A procedure during which a fetus is delivered through the vagina.

cesarean section
The extraction of a fetus through an incision in the abdomen and uterine wall.

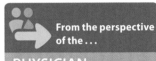
From the perspective of the . . .

PHYSICIAN
Medical problems may occur during pregnancy that are either unrelated to the pregnancy or are related to the pregnancy but require services beyond those usually provided during the prenatal care of a normal pregnancy. These services are reported with E/M codes that describe the level of services provided. The physician should document the reasons for the additional E/M services and the actual services provided.

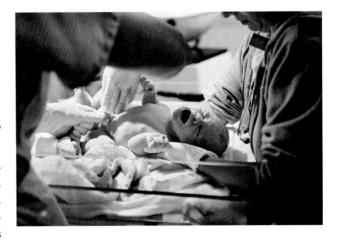
Routine vaginal delivery is reported by one code: 59400.

Cesarean Delivery

CPT code 59510 describes the services typically bundled with cesarean deliveries, including antepartum care, cesarean delivery, and postpartum care. Cesarean delivery alone is reported with code 59514, while cesarean delivery with postpartum care is reported with code 59515. When a hysterectomy is necessary in conjunction with a cesarean delivery, add-on code 59525 is included. Stand-alone antepartum and/or postpartum care are reported with CPT codes 59425, 59426, and 59430.

CODING EXAMPLE

A pregnant woman presents to the hospital in labor. An evaluation shows fetal distress, and the obstetrician makes the decision to perform a cesarean delivery. He has not treated this patient before but sees her for postpartum follow-up care. How should the coder report these services?

Cesarean delivery services are described by codes 59510–59525. Reviewing these codes reveals that cesarean delivery and postpartum care are reported with CPT code 59515.

Delivery after Previous Cesarean Delivery

At times, women who delivered a previous child via cesarean section want to attempt a vaginal delivery. Those procedures, commonly referred to as vaginal birth after cesarean or **VBAC procedures,** are described by several codes, including 59610 (routine obstetric care including antepartum, vaginal delivery after previous cesarean delivery and postpartum care), 59612 (vaginal delivery only), and 59614 (vaginal delivery plus postpartum care).

At times, the attempt at vaginal delivery fails and a repeat cesarean delivery is provided. CPT codes 59618 (antepartum care, cesarean delivery, and postpartum care), 59620 (cesarean delivery only following attempted vaginal delivery), and 59622 (cesarean delivery and postpartum care following attempted vaginal delivery) describe these services. As with CPT codes describing primary cesarean section, stand-alone antepartum and/or postpartum care are reported with CPT codes 59425, 59426, and 59430.

VBAC procedure
Vaginal birth after cesarean section.

CODER'S TIP

The choice of codes reported to describe maternity services depends on the method of delivery. Codes 59400–59410 describe vaginal delivery combined with other components, codes 59510–59515 describe cesarean section combined with other components, and codes 59610–59622 describe vaginal delivery after previous cesarean delivery.

Abortion

Spontaneous abortions treated medically are reported with the appropriate E/M code (99201–99233). Spontaneous abortions treated surgically are reported with CPT code 59812. Missed abortions treated surgically during the first trimester are reported with CPT code 59820, and those treated during the second trimester are reported with CPT code 59821. Separate CPT codes describe different therapeutic abortion procedures, including CPT codes 59840 (Induced abortion, by dilation and curettage) and 59841 (Induced abortion, by dilation and evacuation).

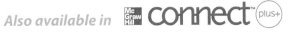
Use the CPT manual and index to select the code for each of the following procedures.

1. Fetal nonstress test _____
2. Amniocentesis _____
3. Surgical treatment of an ectopic pregnancy; abdominal pregnancy _____
4. Laparoscopic treatment of an ectopic pregnancy _____
5. Routine obstetrical care including antepartum care, cesarean delivery, and postpartum care _____
6. Cesarean delivery only following attempted vaginal delivery after previous cesarean delivery _____

12.5.5 Anesthesia for Procedures Described by Codes in the 50000 Series

The codes describing anesthesia for procedures in the 50000 series are located in three main sections of anesthesia codes. Two of these describe anatomical regions: the lower abdomen and the perineum. The third section describes anesthesia for obstetrical procedures. CPT codes describing anesthesia for procedures in the 50000 series of procedure codes include the following ranges of codes:

- Anesthesia for procedures in the lower abdomen (00840–00873)
- Anesthesia for procedures on the perineum and genitalia systems (00904–00952)
- Anesthesia for obstetrical procedures (01958–01969)

CODING EXAMPLE

An anesthesiologist places an epidural for neuraxial labor analgesia. After several hours of labor, the obstetrician makes the decision to perform a cesarean delivery. The anesthesiologist accompanies the patient to the operative suite for this procedure. How are these anesthesia services reported?

Reviewing the obstetrical anesthesia codes shows that the labor epidural is reported with code 01967 and the cesarean delivery is reported with add-on code 01968.

Use the CPT manual and index to select the code that describes the anesthesia for the following procedures.

1. Radical nephrectomy, with regional lymphadenectomy and partial ureterectomy _____
2. Laparoscopic nephrectomy and partial ureterectomy _____
3. Radical orchiectomy, inguinal approach, with abdominal exploration _____
4. Transurethral resection of the prostate (TURP) _____
5. Total abdominal hysterectomy _____
6. Labor epidural for vaginal delivery involving vaginal-rectal tear repair _____

Summary

Learning Outcome	Key Concepts/Examples
12.5.1 Report codes for procedures on the urinary system. **Pages 384–387**	Procedures on the urinary system are organized based on anatomical structures, including the kidneys, ureters, bladder, and urethra. Procedures on the urinary tract structures include incision, excision, introduction, repair, laparoscopy, endoscopy, and kidney transplantation. Many of these may be performed as open or closed procedures (percutaneous, endoscopic, or laparoscopic).
12.5.2 Describe codes for procedures on the male genital system. **Pages 387–389**	Male genitalia procedure codes describe procedures on both external and internal structures, including the penis, testicles, spermatic structures, and prostate. Procedures on the male genital system include incision, excision, introduction, repair, and laparoscopy. Some procedures may be performed open or closed. It is important to understand the type of procedure in order to select the correct code to identify those procedures.
12.5.3 Describe codes for procedures on the female genital system. **Pages 390–392**	Procedures on the female genital system include procedures on internal structures such as the vagina, cervix, uterus, ovaries, and fallopian tubes. Procedures on external structures include those on the vulva, perineum, and introitus. Procedures on the female genitalia include incision, excision, destruction, introduction, repair, endoscopy, laparoscopy, and hysteroscopy. Many of these may be performed as open or closed procedures (percutaneous, endoscopic, or laparoscopic).
12.5.4 Explain codes used to report maternity care services. **Pages 392–394**	Codes describing maternity care include antepartum care, method of delivery (vaginal versus cesarean), postpartum care, and combinations of these services. Combinations of services (e.g., delivery and postpartum care) must be reported with the appropriate combination code. It is incorrect to report these services with separate codes when a combination code exists. This section also includes codes describing specific antepartum tests to assess the condition of the fetus.
12.5.5 Select anesthesia codes for procedures in the 50000 series. **Page 395**	CPT codes describing anesthesia for most of the procedures in the 50000 series are from three major groups of anesthesia codes: anesthesia for procedures on the lower abdomen; anesthesia for procedures on the perineum and genitalia; and obstetrical anesthesia.

Using Terminology

Match each term with its definition.

_____ **1.** L012.5.1 Kidney

_____ **2.** L012.5.1 Ureter

_____ **3.** L012.5.1 Bladder

_____ **4.** L012.5.1 Urethra

_____ **5.** L012.5.1 Rectocele

_____ **6.** L012.5.3 Colposcopy

_____ **7.** L012.5.2 Orchiopexy

A. Surgical fixation of a testis in the scrotum

B. Organ located behind the peritoneum that filters blood to make urine

C. Hernia of the rectum into the vagina

D. Pertaining to the period after delivery

E. Hollow organ where urine collects before being excreted

F. Examination of the vagina by colposcope

_____ **8.** L0.12.5.2 Prostate

_____ **9.** L0.12.5.1 Renal calculus

_____ **10.** L0.12.5.1 Allotransplantation

_____ **11.** L0.12.5.4 Antepartum care

_____ **12.** L0.12.5.4 Postpartum care

_____ **13.** L0.12.5.4 Cesarean section

_____ **14.** L012.5.4 Vaginal delivery

G. Procedure in which a fetus is delivered through an incision in the abdomen and uterine wall

H. Tube connecting the kidney and the urinary bladder

I. Pertaining to the period before delivery

J. Structure leading from the bladder to the outside of the body

K. Implantation of graft

L. Male reproductive gland

M. Procedure in which a fetus is delivered through the vagina

N. Kidney stone

Checking Your Understanding

Select the letter that best completes the statement or answers the question.

1. L012.5.1 The narrow tube that connects the kidney to the urinary bladder is the _____.

  a. Urethra
  b. Ureter
  c. Prostate
  d. Cortex

2. L012.5.1 Another term used to describe kidney stones would be _____.

  a. Cholelithiasis
  b. Renal calculi
  c. Nephrolithiasis
  d. Either renal calculi or nephrolithiasis

3. L012.5.4 If a physician provides antepartum care of a patient for 4–6 visits but does not perform the delivery, what CPT code would be appropriate to report?

  a. 59425
  b. 59426
  c. 59400-52
  d. None of these; evaluation and management codes would be appropriate.

4. L012.5.2 CPT orchiectomy procedures are further defined by which of the following descriptions?

  a. Simple
  b. Partial
  c. Radical
  d. All of these

5. L012.5.4 Obstetrical services provided to a woman who has had a previous cesarean delivery and now wants to attempt a vaginal delivery are reported with which range of CPT codes?

  a. 59618–59622
  b. 59610–59622
  c. 59610–59614
  d. 59400–59430

connect plus+

Enhance your learning by completing these exercises and more at mcgrawhillconnect.com!

6. L012.5.3 Removal of less than 80 percent of the vulvar area describes what type of vulvectomy?
   a. Simple
   b. Radical
   c. Partial
   d. Complete

7. L012.5.1 How is ultrasound imaging guidance reported when used for an ablation of a renal tumor?
   a. 77013
   b. 77022
   c. 76940
   d. It is not coded separately, as it is included in the code.

8. L012.5.1 A cystourethroscopy is performed with irrigation and evacuation of multiple obstructing clots. Which CPT code(s) would be appropriate?
   a. 52000
   b. 52001
   c. 52000, 52001
   d. 52005

9. L012.5.3 The codes in section 58100–58294 describe endometrial sampling, dilation and curettage, excision of fibroids from the uterine myometrium, and a number of hysterectomy procedures. A coder would need to know which of the following in order to accurately code in this range?
   a. The weight of the tumors
   b. Whether a simple or radical hysterectomy was performed
   c. Whether the physician used an abdominal or vaginal approach
   d. All of these

10. L012.5.4 Codes in the range 59000–59076 (Antepartum and Fetal Invasive Services) do not include _____.
    a. Amniocentesis
    b. Fetal nonstress test
    c. Antepartum care of the pregnant woman
    d. Fetal monitoring during labor

Applying Your Skills

Use the CPT manual to determine the correct code to report the following procedures:

1. L012.5.1 Meatotomy, cutting of the meatus, infant _____

2. L012.5.1 Cystourethroscopy with dilation of the bladder for interstitial cystitis with spinal anesthesia _____

3. L012.5.2 Circumcision, surgical, newborn _____

4. L012.5.3 Ligation of the fallopian tube and oviduct with fulguration _____

5. L012.5.1 Adrenalectomy _____

6. L012.5.3 Fimbrioplasty _____

7. L012.5.2 Orchiectomy _____

8. L012.5.2 Ligation of the vas deferens _____

9. L012.5.1 Insertion of a bladder stent _____

10. L012.5.2 Plastic operation of the penis for straightening of chordee _____

11. L012.5.1 Ureterolithotomy, lower one-third _____

12. L012.5.2 Surgical circumcision of a newborn _____

13. L012.5.3 Partial radical vaginectomy _____

14. L012.5.4 Laparoscopic treatment of ectopic pregnancy with salpingectomy _____

15. L012.5.3 Colposcopy of the entire vagina, including the cervix, with biopsies _____

Thinking It Through

Use your critical-thinking skills to answer the questions below.

1. L012.5.3 Review the notes associated with CPT code 58240. Explain why it is important for coders to know the reasons for the surgery (diagnosis) in addition to knowing about the procedure being done. Why is the distinction made with the notes that accompany this code important both to the patient and to reimbursement of the procedure?

   _____
   _____
   _____
   _____

2. L012.5.4 Differentiate between the services included in antepartum care, delivery services, and postpartum care.

   _____
   _____
   _____

3. L012.5.2 A patient with bilateral undescended testes undergoes surgical exploration to locate and place the testes in the scrotal sac. Describe the types of procedures that could be performed and how these would be coded.

   _____
   _____
   _____
   _____

Mc Graw Hill **connect** (plus+)

Enhance your learning by completing these exercises and more at mcgrawhillconnect.com!

MODULE 12.5 | URINARY SYSTEM, MALE AND FEMALE GENITAL SYSTEMS, AND MATERNITY CARE AND DELIVERY   399

Learning Outcomes *After completing this module, students should be able to:*

12.6.1 Differentiate among procedures on the endocrine system.

12.6.2 Contrast procedures on the skull, meninges, and brain.

12.6.3 Explain procedures involving the spine and spinal cord.

12.6.4 Identify procedures on the extracranial nerves, peripheral nerves, and autonomic nervous system.

12.6.5 Describe the major anatomical structures of the eye and surgical procedures performed on those structures.

12.6.6 Explain the major procedures performed on the auditory system.

12.6.7 Code anesthesia services for procedures in the 60000 series.

Key Terms

Adrenal glands

Anterior cranial fossa

Arteriovenous malformation

Carotid body

Craniectomy

Cranioplasty

Craniotomy

Epidural

Extracranial arteries

Frontal bone

Gonads

Infratentorial

Intracranial arteries

Intrathecal

Meninges

Middle cranial fossa

Occipital bones

Pancreas

Parathyroid gland

Parietal bones

Pineal gland

Pituitary gland

Posterior cranial fossa

Supratentorial

Temporal bone

Thymus

Thyroid

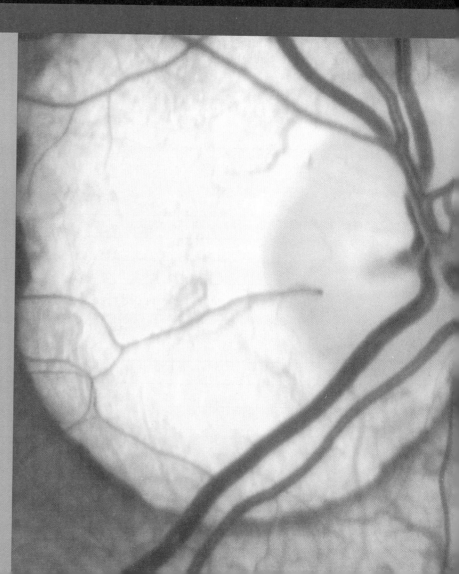

Introduction

The 60000 code series includes procedures on several major systems, including the endocrine system, skull, brain, spine and spinal cord, peripheral nerves, eye, and ear.

12.6.1 Endocrine System (60000–60699)

Endocrine Anatomy

The endocrine system is actually composed of many diverse organs, including the **thyroid, parathyroid, thymus, adrenal glands, pancreas, carotid body, pituitary gland, pineal gland,** and the male and female **gonads** (testes and ovaries).

This section of the CPT only covers the part of the endocrine system that includes the thyroid, parathyroid, thymus, adrenal glands, pancreas, and carotid body. The pituitary and pineal glands are covered under the nervous system. The reproductive endocrine system, including the ovaries and testes, are covered in the male and female genital systems.

CODER'S TIP

Even though procedures on the endocrine system are numbered in the 60000 range, these codes are traditionally included at the end of the 50000 chapter in the CPT manual. These are the only codes that are not included in the chapter that corresponds to the numerical code numbers.

Thyroid

Most of the codes in the code range 60000–60300 describe excision procedures of the thyroid (Figure 12.6.1), including biopsies, excision of cysts and benign tumors, partial or complete thyroid lobectomy (unilateral procedure involving one lobe of the thyroid), and total thyroidectomy. One code (60000) describes incision and drainage of an infected thyroglossal duct cyst, while another code (60300) describes aspiration or injection of a thyroid cyst.

Parathyroid, Thymus, Adrenal Glands, and Carotid Body

Three codes (60500–60505) describe exploration and reexploration procedures of the parathyroid glands. One add-on code (60512) is used when the parathyroid glands are reimplanted after excision from their original site.

Other codes (60520–60605) describe excisions of the thymus, adrenals, and carotid bodies. Three codes (60520–60522) describe thymectomy procedures. Each includes the "separate procedure" parenthetical, indicating that these codes are only used if the thymectomy is the only procedure performed. When this is reported with another procedure on the neck or thorax, the thymectomy is considered to be included in the other procedure.

Open and laparoscopic adrenalectomy procedures are described by separate codes (60540 or 60545 for open adrenalectomies and 60650 for laparoscopic adrenalectomies). A parenthetical note instructs coders not to report these codes with CPT code 50323, which describes the backbench work to prepare a donated kidney for transplant into the recipient. The backbench work includes excision of the adrenal gland from the donor kidney.

thyroid
An endocrine gland in the neck.

parathyroid
Small endocrine glands located on the thyroid that produce parathyroid hormone.

thymus
An endocrine gland located in the mediastinum.

adrenal glands
Endocrine glands located above each kidney that secrete important substances such as epinephrine.

pancreas
A large, curved, elongated gland that lies behind the stomach between the spleen and the duodenum.

carotid body
A small structure on the carotid artery that senses changes in blood pressure and levels of oxygen, carbon dioxide, pH, and temperature and sends regulatory messages to the brain stem.

pituitary gland
A gland that secretes many different hormones that affect the body either directly or by causing other glands to produce hormones.

pineal gland
An endocrine gland, located deep inside the brain, that releases melatonin, a hormone involved in sleep-wake cycles.

gonads
Testes or ovaries.

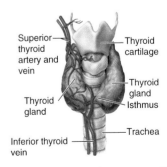

FIGURE 12.6.1 Anatomy of the Thyroid Gland

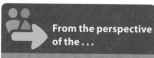

From the perspective of the . . .

CODER

The choice of codes to describe a thyroidectomy (60100–60271) depends on the surgical approach (e.g., sternal split, transthoracic, or cervical). Code selection also depends on whether a radical neck dissection is performed with the thyroidectomy.

CODING EXAMPLE

A patient is found to have abnormal growths on both adrenal glands, and the surgeon schedules an open bilateral adrenalectomy. At the time of surgery, the surgeon finds that the tumors extend into the retroperitoneal region. How should the coder report these procedures?

The coder looks up *adrenal gland* in the index. Under this heading is an "Excision" subheading with an entry identifying retroperitoneal tumor with code 60545. Looking up code 60545, which describes an adrenalectomy with excision of adjacent retroperitoneal tumor, the coder finds a parenthetical note that instructs coders to use modifier 50 for bilateral procedures. Therefore, the coder reports 60545-50.

EXERCISE 12.6.1

Also available in **McGraw Hill** **connect** (plus+)

Use the CPT manual and index to select the best code to describe each procedure.

1. Parathyroidectomy, reexploration _____
2. Adrenalectomy _____
3. Total thyroid lobectomy _____

12.6.2 Procedures on the Skull, Meninges, and Brain (61000–62258)

meninges
Three-layered covering of the brain and spinal cord.

Procedures on the nervous system are divided into three subsections: (1) skull, **meninges**, and brain (61000–62258); (2) spine and spinal cord (62263–63746); and (3) extracranial nerves, peripheral nerves, and autonomic nervous system (64400–64999). This section includes codes describing procedures on the skull (Figure 12.6.2), meninges, and brain. Understanding the anatomy of these structures is crucial to selecting the correct codes to describe the associated procedures.

Procedures on these structures are divided into groups of similar procedures, including:

- Injection, Drainage, or Aspiration (61000–61070)
- Twist Drill, Burr Hole(s), or Trephine (61105–61253)

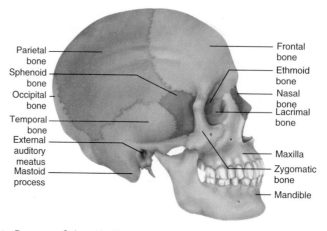

FIGURE 12.6.2 Bones of the Skull

- Craniectomy or Craniotomy (61304–61576)
- Surgery of Skull Base (61580–61619)
- Endovascular Therapy (61623–61642)
- Surgery for Aneurysm, Arteriovenous Malformation, or Vascular Disease (61680–61711)
- Stereotaxis (61720–61791)
- Stereotactic Radiosurgery (Cranial) (61795–61800)
- Neurostimulators (Intracranial) (61850–61888)
- Repair (62000–62148)
- Neuroendoscopy (62160–62165)
- Cerebrospinal Fluid (CSF) Shunt (62180–62258)

CPT codes 61000–61070 describe injection, drainage, and aspiration procedures of the cranial structures. Codes 61105–61215 describe drill or burr holes combined with other procedures. If a burr hole is the only procedure (i.e., it is not followed by another surgical procedure), it is reported with either 61250 or 61253, depending on whether the hole is placed in the supratentorial or infratentorial region. If the burr hole is followed by either a craniectomy or craniotomy, the combined procedures are reported with codes describing those procedures.

The terms *craniotomy* and *craniectomy* describe procedures performed through openings made in the cranium, or upper part of the skull, which is made up of the **frontal, parietal, temporal,** and **occipital bones.** During infancy and early childhood these are separate bones, but they fuse together later to form a solid protective structure in which the brain and other structures are encased. Numerous codes (61304–61576) describe **craniectomy** and **craniotomy** procedures, depending on the underlying reason for the procedure, the location, and the specific procedures performed through the skull opening. It is essential for coders to understand the anatomy to identify the correct code.

CODER'S TIP

Most codes describing craniectomy and craniotomy procedures do not differentiate between the two. A craniotomy is a temporary removal of part of the skull, with the bone replaced at the end of the procedure. A craniectomy removes a portion of the bone either permanently or at least for an extended period of time.

Procedures on the base of the skull are complex and often involve several surgeons of different specialties. One reason for this is the complexity of getting to and through the base of the skull, which is not easily accessible through a simple skin incision. The skull base is like a shelf on which the brain and other intracranial structures rest, protected by the facial bones, jaw, and cranium. Because of this anatomical difficulty, procedures on the base of the skull are not described by a single code. Rather, they are separated into three categories—approach procedures, definitive procedures, and repair/reconstruction procedures—to describe different aspects of the procedures. These codes are grouped together.

CPT codes describing approach procedures (61580–61598) are grouped according to anatomical location—**anterior cranial fossa, middle cranial fossa,** or **posterior cranial fossa.** Definitive procedures (61600–61616) include repair, biopsy, resection, or excision of lesions located within the base of the skull. Similar to the approach procedures, these codes are grouped according to the location of the abnormality. Repair/reconstruction of surgical defects after surgical procedures on the base of the skull are described by two codes. CPT code 61618 describes repair of the dura with free tissue or synthetic grafts. CPT code 61619 describes more extensive closure procedures, such as **cranioplasty,** or myocutaneous pedicle flaps. Complex primary closures are reported with CPT code 15732 or 15756–15758.

frontal bone
The large bone of the forehead.

parietal bones
The two bones forming the side walls and roof of the cranium.

temporal bone
A bone that forms part of the base and sides of the skull.

occipital bones
The back of the skull.

craniectomy
Surgical removal of a portion of the skull, the first stage of most neurosurgical operations on the brain.

craniotomy
Surgical incision of the skull.

anterior cranial fossa
Cranial cavity that houses the frontal lobes.

middle cranial fossa
Cranial cavity that houses the temporal lobes and the hypothalamus

posterior cranial fossa
Cranial cavity that houses the cerebellum, pons, and medulla oblongata.

cranioplasty
Surgical correction of skull defects.

extracranial arteries
Arteries located outside the cranium.

intracranial arteries
Arteries located within the cranium.

arteriovenous malformation
An abnormal communication between an artery and a vein.

supratentorial
The upper part of the brain.

infratentorial
The lower part of the brain.

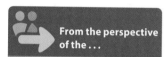
From the perspective of the . . .

CODER

It is important to review code descriptors carefully. Some endovascular therapy codes include radiological supervision and interpretation while others allow for the separate reporting of radiological supervision and interpretation services.

When multiple surgeons perform different aspects of these procedures, each reports the procedures he or she actually performed. If one surgeon performs more than one part of the procedure, modifier 51 is added to the additional procedures performed by that surgeon.

CPT codes 61623–61642 describe endovascular procedures performed on **extracranial arteries** and **intracranial arteries** of the head and neck. These procedures include temporary arterial occlusion, permanent occlusion, angioplasty with or without stent placement, and balloon dilatation. Coders must pay particular attention to any parenthetical notes associated with these codes. Some codes include the radiographic supervision and interpretation necessary to perform the procedure, while other codes allow the radiography services to be reported separately. It also is important for coders to use the latest version of the CPT manual when reporting these codes because the inclusion of associated services, such as radiography, often changes from year to year.

Surgeries for intracranial vascular abnormalities, including aneurysms, **arteriovenous malformations,** or vascular diseases, are described by CPT codes 61680–61711. A series of codes (61680–61692) describes procedures on arteriovenous malformations, also known as A-V malformations. The correct code depends on whether the repair is simple or complex and whether the malformation is located in the upper part of the brain (**supratentorial**), lower part of the brain (**infratentorial**), or within the dural structures.

CODING EXAMPLE

A patient has an intracranial arteriovenous malformation in the infratentorial region. The surgical note describes this as a simple A-V malformation repair. How should the coder report this procedure?

The coder looks up *arteriovenous malformation* in the index and finds a subheading listing cranial repair with codes 61680–61692 and 61705–61708. The coder reviews each code in these ranges and finds that code 61684 describes surgery of a simple infratentorial intracranial arteriovenous malformation. The coder lists this code to report the procedure.

CPT codes 61697–61710 describe procedures on arterial aneurysms. These codes differ from one another by location of the aneurysm (carotid or vertebrobasilar arterial systems) and type of repair. Anastomoses between extracranial and intracranial arteries are described by CPT code 61711. This procedure may be used to bypass arterial occlusions or injuries to connect arteries from outside the skull to those within the skull.

Stereotaxis procedures are described by CPT codes 61720–61791. This series of codes includes three add-on codes that are used with other intracranial or spinal procedures when those procedures are performed using stereotactic assistance. The add-on codes are not used in combination with other stereotaxis procedure codes. Coders must review the guidance included with these add-on codes to determine whether they may be used with specific codes describing other procedures.

Stereotactic radiosurgery (61796–61800) describes distinct procedures involving the use of externally generated radiation beams to eradicate intracranial lesions without making incisions. These codes describe the treatment of a single simple or complex lesion, with add-on codes to describe treatment of additional simple or complex lesions. The codes are used once to describe the treatment of each lesion, even if the treatment involves several sessions. If multiple lesions are treated, the complex code is used if any lesion is considered complex.

Whether a lesion is complex depends on several factors. Any lesion 3.5 cm or greater in any dimension is a complex lesion. Lesions that are within 5 mm of the optic nerve, optic chiasm, or optic tract are complex regardless of size. Lesions within the brain stem are also complex regardless of size. The following lesions are also complex regardless of size: schwannomas, arteriovenous malformations, pituitary tumors, glomus tumors, pineal region tumors, and tumors of the cavernous sinus, parasellar, or petroclival regions. Tumors that are less than 3.5 cm are simple lesions unless they are one of those listed as complex regardless of size. Coders are unlikely to remember all these rules and should review the guidelines when coding these procedures.

Procedures involving intracranial neurostimulator implants are reported with CPT codes 61850–61888. These procedures include implanting simple electrodes (61850–61860) or electrode arrays (61863–61868), as well as revising, replacing, or removing existing neurostimulators (61880–61888).

Repair codes (62000–62148) describe various repairs of bony structures and underlying soft tissues. These codes differ from one another based on the complexity of the repair and the underlying defect that makes the repair necessary. One add-on code describes incision and retrieval of a subcutaneous bone graft used in conjunction with the repair procedure.

CPT codes 62160–62165 describe endoscopic intracranial procedures. These include diagnostic endoscopy if performed in conjunction with the surgical procedure. CPT code 62160 is an add-on code that may be reported with specific procedure codes listed in the parenthetical instructions when those procedures are performed through an endoscope rather than as an open procedure.

At times it is necessary to shunt or divert cerebrospinal fluid (CSF) away from the brain. CPT codes 62180–62258 describe these procedures, differing from one another by the area from which the fluid is shunted (e.g., subarachnoid or subdural space versus from within one of the ventricles of the brain) and by the area to which the fluid is diverted (e.g., the jugular vein or atrium versus the peritoneum, pleural space, or other body cavity). Each code describing placement of a shunt includes a parenthetical instruction to use add-on code 62160 if the shunt is placed via an endoscope rather than through an open procedure.

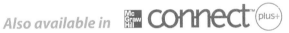

EXERCISE 12.6.2

Also available in

Use the CPT manual and index to select the best code to describe each procedure.

1. Craniectomy for the evacuation of an intracerebral hematoma _____

2. Resection of an intradural infectious lesion of the base of the anterior cranial fossa with dural repair without graft _____

3. Burr hole(s) for implantation of neurostimulator electrodes, cortical _____

12.6.3 Procedures on the Spine and Spinal Cord (62263–63746)

CPT codes describing procedures involving the spine and spinal cord are divided into several distinct code sections, as follows:

- Injection, Drainage, or Aspiration (62263–62319)
- Catheter Implantation (62350–62355)
- Reservoir and Pump Implantation (62360–62368)
- Posterior Extradural Laminotomy or Laminectomy for Exploration or Decompression of Neural Elements or Excision of Herniated Intervertebral Discs (63001–63051)
- Transpedicular or Costovertebral Approach for Posterolateral Extradural Exploration or Decompression (63055–63066)

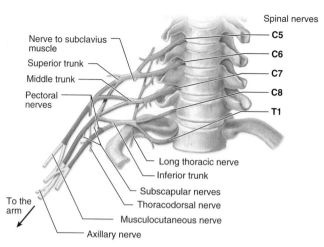

Spinal nerves

Nerve to subclavius muscle
Superior trunk
Middle trunk
Pectoral nerves

C5
C6
C7
C8
T1

To the arm

Long thoracic nerve
Inferior trunk
Subscapular nerves
Thoracodorsal nerve
Musculocutaneous nerve
Axillary nerve

FIGURE 12.6.3 Brachial Plexus

- Anterior or Anterolateral Approach for Extradural Exploration or Decompression (63075–63091)
- Lateral Extracavitary Approach for Extradural Exploration or Decompression (63101–63200)
- Excision by Laminectomy of Lesion Other Than Herniated Disc (63250–63295)
- Excision, Anterior or Anterolateral Approach, Intraspinal Lesion (63300–63308)
- Stereotaxis (63600–63615)
- Stereotactic Radiosurgery (Spinal) (63620–63621)
- Neurostimulators (Spinal) (63650–63688)
- Repair (63700–63710)
- Shunt, Spinal CSF (63740–63746)

Injection, Drainage, or Aspiration

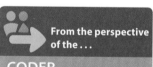

From the perspective of the . . .

CODER

It is necessary to review code descriptors to determine whether fluoroscopy is included in the procedure or not; if it is not included, it must be reported separately.

CPT codes 62263–62319 describe injection, drainage, or aspiration of spinal structures. Many of these codes include parenthetical instructions that provide guidance as to whether the code includes radiological services (e.g., fluoroscopy) or, if reported separately, what code is used to report those services. Injection of contrast material is included in the underlying code if radiological services are included or in the fluoroscopy code if reported separately.

CPT codes 62263 and 62264 describe percutaneous lysis of epidural adhesions utilizing injection of a solution or by mechanical disruption over multiple days (62263) or during multiple sessions during a single day (62264). The code descriptors indicate that these procedures include fluoroscopic guidance and the use of contrast material.

CPT code 62267 describes percutaneous aspiration of the nucleus pulposus, intervertebral disc, or soft tissues surrounding the spinal column for diagnostic purposes. This code does not include fluoroscopic guidance, and the parenthetical note indicates that fluoroscopy, if used, is reported with CPT code 77003.

Coding Distinctions

Spinal puncture and drainage of spinal fluid is reported with CPT code 62270 (diagnostic) or 62272 (therapeutic). Injection of blood into the epidural space (blood patch) at any level of the spine is described by CPT code 62273. Injections of neurolytic substances such as alcohol or phenol are described by three separate codes. CPT code 62280 is reported for subarachnoid injections at any level. In contrast, CPT code 62281 is reported for epidural injections at the cervical or thoracic levels, while CPT code 62282 is used to report epidural injections at the lumbar or sacral levels. Coders must ascertain whether a single code describes procedures at any level or separate codes are used to describe procedures at different levels.

CODING EXAMPLE

A 50-year-old man has severe pain radiating from his neck into his arms. After examining the patient completely, the physician orders a discography of C3–C4, C4–C5, and C5–C6 to determine whether these discs require surgical intervention. How would the coder report the disc injections for these procedures?

The coder looks up *discography* in the index and finds a subheading listing for injection with codes 62290–62291. The coder reviews these two codes in the manual and finds that code 62290 describes lumbar discography injections and code 62291 describes cervical discography injections. The coder reports 62291 X 3.

Another difference between codes is whether they describe a single injection or intermittent injections, which include continuous infusions. For example, CPT codes 62310 and 62311 describe single injections at either the cervical/thoracic or lumbar/sacral levels, whereas CPT codes 62318 and 62319 describe continuous infusions or intermittent boluses through an indwelling catheter at those levels. Coders must know how the substances were injected (single bolus versus intermittent injection) and the level at which they were injected (cervical/thoracic versus lumbar/sacral) to report the correct CPT code.

Implantation of Catheters

CPT codes 62350–62355 describe the implantation of **intrathecal** and **epidural** catheters for long-term infusion of medications through open procedures. Parenthetical notes indicate that percutaneous placement of a catheter is described by other codes. CPT codes 62360–62370 describe implantation, replacement, and removal of reservoirs and pumps often used with implanted catheters for medication infusion.

intrathecal
Situated or occurring under the arachnoid membrane of the brain or spinal cord; the location of spinal fluid.

epidural
Outside the dura.

Procedures on the Spine and Spinal Cord

Spinal structures may be approached from a number of directions, including the posterior, anterior, and lateral approaches as well as combinations such as posterior-lateral and anterior-lateral approaches. CPT codes 63001–63308 describe procedures performed through these approaches, with the codes divided into separate sections based on the particular approach. Each section includes a number of codes describing procedures performed using these approaches, including one or more add-on codes. The most common add-on codes are those used when a procedure described for a single spinal level is performed on additional levels of the spine. Similar to other codes describing procedures on the spine, separate codes are often used to describe procedures on the cervical/thoracic and lumbar/spinal levels. Each code section also includes a number of parenthetical notes instructing coders on which codes may be reported together and, even more importantly, which codes cannot be reported together. Coders must review and understand these instructions to report complex procedures correctly.

Some approaches to the spine, such as an anterior approach, require surgeons to go through the thoracic or peritoneal cavities (or both). Those procedures often involve two surgeons working together as co-surgeons to accomplish the approach and definitive procedure. When two surgeons work together as co-surgeons, each reports the code describing the procedure with modifier 62. Co-surgeons add this modifier to all codes describing procedures they perform together. If one surgeon assists the other on other procedures during the same operative period rather than acting as a co-surgeon, then he or she may report those procedures with modifier 80 or 82.

Stereotaxis and stereotactic radiosurgery procedures on the spine and/or spinal cord are described by CPT codes 63600–63621. As with the stereotactic radiosurgery codes that describe similar intracranial procedures, guidance instructions provide that radiation oncologists use radiation oncology codes 77621–77790 to report clinical treatment planning, treatment delivery, and management. Neurosurgeons reporting the stereotactic radiosurgery codes do not report the radiation oncology codes that describe planning, positioning, or blocking, as these are included in CPT codes 63620–63621. Also, similar to the intracranial stereotactic radiosurgery codes, these are reported only once even if the lesions are treated during multiple sessions. The notes indicate that these codes are only used when the tumor affects neural tissue or abuts dural tissue.

Neurostimulators

CPT codes 63650–63688 describe the placement, replacement, revision, and removal of spinal neurostimulators. These codes are used for both simple and complex stimulators. Separate codes describe percutaneous placement of a catheter with an electrode array (63650) and a laminectomy for the placement of a plate or paddle of electrodes (63655). Similarly, separate codes describe the removal or revision (which includes replacement) of neurostimulators placed percutaneously or via a laminectomy.

CODER'S TIP

CPT codes describing placement, replacement, revision, and removal of neurostimulators describe the surgical procedure, not the electrodes or generator. Those devices are usually reported with HCPCS Level II codes.

Spinal Repairs

CPT codes 63700–63706 describe repairs of meningocele and myelomeningocele defects that are either less than or greater than 5 cm in diameter. These procedures are most often performed in very young individuals, so a parenthetical note instructs coders not to attach modifier 63 to these codes when the procedure is performed on infants weighing less than 4 kg.

CPT codes 63707–63710 describe repairs of cerebrospinal fluid leaks, with different codes describing repairs that either require or do not require a laminectomy as part of the procedure. CPT codes 63740–63746 describe shunts to drain CSF from the spinal subarachnoid space to other locations, such as the peritoneal or pleural cavities. These codes include placement, replacement, revision, and removal of these shunts.

EXERCISE 12.6.3

Also available in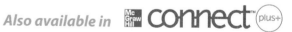

Use the CPT manual and index to select the best code to describe each procedure.

1. Epidural steroid injection, caudal _____
2. Implantation of a programmable pump for epidural drug infusion _____
3. Removal of an entire lumbosubarachnoid shunt system without replacement _____

12.6.4 Procedures on Extracranial Nerves, Peripheral Nerves, and the Autonomic Nervous System (64400–64999)

CPT codes describing procedures performed on various nerves are divided into the following code sections:

- Introduction/Injection of Anesthetic Agent (Nerve Block), Diagnostic or Therapeutic (64400–64530)
- Neurostimulators (Peripheral Nerve) (64550–64595)
- Destruction by Neurolytic Agent (e.g., Chemical, Thermal, Electrical, or Radiofrequency) (64600–64681)
- Neuroplasty (Exploration, Neurolysis, or Nerve Decompression) (64702–64727)
- Transection or Avulsion (64732–64772)
- Excision (64774–64823)
- Neurorrhaphy (64831–64876)
- Neurorrhaphy with Nerve Graft, Vein Graft, or Conduit (64885–64991)

Anesthetic Agents and Nerve Blocks

CPT codes 64400–64530 describe the injection of anesthetic agents for diagnostic or therapeutic blocks of nerves but not the use of neurolytic agents to destroy the nerves. Those procedures are described by other codes. The codes are divided into groups identifying somatic nerves, paravertebral spinal nerves, and autonomic nerves. Most of these blocks may be performed bilaterally. Modifier 50 is attached to the code if the procedure is performed bilaterally.

CPT codes describing blocks of somatic nerves (64400–64455) identify specific nerves or groups of nerves. Some nerve blocks include one code to describe a block that uses a single injection and a second code to describe continuous infusions or intermittent boluses through a catheter to block the same nerve. CPT codes 64479–64484 describe transforaminal epidural injections. These codes are divided by region (cervical/thoracic and lumbar/sacral) and describe the initial level injected and each additional level injected in those two regions. A parenthetical instruction directs coders to use the cervical/thoracic codes when reporting injections at the T12–L1 level. These codes were revised in 2011 with guidance to clarify that imaging must be used when performing these procedures. These codes cannot be reported if imaging (either fluoroscopy or CT) is not used.

> **CODER'S TIP**
>
> CPT codes 64400–64455 describe injections of peripheral nerves. These codes are differentiated from each other by the specific nerve injected and whether the patient undergoes a single injection or continuous infusion.

Blocks of the paravertebral facet (zygapophyseal joint) are described by CPT codes 64490–64495. Imaging guidance (fluoroscopy or CT) is required to report these codes. If imaging guidance is not used during these procedures, they are reported as trigger point injections with CPT codes 20552–20553. As with other spinal injection codes, these are divided into the cervical/thoracic and lumbar/sacral regions. For each region, one code describes the first level injected. An add-on code is used when a second level is injected, and a second add-on code is used when three or more levels are injected. It is important to understand that the second add-on code is reported only once, even if more than three levels are injected.

A patient is seeing a pain physician because he has severe pain in his lower back that radiates into his right leg. The physician decides to inject an anesthetic agent into the facet joints at L3–L4, L4–L5, and L5–S1. He uses fluoroscopic guidance to confirm injections into the facet joints. How are these injections reported?

The coder finds the spinal injection codes by looking up *injection* in the index, then the subheading "Nerve," which has a listing for anesthetic followed by codes 64400–64530. Turning to these individual codes, she finds that lumbar facet joint nerve injections are reported with codes 64493–64495. The first-level injection is reported with 64493, the second-level injection is reported with add-on code 64494, and the third-level injection is reported with add-on code 64495. The fluoroscopy is not separately reported according to the parenthetical notes. The notes also instruct coders not to report these codes if the procedure is not performed with either fluoroscopic or CT guidance.

The coder reports these injections with codes 64493, 64494, and 64495.

CPT codes 64505–64530 describe autonomic nerve blocks, including the sphenopalatine ganglion, carotid sinus, stellate ganglion, superior hypogastric plexus, lumbar or thoracic sympathetic, and celiac plexus nerves.

Nerve Stimulators

Peripheral nerve stimulators are described by CPT codes 64550–64595. These codes include application of transcutaneous neurostimulators (64550), percutaneous implantation, and open procedures to implant stimulators. This series of codes includes procedures involving cranial nerves. This series of codes differentiates between cranial nerves, nonspecific peripheral nerves, and several specific peripheral nerves such as sacral nerves and the posterior tibial nerve. Guidance preceding this series of codes instructs coders to use CPT codes 95970–95975 to describe electronic analysis and programming of neurostimulators. In addition, several parenthetical instructions direct coders to other code sections to describe placement or replacement of generators.

Nerve Destruction

CPT codes 64600–64681 describe the destruction of nerves by neurolytic agents (e.g., chemical, thermal, electrical, or radiofrequency). Specific codes describe procedures on trigeminal nerve branches, facial nerves, and nerves in the neck, trunk, and extremities. Injections of neurolytic agents into the paravertebral facet joint are described by a series of codes (64633–64636). These codes describe a single facet injection at the cervical/thoracic level (64633) and the lumbar/sacral level (64635). Each additional facet joint injection is reported with add-on codes describing cervical/thoracic facet injections (64634) and lumbar/sacral facet injections (64636). Bilateral injections at the same level are reported with the appropriate code and the 50-modifier. Parenthetical Guidance states that fluoroscopic or CT guidance must be used to report code 64634–64636.

Nerve Repairs

Neuroplasty includes decompression of an intact nerve from scar tissue or from other tissue compressing the nerve. CPT codes 64702–64727 describe neuroplasty procedures on various nerves. Some codes describe procedures on specific nerves. One add-on code (64727) is used when an operating microscope is used as part of the procedure.

A series of CPT codes describes transection of certain specific nerves (64732–64772) and the excision of somatic nerves (64774–64795) and sympathetic nerves (64802–64823). Parenthetical notes instruct coders on the use of modifier 50 to describe bilateral procedures and identify those codes that cannot be combined with add-on code 69990 (Microsurgical techniques, requiring use of operating microscope).

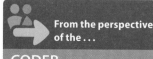

From the perspective of the . . .

CODER

When reporting nerve repairs, it is necessary to know the individual nerve that was repaired as well as the method of repair (e.g., direct repair versus placement of a nerve graft, vein graft, or conduit).

Nerve repairs are described by two series of CPT codes. The first series (64831–64876) describes direct nerve repairs, whereas a second series (64885–64911) describes repairs using nerve grafts, vein grafts, or conduits.

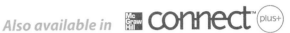
EXERCISE 12.6.4

Use the CPT manual and index to select the best code to describe each procedure.

1. Injection of a facial nerve with an anesthetic agent _____

2. Injection of diagnostic agent, paravertebral facet joint with imaging guidance, L3–L5 _____

3. Revision of a gastric neurostimulator pulse generator _____

12.6.5 Procedures on Ocular Structures (65091–68899)

Procedures on the eye and ocular structures include several broad anatomical divisions:

- Eyeball (65091–65290)
- Anterior Segment (65400–66999)
- Posterior Segment (67005–67299)
- Ocular Adnexa (67311–67999)
- Conjunctiva (68020–68899)

Eyeball

Procedures on the eyeball include removal of the eye, secondary implant procedures, removal of foreign bodies, and laceration repairs. Codes describing removal of the eye (65091–65114) differentiate between evisceration and enucleation as well as whether an ocular implant is used at the time of the original surgery.

CODER'S TIP

Evisceration describes the removal of the contents within the eyeball, leaving the shell of the eye in place. CPT code 65091 describes evisceration without an implant, whereas code 65093 describes the same procedure with placement of an implant. Enucleation describes the removal of the entire eyeball. Three codes describe these procedures: code 65101 describes enucleation without an implant; code 65103 describes the procedure with an implant that does not have the ocular muscles attached; and code 65105 describes the same procedure with the ocular muscles attached to the implant.

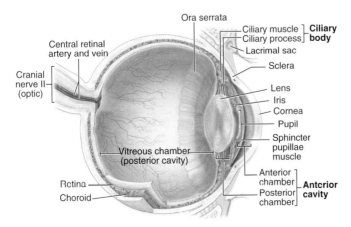

FIGURE 12.6.4 Anatomy of the Eyeball

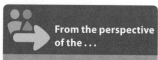
Secondary implant procedures (65125–65175) include placement of initial implants subsequent to the initial procedure, revision or replacement of existing implants, or removal of an ocular implant. These procedures do not include the use of orbital implants. Ocular implants are placed inside the cone formed by the ocular muscles. Orbital implants are those that are outside the muscle cone. A parenthetical instruction directs coders to use CPT code 67550 for the placement of an orbital implant and code 67560 for its removal.

CPT codes 65205–65265 describe removal of foreign bodies from different ocular structures including the conjunctiva, cornea, and anterior or posterior chamber. Parenthetical instructions direct coders to other code sections for removal of various ocular implants.

Laceration repairs described by CPT codes 65270–65290 include repairs of the conjunctiva, sclera, cornea, and extraocular muscles. Repairs of these structures are differentiated by the severity of the underlying laceration.

Anterior Segment

The anterior segment includes the following structures: cornea, anterior chamber, anterior sclera, iris, ciliary body, and lens. Groups of CPT codes describe procedures on each of these structures. Procedures on the cornea (CPT codes 65400–65782) are divided into the following categories: excisions, removal or destruction, keratoplasty, and other procedures. Excisions include excisions of lesions, biopsies, and excisions of pterygiums. Removal or destruction of corneal tissues includes scraping and removal of partial thickness of corneal epithelial tissues.

Corneal transplants, or keratoplasties, are described by several codes, depending on the type of transplant. The backbench preparation of the donor material is included in the code describing the transplant procedure for most transplants. For endothelial transplants (CPT code 65756), the backbench preparation of the endothelial graft prior to transplant is reported separately using add-on code 65757.

Other corneal procedures include radial keratotomy, corneal relaxing incisions, and corneal wedge resections for correction of visual abnormalities. The use of amniotic membrane material as a corneal surface covering for wound healing is described by two codes, one describing the use of the membrane as a self-retaining covering (65778) and the other describing the use of a membrane that is sutured in place (65779).

Procedures on the anterior chamber include incisions on structures within the chamber (65800–65880), removal of material from within the chamber (65900–65930), and injection of air, liquid, or medications into the chamber (66020–66030).

Procedures involving the anterior sclera include numerous procedures for the treatment of glaucoma, including fistulization of the sclera, trabeculectomy, and dilation of the aqueous outflow canal and aqueous shunt (CPT codes 66130–66250). Procedures on the iris and ciliary body include incisions, excisions, repair, and destruction (66500–66770).

Numerous CPT codes (66820–66986) describe intraocular lens procedures, including multiple cataract procedures that involve the removal of the natural lens with and without the insertion of an artificial intraocular lens.

Posterior Segment

The posterior segment consists of the vitreous, retina, choroid, and posterior sclera. Procedures on the vitreous are described by CPT codes 67005–67043, including removal of vitreous (vitrectomy) by several different approaches and methods. Two codes describe implantation of an intravitreal drug delivery system (67027) and injection of a drug into the vitreous (67028). Several codes describe vitrectomy in combination with other procedures (67036–67043).

CPT codes 67101–67121 describe retinal repairs by a variety of different procedures, including cryotherapy, diathermy, photocoagulation, and scleral buckle procedures. Other codes (67208–67229) describe procedures to destroy retinal and/or choroidal lesions.

CODING EXAMPLE

A patient sees her ophthalmologist because of decreased vision over the past few days. The physician examines the patient's eyes and determines that there is an abnormal lesion on the retina that needs to be treated. The physician decides to use photocoagulation to destroy the lesion. How should this be reported?

The coder looks up *retina* in the index and finds the subheading "Lesion" with an indented entry for localized destruction and listings for codes 67208–67218. Looking at these codes in the full list, the coder finds that destruction of a localized lesion of the retina with photocoagulation is reported with code 67210.

Ocular Adnexa

Six extraocular muscles are attached to the eyeball to allow motion in all directions. It is sometimes necessary to move or reconfigure these muscles to correct misalignment of the eyes. CPT codes 67311–67345 describe various procedures on the eye muscles, including procedures involving one or both horizontal muscles, one vertical muscle, two or more vertical muscles, the superior oblique muscle, and muscle transpositions.

Procedures involving the orbit, including the bony structures surrounding the eye, are described by CPT codes 67400–67599. In addition to procedures on the bones of the orbit, these codes describe retrobulbar injections (placing a needle behind the eye to inject medications or neurolytic agents) and orbital implants, which are outside the cone of muscles that attach to the eye.

Procedures on the eyelids include incisions, excisions, destruction of eyelid lesions, tarsorrhaphy (temporary and permanent closure of the upper and lower lids), repairs, and reconstruction of the lids and brow. CPT codes 67700–67999 describe these procedures.

Conjunctiva

CPT codes 68020–68899 describe procedures involving the conjunctiva, including incision and drainage, excision and destruction, injections, and conjunctivoplasties. This section of codes also describes procedures on the lacrimal system (tear ducts), including incisions, repairs, probing to open the ducts, and plugging the ducts to close them off.

EXERCISE 12.6.5

Also available in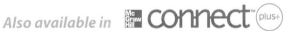

Use the CPT manual and index to select the best code to describe each procedure.

1. Removal of a foreign body, external eye, corneal, without slit lamp _____
2. Removal of lens material, intracapsular _____
3. Release of posterior segment encircling material _____

12.6.6 Procedures on the Auditory System (69000–69979)

CPT codes describing procedures on the auditory system are organized by the anatomical structures that comprise this system:

- External Ear (69000–69320)
- Middle Ear (69400–69799)
- Inner Ear (69801–69949)
- Temporal Bone, Middle Fossa Approach (69950–69979)

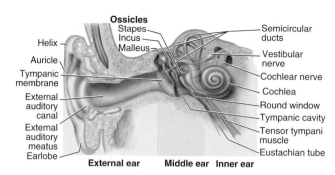

Ossicles
Stapes
Incus
Malleus
Helix
Auricle
Tympanic
membrane
External
auditory
canal
External
auditory
meatus
Earlobe

Semicircular
ducts
Vestibular
nerve
Cochlear nerve
Cochlea
Round window
Tympanic cavity
Tensor tympani
muscle
Eustachian tube

External ear   Middle ear Inner ear

FIGURE 12.6.5 Anatomy of the Ear

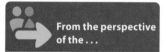

From the perspective of the . . .

CODER

It is extremely important that coders review the parenthetical guidance associated with these codes to properly report removal procedures. For example, these notes instruct coders to use modifier 50 to report bilateral debridement procedures of the mastoidectomy cavity (69220 and 69222). However, when reporting the bilateral removal of impacted cerumen, CPT code 69210 is reported only once without any modifier because the code descriptor includes the phrase "one or both ears."

External Ear

Structures of the external ear include the external ear, the external auditory canal, and the mastoid. Procedures on these anatomical structures include incision, excision, removal, and repair. Incision (69000–69090) describes drainage of abscesses or hematomas of the external ear or external auditory canal. Excision (69100–69155) includes a wide range of procedures from a simple biopsy of the external ear to a radical excision of an auditory canal lesion combined with a radical neck dissection.

Removal procedures include the removal of a foreign body or impacted cerumen (earwax) and debridement of the mastoidectomy cavity. These codes do not describe primary mastoidectomy procedures, only debridement of the contents from the cavity resulting from prior mastoidectomy procedures.

Repair procedures include repair of the external ear (69300) and reconstruction of the external auditory canal (69310 and 69320). Parenthetical notes refer coders to other sections for suture of a wound or injury of the external ear or for reconstruction procedures involving the middle ear.

Middle Ear

The structures of the middle ear include the eardrum (tympanic membrane) and three bones (the malleus, incus, and stapes). Procedures on these structures include introduction, incision, excision, repair, and other procedures.

CODER'S TIP

Some incision codes include the term *myringotomy* in their descriptors, while other codes include the term *tympanostomy* in the descriptor. Both terms describe procedures on the tympanic membrane (eardrum). Myringotomy is used when the membrane is opened but allowed to close and heal after the procedure. Tympanostomy is used when the membrane is opened and kept open by inserting a tube through the membrane to keep it from healing closed until the tube is later removed.

The excision codes (69501–69554) include various mastoidectomy procedures ranging from simple mastoidectomy to radical mastoidectomy. These codes also describe the excision of polyps and certain tumors within the middle ear.

Some repair codes (69601–69676) describe revisions of previous mastoidectomy procedures that result in a more extensive mastoidectomy. The original mastoidectomy would not be described by these codes, but rather with codes from the Excision section. Other repair codes describe tympanoplasty procedures either alone or in combination with a number of other procedures such as surgery on the bones of the middle ear. Coders must understand the complete extent of the procedure to select the correct code to report a tympanoplasty.

Inner Ear

Structures within the inner ear include the semicircular canals, the cochlea, and the vestibulocochlear nerve. CPT codes 69801–69949 describe procedures on these structures, including incision (placing an opening in one of these structures), excision (removal of an anatomical structure), and introduction (placement of a cochlear implant to treat deafness due to specific causes).

CODING EXAMPLE

A patient has a permanent hole in his eardrum as a result of numerous ear infections as a child. The surgeon performs a repair of the tympanic membrane. How should the coder report this procedure?

The coder looks up *ear* in the index and locates the subheading "Drum," which lists a number of codes describing incision, excision, and repair procedures. Under the Repair section, the coder locates code 69610, which includes a tympanic membrane repair in the descriptor. The coder reports code 69610.

Temporal Bone, Middle Fossa Approach

These codes describe procedures on the temporal bone or structures within the middle fossa when approached through the cranium. These include procedures on the vestibular nerve (69950), facial nerve decompression or repair (69955), decompression of the internal auditory canal (69960), and removal of a temporal bone tumor (69970). A parenthetical instruction directs coders to use CPT code 69535 if the temporal bone is resected using an external rather than middle fossa approach.

CODER'S TIP

A parenthetical instruction included in this section directs coders to use CPT code 69535 (Resection temporal bone, external approach) if the procedure is not performed using the middle fossa approach.

Operating Microscope

This section of the CPT manual includes a single add-on code, 69990 (Microsurgical techniques, requiring use of operating microscope [List separately in addition to code for primary procedure]). This code is used when a surgical procedure that may or may not be performed microscopically is, in fact, performed using an operating microscope. Because this is an add-on code, modifier 51 is not appended to this code. Guidance included in this section provides specific instructions regarding the use of this add-on code. The use of magnifying glasses, commonly called magnifying loupes, does not constitute the use of an operating microscope, so this code would not be used. The guidance also includes a number of codes that describe procedures that are almost always performed with the use of the operating microscope, so the add-on code cannot be used with those procedure codes. This list is likely to change from year to year, so it is important for coders to review the list in the current CPT manual when reporting this code.

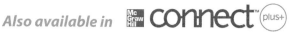
Use the CPT manual and index to select the best code to describe each procedure.

1. Myringoplasty _____

2. Tympanoplasty _____

3. Operating microscope _____

12.6.7 Coding for Anesthesia for Procedures in the 60000 Series

CPT codes describing anesthesia for procedures located in the 60000 series of CPT codes are listed in multiple sections of anesthesia codes because the 60000 codes describe procedures on many different anatomical structures. These range from procedures on the head, neck, and spine to procedures on nerves in every anatomical region of the body. Commonly used anesthesia codes for procedures in the 60000 series are listed in Table 12.6.1.

TABLE 12.6.1 Commonly Used Anesthesia Codes for Procedures in the 60000 Series

Code(s)	Procedure Reported
00120–00148	Anesthesia for procedures on the ears and eyes
00210–00222	Anesthesia for intracranial procedures
00320–00322	Anesthesia for procedures on the thyroid
00540–00541	Anesthesia for procedures on the thorax (approach to thoracic spine)
00600–00670	Anesthesia for procedures on the spine and spinal cord
00866	Anesthesia for adrenalectomy
01180–01190	Anesthesia for obturator neurectomy
01250	Anesthesia for procedures on the nerves of the upper leg
01320	Anesthesia for procedures on the nerves of the knee and popliteal area
01470	Anesthesia for procedures on the nerves of the lower leg
01610	Anesthesia for procedures on the nerves of the shoulder
01710	Anesthesia for procedures on the nerves of the upper arm and elbow
01810	Anesthesia for procedures on the nerves of the forearm, wrist, and hand
01926	Anesthesia for therapeutic interventional radiological procedures involving the arterial system; intracranial
01935–01936	Anesthesia for percutaneous image-guided procedures on the spine and spinal cord
01991–01992	Anesthesia for diagnostic and therapeutic spinal nerve blocks
01996	Daily hospital management of epidural or subarachnoid continuous drug administration

CODING EXAMPLE

A surgeon performs an intracranial vascular procedure with the patient in the sitting position. How should the coder report the anesthesia for this position?

The coder can look up *anesthesia* in the index and locate the subheading "Craniotomy" to find the anesthesia codes for intracranial procedures in the 00210–00222 range. Reviewing each of these codes, the coder finds that only one code describes anesthesia for intracranial procedures in the sitting position, code 00218.

EXERCISE 12.6.7

Also available in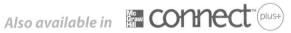

Use the CPT manual to select the best code to describe anesthesia for each procedure.

1. Excision of a neuroma, cutaneous, surgically identifiable _____

2. Injection of an anesthetic agent; trigeminal nerve, any division or branch _____

3. Reinsertion of an ocular implant with or without a conjunctival graft _____

4. Canthoplasty (reconstruction of the canthus) _____

5. Suture of the sciatic nerve _____

6. Revision or removal of a cranial neurostimulator pulse generator or receiver _____

MODULE **12.6** REVIEW

Summary

Learning Outcome	Key Concepts/Examples
12.6.1 Differentiate among procedures on the endocrine system. **Pages 401–402**	This section of codes describes procedures on many, but not all, endocrine glands including the thyroid, parathyroid, thymus, adrenals, and carotid body. Commonly performed procedures include incision and excision. Procedures on the adrenal gland may be open or laparoscopic.
12.6.2 Contrast procedures on the skull, meninges, and brain. **Pages 402–405**	Codes describing procedures on the nervous system are divided into sections based on anatomical structures. Procedures on the skull, meninges, and brain include craniotomy, craniectomy, surgery on the base of the skull, vascular procedures, and the placement of neurostimulators.
12.6.3 Explain procedures involving the spine and spinal cord. **Pages 405–408**	Procedures on the spine and spinal cord include laminotomy, laminectomy, incision, excision, decompression, stereotactic surgery, and the placement of neurostimulators.
12.6.4 Identify procedures on the extracranial nerves, peripheral nerves, and autonomic nervous system. **Pages 409–410**	Codes describing procedures on the peripheral nerves include injection, destruction by neurolytic agent, neuroplasty, neurorrhaphy, and the placement of neurostimulators.
12.6.5 Describe the major anatomical structures of the eye and surgical procedures performed on those structures. **Pages 411–413**	Ocular system procedures include removal of the entire eye, anterior segment surgery, posterior segment surgery, and procedures on the ocular adnexa and conjunctiva. Common procedures include incision, excision, repair, reconstruction, and destruction.
12.6.6 Explain the major procedures performed on the auditory system. **Pages 413–415**	Auditory system procedures are divided according to anatomical location, including external ear, middle ear, and inner ear. The most common procedures include incision, excision, removal, and repair.
12.6.7 Code anesthesia services for procedures in the 60000 series. **Pages 416–417**	Anesthesia codes for procedures in the 60000 series occur in many different sections of anesthesia codes. These codes range from procedures on the head, neck, and spine to procedures on nerves in every anatomical region of the body.

Using Terminology

Match each term with its definition.

_____ **1.** [LO12.6.1] Adrenal glands

_____ **2.** [LO12.6.2] Epidural

_____ **3.** [LO12.6.2] Craniectomy

_____ **4.** [LO12.6.6] Cranioplasty

_____ **5.** [LO12.6.2] Craniotomy

_____ **6.** [LO12.6.2] Gonads

_____ **7.** [LO12.6.3] Meninges

A. Endocrine gland located in the mediastinum

B. A gland that secretes many different hormones that affect the body either directly or by causing other glands to produce hormones

C. Above the dura

D. Upper part of the brain

E. Bone that forms part of the base and sides of the skull

F. Three-layered covering of the brain and spinal cord

_____	**8.** [L012.6.2] Occipital bones	**G.**	Opening of the skull
_____	**9.** [L012.6.4] Pancreas	**H.**	Excision of part of the skull
_____	**10.** [L012.6.5] Pituitary	**I.**	Endocrine gland in the neck
_____	**11.** [L012.6.2] Supratentorial	**J.**	Testes or ovaries
_____	**12.** [L012.6.5] Temporal	**K.**	Organ located on the top of each kidney.
_____	**13.** [L012.6.1] Thymus	**L.**	A large, curved, elongated gland that lies behind the stomach
_____	**14.** [L012.6.2] Thyroid	**M.**	The back of the skull
		N.	Surgical correction of skull defects

Checking Your Understanding

Select the letter that best completes the statement or answers the question.

1. L012.6.1 Portions of the endocrine system covered by CPT codes 60000-60699 include which of the following glands?

  a. Reproductive endocrine system
  b. Pituitary and pineal glands
  c. Thyroid, parathyroid, thymus, adrenal glands, pancreas, and carotid body
  d. All of the above

2. L012.6.2 The medical term _____ means to divert or bypass in order to make an artificial passageway.

  a. Stent
  b. Shunt
  c. Burr hole
  d. Dilation

3. L012.6.5 The code that describes the destruction of a corneal lesion by means of cryotherapy is:

  a. 65400
  b. 65450
  c. 65435
  d. 65410

4. L012.6.3 The code that describes a single epidural steroid injection of the lumbar spine is:

  a. 62310
  b. 62311
  c. 62318
  d. 62319

5. L012.6.2 Codes in the 61304–61576 range describe craniectomy and craniotomy procedures. The selection of the most appropriate code is dependent on which criteria?

  a. The underlying reason for the procedure
  b. Location
  c. The specific procedure performed through the skull opening
  d. All of the above

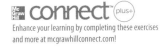

Enhance your learning by completing these exercises
and more at mcgrawhillconnect.com!

6. L012.6.2 CPT code 61711 describes anastomosis between extracranial and intracranial arteries. This procedure is used to:

   a. Bypass arterial occlusions or injuries.
   b. Connect arteries from outside the skull to others within the skull.
   c. Increase or dilate the passage.
   d. Bypass occlusions and connect arteries.

7. L012.6.1 When is add-on code 62160 used with placement of a shunt?

   a. If the shunt is placed via endoscope
   b. If the shunt is placed through an open procedure
   c. Always used with placement of a shunt
   d. Never used with placement of a shunt

8. L012.6.5 What would be the appropriate CPT code to describe the evisceration of ocular contents without an implant?

   a. 65093
   b. 65091
   c. 65101
   d. 65105

9. L012.6.3 For spinal injection codes 62273–62319, what information is necessary to select the correct codes to describe these services?

   a. Whether a single injection or continuous infusion is involved
   b. The spinal level where the injection occurs
   c. Whether a single code describes the injection or multiple codes are needed
   d. All of the above

10. L012.6.6 Which code describes an external approach to the temporal bone rather than through the middle fossa?

    a. 69535
    b. 69955
    c. 69970
    d. 69950

Applying Your Skills

Use the CPT manual to determine the correct code to report the following procedures.

1. L012.6.2 Exploratory infratentorial craniectomy _____

2. L012.6.2 Bifrontal bone flap craniotomy for craniosynostosis _____

3. L012.6.1 Complete adrenalectomy with biopsy and excision of an adjacent retroperitoneal tumor _____

4. L012.6.4 Anesthetic agent injection of the ilioinguinal nerve _____

5. L012.6.6 Repair of the tympanic membrane _____

6. L012.6.5 Sclera repair with glue _____

7. L012.6.3 Single epidural steroid injection at L3–L4 _____

8. L012.6.5 Implantation of an intravitreal drug delivery system _____

9. L012.6.3 Lumbar laminectomy without facetectomy involving three levels with decompression of the spinal cord _____

10. L012.6.3 Transforaminal epidural steroid injection of the lumbar spine with fluoroscopic guidance, two levels _____

11. L012.6.3 Transforaminal epidural steroid injection of the lumbar spine with ultrasound guidance _____

12. L012.6.4 Transposition of the ulnar nerve at the elbow _____

13. L012.6.5 Repair of retinal detachment with vitrectomy and scleral buckling _____

14. L012.6.6 Insertion of a cochlear implant _____

15. L012.6.3 Repair of a 4.0 cm meningocele _____

Thinking It Through

Use your critical-thinking skills to answer the questions below.

1. L012.6.2 Explain why procedures on the base of the skull often involve several surgeons of different specialties and why the procedures often are not described by a single code.

_____

_____

_____

_____

2. L012.6.6 Explain the difference between a myringotomy and a tympanostomy.

_____

_____

_____

_____

3. L012.6.6 Explain the guidelines for the use of CPT code 69990.

_____

_____

_____

_____

connect plus+
Enhance your learning by completing these exercises
and more at mcgrawhillconnect.com!
MODULE 12.6 | ENDOCRINE, NERVOUS, OCULAR, AND AUDITORY SYSTEMS   421

13 PATHOLOGY AND LABORATORY SERVICES

Learning Outcomes *After completing this chapter, students should be able to:*

13.1 Differentiate between organ and disease-oriented panels and the individual codes used to report those tests.

13.2 Explain how to report laboratory tests related to drugs and medicines.

13.3 Identify codes to report laboratory tests.

13.4 Select appropriate codes to describe pathology services.

Key Terms

Anatomic pathology

Chemistry

Complete blood count (CBC)

Drug test

Evocative/suppression testing

Laboratory

Microscopy

Organ/disease panel

Partial thromboplastin time (PTT)

Prothrombin time (PT)

Qualitative

Quantitative

Red blood cell (RBC)

Specimen

Surgical pathology

Therapeutic level

Urinalysis (UA)

White blood cell (WBC)

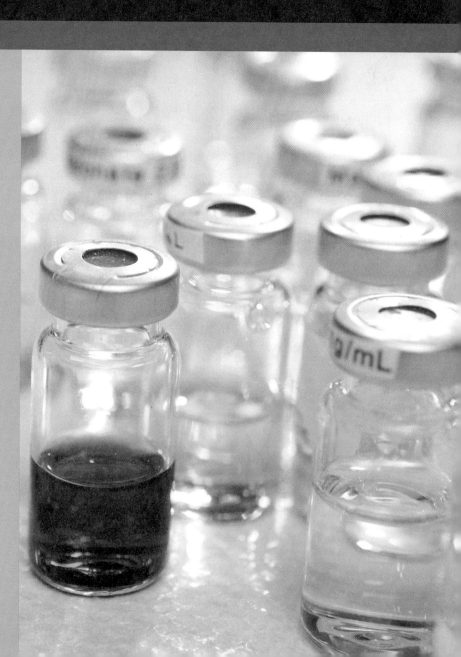

Introduction

Many healthcare professionals rely on laboratory tests to help make or confirm diagnoses, follow patients with known diseases, and monitor the effects of treatments with very potent medications. These tests are not only helpful but may be critical. Laboratory tests and other specialized services provided by pathologists are listed in the Pathology and Laboratory chapter, which is comprised of the 80000 series of CPT codes. These CPT codes are divided into the following types of services:

- Organ or Disease-Oriented Panels (80047–80076)
- Drug Testing (80100–80103)
- Therapeutic Drug Assays (80150–80299)
- Evocative/Suppression Testing (80400–80440)
- Consultations (Clinical Pathology) (80500–80502)
- Urinalysis (81000–81099)
- Chemistry (82000–84999)
- Hematology and Coagulation (85000–85999)
- Immunology (86000–86849)
- Transfusion Medicine (86850–86999)
- Microbiology (87001–87999)
- Anatomic Pathology (Postmortem Examination) (88000–88099)
- Cytopathology (88104–88199)
- Cytogenetic Studies (88230–88299)
- Surgical Pathology (88300–88399)
- In Vivo Laboratory Procedures (e.g., Transcutaneous) (88720–88741)
- Other Procedures (89049–89240)
- Reproductive Medicine Procedures (89250–89398)

Many code sections have guidance materials preceding the list of specific codes. It is important for coders to review these materials. Instructions in the guidance material may change from year to year, so over time even the most experienced coders may no longer be correctly reporting services.

Parenthetical notations follow some code descriptors. These instruct coders on how to correctly report situations that may be similar to, but not exactly the same as, the one described in the code descriptor. If present, it is imperative that coders review the comments before reporting the code to ascertain whether the situation being reported is accurately reflected in the code selected or if another code might be more appropriate.

To locate the CPT code for a specific test, it is best practice to use the index to find one or more codes for tests involving the particular substance in question. The coder then reviews each listed code to determine which is the most appropriate for the specific test performed. Some index listings do not have a code associated with them, but instead refer to other listings that include specific codes.

13.1 Organ or Disease-Oriented Panels (80047–80076)

There are ten **organ panels** or **disease-oriented panels** of **laboratory** tests described in the CPT manual. According to the CPT guidance, these panels were developed for coding purposes only and are not clinical guidelines as to which tests are appropriate for specific clinical settings. Physicians commonly use these panels to screen for or diagnose various diseases. Physicians may also use these tests to follow a patient who has a number of different diseases. The panel components do not limit whether other tests may be performed. If additional tests are performed, they should be reported separately using the appropriate CPT codes. Organ or disease-oriented panels listed in the CPT are shown in Table 13.1.

organ/disease-oriented panel
A predefined cluster of laboratory tests to evaluate a diseased organ, organ system, or disease.

laboratory
A facility designed to perform tests on specimens.

TABLE 13.1 Organ or Disease-Oriented Panels (80047–80076)

CPT Code	Panel	Tests in Panel
80047	Basic metabolic panel (ionized calcium)	Calcium, ionized Carbon dioxide Chloride Creatinine Glucose Potassium Sodium Urea nitrogen (BUN)
80048	Basic metabolic panel (total calcium)	Calcium, ionized Carbon dioxide Chloride Creatinine Glucose Potassium Sodium Urea nitrogen (BUN)
80050	General health panel	Comprehensive metabolic health panel Complete blood count (CBC) with either an automated or manual differential white blood count (WBC) Thyroid-stimulating hormone
80051	Electrolyte panel	Carbon dioxide Chloride Potassium Sodium
80053	Comprehensive metabolic health panel	Albumin Bilirubin, total Calcium, total Carbon dioxide Chloride Creatinine Glucose Phosphatase, alkaline Potassium Protein, total Sodium Transferase, alanine amino (ALT or SGPT) Transferase, aspartate amino (AST or SGOT) Urea nitrogen (BUN)
80055	Obstetric panel	Complete blood count (CBC) with either an automated or manual differential white blood count (WBC) Hepatitis B surface antigen (HBsAg) Antibody, rubella Syphilis test, nontreponemal antibody; qualitative Antibody screen, red blood cell (RBC) Blood typing, ABO and Rh(D)
80061	Lipid panel	Cholesterol, serum, total Lipoprotein, direct measurement, high-density cholesterol (HDL) Triglycerides

(Continued)

TABLE 13.1 *(Concluded)*

CPT Code	Panel	Tests in Panel
80069	Renal function panel	Albumin Calcium, total Carbon dioxide Chloride Creatinine Glucose Phosphorus inorganic (phosphate) Potassium Sodium Urea nitrogen (BUN)
80074	Acute hepatitis panel	Hepatitis A antibody (HAAb), immunoglobulin M (IgM) antibody Hepatitis B core antibody (HBcAb), IgM antibody Hepatitis B surface antigen (HBsAg) Hepatitis C antibody
80076	Hepatic function panel	Albumin Bilirubin, total Bilirubin, direct Phosphatase, alkaline Protein, total Transferase, alanine amino (ALT or SGPT) Transferase, aspartate amino (AST or SGOT)

CODER'S TIP

Coders cannot report a code for a laboratory panel if any of the component tests for that panel were not performed. Coders cannot add modifier 52 (reduced services) to a code identifying a panel to indicate that not all the tests were performed. If not all the tests were performed, report the codes that describe the individual tests that were provided.

CODING EXAMPLE

A laboratory performs carbon dioxide, chloride, creatinine, glucose, potassium, sodium, and urea nitrogen tests but does not perform an ionized calcium test. How should the lab coder report these tests?

It is incorrect to report this with CPT code 80047 (Basic metabolic panel [Calcium, ionized]) because the ionized calcium test was not performed. It is also incorrect to report each of these tests individually because there is a panel that includes most of them.

The coder uses CPT code 80051 to report this series of tests (electrolyte panel, which includes the carbon dioxide, chloride, potassium, and sodium tests) and separately reports CPT codes 82565 (creatinine), 82947 (glucose), and 84520 (urea nitrogen) to describe those tests.

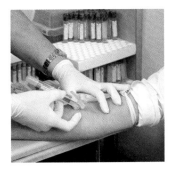

Many laboratory tests begin with the drawing of a patient's blood.

In some instances, two or more panels may describe some of the tests performed. It is not appropriate to report more than one panel when the tests overlap. Coders should report the largest panel that describes some or all of the tests performed. Any additional tests are reported separately.

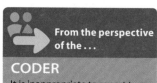

From the perspective of the . . .

CODER

It is inappropriate to report two lab panels if the tests in those panels overlap.

CODER'S TIP

It is incorrect to report both 80047 and 80051 to describe the same series of tests. The tests described by code 80051 are all included in code 80047, which is a larger panel, so that code is used and any additional tests, if performed, are reported separately.

Similarly, the general health panel (80050) includes all the tests listed in the comprehensive metabolic panel (80053) plus additional tests.

EXERCISE 13.1

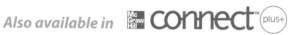
Also available in

Use the CPT manual and index to answer the following questions.

1. Which code(s) would a laboratory report if the physician orders a lipid panel? _____

2. List one way to locate the code(s) for a lipid panel in the index. _____

3. What codes would the laboratory report if it performed an SGOT, SGPT, BUN, and urinalysis? _____

4. A physician orders almost all of the tests contained in a metabolic panel but not all of them. Can the laboratory report the code for the metabolic panel because they did most of the tests? Explain your answer. _____

5. Can a comprehensive metabolic panel and a general health panel be reported at the same time? Explain your answer. _____

13.2 Lab Tests Involving Drugs or Medicines (80100–80440)

Drug Testing

qualitative

Indicates whether or not a particular substance is present in a sample.

drug test

A chemical test used to evaluate the presence of a particular drug.

quantitative

Determines how much (quantity) of a substance is present in a sample.

Many individual drugs or drug classes can be detected in a biological sample such as blood or urine. These are usually detected through a **qualitative** screen. If that screen is positive, a second confirmation procedure is performed. Both the initial screening **drug test** and the second confirmation test are qualitative. Neither of these tests would indicate the amount of the drug present in the sample. These qualitative tests are reported using CPT codes 80100–80104. Although the CPT manual lists 13 drug classes for which these tests may be performed, each of which may include a number of specific drugs, there are only five codes to describe these qualitative drug tests. If a **quantitative** test of a particular drug is necessary, those tests are reported using the therapeutic drug assay codes (80150–80299) or the chemistry codes (82000–84999) discussed below.

CODER'S TIP

It is important to understand the difference between a qualitative test and a quantitative test, as this often makes a difference when it comes to code selection.

A qualitative test only shows that a substance is present in the sample, not how much is there. A quantitative test reports the amount of the substance present in the sample. If the results of the test are reported with an amount (quantity), the test is by definition a quantitative test. Some test results are reported as positive or negative. These are qualitative tests because no amount or quantity is reported with the test results.

A laboratory performs a test to determine the amount of human chorionic gonadotropin, or hCG, present in a patient's blood sample. How is this test reported?

To determine the correct code to report this test, the coder can look up either *human chorionic gonadotropin* or *hCG* in the index. Both appear in the alphabetical listing, but instead of providing CPT codes, each of these entries refers to the listing for chorionic gonadotropin. Turning to that listing, several code options appear, including 84702 (Gonadotropin, chorionic [hCG], quantitative) and 84703 (Gonadotropin, chorionic [hCG], qualitative). Because the test provided an amount of this substance present in the blood sample, the quantitative code (84702) is the appropriate code.

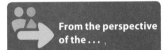

From the perspective of the . . .

CODER

If a qualitative test is performed to determine whether a particular drug is present in the sample, followed by a quantitative test to determine the amount of that drug present in the sample, both codes are reported as separate services. These are separate tests and, as such, they are reported separately.

Therapeutic Drug Assay

It is sometimes necessary to determine whether a particular medication is at a **therapeutic level,** meaning that it is present in sufficient quantity to have the desired effect, but the amount is not so high that it is dangerous. The range between "enough" and "not too much" is often referred to as the therapeutic range. Determining whether a patient is taking enough or too much of a particular drug usually involves performing a quantitative test to determine how much of the drug is in the patient's blood. These tests are reported with CPT codes 80150–80299.

An individual may ingest one of the drugs listed in the Therapeutic Drug Assay section for nontherapeutic reasons. If a laboratory performs a quantitative test to determine the amount of that drug present, the lab would report the appropriate therapeutic drug assay code even though there is no therapeutic reason for taking the drug.

therapeutic level
Present in sufficient quantity to have the desired effect but not in an amount high enough to be dangerous.

Therapeutic drug assays are not used to screen for the presence of illegal substances. If performed, such tests are described by the codes in the Drug Testing section.

From the perspective of the . . .

LAB CODER

To report CPT code 80412 (Corticotropin-releasing hormone [CRH] stimulation panel), the laboratory must test for two separate chemicals, and each one must be tested for six times. These are listed as cortisol (82533 X 6) and adrenocorticotropic hormone (82024 X 6) in the CPT code descriptor for 80412. If even one of these tests is performed less than the required six times, code 80412 cannot be reported.

Evocative/Suppression Testing

Sometimes it is necessary to perform a series of tests to determine whether a patient has responded appropriately to particular agents or chemicals. This usually involves taking a baseline test of a particular substance that is present in the patient, giving an evocative agent (intended to increase the amount of the substance) or suppressive agent (intended to decrease the amount of that substance), and then retesting to determine whether the amount of that substance changed as expected.

Some **evocative/suppression testing** codes (80400–80440) list which laboratory tests must be performed and how many times each must be performed to report that code. This is indicated by naming the particular test followed by the CPT code for that test and the number of times the test must be performed by adding "X" (times) and a number following the CPT code. If the required number of tests is not performed, it is incorrect to report the CPT code that describes the evocative or suppression testing procedure.

These codes only describe the test procedures. Other CPT codes describe administration of the evocative/suppression agents by a physician. If the physician remains with the patient during the test, this may be reported with the appropriate E/M codes, including the prolonged services codes as appropriate.

evocative/suppression testing
Testing that determines a patient's reaction to a substance by using an agent to increase or decrease the patient's level of that substance.

Use the CPT manual and index to answer the questions below.

1. What code(s) are reported to describe testing for the presence of cocaine, opiates, and amphetamines, assuming these can be tested together in one chromatographic procedure? _____

2. When the test for cocaine, opiates, and amphetamines is run, the report shows positive for cocaine and opiates, and a separate confirmatory test is performed for each drug. What code(s) are reported to describe the confirmatory tests? _____

3. What code is reported if another test is performed in the above scenario to quantify the amount of cocaine present in the sample? _____

4. A patient goes to the lab for a breath test for the presence of alcohol. What code should the lab report for this test? _____

5. What code is reported to describe a test to determine whether a patient has a therapeutic level of nortriptyline? _____

6. A laboratory performs a glucagon tolerance panel for insulinoma. What tests must be performed, how many times must they be performed, and which codes describe these tests? _____

13.3 Reporting Other Lab Tests (80500–87999)

Consultations (Clinical Pathology)

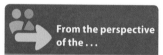

From the perspective of the . . .

PATHOLOGIST
To select the correct consultation codes from the Pathology and Laboratory section of the CPT manual, it is imperative to know which services the physician provided.

On occasion, the treating physician may request a pathology consultation when it is necessary to have additional medical expertise and judgment to correctly interpret a particular test result. The pathologist reporting this service must provide a written report to the requesting physician that includes the pathologist's medical interpretation. Merely reporting a test result is not considered a clinical pathology consultation.

CPT code 80500 is used to report a limited consult that does not require the pathologist to review the patient's history and medical records. CPT code 80502 indicates that the pathologist performed a comprehensive consult, including a review of the patient's history and medical records.

Urinalysis

urinalysis (UA)
Examination of the urine, typically by chemical or microscopic means.

microscopy
The use of a microscope to examine very small objects.

Laboratories can perform tests on urine samples using dipsticks or reagents to detect a number of different chemicals, including bilirubin, glucose, hemoglobin, ketones, leukocytes, nitrite, pH, protein, and urobilinogen, or to determine the specific gravity of the urine sample. These **urinalysis** tests may be either nonautomated or automated and can be performed with or without **microscopy** (manually looking at a sample under a microscope to determine whether other substances, such as red or white blood cells, are present in the sample). There are four CPT codes to describe the possible combinations of these two factors, as follows:

- 81000: Nonautomated with microscopy.
- 81001: Automated with microscopy.
- 81002: Nonautomated, without microscopy.
- 81003: Automated, without microscopy.

Laboratories may also test urine samples to detect the presence of bacteria (81007) or to determine whether a patient is pregnant (81025).

Chemistry

The CPT manual lists codes for several hundred specific chemical substances that may be measured. Each **chemistry** test is described by an individual CPT code in the 82000–84999 range and, unless otherwise specified, each test is quantitative. Unless the code descriptor states that it is for a particular sample type (e.g., blood, urine, or feces), the code is used to describe a test performed on a sample from any source. If the same substance is measured in multiple specimens from different sources or in multiple specimens collected from the same source at different times, the CPT code describing that chemical test is reported separately for each **specimen.**

Molecular Pathology

Beginning in 2012, a number of new CPT codes (81200–81408) have been developed to describe molecular pathology tests. CPT codes 81200–82355, collectively referred to as Tier 1 Molecular Pathology Procedures, describe tests to detect gene-specific abnormalities. Guidelines preceding this section describe the various tests and possible abnormalities that may be detected. This section is likely to expand significantly over the next several years as the CPT expands the list of individual gene-testing procedures.

CPT codes 81370–81383 describe human leukocyte antigen (HLA) testing to assess donor and recipient compatibility for patients undergoing solid organ and hematopoietic stem cell (bone marrow) transplants. CPT codes 81400–81408, commonly referred to as Tier 2 Molecular Pathology Procedures, describe nine levels of molecular pathology procedures, each of which describes tests for multiple different gene abnormalities. These are not likely to be performed as frequently as tests in the Tier 1 code section. Tests for genetic abnormalities that are not specifically listed in these code groups should be reported with the appropriate code in the 83890–83914 and 88384–88386 code series.

Hematology and Coagulation

Code range 85002–85999 lists specific tests performed on blood samples. These tests are specific to blood components, not chemistry or other tests performed on a blood sample. Some tests measure a number of different blood components. For example, a **complete blood count (CBC)** measures hemoglobin (Hgb), hematocrit (Hct), **red blood cells** (RBCs), **white blood cells** (WBCs), and platelets. Other tests only measure one blood component, such as Hgb or Hct.

Other tests measure specific clotting factors necessary for the proper formation of blood clots (Figure 13.1) and other factors that break down blood clots. The ability to form blood clots is often measured by the **prothrombin time (PT)** and the **partial thromboplastin time (PTT).** Some codes describe groups of individual tests that are performed together. If a bundled code describes the tests performed, it is incorrect to report those tests using individual codes.

chemistry
Type of tests that measure chemical substances in a specimen.

specimen
A sample, as of tissue, used for examination.

complete blood count (CBC)
One of the most common diagnostic laboratory tests that measures red blood cells, white blood cells, hematocrit, hemoglobin, platelets, and other elements in a certain volume of blood.

red blood cell (RBC)
A cell that contains hemoglobin that carries oxygen to body tissues.

white blood cell (WBC)
A cell that helps protect the body from infection and disease.

prothrombin time (PT)
A test that measures the time needed for clot formation in blood plasma.

partial thromboplastin time (PTT)
A measurement of certain coagulation factors in blood plasma.

CODING EXAMPLE

A laboratory performs a series of automated blood count tests on a patient's blood sample, including hematocrit, hemoglobin, red blood cell count, white blood cell count, platelet count, and differential white blood cell count. How should a coder report this series of tests?

The coder should look in the index under the term *blood cell count,* which includes a series of individual tests and a listing under "Hemogram" for automated tests 85025 and 85027. Reviewing these codes shows that code 85025 lists all of the automated tests performed by the laboratory. Code 85027 includes all of the automated tests except an automated differential white blood count. The coder reports code 85025.

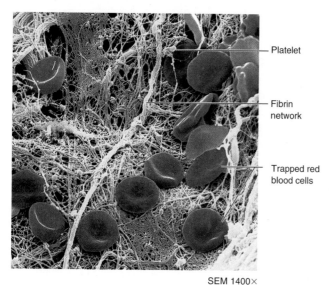

- Platelet

- Fibrin network

- Trapped red blood cells

SEM 1400×

FIGURE 13.1 Blood Clot

Immunology

Code range 86000–86849 describes laboratory tests to detect specific antigens, toxins, peptides, or antibodies by a variety of methods. Codes in this section also describe tests to determine the number of certain immune system cells present in a sample, including lymphocytes, B cells, natural killer cells, T cells, and stem cells.

A separate family of codes (86602–86804) describes multiple-step qualitative or semiquantitative immunoassay tests to detect antibodies to agents causing infectious diseases. Guidance information in this section directs coders to report a particular code multiple times if the test is performed more than once to detect different types of infectious agents within that general classification. If multiple assays are performed to detect antibodies of different immunoglobulin classes (e.g., IgG or IgM), the CPT code describing that assay is reported multiple times. In some cases, different codes describe assays for IgM and other antibodies. When different codes exist, report both codes when the lab performs one test for IgM antibodies and another for IgG or other antibodies to the same antigen.

CODER'S TIP

CPT codes 86602–86804 are only used to report multiple-step tests. CPT code 86318 (Immunoassay for infectious agent antibody, qualitative or semiquantitative, single-step method [e.g., reagent strip]) is reported if a single-step immunoassay test is performed.

Transfusion Medicine

Transfusion medicine codes (86850–86899) describe services associated with blood transfusions. Transfusion services include tests such as antibody screen, determination of ABO blood type, and Rh factor. These services also include preparation of blood products—including freezing and thawing units of whole blood, serum, and fresh frozen plasma—and other services associated with transfusions.

Laboratory tests determine whether an individual has blood type A, B, AB, or O. This designation indicates what antigens are on the surface of the individual's red blood cells. Other tests determine whether the individual is Rh(D) positive or negative. Determining an individual's blood type involves both ABO typing and determining whether the blood is Rh(D) positive or negative.

Microbiology

Microbiology is the identification of specific bacteria, viruses, parasites, and fungi. Specific codes differentiate between presumptive and definitive identification. Definitive identification is based on special testing that identifies the organism down to the genus or species level. Presumptive identification is more general in nature and is based on colony morphology, growth on specific media, appearance under a microscope with Gram stain techniques, or up to three specific tests.

Tests to identify specific organisms may be performed on primary samples or on cultured samples where a small number of organisms are grown on specific growth media. Tests performed on cultured samples are described by CPT codes 87140–87158, whereas those performed on primary samples are described by codes 87260–87905.

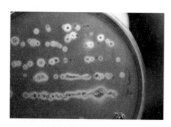

FIGURE 13.2 Blood Agar Plate Growing Bacteria from a Human Throat

These codes describe various tests, including gas chromatography, liquid chromatography, immunofluorescent techniques, multiple-step qualitative and semiquantitative enzyme immunoassay tests, nucleic acid detection (DNA or RNA), and immunoassay with direct optical observation. If the lab performs tests to detect multiple organisms, each test is reported separately. Modifier 59 is added when reporting the same code more than once to describe tests for more than one type of organism (different species or strain) identified by a single code.

CODER'S TIP

If a laboratory test is repeated on the same day as the original test, modifier 91 is added to the code for the additional tests. This modifier is only used for laboratory tests, not other diagnostic tests such as x-rays or other diagnostic imaging tests. If a urinalysis is performed three times, those tests are reported as 81000, 81000-91, and 81000-91. If a microbiology test is repeated to detect a different organism, modifier 91 is not added to the code. Rather, modifier 59 is added to the code for the particular microbiology test.

CODER'S TIP

Codes in the Microbiology section describe procedures that identify the infectious agent itself. Tests that identify antibodies to these agents are reported with CPT codes 86602–86804.

EXERCISE 13.3

Also available in 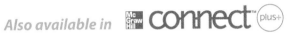 connect plus+

Use the CPT manual and index to answer each question below.

1. What is the appropriate code to report an automated complete blood count (CBC)? _____

2. What code indicates that the laboratory performed a total prostate-specific antigen (PSA) test? Can this test be performed on a laboratory specimen from a woman? _____

3. What code appropriately reports the testing of human growth hormone (HGH) antibody? _____

4. A laboratory performs a throat culture with isolation and presumptively identifies the isolate. What CPT code would the laboratory report for this service? _____

5. What CPT code would appropriately report detection of cytomegalovirus using a direct fluorescent antibody technique? _____

6. A laboratory uses a multiple-step qualitative or semiquantitative enzyme immunoassay technique to detect the antigen of the respiratory syncytial virus infectious agent. What code should be used to report this test? What code would be reported if the same infectious agent were detected using the immunofluorescent technique? _____

13.4 Coding for Pathology Services (88000–89398)

Anatomic Pathology

Anatomic pathology codes describe professional services associated with postmortem examinations (autopsies). Separate families of codes describe gross examinations only (visual inspection of the organs) and gross and microscopic examinations (both visual inspection and studying tissue samples under a microscope). Each

anatomic pathology
Examination of tissue to determine the presence or cause of illness.

family is divided into individual codes to designate anatomic pathology services on an infant or newborn and whether or not central nervous system (CNS) tissue was examined.

CODING EXAMPLE

A pathologist performs an autopsy on an adult with known severe diseases. He performs a gross examination only that includes all internal organs and the brain, but he does not include examination of the spinal cord. How should the coder report this service?

The coder looks up *autopsy* in the index. One of the subheadings is "Gross Exam," which lists a range of codes from 88000–88016. Looking at these individual codes shows that the appropriate code to report an autopsy on an adult that includes the brain but not the spinal cord is 88005.

Later, the same pathologist examines an infant who suffered an unexplained death. He examines all the organs including the brain but not the spinal cord. He also performs microscopic examinations of the organs. How does the coder report this service?

The coder looks up *autopsy* in the index and finds a "Gross and Microscopic" subheading with a code range of 88020–88029. Looking at the individual codes, the coder finds that code 88028 describes a gross and microscopic autopsy of an infant, including the brain but not the spinal cord.

Cytopathology and Cytogenetic Studies

Cytopathology codes (88104–88199) report tests on cells obtained through a variety of methods, including washings, brushings, lavage, scraping, and the use of swabs. Codes in the first group (88104–88140) describe tests from sources other than cervical or vaginal specimens (Pap smears). Other codes also describe tests from sources other than cervical or vaginal specimens, including 88160–88162, 88172–88173, and 88184–88189.

Pap smear tests are reported with CPT codes 88141–88155, 88164–88167, and 88174–88175. These tests have evolved over the years, and there are various methods available to perform these tests in physician offices or in fully certified laboratories. To select the correct code, coders must know the method used to examine the cervical or vaginal specimen during the Pap test.

Cytogenetic tests are performed on cells to detect genetic abnormalities or neoplastic conditions. These tests include various tissue cultures, chromosomal analysis, and molecular cytogenetics. The specific diseases for which the tests are performed may be identified using genetic testing modifiers found in Appendix I.

Surgical Pathology

Pathologists often examine tissue samples removed during surgery to determine the cause of underlying disease or whether any disease is present in the tissue, a process known as **surgical pathology.** If this only requires a gross examination (visual inspection), the service is reported with CPT code 88300 (Level I - Surgical pathology, gross examination only). If a microscopic examination is also performed, the specific organ or tissue sample examined determines which CPT code is used to report the service (88302–88309). These codes identify Level II–VI surgical pathology services. Additional services that may be performed on a particular tissue sample or organ are listed using codes 88311–88399 and are reported separately if performed.

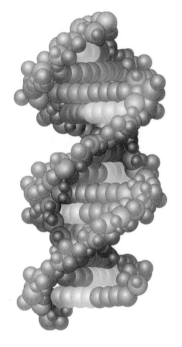

Cytogenetic tests use the knowledge of DNA structure to detect genetic abnormalities or neoplastic conditions.

surgical pathology
The examination of tissue samples removed during surgery to determine the presence or cause of a disease.

The five levels of surgical pathology codes that include microscopic tissue examination represent increasing probabilities of diseases or malignancies in the tissues. While almost any tissue could develop a malignancy, some tissues are more likely to do so. For example, an appendix that is removed incidental to another operation, fallopian tubes removed during a tubal ligation, fingers, and toes are all very unlikely to have developed malignancies. Microscopic examination of these tissues is usually performed for the purpose of confirming that it is the correct tissue and that there is no disease present. These examinations are categorized under Level II (88302). In contrast, a colon removed for reasons other than for tumor is more likely to have an unsuspected tumor and is grouped in Level V (88307), whereas a colon resected for a known tumor is assigned to Level VI (88309).

The Surgical Pathology section also includes codes to report pathology consults regarding tissue specimens. These may be for the purpose of consulting and reporting findings on slides prepared elsewhere (88321), consulting and reporting on specimens that require slide preparation (88323), or consultation by the pathologist during surgery before the surgeon continues the surgical procedure (88329). Surgical consults during a surgical procedure may involve frozen section examinations, during which a microscopic examination is performed on a specimen before the surgeon continues.

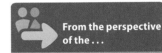

From the perspective of the . . .

PATHOLOGIST

It is important that coders know there are professional and technical components of some pathology codes. Coders must know whether the entity reporting the service is a pathologist reporting the professional services only (reported with modifier 26 added to the code); a laboratory reporting the technical component only (reported with the TC modifier added to the code); or a single entity reporting both the professional and technical components as a global code (reported without any modifier).

In Vivo Laboratory Procedures

Codes 88720–88741 describe in vivo transcutaneous laboratory tests performed with transducers, including bilirubin, hemoglobin, carboxyhemoglobin, and methemoglobin. These tests may be performed in locations outside of the laboratory.

Reproductive Medicine Procedures

Laboratory services associated with reproductive medicine (e.g., in vitro insemination, preparation of embryos for in vitro fertilization procedures, cryopreservation of embryos, etc.) are reported with codes 89250–89398.

EXERCISE 13.4   *Also available in*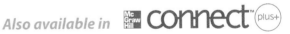

Use the CPT manual and index to answer the following questions.

1. A pathologist performs a postmortem examination on a 25-year-old man who died in a motor vehicle accident. The autopsy included gross and microscopic exams of all tissues, including the brain and spinal cord. What is the correct code to report this examination? _____

2. A surgeon performs a hysterectomy for suspected malignant tumor and sends the specimen to the pathology laboratory for gross and microscopic examination and determination of the tumor type. What code describes these services? _____

3. A surgeon requests a pathology consult during surgery to determine whether a surgical specimen is malignant. The pathologist performs frozen section examinations on three separate tissue blocks. What code(s) would be used to report the pathology consult? _____

CHAPTER **13** REVIEW

Summary

Learning Outcome	Key Concepts/Examples
13.1 Differentiate between organ and disease-oriented panels and the individual codes used to report those tests. **Pages 423–426**	Organ and disease-oriented panels are groups of tests commonly ordered by providers to screen for, diagnose, or follow the progress of certain diseases. CPT codes identifying these panels may only be reported if all the tests listed in the panel are performed. If additional tests are performed, they are reported separately. Two or more panels may not be reported if the tests performed overlap multiple panels. If two or more panels list some of the tests, the largest panel in which all the listed tests were performed is reported, with any other tests reported separately.
13.2 Explain how to report laboratory tests related to drugs and medicines. **Pages 426–427**	Qualitative tests determine whether a certain substance is present in the test sample, but they do not measure how much of that substance is present. Quantitative tests determine how much of a substance is present in a test sample. Drug testing involves qualitative tests to detect the presence of one or more specific drugs. If a quantitative test is performed to determine how much of a drug is present, the test is reported with the appropriate code from the Chemistry section. Therapeutic drug assays are quantitative tests to measure the amount of a specific medication present in the test sample. Most often, these tests are used to determine whether a particular medication is in the therapeutic range, which is defined as the amount necessary to achieve the desired results. Evocative/suppression tests involve measuring the amount of a particular substance in the patient, giving the patient a drug or agent to either increase or decrease that substance in the patient, and then measuring that substance in the patient after giving the drug or agent. A single CPT code describes all required measurements, which are listed as part of the code descriptor.
13.3 Identify codes to report laboratory tests. **Pages 428–431**	Laboratory tests include urinalysis, chemistry, hematology and coagulation, immunology, and microbiology tests. Coders should be able to determine the correct CPT code to report laboratory tests by using the index to determine a complete list of codes that describe a particular test and then reviewing those codes in detail to determine which one best describes the services provided.
13.4 Select appropriate codes to describe pathology services. **Pages 431–433**	Anatomic pathology codes describe postmortem examinations (autopsies) of tissues and/or organs. These families of codes describe gross examination only, limited gross and microscopic examination, and complete gross and microscopic exams. Surgical pathology examinations are divided into six levels, depending on the complexity of tissue examination. A Level I examination involves gross examination only, while Levels II–VI include gross and microscopic examination of tissues.

Using Terminology

Match the key terms with their definitions.

_____ **1.** [LO13.1] Laboratory

_____ **2.** [LO13.2] Organ/Disease Panel

_____ **3.** [LO13.4] Anatomic Pathology

_____ **4.** [LO13.4] Surgical Pathology

A. A quantity of biological material or tissue for use in testing, examination, or study

B. The study of tissue removed during surgery for structure, disease, and abnormality

_____ 5. [L013.2] Quantitative
_____ 6. [L013.2] Qualitative
_____ 7. [L013.3] Complete Blood Count
_____ 8. [L013.3] Red blood cell
_____ 9. [L013.3] White blood cell
_____ 10. [L013.3] Urinalysis
_____ 11. [L013.3] Prothrombin time
_____ 12. [L013.3] Chemistry Test
_____ 13. [L013.2] Drug Test
_____ 14. [L013.2] Therapeutic Level
_____ 15. [L013.2] Evocative/Suppression Testing
_____ 16. [L013.1] Specimen

C. The desired level of a drug in the body for the intended effect, neither too high or too low
D. The postmortem study of changes in the function, structure, or appearance of organs or tissues upon autopsy
E. A quantitative test measurement of the several blood cell types in circulation
F. Test that measures presence of a chemical substance
G. Coagulation study
H. Results are expressed as a numerical value
I. The cell that carries oxygen in the blood
J. Testing to determine whether a patient responds appropriately to particular agents or chemicals
K. Location where tests and experimental work are performed
L. The circulating immune-system cells involved in defending the body against infectious disease and foreign materials
M. A predefined cluster of laboratory tests to evaluate a diseased organ, organ system, or disease
N. Tests for presence or absence of a substance
O. Test performed on urine as a common method of diagnosis
P. Test that determines presence or absence of a particular drug or drug class

Checking Your Understanding

Select the letter that best completes the statement or answers the question.

1. L013.2 Testing for the presence of an antiseizure medication in a patient is an example of what type of test?
   a. Chemical
   b. Qualitative
   c. Quantitative
   d. Evocative

2. L013.2 The CPT manual's list of drug classes can be found at the beginning of which section?
   a. Phlebotomy
   b. Chemistry Testing
   c. Urinalysis
   d. Drug Testing

3. L013.4 When coding for _____ services, coders must know the site from which the specimen was taken.
   a. Drug testing
   b. Surgical
   c. Anatomic pathology
   d. Surgical pathology

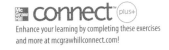

Enhance your learning by completing these exercises and more at mcgrawhillconnect.com!

CHAPTER 13 | PATHOLOGY AND LABORATORY SERVICES   435

4. L013.1 Organ or disease-oriented panels may only be reported if _____ tests in the panel have been performed.

   a. Some
   b. All
   c. Reduced
   d. Drug

5. L013.3 The basic renal function panel includes 10 tests such as _____ and _____.

   a. BUN, creatinine
   b. Cholesterol, triglycerides
   c. Blood type and Rh factor
   d. Alkaline phosphatase, bilirubin

6. L013.2 Other than the lab panels identified with CPT codes 80047–80076, there are additional test panels to report _____, described by codes _____.

   a. Evocative/suppression testing, 80400–80440
   b. Drug testing, 80800–80880
   c. Urinalysis, 80210–80310
   d. Qualitative testing, 84000–84440

7. L013.3 CPT code 81025, which describes a visual color pregnancy test, is an example of what type of test?

   a. Quantitative
   b. Microscopic
   c. Qualitative
   d. Chemistry

8. L013.4 A gross and microscopic examination of a surgically excised (enucleated) eye is an example of what level of surgical pathology?

   a. Level III
   b. Level IV
   c. Level V
   d. Level VI

9. L013.3 Clinical pathology consultations are described by which CPT codes?

   a. 80500 and 80502
   b. 80400 and 80440
   c. 88000 and 88005
   d. 88300 and 88305

10. L013.4 When coding for molecular diagnostic procedures to test for specific diseases, modifiers located in _____ must be added to the code.

    a. Appendix A
    b. Appendix B
    c. Appendix I
    d. Appendix II

11. L013.3 Which of the following code ranges corresponds to tests that determine the specific gravity of a urine sample?

    a. 82000–82030
    b. 84315–84375
    c. 80400–80440
    d. 81000–81003

12. L013.3 To report a dipstick urinalysis, it is necessary to know whether the test was _____.

    a. Professional or technical
    b. Manual or automated
    c. Compulsory or voluntary
    d. Qualitative or quantitative

13. L013.3 Which code is used to report an unlisted chemistry test?

    a. 84900   **c.** 84999
    b. 85999   **d.** 86849

14. L013.1 The lab performs all of the components of a basic metabolic panel (total calcium) (code 80048) plus a total bilirubin (code 82247), which is a component of the comprehensive metabolic panel (code 80053). What is the correct way to code this set of tests?

    a. Codes 80048 and 80053
    b. Code 80048 or 80053
    c. Code 80053 with modifier 52
    d. Codes 80048 and 82247

15. L013.4 The pathology codes differ from other laboratory codes in that they have both _____ and _____ components.

    a. Professional, technical
    b. Manual, automated
    c. Compulsory, voluntary
    d. Chemistry, drug

16. L013.4 The surgical pathology codes are divided into how many different levels?

    a. 5   **c.** 2
    b. 6   **d.** 13

17. L013.4 Medical examiners report their services for postmortem examinations with CPT codes _____ from the Pathology and Laboratory section of the CPT manual.

    a. 88000–88099   **c.** 88300–88309
    b. 80500–80502   **d.** 82000–83000

18. L013.3 Quantitative tests for drugs are reported with CPT codes from the _____ section or _____ section.

    a. Chemistry, Therapeutic Drug Assay
    b. Urinalysis, Chemistry
    c. Pregnancy, Drug Testing
    d. Evocative/Suppression Testing, Therapeutic Drug Assay

connect plus+

Enhance your learning by completing these exercises and more at mcgrawhillconnect.com!

CHAPTER 13 | PATHOLOGY AND LABORATORY SERVICES   **437**

19. L013.3 If the tests listed in two lab panels overlap, the coder should not report both panels, but should report _____.

    a. The panel that is more expensive

    b. The panel that includes the largest number of the tests performed

    c. The panel that produces qualitative results

    d. The panel that includes all overlapping tests only

20. L013.2 An emergency room patient has a positive visual urine pregnancy test followed by a quantitative blood pregnancy (gonadotropin, chorionic, or hCG) test. How should this be coded?

    a. Use code 81025 alone because the second test is confirmatory.

    b. Use code 84702 alone because it is more specific.

    c. Use code 81025 or 84702 because both are pregnancy tests.

    d. Use codes 81025 and 84702.

Applying Your Skills

Use the CPT manual to select the correct code to report each of the following procedures.

1. L013.1 Panel that tests for total protein, bilirubin (total and direct), albumin, phosphatase, alkaline, SGOT, and SGPT _____

2. L013.3 Throat culture in the laboratory _____

3. L013.3 Alcohol breath test _____

4. L013.3 Manual count of blood cells _____

5. L013.3 Physician interpretation of a peripheral blood smear with a written report _____

6. L013.1 Basic metabolic panel with total calcium _____

7. L013.3 Total PSA test _____

8. L013.3 Automated platelet count _____

9. L013.3 Chromosome analysis for 20–25 cells _____

10. L013.3 Lab test for the level of carbon dioxide (not part of a blood gas analysis) _____

11. L013.3 Test for total estrogen _____

12. L013.3 Test for dipropylacetic acid _____

13. L013.4 Pathology of a testicular biopsy _____

14. L013.4 Pathological evaluation of a specimen from a patient who had his finger amputated _____

15. L013.4 Preparation and screening of a cytopathology smear with interpretation _____

16. L013.4 Technical component of the cytometry flow for five markers _____

17. L013.4 Cervical cytopathology with physician interpretation _____

18. L013.4 Surgical pathology of a biopsy of the fallopian tube _____

19. L013.4 Cryopreservation of four embryos _____

20. L013.4 Yearly storage of semen _____

21. L013.4 Insemination of oocytes _____

22. L013.3 Macroscopic exam for a parasite _____

23. L013.3 Intradermal skin test for tuberculosis _____

24. L013.3 Antibodies to an enterovirus _____

25. L013.3 Fetal lung maturity assessment; L/S ratio _____

26. L013.4 Autopsy of a stillborn with examination of the brain _____

27. L013.4 Unlisted autopsy procedure _____

28. L013.3 Assay for group A streptococcus using the amplified probe technique _____

29. L013.3 Confirmatory tests of the hepatitis C antibody _____

30. L013.3 CBC (complete blood count) with automated differential _____

Thinking It Through

Use your critical-thinking skills to answer the questions below.

1. L013.4 Explain the differences between the type of specimen used for cytopathology studies (codes 88104–88140) and surgical pathology studies (codes 88300–88309).

_____

_____

2. L013.2 Explain what is unique about codes in the Evocative/Suppression Testing section, compared to other Pathology and Laboratory codes, with respect to repeat tests.

_____

_____

3. L013.1 Can a laboratory report codes describing a test for acid phosphatase and a comprehensive metabolic panel together if both are performed at the same time? Explain your answer.

_____

_____

4. L013.1 Is it correct to report a comprehensive metabolic panel and an electrolyte panel for the same patient at the same time? Can they be reported on the same date of service if provided at different times during the day? Explain your answers.

_____

_____

Enhance your learning by completing these exercises and more at mcgrawhillconnect.com!

CHAPTER 13 | PATHOLOGY AND LABORATORY SERVICES   439

14 MEDICINE SERVICES

Learning Outcomes
After completing this chapter, students should be able to:

14.1 Explain the structure of the Medicine chapter and its general guidelines.

14.2 Select codes to report the administration of immune globulins and vaccines.

14.3 Identify codes to report psychiatry, dialysis, gastroenterology, ophthalmology, and otorhinolaryngologic services.

14.4 Select codes to report cardiovascular, immunological, and neurological procedures.

14.5 Identify codes to report injections, infusions, therapeutic procedures, rehabilitation, moderate sedation, home health services, and medication therapy management.

Key Terms

Administration

Aphakia

Bronchodilator

Cardiac catheterization

Cardiography

Congenital

Coronary artery stent

Electroencephalogram (EEG)

Human papillomavirus (HPV)

Immune globulin

Measles, mumps, and rubella (MMR)

Moderate sedation

Refractive state

Vaccine

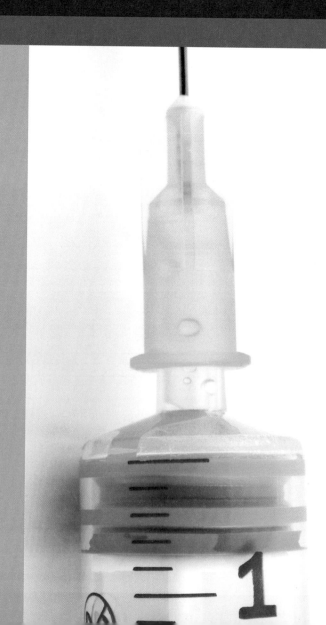

Introduction

The Medicine chapter comprises most of the 90000 series of CPT codes. The exception is the Evaluation and Management (E/M) code series (99201–99499), which is located in the first chapter of the CPT manual. The Medicine chapter is the most diverse chapter in the CPT manual, with over 30 separate code sections and approximately 100 subsections of nonoverlapping services. Many of these codes describe invasive procedures that are commonly performed by nonsurgical specialists, such as physicians who are medicine specialists.

14.1 Medicine Chapter Structure and General Guidelines

The major medical areas described by codes in the 90000 series appear in the following sections:

- Immune Globulins, Serum or Recombinant Products (90281–90399)
- Immunization Administration for Vaccines/Toxoids (90460–90474)
- Vaccines, Toxoids (90476–90749)
- Psychiatry (90801–90899)
- Biofeedback (90901–90911)
- Dialysis (90935–90999)
- Gastroenterology (91010–91299)
- Ophthalmology (92002–92499)
- Special Otorhinolaryngologic Services (92502–92700)
- Cardiovascular (92950–93799)
- Noninvasive Vascular Diagnostic Studies (93880–93998)
- Pulmonary (94002–94799)
- Allergy and Clinical Immunology (95004–95199)
- Endocrinology (95250–95251)
- Neurology and Neuromuscular Procedures (95800–96020)
- Medical Genetics and Genetic Counseling Services (96040)
- Central Nervous System Assessments/Tests (96101–96125)
- Health and Behavior Assessment/Intervention (96150–96155)
- Hydration, Injections and Infusions, Chemotherapy (96360–96549)
- Photodynamic Therapy (96567–96571)
- Special Dermatological Procedures (96900–96999)
- Physical Medicine and Rehabilitation (97001–97799)
- Medical Nutrition Therapy (97802–97804)
- Acupuncture (97810–97814)
- Osteopathic Manipulative Treatment (98925–98929)
- Chiropractic Manipulative Treatment (98940–98943)
- Education and Training for Patient Self-Management (98960–98962)
- Non-Face-to-Face Nonphysician Services (98966–98969)
- Special Services, Procedures and Reports (99000–99091)
- Qualifying Circumstances for Anesthesia (99100–99140)
- Moderate (Conscious) Sedation (99143–99150)
- Other Services and Procedures (99170–99199)
- Home Health Procedures/Services (99500–99602)
- Medication Therapy Management Services (99605–99607)

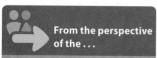
Codes within each category often describe many unrelated services. It is very important that coders understand how to use the index to identify codes describing the services that must be reported. In many cases, there are a number of CPT codes that generally describe a service listed in the index. Coders must review all the listed codes to determine which one best describes the service(s) provided.

The Medicine section of the CPT includes guidelines that are generally applicable to other code sections but may have slightly different applications to this section than to surgical procedure codes. These guidelines are found at the beginning of the 90000 series and are summarized below.

Multiple Procedures

Multiple procedures provided to an individual patient by a single provider on the same day should be reported with separate codes. For example, if an ophthalmologist provides E/M services and other separately identifiable services not typically included in the E/M visit, both the E/M visit and the other services should be reported.

Additional procedures may be paid differently than primary procedures. Many payers pay less for additional procedures than they would pay for the same procedure if it were the primary procedure provided. The logic behind this payment differential is that much of the work of the second procedure duplicates work included in the payment for the primary procedure. Payers often will not pay for this duplicative work. Medicare, for example, generally pays 50 percent of its usual fee schedule amount for additional procedures.

In addition to the discounted payment for secondary procedures, payers often bundle some procedures with others, paying only for the primary procedure. These bundling rules are complex and often differ from payer to payer. Regardless of the payment or bundling rules applied by payers, coders should report all services provided.

CODER'S TIP

Coders should report the services provided. Some payers, including federal programs like Medicare, do not pay for every service reported. Payers often have payment bundling rules that differ from the coding rules that determine which codes are reported. Payment rules should not determine how coders report the services provided.

Add-on Codes

Procedures designated by add-on codes, identified in the CPT manual by a plus (+) sign, are never reported as a primary service. These can only be reported with the "parent" code. Most often there is only one parent code for each add-on code, but in some instances there are several parent codes associated with an individual add-on code. In other cases, there are multiple add-on codes associated with a single parent code.

In addition to the plus-sign designation, add-on codes are listed in Appendix D and often contain phrases such as "each additional" or the parenthetical "(List separately in addition to primary procedure)" in their code descriptors. Coders should not add modifier 51 (additional procedure) to add-on codes when reporting those services. These codes should not be confused with CPT codes listed in Appendix E that are exempt from modifier 51 for other reasons. These codes are not add-on codes but, similar to add-on codes, coders should not add modifier 51 to them.

Separate Procedures

Some CPT codes include the term "separate procedure" as part of their code descriptors. These procedures are often performed as part of another procedure. When that occurs, the code for the procedure should not be reported separately. The separate procedure code descriptor designation indicates that the code is reported separately when the larger procedure is *not* performed, indicating that this procedure was performed separately.

CODER'S TIP

Even experienced coders sometimes confuse the *separate procedure* designation and concept. This designation does not mean that the procedure described by this code is always reported as a separate procedure. Indeed, this designation indicates that the procedure described by the code often is *not* performed as a separate procedure and the code should not be reported separately *unless* this procedure was not performed as part of a larger procedure.

Unlisted Services or Procedures

The introductory guidelines include a list of 19 unlisted codes from the Medicine section of CPT codes. These codes also appear in the appropriate code sections, but they are listed together at the beginning of the chapter for convenience.

Materials Supplied by Physician

Many procedures listed in the Medicine code sections require separate supplies or other materials such as sterile surgical equipment or drugs. When a provider supplies these items, the items should be listed separately in addition to the procedure code describing the procedure. These supplies are designated with CPT code 99070 (Supplies and materials [except spectacles], provided by the physician over and above those usually included with the office visit or other services rendered [list drugs, trays, supplies, or materials provided]) or by other specific codes identifying the supplies provided. Payers may not always pay for these supplies, but coders should report them regardless of those policies.

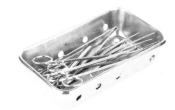

CPT code 99070 describes supplies, such as trays or sterile equipment, that are provided by the physician and are beyond what is usually included in an office visit or service. Use code 99070 to report these kinds of supplies, even if they will not be reimbursed by the payer.

EXERCISE 14.1

Also available in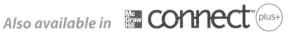

Use the CPT manual and general guidelines to answer the following questions.

1. The introductory guidance to the Medicine chapter lists _____ unlisted codes that appear throughout the chapter.
   a. 34 (1 in each main section)
   b. 19
   c. 54
   d. 1

2. Which of the following CPT codes can be reported on its own?
   a. 92978
   b. 92979
   c. 92980
   d. 92981

3. All add-on codes are exempt from reporting which of the following modifiers?
   a. 25
   b. 51
   c. 26
   d. All of these

(Continued)

4. Does the following summary accurately describe the general guidance that applies to codes from the Medicine chapter? Explain why you think it is or is not accurate.

Summary: The term "separate procedure" in a code descriptor means the code can always be reported in addition to other codes describing the services provided.

_____

_____

_____

5. Evaluate whether the following statement is accurate and discuss the reasons for your answer: Coders should only report the procedures that the provider will be paid for, not the ones that payers will not cover. Agree or disagree? Why?

_____

_____

_____

14.2 Immune Globulins; Immunization Administration for Vaccines/Toxoids; Vaccines, Toxoids (90281–90749)

Immune Globulins

immune globulins
Any in the family of glycoproteins (molecules consisting of a simple sugar attached to an amino acid) that function as antibodies in immune response.

CPT codes 90281–90399 identify serum **immune globulins** (those extracted from human blood) or recombinant immune globulins produced in a laboratory through genetic modifications of human or animal proteins. The code descriptors identify specific immune globulins and may include the specific route of administration. CPT code 90399 is used to report unlisted immune globulins.

These codes only report the immune globulin itself. The administration of these immune globulins is reported with CPT codes 96365–96368, 96372, 96374, or 96376, depending on the route of administration.

Immunization Administration for Vaccines/Toxoids

administration
Giving a drug directly by injection, by mouth, or by any other route that introduces the drug into the body.

CPT codes 90460 and 90461 describe the **administration** of vaccines and toxoids to patients 18 years of age and younger only when a physician or other professional provides face-to-face counseling to the patient and family. If counseling is not provided to the patient/family or if the vaccine is administered to a patient over 18 years of age, the administration should be reported with CPT codes 90471–90474.

CODER'S TIP

These administration codes are only reported with vaccines and toxoids. The administration of other medications, including immune globulins, is reported with CPT codes listed in the guidance associated with those codes (96365–96368, 96372, 96374, or 96376).

There is only one initial administration code reported for a single route of administration during a visit. If multiple vaccines are administered by the same route, add-on codes are used to designate the additional administrations.

To select the correct code describing the vaccine administration, it is necessary to identify the route of administration.

When a provider performs other services beyond the administration of the vaccine, such as a separate E/M visit, the CPT code describing those other services may be reported separately.

Vaccines, Toxoids

CPT codes 90476–90749 identify individual **vaccines** and/or toxoids. Some CPT codes describe individual vaccines, such as the vaccine for **human papillomavirus (HPV)**, whereas others describe combination vaccines, such as the vaccine for **measles, mumps, and rubella (MMR)**. Individual vaccine codes may not be reported for each component of a combination vaccine. When a combination vaccine is given, it is only appropriate to report the code describing the combination vaccine.

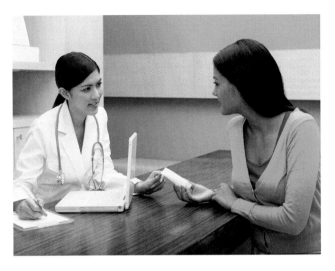

These codes only identify the vaccine itself, not the administration of the vaccine. Administration of the vaccine is reported with one of the vaccine administration codes (90460–90474). The administration of a vaccine is not subject to the multiple-procedure reduction, and modifier 51 is not added to these codes. Similarly, separately identifiable E/M services may be reported in addition to the vaccine and vaccine administration codes when those services are provided.

New vaccines are introduced on a regular basis. In an effort to keep the CPT manual current, new vaccines are sometimes identified in the manual before the FDA releases the vaccine for general use. Those vaccine CPT codes are identified with a lightning bolt symbol in the CPT manual. Coders should be aware that even though these codes are listed, they should not be reported until the FDA approves the vaccine.

When other services are provided in addition to the administration of a vaccine, such as a separate consultation, report these services with separate CPT codes.

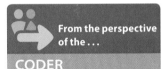
From the perspective of the . . .

CODER

To report administration codes, it is necessary to know the route of administration (e.g., intramuscular, subcutaneous, intranasal, etc.).

CODING EXAMPLE

A child is given two vaccines in her pediatrician's office without any associated counseling. One vaccine is a subcutaneous injection of live varicella virus, and the other is an oral administration of live poliovirus. How should the coder report these services?

The coder looks under the heading "Vaccines" in the index and locates code 90716 to describe the live varicella virus vaccine for subcutaneous use and code 90712 to describe the live poliovirus vaccine for oral use.

The coder also must report the administration codes for the two vaccines. Because the pediatrician did not provide counseling to the patient or family, administration codes 90460 and 90461 cannot be reported. Instead, the administration is reported with codes 90471–90474. Reviewing the descriptors of these codes shows that the first vaccine administration is reported with code 90471, which describes a subcutaneous vaccine administration. The second vaccine is administered orally, which is reported with either code 90473 or code 90474. The parenthetical note with these codes instructs coders not to report code 90473 with code 90471. Instead, add-on code 90474 is used to indicate that the oral vaccine was administered in addition to another vaccine.

The correct coding for these services is:
- 90716 Varicella virus vaccine, live, for subcutaneous administration
- 90471 Immunization administration (percutaneous, intradermal, subcutaneous, or intradermal), 1 vaccine
- 90712 Poliovirus, live, for oral administration
- 90474 Immunization administration by intranasal or oral route, each additional vaccine

vaccine
A preparation that provides immunity to a specific infectious disease by stimulating the body to produce antibodies, usually given by injection.

human papillomavirus (HPV)
A group of over 100 viruses that cause a range of afflictions, such as warts and cervical cancer.

measles, mumps, and rubella (MMR)
A vaccine against measles, mumps, and rubella that is administered in two doses: the first between 12 and 15 months, and the second between 4 and 6 years.

Use the CPT manual to select the codes for the following vaccines and administrations.

1. Measles, mumps, and rubella (MMR) given subcutaneously for a 2-year-old toddler after advising parents of the risks and benefits _____

2. Influenza vaccine, split virus, preservative free, given intramuscularly to a 19-year-old woman _____

3. Human papillomavirus (HPV), quadrivalent, 3-dose schedule, given intramuscularly to a 26-year-old woman _____

4. A 21-year old mother takes her 6-month-old daughter to the pediatrician's office to get her scheduled series of immunizations. According to the schedule, she should receive the following vaccines: Hepatitis B (HepB); Diphtheria, tetanus toxoids, and acellular pertussis (DTaP); inactivated polio virus (IPV); and intranasal influenza. What codes report both administration and the vaccines listed above? _____

5. A 7-month-old baby who was born prematurely is given 50 mg of recombinant monoclonal antibody against respiratory syncytial virus intramuscularly. How is this coded? _____

14.3 Psychiatry; Biofeedback; Dialysis; Gastroenterology; Ophthalmology; and Otorhinolaryngologic Services (90801–92700)

Psychiatry

Psychiatric services may be provided to patients in addition to other outpatient or hospital services. CPT codes 90801 and 90802 describe psychiatric diagnostic interviews. CPT code 90801 describes a verbal diagnostic interview, whereas code 90802 describes an interactive interview using play equipment, physical devices, language interpreter, or other methods of communication. This is used when the subject is too young or impaired to provide information using adult language skills.

CPT codes 90804–90829 describe psychotherapy services in both office and facility settings. Services in each location are further divided between insight-oriented and interactive psychotherapy. The codes within each section are subdivided by the length of time the services are provided. Each code describing psychotherapy services alone is paired with a corresponding code describing the same psychotherapy service combined with medical evaluation and management services. When the combined codes are reported, the total times of both services are combined to determine the correct code, even if the two services are not provided concurrently. If medical E/M services are provided on a day that psychotherapy services are not, the appropriate E/M code should be reported.

Choosing the correct psychotherapy code requires coders to determine the following:

1. Type of psychotherapy (insight oriented vs. interactive).
2. Place of service (office vs. facility).
3. Face-to-face time spent providing the service.
4. Whether E/M services were furnished on the same date of service.

CODER'S TIP

When psychotherapy services and E/M services are provided on the same day, the combined codes should be used, not separate psychotherapy and E/M codes. The medical E/M services need not be provided during the same session as the psychiatric services, but the combined times of both are used to determine the most appropriate code.

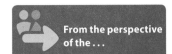

From the perspective of the . . .

PSYCHIATRIST

It is important that coders understand that most psychiatric visit codes are based on the time the physician spends with the patient. Coders must review the chart to determine the length of time so the correct code is reported.

CPT codes 90845–90899 describe other psychiatric services, such as psychoanalysis, family psychotherapy, group therapy, pharmacologic management, electroconvulsive therapy (ECT), hypnotherapy, and individual psychophysiological therapy.

CODER'S TIP

When selecting codes to describe psychotherapy services, coders must consider the place of service (outpatient vs. inpatient location); the type of psychotherapy (insight oriented vs. interactive); the total time of the procedure; and whether E/M services are provided in conjunction with the psychotherapy services.

For example, individual, insight-oriented psychotherapy services provided for a total of 80 minutes would be reported with CPT code 90808. If the same services were provided with medical E/M services, they would be reported with code 90809.

Biofeedback

CPT codes 90901 and 90911 describe biofeedback training. Code 90911 is reserved for training of the perineal muscles, anorectal or urethral sphincter. If biofeedback is part of psychophysiological therapy, it is reported with CPT codes 90875–90876.

Dialysis

CPT codes 90935 and 90937 describe individual hemodialysis procedures combined with E/M services related to the renal disease provided on the same day as the hemodialysis services. Code 90935 is reported if only one evaluation is necessary on that day, whereas code 99037 is reported if more than one evaluation is necessary. These codes are used to report inpatient end-stage renal disease (ESRD) and non-ESRD-related dialysis services or outpatient non-ESRD-related dialysis services.

CPT codes 90945 and 90947 report services when a dialysis technique other than hemodialysis is used (e.g., peritoneal dialysis, hemofiltration, or continuous renal replacement therapies). CPT code 90945 describes dialysis with one evaluation; CPT code 90947 describes dialysis with more than one evaluation.

CPT codes 90951–90962 describe outpatient ESRD services that are provided on a monthly basis. These codes are divided into four code series depending on the patient's age—younger than 2 years, 2–11 years, 12–19 years, and 20 years of age and older. Each series is subdivided based on the number of physician face-to-face visits that occur during the month—four or more visits, two to three visits, or one visit.

ESRD services include establishing the dialysis protocol, E/M services, telephone calls, and patient management during the month. If a patient is assessed for dialysis but doesn't receive dialysis services for the entire month, the services are reported with these codes based on the number of actual face-to-face visits that occur. If the patient is not assessed for dialysis but receives dialysis services for less than a full month, those services are reported with CPT codes 90967–90970, depending on the patient's age (see next page).

Home dialysis services are reported on a monthly basis with the age-specific CPT codes 90963–90966. The age divisions are the same as those for the ESRD services provided in outpatient centers (i.e., younger than 2 years, 2–11 years, 12–19 years, and 20 years of age and older).

CPT codes 90967–90970 describe *daily* dialysis services rather than monthly services. These codes describe age-specific dialysis services provided under certain circumstances: home dialysis for less than a full month; outpatient dialysis services with face-to-face visits but without a full assessment; dialysis stopped due to recovery or death; or patient receipt of a kidney transplant during the month.

CODING EXAMPLE

A 34-year-old male with ESRD has been undergoing regular outpatient hemodialysis services. During one month of these services, he was admitted to the hospital for acute cholecystitis, had his gallbladder removed, and remained in the hospital for a total of six days. During this hospitalization, he had dialysis treatments three times. During the first procedure, he saw the hospital dialysis physician twice; during the other two procedures, he saw the physician once. In spite of the fact that he was hospitalized for part of the month, he had three face-to-face visits with his regular dialysis physician in that time. Report the outpatient and inpatient dialysis services.

The monthly outpatient hemodialysis treatments are reported based on the patient's age (over 20 years) and the number of face-to-face visits with the physician (three visits). The appropriate code is 90961. The first inpatient dialysis procedure is reported with code 90937, whereas the other two are reported with code 90935.

Gastroenterology

Code range 91010–91299 describes measurement techniques for gastroenterology studies. These include esophageal, gastric, duodenal, and colon motility studies using manometry; reflux tests; gastrointestinal tract imaging utilizing capsule endoscopy devices; rectal tone tests; and anorectal manometry.

Ophthalmology

The General Ophthalmological Services section codes (92002, 92004, 92012, and 92014) describe intermediate and comprehensive professional services provided to new and established patients. Each of these codes includes a medical examination, evaluation, and initiation of diagnostic and treatment programs. The comprehensive services codes are reported only once even if the services are provided during multiple visits.

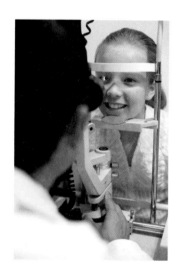

Ophthalmologists can report eye examinations with either general E/M codes or general ophthalmological services codes.

CODER'S TIP

Ophthalmologists may use either the general E/M codes (99201–99215) or the general ophthalmological services codes (92002–92014) to report examinations provided to new and established patients.

Codes in the Special Ophthalmological Services section (92015–92287) describe evaluations of the visual system that are not included under a general ophthalmological examination. These include services such as determination of **refractive state**; examination under anesthesia; gonioscopy; corneal topography; visual field examinations; serial tonometry with multiple measurements; computerized diagnostic imaging; extended ophthalmoscopy beyond that included in a general examination; retinal imaging; and ocular photography.

refractive state
The eye's ability to form recognizable images.

Remote imaging for either the detection of retinal disease (code 92227) or the monitoring and management of known retinal disease (code 92228) may not be reported with any E/M codes (92002–92014 or 99201–99350) or with codes describing other retinal imaging procedures (92133, 92134, or 92250).

CPT codes 92310–92326 describe contact lens services. These services are not part of the general ophthalmological examination. These services include all fitting services, patient instruction, and refitting of the contact lenses during the training period, as necessary. Follow-up care of contact lenses is included in the general ophthalmological services after the initial training and fitting.

A prescription for glasses is included in the services under CPT code 92015 (Determination of refractive state), including prescriptions for monofocal, bifocal, and trifocal lenses. Fitting of spectacles (99340–99371) is a separate service that involves measuring anatomical characteristics, providing instructions regarding lenses and frames, and adjusting the glasses after fabrication. Separate codes describe services for patients with **aphakia** (an absence of the natural lens in the eye, usually due to surgical excision for cataract or trauma). These codes do not include supplies such as frames and lenses.

aphakia
The absence of the natural lens in the eye, usually due to surgical excision for cataract or trauma.

Special Otorhinolaryngologic Services

Routine diagnostic and treatment procedures are included in evaluation and management services and are not separately reported when an E/M service is reported on the same day. Routine services include otoscopy, rhinoscopy, tuning fork tests, and the removal of nonimpacted cerumen. Special otorhinolaryngologic services described by CPT codes 92502–92700 are diagnostic and treatment services that are not included in an E/M service. These services may be reported separately.

The codes in this section describe a variety of services, including evaluation of speech and language, vestibular function, audiologic function, diagnostic evaluation of cochlear implants, speech-generating devices, swallowing function tests, hearing aid evaluation, and auditory rehabilitation.

Audiologic function tests include both ears unless otherwise indicated in the code descriptor. If only one ear is tested during a test that is typically performed on both ears, modifier 52 (reduced services) is added to the CPT code that describes the test performed.

When a service described by CPT codes 92502–92700 is provided during the same visit as an E/M service, both services may be reported.

EXERCISE 14.3

Also available in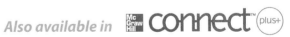

Use the CPT manual to select the correct code to report the following services.

1. Individual psychotherapy, interactive, using play toys or other forms of nonverbal communication, in the hospital, with 78 minutes of patient care _____

2. Single physician evaluation of a hemodialysis procedure _____

(Continued)

3. Dialysis for end-stage renal disease for 13 days for a 7-year-old patient _____

4. Gastric motility study with manometry _____

5. Gastrointestinal tract imaging, intraluminal, esophagus, with physician interpretation and report _____

_____

6. Ophthalmological service, new patient medical exam and evaluation with initiation of diagnostic and treatment program, intermediate _____

7. CPT codes 92601–92604 describe initial and subsequent programming of a cochlear implant device. Placement of the device is described by code _____ .

8. Which factor determines how vestibular function tests are classified? _____

14.4 Cardiovascular, Pulmonary, Immunological, and Neurological Services (92950–96155)

Cardiovascular

The Cardiovascular section (92950–93799) contains a variety of subsections describing nonsurgical procedures on the heart and major vessels, including:

- Therapeutic Services and Procedures
- Cardiography
- Cardiovascular Monitoring Services
- Implantable and Wearable Cardiac Device Evaluations
- Echocardiography
- Cardiac Catheterization
- Intracardiac Electrophysiological Procedures/Studies
- Peripheral Arterial Disease Rehabilitation
- Noninvasive Physiologic Studies and Procedures
- Other Procedures

coronary artery stent
A slender device used to hold open one of several arteries branching from the aorta that supply blood to the heart muscle.

Therapeutic Services and Procedures Therapeutic services and procedures include cardiopulmonary resuscitation (CPR), temporary transcutaneous pacing, cardioversion, and intravascular procedures on coronary vessels.

CPT codes 92980 and 92981 describe the placement of **coronary artery stents**, with 92980 describing the first vessel and 92981 reporting each additional vessel. These codes include the phrase "with or without other therapeutic intervention" as part their descriptors. When coronary angioplasty (92982, 92984) or atherectomy (92995, 92996) procedures are performed in the same artery in addition to stent placement, those procedures are considered other therapeutic interventions with the stent procedure and are not separately reported. If these procedures are performed alone without stent placement, those codes are reported as the primary procedure codes. When angioplasty or atherectomy procedures are performed on vessels other than the vessels undergoing stent placement, those procedures are reported with add-on code 92984 or 92996.

Percutaneous transluminal coronary thrombectomy and coronary brachytherapy are described by add-on codes 92973 and 92974. These services are reported in addition to CPT codes describing stent placement, angioplasty, and atherectomy procedures and are not considered therapeutic interventions associated with CPT codes 92980 and 92981.

Other procedures reported with codes from this section include valvuloplasty, atrial septectomy or septostomy, and pulmonary artery angioplasty.

Cardiography CPT codes 93000, 93005, and 93010 describe electrocardiograms (ECGs) with at least 12 leads, while codes 93040, 93041, and 93042 describe rhythm strips with 1–3 leads. The first code in each series includes the tracing, interpretation, and report; the second code describes the tracing only without interpretation and report; and the third code describes the interpretation and report only. CPT codes 93015–93018 describe an entire cardiovascular stress test or parts of that test.

cardiography
A recording of the heart in order to examine it.

CODING EXAMPLE

A cardiologist is called to evaluate a patient with a rapid heart rate who has been in the hospital for other reasons. He orders a 12-lead ECG and provides the interpretation and report for this examination. After evaluating the ECG, he orders medications for the patient and a rhythm strip ECG to be performed six hours later. He provides an interpretation and report for the second ECG. How should the ECG services be reported?

The coder looks up *ECG* in the index and is directed to the "Electrocardiography" entry for these services. Several subheadings appear under this main listing. Reviewing these codes in the tabular list of codes shows that code 93010 describes the interpretation and report of a 12-lead ECG, and code 93042 describes the interpretation and report of a rhythm strip. The ECG services provided by the cardiologist are described by codes 93010 and 93042.

Cardiovascular Monitoring Services These are diagnostic procedures using various technologies to assess the cardiac rhythm. CPT codes 93224–93227 describe external ECG monitors (sometimes referred to as Holter monitors) that provide up to 48 hours of recorded and stored information for later interpretation. In contrast, CPT codes 93228–99329 are external recording devices that automatically transmit event-triggered data in real time to remote surveillance centers for up to 30 days. These codes can only be reported once per 30 days. CPT codes 93268–93278 describe external recording devices that can be downloaded for up to 30 days but do not transmit data in real time.

Implantable and Wearable Cardiac Device Evaluations Implantable and wearable cardiac devices include cardiovascular monitors, pacemakers, cardioverter-defibrillators, and loop recorders. These devices may have a single lead, dual leads, or multiple leads. These devices require periodic evaluation and programming to test device function and select optimum values.

CPT codes 93279–93292 describe individual in-person services. Separate codes describe programming and interrogation for pacemakers, cardioverter-defibrillators, and loop recorders with various numbers of leads. Two CPT codes (93286 and 93287) describe device evaluations in the perioperative period (before and after surgery) to determine correct device functioning. These codes are reported twice when the services are performed both before and after the surgical procedure.

CPT codes 93293–93299 describe remote monitoring and interrogation of these devices. Several codes are reported only once per 90 days and cannot be reported if services are provided for less than 30 days. Other codes are only reported once per 30 days and cannot be reported if services are provided for less than 10 days.

CODER'S TIP

Coders should recognize which CPT codes describe services that are reported each time they are provided (93279–93292), reported once for each 90-day service period (93293–93296), or reported once per 30-day service period (93297–93298). The 90- and 30-day codes have a minimum number of days of service associated with them.

Echocardiography Transthoracic and transesophageal echocardiography are diagnostic tests that use ultrasonic signals to assess cardiac function, intracardiac blood flow, and hemodynamics. CPT codes 93303–93352 describe individual and combinations of echocardiography exams. Some codes describe complete procedures (probe placement, interpretation, and report) with associated codes describing individual aspects of the procedure, such as probe placement only or interpretation and report only.

cardiac catheterization

Insertion of a catheter into a vein, usually of the leg or arm, to investigate the condition of the heart, the coronary arteries, and surrounding blood vessels; to take blood samples; and to plan for surgery.

congenital

Present at birth, either inherited or due to an event during gestation up to the moment of birth.

Cardiac Catheterization

Cardiac catheterization (93451–93581) procedures include inserting catheters in a peripheral vein or artery; threading the catheter to the heart and great vessels; measuring pressures within those structures; and reporting those findings. Right heart catheterization measures pressures in the right atrium, right ventricle, pulmonary artery, and may include blood gas and/or cardiac output measurements. Left heart catheterization measures pressures in the left atrium and left ventricle.

Beginning in the 2011 version of the CPT manual, a new series of codes (93451–93461) describes various cardiac catheterization procedures or combinations of procedures performed for conditions other than **congenital** cardiac anomalies. This series of codes includes all portions of the catheterization procedure, such as catheter placement, injection of contrast material, and supervision and interpretation of angiogram imaging procedures during catheterization. To select the correct code to describe these catheterizations, it is necessary to understand all the procedures performed through the catheter. Once these have been identified, the individual code or codes are selected to describe those procedures, including:

- Right heart catheterization (93451)
- Left heart catheterization (93452)
- Combined right and left heart catheterization (93453)
- Coronary artery angiography of one or more coronary vessels (93454)
- Coronary artery angiography with bypass graft angiography (93455)
- Coronary artery angiography with right heart catheterization (93456)
- Coronary artery angiography with bypass graft angiography and right heart catheterization (93457)
- Coronary artery angiography with left heart catheterization (93458)
- Coronary artery angiography with left heart catheterization and bypass graft angiography (93459)

- Coronary artery angiography with right and left heart catheterization (34560)
- Coronary artery angiography with right and left heart catheterization and bypass graft angiography (93461)

When selecting the codes to describe these procedures, it is incorrect to report separate codes for procedures that are described together in one code. For example, if a left heart catheterization is performed with coronary artery catheterization, it must be reported with code 93458. It is not correct to report code 93452 for the left heart catheterization and code 93454 for the coronary artery catheterization.

Coders also must understand that these codes are only reported once, even if multiple arteries are catheterized. For example, code 93454 is only reported once for selective catheterization of the coronary arteries, even if multiple coronary arteries are individually catheterized. This is very different than reporting codes to describe peripheral artery catheterization procedures. In those procedures, separate codes are reported to describe the farthest portion of each artery into which the catheter tip is placed.

Several add-on codes describe additional procedures that may be performed with any of the catheterization and/or angiography procedures listed above, including a left heart catheterization by puncture through the septum or atrial wall from the right side of the heart (93462), administration of pharmacologic agents during the catheterization (93463), and physiological exercise during the catheterization (93464). These codes are reported in addition to the underlying catheterization procedure codes. CPT code 93503 describes placement of a flow-directed catheter (e.g., a Swan-Ganz catheter) for monitoring.

A separate series of codes (93530–93533) describes catheterization procedures for congenital cardiac conditions. One code (93530) describes right heart catheterization only. Codes 93531–93533 describe right heart catheterization with left heart catheterization for congenital anomalies. The difference between these three codes is the method of left heart catheterization.

This series of codes is very different than the series describing catheterization procedures for conditions other than congenital heart disease. Catheterization for conditions other than congenital heart disease include placement of catheters, injection of contrast material, imaging supervision, interpretation, and report. These are not reported separately. In contrast, catheterization procedures for congenital cardiac anomalies do not include contrast injections; injection procedures are reported separately with add-on codes 93563–93568. These codes describe injections of:

- One or more coronary arteries (93563)
- Coronary artery bypass grafts (93564)
- Left ventricle or left atrium (93565)
- Right ventricle or right atrium (93566)
- Aorta (93567)
- Pulmonary artery (93568)

These injection codes describe individual injections and are reported in addition to the code describing the catheterization procedure for congenital cardiac anomalies. When multiple injections are performed during a catheterization procedure for congenital anomalies, all appropriate add-on codes describing those injections are reported together.

In addition to catheterization to evaluate congenital anomalies or for diagnoses other than congenital anomalies, a Doppler probe may be placed in each coronary artery or coronary artery bypass graft to measure the velocity of blood flow within that vessel. These procedures are reported with two add-on codes, 93571 and 93572. Code 93571 is reported for the initial coronary artery or graft, and code 93572 is reported for each additional coronary artery or graft in which Doppler measurements are performed.

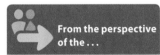

From the perspective of the . . .

CODER

In order to correctly report cardiac catheterization procedures, it is necessary to know the underlying diagnosis (i.e., whether the patient has a congenital cardiac anomaly or a diagnosis other than congenital anomaly). The next step is to identify all catheterization procedures performed to identify the code or codes to describe those procedures.

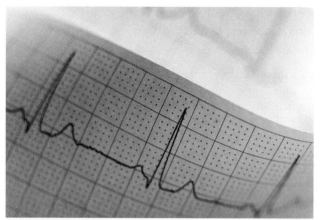

ECG recordings, like the one shown here, are performed by placing catheters in specific locations within the heart.

Intracardiac Electrophysiological Procedures/Studies Intracardiac electrophysiological studies are invasive diagnostic procedures that include ECG recording, arrhythmia induction, mapping, ablation of abnormal cardiac tissues, and combinations of these procedures.

ECG recordings (93600–93603) are performed with intracardiac catheters placed in specific locations within the heart. Arrhythmia induction (93610, 93612, and 93618) involves stimulating various areas of the heart through the catheters in an attempt to cause arrhythmias. Other codes (93620–93624 and 93640–93642) include recording, pacing, and arrhythmia induction from one or more intracardiac sites.

CPT codes 93609 and 93613 are add-on codes that describe mapping procedures. These are never reported as primary procedures; instead, they are reported in addition to the primary procedure codes. When abnormal cardiac tissues causing arrhythmias are identified, those areas of tissue are ablated using radio-frequency to destroy the tissues (93651 and 93652).

Noninvasive Physiologic Studies and Procedures CPT code range 93701–93790 includes several physiological measurements, such as bioimpedance-derived cardiovascular analysis, electronic analysis of an antitachycardia pacemaker system, temperature gradient measurements, programming of a wearable cardioverter-defibrillator, interrogation of a ventricular assist device, and measurement of venous pressure.

Noninvasive Vascular Diagnostic Studies

Vascular studies include patient care, supervision of the studies, interpretation of the results with copies for patient records, and analysis of all data. When flow is analyzed as part of these procedures, hard copies of the data and recordings must be included in the patient records, including measurements of bidirectional flow. Use of simple devices that do not produce hard copies or measure bidirectional flow is considered to be part of the physical exam and cannot be reported separately.

Guidance at the beginning of this code section describes limited and complete studies based on the number of measurements at various anatomical locations. The major arterial studies include cerebrovascular arterial studies (93880–93893), extremity arterial studies (93922–93931), extremity venous studies (93965–93971), visceral and penile vascular studies (93975–93982), and extremity arterial-venous studies (93990).

Pulmonary

Pulmonary medicine includes a series of codes describing ventilator management (94002–94005). These codes describe the initial day and subsequent days of hospital ventilator management, services in a nursing facility on a daily basis, and home ventilator management services provided over a calendar month.

bronchodilator
A drug that opens the breathing tubes in the lungs.

Other procedures (94010–94799) include laboratory measurements of pulmonary function and lung capacity; administration of medications such as **bronchodilators** with measurement of responsiveness to these medications; aerosol inhalation treatments; oxygen uptake and expired gas analysis; and various other tests.

Allergy and Clinical Immunology

CPT codes 95004–95075 describe allergy testing procedures (e.g., percutaneous, intradermal, and inhalation tests) to determine substances causing allergic reactions.

Most codes provide instructions to indicate the number of tests performed by each method.

Professional services associated with allergen immunotherapy are described by CPT codes 95115–95199. These codes describe injection of allergen immunotherapy agents only, providing and injecting allergenic extracts, and preparation of allergenic extracts. Coders must understand the full range of services provided during the visit to select the correct code to describe these services.

Endocrinology

Codes 95250 and 95251 describe continuous glucose monitoring of a patient using a subcutaneous sensor. Continuous glucose monitoring involves an implantable sensor that measures the blood glucose level. These measurements are used to adjust patient insulin therapy.

CPT code 95250 includes placement of the sensor, monitor adjustments, print-out of the data, and removal of the sensor. CPT code 95251 describes the interpretation and report associated with reviewing the data. The measurement period must be at least 72 hours to report these codes. The codes are only reported once a month, even when the measurement period is much longer than the 72-hour minimum time.

Neurology and Neuromuscular Procedures

Code range 95800–96020 consists of multiple subsections that describe neurological test procedures, including:

- Sleep Testing (95800–95811)
- Routine Electroencephalography (95812–95830)
- Muscle and Range of Motion Testing (95831–95857)
- Electromyography (95860–95872 and 95885–95887)
- Guidance for Chemodenervation and Ischemic Muscle Testing (95873–95875)
- Nerve Conduction Tests (95900–95905)
- Intraoperative Neurophysiology (95920)
- Autonomic Function Tests (95921–95923)
- Evoked Potentials and Reflex Tests (95925–95939)
- Special EEG Tests (95950–95967)
- Neurostimulators, Analysis-Programming (95970–95982)
- Other Procedures (95990–95999)
- Motion Analysis (96000–96004)
- Functional Brain Mapping (96020)

E/M services sometimes are provided in addition to these procedures and may be reported separately. Some tests (e.g., **electroencephalograms** [EEGs], autonomic function, evoked potential, reflex tests, electromyelogram [EMG], nerve conduction velocity [NCV], and magnetoencephalography [MEG]) described in this section include the test procedure plus the physician interpretation and report. If only the interpretation and report are provided, the code should be reported with modifier 26 to identify the professional component. Some tests, including EEG and intraoperative testing, include recording time as part of the code descriptors. Recording time only includes the time that the actual recording is occurring, not the time to set up the test or to remove the equipment after the recording is done.

electroencephalogram (EEG)
A record of the electrical activity of the brain.

CPT code 95920 is an add-on code describing intraoperative neurophysiology services, which are reported in addition to the CPT code describing the underlying test performed. This code is reported when the test is performed in the operating room during a surgical procedure. It is reported on a per-hour basis. This code is not reported if the recording time is less than 30 minutes. This time does not include performing a baseline study for comparison. CPT code 95920 is only reported once per hour, even if more than one neurophysiological test is performed during the operative session.

Medical Genetics and Genetic Counseling Services

CPT code 96040 describes genetic counseling services to a patient and family by trained genetic counselors. This code is reported for each 30 minutes of face-to-face time but is not reported if face-to-face time is less than 15 minutes. If a physician provides the genetic counseling, the appropriate E/M code is reported to describe those services.

Central Nervous System Assessments/Tests

CPT codes 96101–96125 describe tests of central nervous system cognitive functions, including cognitive processes, visual motor responses, and abstractive abilities. These tests are reported on a per-hour basis but must include a minimum of 31 minutes. Most of these codes can only be reported on the basis of face-to-face time. Several codes, including 96101, 96116, 96118, and 96125, include the time spent interpreting the tests and preparing the reports.

Health and Behavior Assessment/Intervention

CPT codes 96150–96155 describe assessments and interventions that focus on the psychosocial factors related to the patient's physical health status. These codes do not describe preventive medicine counseling or psychiatric services, each of which would be reported with CPT codes describing those services. These codes describe each 15-minute interval of face-to-face time by nonphysician providers. They are not used to report services provided by physicians. If a physician provides these services, the appropriate E/M code is reported to describe those services.

EXERCISE 14.4

Also available in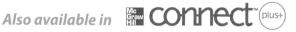

Use the CPT manual to select the correct code to report the following services.

1. Routine 12-lead ECG, tracing only _____

2. Interrogation and evaluation of an implantable loop recorder system device with physician analysis, review, and report, including heart rhythm derived data analysis _____

(Continued)

3. Left heart catheterization, including intraprocedural injection for left ventriculography _____

4. Bronchodilation responsiveness, spirometry, before and after bronchodilator administration _____

5. A physician applies a patch containing 15 specific allergenic substances to a patient's arm to determine the patient's specific allergies _____

6. Electroencephalogram (EEG); including recording while the patient is awake and asleep _____

7. Nerve velocity conduction test of ulnar and radial nerves, amplitude and latency/velocity, with F-wave study

_____

8. Interrogation device evaluation and analysis of a multiple-lead cardioverter-defibrillator _____

14.5 Injections and Infusions; Therapeutic Services; Rehabilitation; Moderate Sedation; Home Health and Medication Therapy Management Services (96360–99607)

Hydration, Therapeutic Injections and Infusions, and Chemotherapy

These three families of codes describe:

- Hydration therapy with intravenous (IV) fluids only.
- Injecting or infusing IV drugs for therapeutic, prophylactic, or diagnostic purposes.
- Injecting or infusing chemotherapy and other highly complex drugs or biologic agents.

These codes describe physician oversight of the preparation and administration of fluids and/or drugs. These codes are not reported when the substances are administered in the facility setting, even when the physician orders the administration of those fluids, drugs, or other substances.

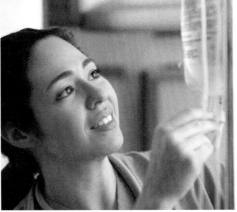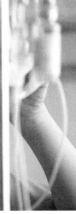

Hydration Codes 96360–96361 describe the infusion of IV fluids only. They do not include injection or infusion of drugs or other substances. CPT code 96360 describes the first hour of IV hydration and cannot be reported for infusions of less than 30 minutes. Code 96361 is an add-on code reported for each additional hour, but it must include at least 30 minutes of each additional hour reported.

Therapeutic, Prophylactic, and Diagnostic Injections and Infusions Codes 96365–96379 describe the intravenous, subcutaneous (SC), intramuscular (IM), or intra-arterial (IA) injection and/or infusion of drugs or other substances. Each series of codes includes a primary code that describes the initial drug injection or the first hour of drug infusion. Add-on codes describe additional time of infusion beyond the first hour. Other add-on codes describe the injection/infusion of additional substances either sequentially (one after the other) or concurrently (two or more drug infusions occurring at the same time). These codes are not used when the injection or infusion includes chemotherapeutic or highly complex biologic agents.

Intravenous hydration is described by codes 96360–96361. The first code describes the first hour of hydration, while the second code is an add-on code reported for each additional hour of hydration. Note the time limits associated with each of these codes.

Chemotherapy and Complex Drug or Biologic Agent Administration Chemotherapy agents or highly complex drugs require a higher degree of physician supervision over the preparation of the solutions and their administration. Separate families of codes within the 96401–96549 range describe injections or infusions of these agents, with primary codes for the initial hour or substance given and add-on codes describing additional time or additional substances given.

CODER'S TIP

Services necessary to perform IV hydration, injections, or infusions are included in those services and are not reported separately. These include the use of local anesthesia; starting the IV or accessing an indwelling IV catheter; flushing the IV catheter after the injection or infusion; and standard supplies necessary to perform the procedure, such as IV tubing, syringes, and needles.

Add-on code 96361 (instead of code 96360) is used to report IV hydration provided after IV injections or infusions of therapeutic or chemotherapy agents, including the first hour.

If time is a factor for a particular code, the time is the actual time the infusion is administered. Injections include infusions of less than 15 minutes.

CODING EXAMPLE

A physician starts an IV to give medications to a patient in his office. He begins a concurrent infusion of drugs A and B, which runs for a total of 1 hour and 45 minutes. After this, the physician begins a sequential infusion of drug C, which runs for 2 hours. After these infusions are finished, the physician runs an infusion of normal saline for one hour without any drugs. How are these services reported?

The first infusion of drug A is reported with code 96365 for the first hour and add-on code 96366 for the additional 45 minutes of infusion time. The concurrent infusion of drug B is reported with code 96368. The parenthetical note with this code instructs coders to report this code only once per encounter, so it is not time dependent. The infusion of drug C is reported with add-on code 96367 to describe the first hour, with add-on code 96366 for the additional hour. The one-hour infusion of normal saline following the drug infusions is reported with add-on code 96361. The hydration add-on code is used even though there is no initial hour of hydration because this is considered an additional service to the initial infusion of drug A. The parenthetical note with code 96361 provides this instruction.

Would this be reported differently if the drug infusions were given in the hospital outpatient setting? Yes, because physicians do not report these codes if the infusions are given in a facility setting.

Photodynamic Therapy

CPT code 96567 describes the use of external light to activate photosensitive drugs to treat malignant lesions in the skin or adjacent mucosa. This code is reported once per session, regardless of the total time the phototherapy is provided.

CPT codes 96570 and 96571 are add-on codes that describe photodynamic therapy provided in conjunction with endoscopy and/or bronchoscopy. These codes are reported in addition to the underlying codes describing the particular endoscopy/bronchoscopy procedure. Code 96570 describes the first 30 minutes of photodynamic therapy but must include at least 23 minutes of time for the service. Code 96571 is used to report each additional 15-minute period of photodynamic therapy but must include at least 8 minutes of time beyond the previous 15-minute period.

Special Dermatological Procedures

Most services provided by dermatologists are reported with E/M office visit or consultation codes. CPT codes 96900–96999 describe therapies typically provided by dermatologists that may be reported separately, including actinotherapy using ultraviolet light, microscopic examination of hair, whole-body photography, photochemotherapy, and laser therapy.

Physical Medicine and Rehabilitation

CPT codes 97001–97799 describe services provided by physicians, therapists (physical or occupational), and other nonphysician healthcare providers. These services include:

- Evaluations by nonphysician healthcare providers.
- Application of modalities (heat, cold, acoustic, light, mechanical, or electrical energy) to tissues or anatomical locations.
- Therapeutic procedures.
- Active wound care management.
- Tests and measurements.
- Orthotic and prosthetic management.

CODER'S TIP

Physical medicine and rehabilitation services require face-to-face time by the provider. If face-to-face services are provided in incremental intervals during the same visit, the times may be accumulated to determine the total face-to-face time. When providers perform multiple services, each service is reported separately without modifier 51 added to the code.

Medical Nutrition Management

Codes 97802–97804 describe nutrition management by nonphysicians (such as dieticians), including initial assessments, reassessments, and group sessions.

Acupuncture

Two primary codes (97810 and 97813) describe the initial 15 minutes of acupuncture therapy either with or without electrical stimulation of the acupuncture needles. Two add-on codes (97811 and 97814) describe additional 15-minute time increments with or without electrical stimulation. These add-on codes include repositioning of the acupuncture needles.

If the patient requires a significant, separately identifiable E/M service beyond that usually associated with an acupuncture service, it is reported with the appropriate E/M code with modifier 25 attached.

CODER'S TIP

Only one primary code describing an initial 15-minute service may be reported per day. If a provider performs acupuncture with and without electrical stimulation on the same day, only one initial period is reported. All additional time is reported with the appropriate add-on code.

Osteopathic Manipulative Treatment

CPT codes 98925–98929 describe osteopathic manipulative treatment. These procedures are most often provided by a doctor of osteopathic medicine (DO). These codes differ from one another based on the number of body regions manipulated (1–2 regions, 3–4 regions, 5–6 regions, 7–8 regions, or 9–10 regions). For purposes of these codes, body regions include the head, cervical (neck), thoracic, lumbar, sacral, and pelvic regions; lower extremities; upper extremities; rib cage region; and abdominal region.

Chiropractic Manipulative Treatment

Three CPT codes (98940–98942) describe chiropractic treatments of various numbers of spinal regions (cervical, thoracic, lumbar, sacral, and pelvic), with one code (98943) describing chiropractic treatments of one or more extraspinal regions. These services are most often provided by a doctor of chiropractic medicine (DC).

Education and Training for Patient Self-Management

Codes 98960–98962 describe education and training by nonphysicians that is intended to improve patient self-management of disease processes. Physicians usually order this education as part of their professional services, but other healthcare professionals provide the actual training.

Non-Face-to-Face Nonphysician Services

Codes 98966–98969 describe services that are similar to non-face-to-face services by physicians (e.g., phone calls or online evaluation) but are provided by other healthcare professionals.

Special Services, Procedures and Reports

Codes 99000–99091 describe a variety of services not included in other CPT code sections, including:

- Handling of specimens for laboratory studies.
- On-call hospital services.
- Services provided at times other than usual office hours.
- Office supplies not described by specific codes.
- Preparation of special reports.
- Analysis of clinical data stored in computers.

Qualifying Circumstances for Anesthesia

Add-on codes 99100, 99116, 99135, and 99140 are used in conjunction with CPT codes describing specific anesthesia services (00100–01999). The use of these codes is described in detail in the chapter on anesthesia services. Briefly, these codes describe extremes of age (99100), the use of total body hypothermia (99116), the use of controlled hypotension (99135), and anesthesia complicated by emergency conditions (99140).

Moderate (Conscious) Sedation

Moderate sedation is not an anesthetic or anesthesia service. Moderate sedation codes (99143–99150) describe a state of depression induced by drugs during which patients respond purposefully to verbal commands. It is not necessary for the provider to support the patient's airway. Spontaneous ventilation and cardiovascular function are usually adequate throughout the procedure without intervention. Moderate sedation is more than minimal sedation (anxiolysis) and less than deep

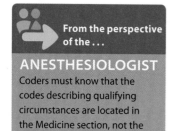

From the perspective of the . . .

ANESTHESIOLOGIST

Coders must know that the codes describing qualifying circumstances are located in the Medicine section, not the Anesthesia section.

moderate sedation
A state of depression induced by drugs during which patients respond purposefully to verbal commands.

sedation. Moderate sedation does not include monitored anesthesia care, which is reported with specific anesthesia CPT codes 00100–01999.

The six moderate sedation codes are divided into two groups of three codes, one group describing moderate sedation by the provider performing the underlying procedure that makes the sedation necessary (99143–99145) and the other describing moderate sedation by another provider (99148–99150). Within each group, there are two primary codes describing the first 15 minutes of moderate sedation—one for patients younger than 5 years of age and the other for patients 5 years of age and older. Each group includes an add-on code describing each additional 15 minutes of moderate sedation for patients of any age.

CODER'S TIP

Some CPT codes describe procedures in which it is assumed the patient will be provided moderate sedation. These codes are identified with a bull's-eye symbol and listed in Appendix G of the CPT manual. Specific rules determine when moderate sedation codes may be reported in conjunction with those services. CPT codes 99143–99145 (moderate sedation by the same provider) cannot be reported with codes listed in Appendix G, regardless of where the services are provided. CPT codes 99148–99150 (moderate sedation by a second provider) may be reported with codes listed in Appendix G if the services are provided in the facility setting but not if the services are provided in a nonfacility setting.

Home Health Procedures/Services

CPT codes 99500–99600 describe services provided by nonphysicians in a patient's residence, including assisted living facilities, group homes, custodial care facilities, or schools. Physicians providing care at the patient's home should report those services with the home visit E/M codes (99341–99350) and report other services with the appropriate CPT codes. Nonphysician healthcare providers reporting home health services may also report an E/M service with modifier 25 if they provide a significant, separately identifiable E/M service and are authorized to report E/M codes.

CPT code 99601 and add-on code 99602 describe home infusion procedures. Code 99601 describes the first two hours of infusion time, and code 99602 reports each additional hour.

Medication Therapy Management Services

CPT codes 99605–99607 describe medication therapy management services (MTMS) provided by a pharmacist in face-to-face interactions with the patient to optimize the treatment response to medications or to manage medication interactions or complications. CPT code 99605 is for the first 15 minutes of services provided to a new patient. Code 99606 describes the first 15 minutes of MTMS provided to an established patient. Add-on code 99607 describes each additional 15 minutes of MTMS to either new or established patients.

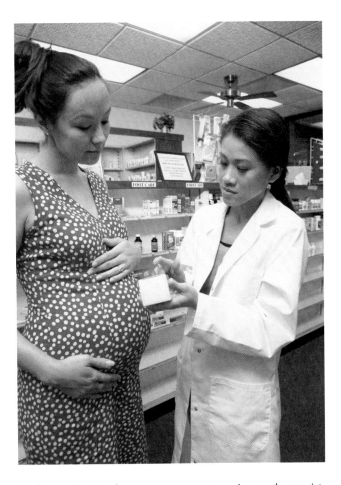

During medication therapy management services, a pharmacist interacts face to face with a patient to optimize the patient's response to medication or to help manage medication interactions or complications.

Also available in McGraw Hill **connect**™ plus+

Use the CPT manual to select the correct code to report the following services.

1. Concurrent infusion of an additional drug during intravenous infusion of a primary therapeutic agent _____

2. Injection of a chemotherapy agent directly into three lesions _____

3. Injection of two chemotherapy agents into the subarachnoid space via a subcutaneous reservoir _____

4. Reevaluation for athletic training _____

5. Debridement of an open wound with wound assessments and whirlpool _____

6. Osteopathic manipulative treatment of the head, neck, and both shoulders _____

7. Conscious sedation for 55 minutes of a 4-year-old child _____

8. Medication therapy management provided by a pharmacist to a new patient _____

Summary

Learning Outcome	Key Concepts/Examples
14.1 Explain the structure of the Medicine chapter and its general guidelines. **Pages 441–443**	The Medicine chapter consists of over 100 sections and subsections of codes describing procedures that are not typically considered surgical procedures. Broad categories of medicine codes include vaccines and administration; psychiatric services; dialysis; ophthalmology; otorhinolaryngologic services (ear, nose, and throat nonsurgical services); cardiology procedures; pulmonary procedures; neurological studies; IV infusions and chemotherapy; physical medicine and rehabilitation; and many other services described by these series of codes. The introductory material to this chapter includes general guidelines that apply to all code sections in the chapter, including reporting multiple procedures, the use of add-on codes, the meaning of "separate procedure" notations in code descriptors, the use of unlisted procedure codes, and reporting supplies used during these services.
14.2 Select codes to report the administration of immune globulins and vaccines. **Pages 444–445**	Individual vaccines are identified by CPT codes in the 90000 series. Vaccines that are manufactured in combination are identified with one code for the combined vaccine. If physicians combine two or more vaccines in one injection, both may be identified with separate codes. Immune globulins also may be identified by CPT codes from this chapter. Vaccine administration is identified with one set of CPT codes, but immune globulin administration is identified with another set of codes.
14.3 Identify codes to report psychiatry, dialysis, gastroenterology, ophthalmology, and otorhinolaryngologic services. **Pages 446–449**	Psychiatrists may report psychotherapy with codes from the 90000 series or with E/M codes. Psychotherapy may be combined with other services and both reported. CPT codes are used to describe a month of dialysis services, with separate codes describing dialysis based on patient age, type of dialysis, and whether or not evaluation services are performed during the month. Ophthalmologists may report general exams on new or established patients with CPT codes from the 90000 series or with E/M codes, but not both. Eye exams include some routine services, but other services may be reported separately. Otorhinolaryngologic codes include services that may be provided by physicians and nonphysicians, including audiologists and other providers.
14.4 Select codes to report cardiovascular, immunological, and neurological procedures. **Pages 450–456**	Codes in the Cardiology section of the 90000 code series describe both cardiology studies and procedures, including ECG; echocardiography; cardiac catheterization; angiography, angioplasty, and stent placement; electrophysiology studies; and evaluation of pacemakers and defibrillators. Pulmonary procedures include ventilator management and pulmonary function studies that may be performed in conjunction with therapeutic measures to determine the efficacy of the treatments provided. Allergy and immune therapy codes describe both allergy testing to determine specific allergens to which an individual is allergic as well as therapeutic measures to treat the allergy symptoms on a systemic basis. Neurology and neuromuscular testing includes a number of different procedures, including electroencephalograms, neuromuscular testing, nerve conduction studies, evoked potentials, intraoperative testing procedures, and functional brain mapping.

(Continued)

Learning Outcome	Key Concepts/Examples
14.5 Identify codes to report injections, infusions, therapeutic procedures, rehabilitation, moderate sedation, home health services, and medication therapy management. **Pages 457–461**	Hydration codes describe the administration of IV fluids for purposes of hydration only. Injection and infusion codes describe the administration of drugs and other substances via multiple routes of administration such as intramuscularly, intravenously, or subcutaneously. Chemotherapy codes describe the administration of substances requiring a high degree of supervision due to the risks involved. Physical medicine and rehabilitation codes describe numerous services, including the evaluation of patients by physical therapists, occupational therapists, and athletic trainers. These codes also describe therapeutic procedures, wound care, and the fitting of orthotic and prosthetic devices. Codes from the Medicine chapter may be used as add-on codes to identify qualifying circumstances with codes describing anesthesia services (00100–01999). Medicine codes are also used to describe moderate (conscious) sedation, which helps make patients more comfortable during uncomfortable procedures but is not considered an anesthesia service.

Using Terminology

Match the key terms with their definitions.

_____ **1.** L014.2 Immune globulins
_____ **2.** L014.2 Administration
_____ **3.** L014.2 Vaccine
_____ **4.** L014.2 Measles, mumps, and rubella (MMR)
_____ **5.** L014.2 Human papillomavirus (HPV)
_____ **6.** L014.3 Refractive state
_____ **7.** L014.3 Aphakia
_____ **8.** L014.4 Coronary artery stent
_____ **9.** L014.4 Cardiography
_____ **10.** L014.4 Cardiac catheterization
_____ **11.** L014.4 Congenital
_____ **12.** L014.4 Bronchodilator
_____ **13.** L014.4 Electroencephalogram
_____ **14.** L014.5 Moderate sedation

A. Serum extracted from human blood or produced in a lab through genetic modifications of human or animal proteins

B. Establishes whether a prescription is required for vision correction

C. Vaccine given subcutaneously to prevent three common childhood diseases

D. An invasive diagnostic medical procedure that includes inserting a catheter in the heart

E. A diagnostic medical procedure that records the heart's electronic activity

F. CPT codes that describe substances that prevent diseases, some of which are identified with a lightning bolt symbol indicating pending FDA approval

G. A condition in which the crystalline lens of the eye is absent

H. A rod or threadlike device for supporting tubular structures during surgical anastomosis or for holding arteries open during angioplasty

I. Present at birth

J. A graphic chart on which is traced the electric potential produced by the brain cells as electrodes are placed on the scalp

K. Virus that is the cause of common warts of the hands and feet as well as lesions of the mucous membranes of the oral, anal, and genital cavities

L. The act of giving medicine

M. A substance, especially a drug, that relaxes contractions of the smooth muscle to improve ventilation to the lungs

N. A state of quiet calmness induced by the use of medication while the patient is conscious

Checking Your Understanding

Select the letter that best completes the statement or answers the question.

1. L014.5 Which face-to-face time increment is reported when performing acupuncture?

   a. 10 minutes
   b. 15 minutes
   c. 20 minutes
   d. 30 minutes

2. L014.2 Which modifier is not added to immune globulin codes 90281–90399?

   a. 26
   b. 47
   c. 51
   d. 22

3. L014.1 Some procedures and services classified in the Medicine section are generally considered an integral component of a larger or more complete procedure or service. At times, however, these services may be provided on their own. These are identified by the following term in the code descriptor:

   a. Add-on codes.
   b. Special report.
   c. Home health procedures and services.
   d. Separate procedure.

4. L014.3 Code 96374 is reported each day when less than a full month of ESRD services are provided on a patient aged _____.

   a. 2–11 years
   b. 11–16 years
   c. 0–2 years
   d. 5–10 years

5. L014.1 When no surgical incision or excision is required to perform a procedure, it is considered _____.

   a. Minimally invasive
   b. Noninvasive
   c. An add-on code
   d. A separate procedure

6. L014.1 The Medicine chapter comprises most of the 90000 series of CPT codes. The exception to this is the section of codes that describe the _____ code series.

   a. Anesthesia
   b. Evaluation and Management
   c. Pathology and Laboratory
   d. Radiology

Mc Graw Hill connect plus+

Enhance your learning by completing these exercises
and more at mcgrawhillconnect.com!

CHAPTER 14 | MEDICINE SERVICES   465

7. L014.1 Procedures designated by add-on codes, identified by a plus (+) sign, can only be reported with a(n) _____.

   a. Parent code
   b. Separate procedure code
   c. HCPCS code
   d. Unlisted service or procedure code

8. L014.2 If counseling is not provided during administration of a vaccine to an 18-year-old, the administration should be reported with CPT codes _____.

   a. 90471–90474
   b. 90460–90461
   c. 96365–96368
   d. 96372, 96374

9. L014.3 CPT codes describing ESRD services are reported _____.

   a. Weekly
   b. Monthly
   c. Every three months
   d. Quarterly

10. L014.2 There are two codes reported for each vaccine given. These codes describe _____.

    a. The vaccine and administration
    b. The vaccine and E/M service
    c. The vaccine and materials supplied by the physician
    d. The vaccine and the allergy extract

11. L014.4 A nurse administers a single allergy injection using allergenic extract that was previously prepared by an allergist and brought to the office by the patient. Report code _____.

    a. 95130
    b. 95144
    c. 95145
    d. 95115

12. L014.4 A patient undergoes a sleep study with a technologist in attendance and simultaneous recording of ECG, ventilation, respiratory effort, and oxygen saturation. This is reported with the following CPT code:

    a. 95806
    b. 95807
    c. 95808
    d. 95811

13. L014.4 A trained genetic counselor met for the first time with a couple, who was referred by their doctor, and conducted medical genetic counseling for 90 minutes. Report code(s) _____.

    a. 96040 X 3
    b. 96040-22
    c. 99215, 96040, 96040, 96040-52
    d. 99201, 96040

14. **L014.4** When a functional MRI (fMRI) is performed by a provider other than a physician or a psychologist, report code(s) _____.

   a. 96020, 70554
   b. 70555-51
   c. 70554
   d. 96020, 70555

15. **L014.4** A patient sees her ophthalmologist for a refractive state determination. The ophthalmologist would report the following code:

   a. 92025
   b. 92014
   c. 99214
   d. 92015

16. **L014.5** An established patient of Dr. John's underwent routine insertion of an IV catheter and a one-hour IV infusion of 1,000 ml of normal saline with potassium chloride and magnesium sulfate. This is reported with code _____.

   a. 96365
   b. 36000
   c. 36410
   d. 36556

17. **L014.4** CPT codes describing ESRD-related services for dialysis provided for less than a full month are differentiated by the patient's _____.

   a. Diagnosis
   b. Age
   c. Symptoms
   d. Treatment

18. **L014.4** A patient undergoes transtelephonic pacemaker evaluation of her multiple-lead pacemaker system for 60 days. This procedure includes the physician analysis, review, and his documented report. This code is reported as _____.

   a. 93293 just once
   b. 93293 just twice in 60 days
   c. 93293 X 60
   d. 93279

19. **L014.4** A radiologist in the hospital performs a Doppler analog waveform analysis, a photoplethysmography and a flow velocity signal of the arteries of both arms, and a duplex scan of both arms. The patient was referred to the radiologist because of numbness and tingling in the arms that were suspected to be related to thoracic outlet syndrome. What procedure code(s) should be used to report this scenario?

   a. 93922-50-TC, 93939-50-TC
   b. 93922-26, 93930-26
   c. 93922-TC, 93930-26
   d. 93922

connect™ plus+
Enhance your learning by completing these exercises
and more at mcgrawhillconnect.com!

CHAPTER 14 | MEDICINE SERVICES   467

20. L014.5 Add-on codes used in conjunction with CPT codes describing specific anesthesia services are
_____.

    a. 99100, 99116, 99135, 99140
    b. 00100–01999
    c. 99100, 99116, 00100, 01999
    d. None of these

Applying Your Skills

Use your CPT manual to determine the correct code(s) to report each of the following services.

1. L014.3 Auditory evoked potentials for testing of the central nervous system, comprehensive exam
_____

2. L014.2 Diphtheria, tetanus toxoid, acellular pertussis vaccine, and inactivated poliovirus vaccine (DTaP-IPV) administered to a 5-year-old after discussing this vaccine with the child's mother _____

3. L014.3 Outpatient ESRD-related services provided over a one-month period to a 25-year-old patient, including four face-to-face physician visits _____

4. L014.3 Hemodialysis services provided to an inpatient, including two physician visits on the day of dialysis
_____

5. L014.3 Gastric intubation and aspiration for treatment _____

6. L014.3 Fifty minutes of individual psychotherapy with medical evaluation and management services
_____

7. L014.3 Binaural hearing aid check _____

8. L014.4 Programming evaluation of implantable dual-lead pacemaker system with report
_____

9. L014.4 Perioperative evaluation of dual-lead implantable cardioverter-defibrillator, before and after surgical procedure _____

10. L014.4 Real-time transesophageal echocardiography with image documentation, including probe placement, image acquisition, interpretation, and report _____

11. L014.4 Placement of a Swan-Ganz catheter _____

12. L014.4 Inhalation bronchial challenge testing with histamine _____

13. L014.3 Psychiatric diagnostic interview of a 4-year-old patient, interactive technique _____

14. L014.5 Physical therapy reevaluation _____

15. L014.5 Intravenous administration of substances designed to treat malignant tumors, 1 hour and 45 minutes
_____

16. L014.2 Routine diphtheria/tetanus immunization injection by the medical assistant _____

17. L014.3 Biofeedback training of the perineal muscles and urethral sphincter _____

18. L014.5 Chemotherapy injections directly into three lesions _____

19. L014.5 (a) Hydration infusion therapy, 45 minutes _____

  (b) Hydration therapy, 20 minutes _____

20. L014.5 Therapy with hot and cold packs _____

21. L014.4 Percutaneous transluminal coronary angioplasty (PTCA) procedure on three vessels

_____

22. L014.4 Three-hour encephalogram while awake _____

23. L014.2 Quadrivalent HPV vaccine, intramuscular administration, and preservative-free split-virus influenza virus vaccine, intramuscular administration, to a 22-year-old _____

24. L014.2 Immune globulin, intramuscular injection _____

25. L014.3 Initial extended ophthalmoscopy with retinal drawings _____

26. L014.5 Conscious sedation for 4-year-old child for 1 hour and 43 minutes_____

27. L014.5 Medication therapy management for a new patient by a pharmacist _____

28. L014.4 Neurobehavioral status exam, including interpretation and report, 107 minutes total time

_____

29. L014.5 Thirty minutes of sedation for a 7-year-old undergoing an uncomfortable procedure

_____

30. L014.5 Assessment of aphasia with interpretation and report, per hour _____

Thinking It Through

Use your critical-thinking skills to answer the questions below.

1. Describe the factors that coders must consider when reporting dialysis services for patients with ESRD, including services provided on a monthly basis in a dialysis center as well as inpatient or outpatient individual dialysis services provided in a hospital. Describe when the individual dialysis service codes are reported.

_____

_____

2. Describe the families of codes used to report cardiac catheterization procedures for noncongenital and congenital anomalies. Explain which additional services associated with the catheterization procedure may be reported separately for either or both of these catheterization procedures.

_____

_____

3. Explain the differences between hydration therapy with IV fluid; therapeutic, prophylactic and diagnostic injections and infusions; and administration of chemotherapy or other highly complex drugs or biologic agents. Include a brief explanation of the reporting conventions for these services.

_____

_____

connect plus+

Enhance your learning by completing these exercises
and more at mcgrawhillconnect.com!

CHAPTER 14 | MEDICINE SERVICES   469

15

INTRODUCTION TO THE HEALTHCARE COMMON PROCEDURE CODING SYSTEM (HCPCS)

Learning Outcomes *After completing this chapter, students should be able to:*

15.1 Explain HCPCS codes.

15.2 Identify services described by A-, B-, C-, and E-codes.

15.3 Select codes to report services described by G-, H-, J-, K-, L-, and M-codes.

15.4 Determine codes to report services described by P-, Q-, R-, S-, T-, and V-codes.

15.5 Use HCPCS modifiers.

Key Terms

Advanced life support (ALS)

Basic life support (BLS)

Durable medical equipment (DME)

Emergency transportation

Enteral and parenteral therapy

Level I HCPCS codes

Level II HCPCS codes

Medical supplies

Non-emergency transportation

Orthotic

Physician Quality Reporting Initiative (PQRI)

Prosthetic

Table of Drugs

Unit of service

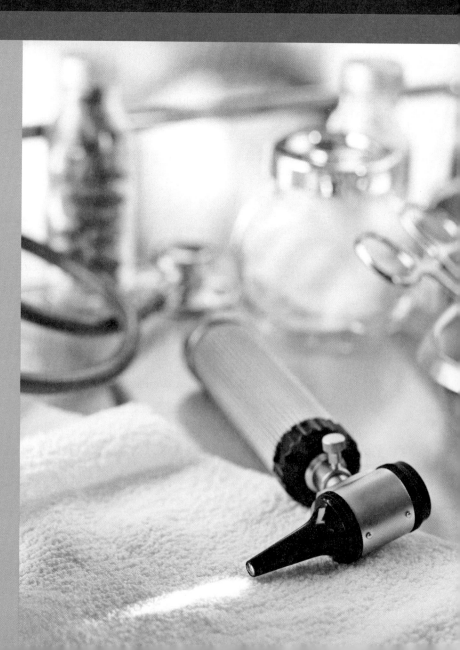

Introduction

In 1983, the Centers for Medicare and Medicaid Services (CMS) created a coding system known as the Healthcare Common Procedure Coding System (HCPCS). This procedural coding system was developed to meet the needs of Medicare and Medicaid, as well as other healthcare participants. CPT codes generally describe services provided by physicians and other licensed professionals. Other services, such as devices or supplies, are often provided as part of those services. Since those services are not described by CPT codes, CMS created the HCPCS system to describe them. Examples of services and supplies described by HCPCS codes include emergency and non-emergency transportation, medical supplies, durable medical equipment, prosthetics, orthotics, and supplies used when performing professional services. Coders must become as familiar with reporting HCPCS codes as they are with reporting CPT codes, including when HCPCS codes should be reported and which modifiers to assign with them to provide additional detail.

15.1 HCPCS Codes

Functions of HCPCS Codes

The HCPCS is divided into Level I and Level II HCPCS codes. **Level I HCPCS codes** are the Current Procedural Terminology (CPT) codes that have been discussed in detail in other chapters. These are maintained by the American Medical Association and primarily describe services provided by physicians and other healthcare professionals. Because Medicare and other insurers cover a variety of services, supplies, and equipment that are not identified by CPT codes, CMS established the **Level II HCPCS codes** to report these other services.

Representatives from CMS, the Health Insurance Association of America (HIAA), and the Blue Cross and Blue Shield Association (BCBSA) update the HCPCS Level II codes on a quarterly basis. The American Dental Association (ADA) establishes and maintains the Current Dental Terminology (CDT) codes, which describe dental procedures. The CDT codes are updated every two years and up until 2011 were incorporated into the HCPCS Level II codes. HCPCS Level II codes change from year to year, so it is important that coders keep up with the additions, deletions, and revisions.

Level II HCPCS codes are in the public domain and are free to use. They are available from:

- The CMS website (public use files).
- The *Federal Register.*
- Medicare carriers.
- Commercial publishers.

Level I HCPCS codes
Current Procedural Terminology (CPT) codes that primarily describe services provided by physicians and other healthcare professionals.

Level II HCPCS codes
Codes that report services, supplies, and equipment not identified by CPT codes that are covered by Medicare and other insurers.

CODER'S TIP

Occasionally a CPT code and HCPCS code may each describe a similar service. Usually the HCPCS code has a greater level of specificity. For example, CPT code 99070 generically describes miscellaneous supplies provided by a physician. HCPCS codes, however, often describe these supplies in more specific detail.

This chapter focuses on the Level II HCPCS codes and some of their modifiers. The Level II HCPCS includes many more modifiers than the CPT. These modifiers and definitions are available from many sources and, like the HCPCS codes, are part of the public domain.

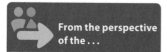

Uses of HCPCS Codes

HCPCS codes should generally be used:

- When there is no CPT code that describes the item or service provided.
- When the HCPCS code is more specific than the CPT code.
- When instructed to do so by a particular payer.

The CPT primarily describes professional services. Other healthcare-related services, such as durable medical equipment, drugs, transportation, and many others, are not included in the CPT. These services, however, are described by HCPCS codes and will be discussed in detail in this chapter.

Some services are described by both CPT and HCPCS codes. In this situation, Medicare often instructs coders to use the HCPCS codes. Other payers may instruct otherwise. Coders should be familiar with the requirements for each entity to which they report coding information.

Index and Tabular List of Services

In order to use the HCPCS manual effectively, coders must use the index (usually found at the front of the manual) to identify the range of codes that describes the service or supply. Depending on the type of service reported, the index might list a single code, a family of codes, or families of codes in a single HCPCS category or multiple codes in more than one HCPCS category.

Once all possible codes are located in the index, the coder must locate each code in the tabular list of services to determine which is the most appropriate code to describe the service or item provided. After identifying the best HCPCS code to describe the service provided, the coder must then determine how many units of the code should be reported.

The **Table of Drugs** is used to identify specific codes that describe medications provided to patients in physician offices or medical facilities. These codes are not used to identify prescription medications provided by a pharmacy. The Table of Drugs lists medications by their generic and brand names, the particular HCPCS code identifying the medication, the most common routes of administration, and the unit value for the HCPCS code. Once a code for a particular medication has been identified, coders still must review the actual HCPCS code in the tabular list of codes to determine that the code listed in the Table of Drugs is the most appropriate code to report use of that medication.

Table of Drugs
Table in the HCPCS manual used to identify specific codes that describe medications provided to patients in physician offices or medical facilities.

Calculating Multiple Units of Service

Many HCPCS code descriptors include a particular amount of the described service. This amount is a **unit of service** described by the code. The actual amount provided is often greater than the unit value. If so, the coder should list the HCPCS code that describes the service followed by a sufficient number of units to account for the total services provided.

unit of service
A particular amount of a described service included in a HCPCS code descriptor.

CODER'S TIP

Coders must pay particular attention to the definitions and unit values of HCPCS codes. Many HCPCS codes have specific quantities in each description. Coders must be extremely mindful of terms such as "each," "per pair," "per ounce," "per cc," "per 100 calories," and "per square inch." Unit values in the code descriptors are important when calculating the number of units provided.

CODING EXAMPLE

A physician gives her patient 1,000 mg of Rocephin, an antibiotic, in her office. How should the coder report this medication?

(Continued)

Because Rocephin is a drug, the coder turns to the Table of Drugs and finds that Rocephin is listed with HCPCS code J0696. The coder then looks up that code in the tabular list, where the generic name for Rocephin (ceftriaxone sodium) is also listed. HCPCS code J0696 describes 250 mg of Rocephin as the unit dose. To appropriately report the amount of drug provided, the coder would list J0696 HCPCS with four units following the code (J0696 X 4).

Rocephin is commonly administered in 500, 750, or 1,000 mg doses. These would be reported with J0696 X 2, J0696 X 3, or J0696 X 4.

Identifying Services Described by Each Category of HCPCS Codes

Level II HCPCS codes are grouped according to types of services or supplies. HCPCS codes are alphanumeric consisting of a single letter (A–V) followed by four numerical digits. This is in contrast to CPT Category I codes, which are identified using five numerical digits or CPT Category II and Category III codes, which are identified with four numerical digits followed by a single letter. Understanding the specific types of services, supplies, equipment, devices, and medications included in each section is necessary for accurate coding. In the HCPCS manual, instructions and information applicable to a specific category of codes are found at the beginning of each major category. Coders should be familiar with this information and review it frequently as these instructions and guidance often change with each new edition of the HCPCS manual.

Level II HCPCS codes are divided into the categories shown in Table 15.1.

TABLE 15.1 Categories of Level II HCPCS Codes

Code Category	Services Described
A	Transportation services including ambulance; medical and surgical supplies; administrative, miscellaneous, and investigational
B	Enteral and parenteral therapy
C	Outpatient prospective payment system (OPPS)
E	Durable medical equipment
G	Procedures/professional services (temporary); Physician Voluntary Reporting Program codes; last-minute additions
H	Alcohol and drug abuse treatment services
J	Drugs administered other than oral method
K	Codes assigned to the DME Medicare administrative contractors
L	Orthotic and prosthetic procedures
M	Other medical services
P	Pathology and laboratory services
Q	Miscellaneous services (temporary)
R	Diagnostic radiology services
S	Temporary national codes (non-Medicare)
T	National T-codes established for state Medicaid agencies
V	Vision, hearing, and speech-language pathology services

Also available in **Mc Graw Hill** **connect** (plus+)

Answer the questions below.

1. Which regulatory agency maintains the HCPCS codes? _____

2. HCPCS codes beyond those in the CPT system are also known as what type of code? _____

3. If a CPT code and HCPCS code have exactly the same code descriptions, which one should be reported for non-Medicare patients? _____

4. In the HCPCS system, CPT codes are also known as _____.

5. When reporting services identified with HCPCS codes, it is important for coders to identify the _____ value included in the definition to determine how many times to report the service.

15.2 HCPCS A-, B-, C-, and E-Codes

A-Codes: Transportation Services Including Ambulance; Medical and Surgical Supplies; Administrative, Miscellaneous and Investigational

HCPCS A-codes describe transportation services; supplies commonly used by physicians and facilities to treat patients; and nonprescription drugs and radiopharmaceutical diagnostic imaging agents. The transportation and medical supplies sections are further subcategorized to provide a greater level of specificity for more precise coding.

emergency transportation
Transportation used to bring a critically ill patient to a hospital.

non-emergency transportation
Transportation used to move a patient who is not in immediate, critical need of medical care.

basic life support (BLS)
The level of medical care given to a patient with life-threatening illnesses or injuries until the patient reaches a hospital.

advanced life support (ALS)
A higher level of medical care that supports circulation and breathing while the patient is being transported.

Transportation Transportation codes are divided into two broad categories—**emergency transportation** and **non-emergency transportation.** Some transportation services are reported on a per-mile basis, and coders must pay attention to the unit values of these codes when reporting services.

Emergency transportation is most often provided by an ambulance service. There are two types of ground ambulance services—**basic life support (BLS)** and **advanced life support (ALS).** These designations refer to the equipment available on the ambulance and the personnel manning the vehicle. At times an ALS vehicle may be used to provide a BLS-level transport, but a BLS vehicle is not generally equipped to provide an ALS-level transport. Both types of vehicles may be used at times to provide non-emergency transportation services. Coders must be careful to identify the type of transportation as well as the type of vehicle used during transport.

The following are examples of transportation HCPCS codes commonly used by coders:

- A0426: Ambulance service, advanced life support, non-emergency transport, level 1
- A0427: Ambulance service, advanced life support, emergency transport, level 1
- A0428: Ambulance service, basic life support, non-emergency transport (BLS)
- A0425: Ground mileage, per statute mile
- A0100: Non-emergency transportation; taxi
- A0130: Non-emergency transportation; wheelchair van
- A0180: Non-emergency transportation: ancillary: lodging, recipient
- A0190: Non-emergency transportation: ancillary: meals, recipient

Reports for ambulance transportation services also should include a separate HCPCS code to identify the number of miles the ambulance transported the patient. The mileage code is listed separately with the number of units attached to the code to indicate the number of miles traveled.

HCPCS modifiers were discussed in detail in Chapter 7 and will be reviewed in Section 15.5 of this chapter. Ambulance modifiers are different than other modifiers. When ambulance services are reported, special modifiers must be used to identify the pick-up point and destination of the ambulance trip. Single-digit characters identify each of these locations and are combined to form a two-digit character that accurately describes the two location points. The most common locations are:

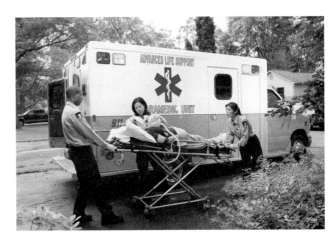

D   Diagnostic or therapeutic site other than a hospital or physician's office

H   Hospital

J   Freestanding end-stage renal disease (ESRD) facility

N   Skilled nursing facility (SNF)

P   Physician's office

R   Residence

S   Scene of an accident

Coders often must assign codes for a patient's medical transportation. When choosing a code to report this service, note factors such as the type of transportation, whether life support was provided, and whether the transportation was an emergency.

These location identifiers are combined to create the two-digit modifier that specifically describes the pick-up and destination points of the ambulance trip. It is possible that an ambulance modifier could be the same as another HCPCS modifier. The meaning of the modifier depends on the code to which it is attached.

CODING EXAMPLE

An ambulance transports an injured individual from the scene of an accident to the hospital after a severe automobile accident. This trip is a total of 18 miles. Which codes and modifier describe this service?

Reviewing the ambulance codes, the coder finds that HCPCS code A0427 describes the ambulance transport. The code is reported with modifier SH, indicating that the trip started at the accident scene and ended at the hospital. HCPCS code A0425 (Ground mileage, per statute mile) is reported to indicate the total miles. The coder reports A0427-SH and A0425 X 18.

CODER'S TIP

The pick-up/destination modifiers may be the same as other HCPCS modifiers, but they may have completely different meanings when used with an ambulance code. For example, ambulance modifier HN indicates transportation between a hospital and a skilled nursing facility. However, when used with other codes, HN indicates that the provider has received training at the bachelor's degree level. Even though the modifiers are the same, they have different meanings.

Non-emergency transportation codes distinguish between different types of vehicles (e.g., bus, minivan, wheelchair van, taxi, or air travel). This section also includes codes for meals and lodging provided during these transports.

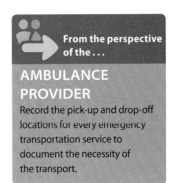

From the perspective of the . . .

AMBULANCE PROVIDER

Record the pick-up and drop-off locations for every emergency transportation service to document the necessity of the transport.

CODER'S TIP

State Medicaid programs often provide non-emergency transportation and use these codes to identify those services.

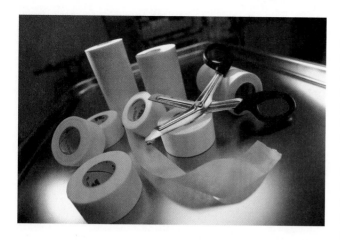

Medical and Surgical Supplies This section includes hundreds of codes used to identify various **medical supplies** provided to patients as part of their treatment. Most of these supplies are single-use disposable items, in contrast with items that are used repeatedly over a long period of time. Examples of the latter types of supplies are **durable medical equipment** (described by E-codes) and wheelchairs (described by K-codes).

Supplies described by A-codes are organized into numerous categories, ranging from syringes to diabetic testing supplies; from contraceptives to ostomy supplies; from wound dressings to diabetic shoes. There are simply too many different categories of codes to cover individually. As discussed above, coders must effectively use the index to locate ranges of codes for the services provided and then use the tabular listing of individual codes to select the correct code from that range.

Medical and surgical supplies are classified by whether they are single-use items (e.g., bandages) or durable items (e.g., crutches).

medical supplies
Items provided to patients as part of their treatment; generally used once and then disposed of.

durable medical equipment (DME)
Reusable medical equipment bought or rented for use in the home.

CODING EXAMPLE

A physician provides five 6″ × 4″ (24 sq. in.) nonimpregnated, sterile gauze pads with an adhesive border to a patient to change a wound dressing daily. How should the coder report these supplies?

The coder looks up *gauze pads* in the index and is directed to the A6216–A6230 range of HCPCS codes. The coder then refers to the tabular listing of codes and locates HCPCS code A6220 (Gauze, nonimpregnated, sterile, pad size more than 16 sq. in. but less than or equal to 48 sq. in., with any size adhesive border, each dressing), which correctly describes the gauze pads provided. The coder lists this code with five units of service to identify the number of pads provided to the patient. The coder reports these supplies as A6220 X 5.

Administrative, Miscellaneous, and Investigational This section of HCPCS A-codes includes codes for several types of products. Many of these are related to radiopharmaceutical diagnostic imaging agents used during radiology imaging studies. Numerous imaging agents are currently in use, and new codes are frequently added. Coders should be able to locate codes for these imaging agents by using the index and then choose the single best code by using the tabular section.

B-Codes: Enteral and Parenteral Therapy

enteral and parenteral therapy
The provision of nutrients to prevent or treat malnutrition.

HCPCS B-codes describe **enteral and parenteral therapy.** This section includes codes for different types of formulas and the supplies necessary to administer them, including infusion pumps. Many payers, including Medicare, require certification of the medical necessity of these therapies.

Many of these codes have units measured in calories, grams, or milliliters. The codes are reported with the number of units necessary to describe the total amounts provided to the patient.

Examples of enteral and parenteral supplies include:

- B4035: Enteral feeding supply kit; pump fed, per day
- B4087: Gastrostomy/jejunostomy tube, standard, any material, any type, each
- B4149–B4162: Enteral formulas, various solutions, 100 calories = 1 unit
- B4185: Parenteral nutrition solution, per 10 grams lipids
- B9002: Enteral nutrition infusion pump, with alarm

C-Codes: Outpatient Prospective Payment System (OPPS)

HCPCS C-codes describe some services, drugs, biologicals, radiopharmaceuticals, devices, and supplies provided in the outpatient hospital setting. Medicare uses these codes to determine payments for outpatient services. These codes are not used when these products or services are provided in an inpatient or office setting. Most C-codes describe products and services that do not have other HCPCS codes assigned to them.

A few examples of C-codes describing services provided in an outpatient hospital include:

- C1717: Brachytherapy source, nonstranded, high dose rate iridium-192, per source
- C1721: Cardioverter-defibrillator, dual chamber (implantable)
- C1756: Catheter, pacing, transesophageal
- C1785: Pacemaker, dual chamber, rate-responsive (implantable)
- C8900: Magnetic resonance angiography with contrast, abdomen

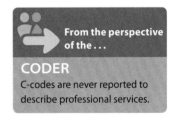

From the perspective of the . . .

CODER
C-codes are never reported to describe professional services.

D-Codes: Dental Procedures

The American Dental Association maintains and copyrights the Current Dental Terminology (CDT), which was incorporated into the HCPCS Level II code set and HCPCS manual until 2011. These codes were not included in the 2011 HCPCS manual. It is unclear whether CMS will include CDT codes in future editions of the HCPCS manual. Because of this uncertainty, this text will not address CDT codes in detail.

E-Codes: Durable Medical Equipment

HCPCS E-codes describe durable medical equipment (DME), which generally includes equipment that is meant to be long lasting, can withstand repeated use, may be used in the home, and typically is not used by individuals who do not have a medical condition. Examples of DME include but are not limited to canes, crutches, commodes, decubitus care equipment, bath and toilet aids, hospital beds and accessories, oxygen and respiratory equipment, monitoring equipment, traction devices, and wheelchairs.

E-codes also include numerous individual replacement parts for DME that require routine repair or maintenance. Coders should use the index to locate sections of codes applicable to specific devices, then go to the tabular section and choose the correct code from among the codes within that section. E-codes are highly specific and detailed. Each section contains multiple codes that have small differences between them. Coders should understand that minor changes in the device descriptors affect the choice of the correct code.

CODER'S TIP

Coders should ensure that the chosen code best describes the particular equipment to the greatest level of specificity. This is especially important when selecting a code from among the numerous codes describing accessories or replacement items for DME products.

E-codes require the use of modifiers to indicate whether the equipment is new or used and whether it is rented or purchased. These modifiers include NU (new), UE (used), and RR (rented). To code for DME, coders must understand the use of each of these modifiers.

EXERCISE 15.2

Also available in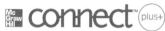

Use the HCPCS manual to select the HCPCS codes for the following services.

1. An emergency helicopter landing at the scene of an accident and transporting the patient to the nearest hospital heliport _____ *(Include the ambulance modifier.)*

2. Transportation of a patient from the doctor's office back to the skilled nursing facility for a non-emergency wheelchair van _____ *(Include the ambulance modifier.)*

3. A disposable external urethral clamp or compression device that is not used with a catheter clamp _____

4. The use of 10 nonreusable surgical dressing holders _____

5. The use of a one-way chest drain valve _____

6. Five hundred calories of a nutritionally complete, calorically dense enteral formula with intact nutrients, including proteins, fats, carbohydrates, vitamins, and minerals and may include fiber that is administered through an enteral feeding tube, 100 calories = 1 unit _____

7. An adjustable, folding, wheeled walker _____

8. A fixed-height hospital bed with side rails, without a mattress _____

15.3 HCPCS G-, H-, J-, K-, L-, and M-Codes

G-Codes: Procedures/Professional Services (Temporary); Physician Voluntary Reporting Program Codes; Last-Minute Additions

HCPCS G-codes are created by CMS and are under Medicare's jurisdiction. In general, G-codes identify professional healthcare procedures and services that would otherwise be coded by CPT codes but for which there are no CPT codes. In some cases, however, CMS creates a G-code that has the same meaning as an existing

CPT code. When both a CPT code and HCPCS G-code describe the same service, CMS generally requires the use of G-codes to describe services provided to Medicare members.

G-codes also include **Physician Quality Reporting Initiative (PQRI)** measures, which were created by CMS for physicians to use when reporting their performance of certain services or the reason a particular service was not performed. They are reported for purposes of Medicare monitoring of physician quality.

The following are examples of common types of G-codes to report services to Medicare:

- G0009: Administration of pneumococcal vaccine
- G0105: Colorectal cancer screening; colonoscopy on individual at high risk
- G0337: Hospice evaluation and counseling services, pre-election
- G8006: Acute myocardial infarction: patient documented to have received aspirin at arrival
- G8007: Acute myocardial infarction: patient not documented to have received aspirin at arrival
- G8115: Patient documented to have received pneumococcal vaccination
- G8116: Patient not documented to have received pneumococcal vaccination

CODER'S TIP

For Medicare patients, G-codes take precedence over the use of similar CPT codes. CPT codes are used when no G-code exists to describe the services provided to the Medicare patient. For non-Medicare patients, CPT codes generally are used when a CPT and HCPCS code have essentially identical descriptors.

H-Codes: Alcohol and Drug Abuse Treatment Services

HCPCS H-codes describe alcohol and drug abuse treatment services. These codes are used by state Medicaid agencies that are mandated by state law to have separate codes for identifying mental health services that include alcohol and drug abuse treatment services as well as at-risk prenatal care. Medicare, however, does not accept H-codes to report services. Some H-codes differentiate between services provided by physicians and those provided by nonphysicians.

Examples of H-codes used to report alcohol and drug abuse treatment services include:
- H0001: Alcohol and/or drug assessment
- H0014: Alcohol and/or drug services; ambulatory detoxification
- H0031: Mental health assessment, by nonphysician
- H1000: Prenatal care, at-risk assessment
- H2011: Crisis intervention services, per 15 minutes

CODER'S TIP

Some H-codes include a specific time increment within the code descriptor. Coders must be aware of the time element in the descriptor and the documented amount of time the service was provided to correctly code for the services. For example, if the code descriptor is "per 15 minutes" and the medical record indicates that the provider spent one hour providing the service, the claim would include the code with four units.

J-Codes: Drug Administered Other Than Oral Method

HCPCS J-codes identify drugs that are not self-administered, including injectable, inhalation solution drugs, and some drugs given orally. This section includes chemotherapy and immunosuppressive drugs. The HCPCS manual includes a Table of Drugs that includes the code, drug name, route of administration, and the amount of drug considered to be a unit dose. This is not to be confused with a recommended dose, but rather is used to calculate the number of units of the drug provided.

A few examples of J-codes describing medications administered by physicians or other professionals include:

- J0285: Injection, amphotericin B, 50 mg
- J0290: Injection, ampicillin sodium, 500 mg
- J0360: Injection, hydralazine HCl, up to 20 mg
- J0694: Injection, cefoxitin sodium, 1 g
- J7040: Infusion, normal saline solution, sterile (500 ml = 1 unit)
- J7070: Infusion D5W, 1000 cc
- J9217: Leuprolide acetate (for depot suspension), 7.5 mg
- J9265: Paclitaxel, 30 mg (Use this code for Taxol, Nov-Onxol.)

CODING EXAMPLE

A patient is given 50 mg of amphotericin B and 1,000 mg of ampicillin, each diluted in a separate 500 ml bag of normal saline. How would the coder report these services? The coder would first turn to the Table of Drugs to find the code for amphotericin B (J0285), which has a unit value of 50 mg, and ampicillin (J0290), which has a unit value of 500 mg. The coder also finds that each 500 ml bag of normal saline is reported with code J7040.

Therefore, the coder reports the following codes and units:

- J0285   1 unit (50 mg is the unit dose for this code)
- J0290 X 2   2 units (500 mg per unit X 2 equals 1,000 mg)
- J7040 X 2   2 units (1 unit for each 500 ml bag of normal saline)

CODER'S TIP

When selecting J-codes to identify drugs given by injection, infusion, or inhalation, coders should begin by looking up the drug in the Table of Drugs in the HCPCS manual. If more than one code describes the drug, the coder should review all the codes in the J-code section to determine the most appropriate code. Once the correct code is identified, the coder must calculate the number of units based on the unit value in the code descriptor and the actual dose given. This is a critical step that can result in coding errors if the calculations are inaccurate.

K-Codes: Temporary Codes

HCPCS K-codes are temporary codes used by special Medicare contractors responsible for claims involving DME products. This section contains numerous codes, primarily describing standard and power wheelchairs, wheelchair accessories, and replacement parts necessary for maintenance.

A few examples of K-codes include:

- K0001: Standard wheelchair
- K0010: Standard-weight frame motorized/power wheelchair
- K0071: Front castor assembly, complete with pneumatic tire, each
- K0733: Power wheelchair accessory, 12 to 24 amp hour sealed lead acid battery, each

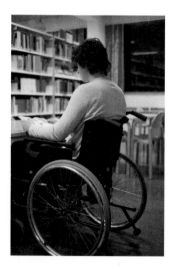

Wheelchairs are classified as durable medical equipment, as are their replacement parts.

L-Codes: Orthotic and Prosthetic Procedures (L0112–L9900)

HCPCS L-codes describe orthotic and prosthetic devices. These codes are categorized by body area and subdivided for a greater level of specificity. An **orthotic** is a device that supports an impaired body part. Orthotics range from simple wrist splints to complex custom-fabricated knee braces designed to provide support during strenuous physical activities. A **prosthetic** generally replaces a missing body part. Like orthotics, prosthetics range from simple devices to very complex ones that use microprocessor computers to control joint motion.

orthotic
A device that supports an impaired body part.

prosthetic
A device that generally replaces a missing body part.

Orthotic devices are either custom-fabricated, prefabricated, or off-the-shelf devices. A custom-fabricated orthotic device is individually made for a particular patient. Usually these are fabricated by an orthotist, who begins with raw materials such as sheets of plastic materials that are molded and shaped into the custom-fabricated device.

Prefabricated orthotic devices are made in various sizes in a factory. The appropriate device is selected for the patient, and then it is modified as necessary to fit the patient. Examples of prefabricated devices include walking boots, often prescribed for patients with severe ankle sprains or minor fractures in the later stages of healing. Off-the-shelf orthotic devices are purchased and used just as they are. Examples of these might include slings or wrist splints purchased in a retail drugstore.

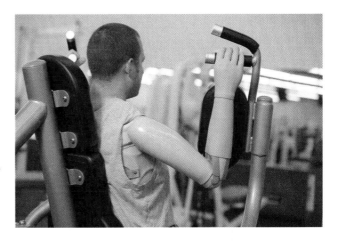

A prosthetic is a device that replaces a missing body part. It can be anywhere on the spectrum from very simple to very complex and computerized.

A few examples of L-codes include:

- L0140: Cervical, semi-rigid, adjustable (plastic collar)
- L0430: Spinal orthotic, anterior-posterior-lateral control, with interface material, custom fitted (DeWall Posture Protector only)
- L1832: Knee orthotic (KO), adjustable knee joints (unicentric or polycentric), positional orthotic, rigid support, prefabricated, includes fitting and adjustment
- L1840: Knee orthotic (KO), derotation, medial-lateral, anterior cruciate ligament, custom fabricated
- L6100: Below elbow, molded socket, flexible elbow hinge, triceps pad (prosthetic)
- L6711: Terminal device, hook, mechanical, voluntary opening, any material, any size, lined or unlined, pediatric

M-Codes: Other Medical Services

HCPCS M-codes describe a few miscellaneous medical services. There are only six codes in this section. Medicare does not accept five of these six codes.

The following six codes are the entire list of HCPCS M-codes:

- M0064: Brief office visit for the sole purpose of monitoring or changing drug prescriptions used in the treatment of mental psychoneurotic and personality disorders (may be covered by Medicare)
- M0075: Cellular therapy (not covered by Medicare)
- M0076: Prolotherapy (not covered by Medicare)
- M0100: Intragastric hypothermia using gastric freezing (not covered by Medicare)
- M0300: IV chelation therapy (chemical endarterectomy) (not covered by Medicare)
- M0301: Fabric wrapping of abdominal aneurysm (not covered by Medicare)

EXERCISE 15.3

Also available in **McGraw Hill connect** (plus+)

Use the HCPCS manual to select the HCPCS code for the following services.

1. Administration of the pneumococcal vaccine to a Medicare patient _____
2. Glaucoma screening for a high-risk Medicare patient _____
3. Forty-five minutes of therapeutic behavioral service for a Medicaid patient _____
4. An injection of penicillin G benzathine, 1.2 million units _____
5. An injection of Cipro, 600 mg _____
6. A lightweight wheelchair _____
7. A heavy-duty power wheelchair with a solid seat back for a person who weighs 372 pounds _____
8. An extra-heavy-duty power wheelchair designed to accommodate a patient who weighs 622 pounds _____
9. A cervical collar molded to a patient model _____

15.4 HCPCS P-, Q-, R-, S-, T-, and V-Codes

P-Codes: Pathology and Laboratory Services (P2028–P9615)

HCPCS P-codes are used to report pathology and laboratory services. This code section is subdivided into four sections: Chemistry and Toxicology Tests, Pathology Screening Tests, Microbiology Tests, and Miscellaneous Tests (for all other services).

Examples of HCPCS P-codes include the following:

- P2031: Hair analysis (excluding arsenic)
- P3001: Screening Papanicolaou smear, cervical or vaginal, up to three smears, requiring interpretation by physician
- P7001: Culture, bacterial, urine; quantitative, sensitivity study
- P9010: Blood (whole), for transfusion, per unit
- P9031: Platelets, leukocytes reduced, each unit

Q-Codes: Miscellaneous Services (Temporary)

HCPCS Q-codes are temporary codes originally used by CMS to report cast and splint supplies. However, this section of temporary codes has been expanded to encompass supplies, procedures, and services that include contrast material, screening Papanicolaou smears, chemotherapy administration, lab tests, and oral pharmaceuticals.

The following are some examples of Q-codes:

- Q0091: Screening Papanicolaou smear; obtaining, preparing and conveyance of cervical or vaginal smear to laboratory
- Q0144: Azithromycin dihydrate, oral, capsules/powder, 1 g (Use this code for Z-Pak.)
- Q0496: Battery, other than lithium-ion, for use with electric or electric/pneumatic ventricular assist device, replacement only
- Q4005: Cast supplies, long arm cast, adult (11 years +), plaster
- Q4008: Cast supplies, short arm cast, pediatric (0–10 years), fiberglass
- Q4101: Apligraf, per square centimeter
- Q9967: Low osmolar contrast material, 300–399 mg/ml iodine concentration, per ml

R-Codes: Diagnostic Radiology Services

The three HCPCS R-codes describe the transportation and setup of equipment from a facility to a home or nursing home for the purpose of performing diagnostic tests such as x-rays or ECGs. These codes are used in addition to the most appropriate CPT or HCPCS code that describes the services provided.

The three R-codes are:

- R0070: Transportation of portable x-ray equipment and personnel to home or nursing home, per trip to facility or location, one patient seen
- R0075: Transportation of portable x-ray equipment and personnel to home or nursing home, per trip to facility or location, more than one patient seen
- R0076: Transportation of portable ECG to facility or location per patient

S-Codes: Temporary National Codes (Non-Medicare)

HCPCS S-codes are developed by the Blue Cross and Blue Shield Association and HIAA to report drugs, supplies, or services for which there are no national codes. These codes are designed to meet the needs of the private sector but state Medicaid agencies may use these codes as well. Medicare does not recognize the use of S-codes to describe services provided to Medicare beneficiaries. S-codes may be established for a number of reasons, such as to set case rates, identify new surgical services, describe laboratory testing in greater detail, or add specificity to the description of mental health services.

The following are a few examples of HCPCS S-codes:

- S0610: Annual gynecological examination, new patient
- S0612: Annual gynecological examination, established patient
- S2053: Transplantation of small intestine and liver allografts
- S5520: Home infusion therapy, all supplies (including catheter) necessary for a peripherally inserted central venous catheter (PICC) line insertion
- S9083: Global fee urgent care centers
- S9141: Diabetic management program, follow-up visit to MD provider
- S9991: Services provided as part of a Phase III clinical trial

CODER'S TIP

Medicare does not recognize S-codes. Many state Medicaid programs, however, recognize the use of S-codes to describe services provided through those programs. Coders should be aware of the differences between Medicare and the state Medicaid program in their area. Although both are government health payment systems, the differences may be significant.

T-Codes: National T-Codes Established for State Medicaid Agencies

HCPCS T-codes are national codes established for use by state Medicaid agencies. These codes were established when the Health Insurance Portability and Accountability Act (HIPAA) eliminated the use of HCPCS Level III codes, which were also known as "local codes." Many of these codes describe nursing and home health-related services, substance abuse treatment, and training-related procedures. Only state Medicaid directors can submit requests for new T-codes. Medicare does not recognize T-codes.

Following are a few examples of HCPCS T-codes:

- T1002: RN services, up to 15 minutes
- T1021: Home health aide or certified nurse assistant, per visit
- T2030: Assisted living, waiver; per month
- T4523: Adult-sized disposable incontinence product, brief/diaper, large, each
- T4538: Diaper service, reusable diaper, each diaper

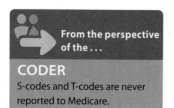

From the perspective of the . . .

CODER

S-codes and T-codes are never reported to Medicare.

CODING EXAMPLE

A supply company provides incontinence supplies to a Medicaid patient. The patient uses eight large adult-sized disposable diapers per day, and the company arranges delivery once per week. The supply company sends a claim each week to the Medicaid agency. How should the coder report these supplies?

The coder looks up *incontinence* in the index and finds several subheadings, including "brief or diaper" with a listing for codes T4521–T4524. Reviewing these codes shows that code A4523 describes large disposable diapers with the word "each" indicating that the code is reported once for each diaper provided. On a weekly basis, the coder would report A4523 X 56 (eight diapers per day times seven days per week).

V-Codes: Vision Services, Hearing Services, and Speech-Language Pathology Services

HCPCS V-codes describe vision, hearing, and some speech-language pathology services. Services described by V-codes include lenses, contacts, vision aids, ocular prosthetics, speech-language pathology, and various hearing services.

Examples of HCPCS V-codes include:

- V2100: Sphere, single vision, plano to plus or minus 4.00, per lens
- V2500: Contact lens, PMMA, spherical, per lens
- V5008: Hearing screening
- V5050: Hearing aid, monaural, in the ear
- V5362: Speech screening
- V5364: Dysphagia screening

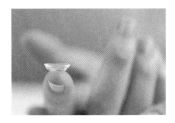

HCPCS V-codes describe services related to vision, hearing, and speech pathology.

EXERCISE 15.4

Also available in **connect** (plus+)

Use the HCPCS manual to select the HCPCS code and, when appropriate, the HCPCS modifier for the following services.

1. An infusion of 25 percent human albumin, 40 ml _____
2. Fiberglass cast supplies for a short arm splint for a child 4 years of age _____
3. Genetic testing for Gaucher's disease _____
4. Forty-five minutes of case management services provided to a Medicaid patient _____
5. Oversize lenses for both eyes _____
6. Speech screening _____
7. A monaural hearing aid worn in the ear _____

15.5 HCPCS Modifiers and HCPCS Manual Appendices

HCPCS Level II codes include two-character alphanumeric modifiers that provide additional information but do not change the definition of the code. HCPCS Level II modifiers may be used with both CPT and HCPCS Level II codes. There are many more HCPCS modifiers than CPT modifiers, and under certain circumstances a CPT modifier and HCPCS Level II modifier may both be used with the same code. The HCPCS Level II manual includes a complete list of modifiers and their descriptions. Refer to Chapter 7 of this text for a more complete discussion of modifiers.

The ambulance modifiers have been discussed earlier in this chapter. Other commonly used modifiers are listed below, but this should not be used as a reference for modifiers. Coders should use a complete list of modifiers when selecting the appropriate modifiers to add to any HCPCS code.

Anatomical Modifiers

E1–E4	Used to identify specific eyelids.
FA, F1–F9	Used to identify specific fingers.
TA, T1–T9	Used to identify specific toes.
RC, LC, and LD	Used to identify specific coronary arteries.
RT and LT	Used to identify right and left sides.

DME and Other Equipment Modifiers

NU   Equipment is new.

NR   Equipment is new when rented and subsequently purchased.

RR   Equipment is rented.

UE   Equipment is used.

Radiology Modifiers

GG   Screening mammogram and diagnostic mammogram performed on the same patient on the same day.

GH   Screening mammogram converted to a diagnostic mammogram.

Place of Service Modifier

SG   Service provided at an ambulatory surgery center.

New modifiers are frequently added, so coders must use the most current HCPCS manual (with its list of current modifiers) when selecting HCPCS codes.

CODING EXAMPLE

A DME supplier delivers several pieces of equipment to a patient's home, including an adjustable electric hospital bed with side rails and mattress, a trapeze bar (Patient Helper) attachment for the bed to allow the patient to move, a commode chair with detachable arms for bedside use, and a standard wheelchair. The bed and trapeze are supplied on a rental basis, the commode is purchased new, and the wheelchair is purchased as used equipment. How should the coder report this equipment?

The coder looks in the index to determine which codes describe the equipment supplied. HCPCS code E0265 describes the hospital bed; E0910 describes the trapeze; E0165 describes the bedside commode; and K0001 describes the wheelchair. Equipment purchased new is identified with the NU modifier, equipment purchased used is identified with the UE modifier, and rented equipment is identified with the RR modifier.

The coder would report the equipment with the following HCPCS codes: E0265-RR, E0910-RR, E0165-NU, and K0001-UE.

Appendices

Most HCPCS manuals have several appendices attached to the publication. Although there may be some variation, Appendix 1 is usually the Table of Drugs. Appendix 1 is used in place of the general index when trying to identify the correct code to use when reporting drugs provided to patients in a doctor's office or healthcare facility. It is not used to report medications dispensed by a pharmacy.

Appendix 2 lists all of the HCPCS modifiers. There are more than 250 HCPCS modifiers, many more than the number of CPT modifiers. Appendix 3 is a list of HCPCS abbreviations and acronyms, some of which are listed in Table 15.2. Appendix 4 reprints some of the Medicare publications and guidance documents. Appendices 2, 3, and 4 are included as convenient references for coders.

TABLE 15.2 Selection of Common Abbreviations Used in HCPCS Coding

Abbreviation or Acronym	Meaning
ADA	American Dental Association
ALS	Advanced life support
BLS	Basic life support
CPT	Current Procedural Terminology
CMS	Centers for Medicare and Medicaid Services
DME	Durable medical equipment
HCPCS	Healthcare Procedure Coding System
HIAA	Health Insurance Association of America
IM	Intramuscular
IV	Intravenous
Inj	Injection
mg	Milligram
ml	Milliliter
Sub Q, SQ	Subcutaneous

EXERCISE 15.5

Also available in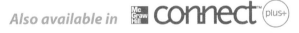

Use the HCPCS manual to select the appropriate modifiers that should be added to HCPCS codes in the following scenarios.

1. A surgical procedure on the fourth and fifth digits of the left hand _____
2. Anesthesia services personally provided by an anesthesiologist _____
3. A wheelchair rented on a month-to-month basis _____
4. Ambulance transportation from a physician's office to the patient's home _____
5. Left side of the body _____
6. Durable medical equipment purchased used _____
7. Upper right eyelid _____
8. Right foot, great toe _____
9. Services to report facility charge at an ambulatory surgical center _____

Summary

Learning Outcome	Key Concepts/Examples
15.1 Explain HCPCS codes. **Pages 471–473**	The Healthcare Common Procedure Coding System (HCPCS) was developed by CMS to report services not usually found in the CPT coding system. HCPCS codes typically describe services or supplies not usually considered professional services, such as durable medical equipment, drugs, transportation, and other services.
	HCPCS codes are used to report services when: (a) there is no CPT code to describe that service, (b) the HCPCS code is more specific than the CPT code, or (c) when instructed to do so by the payer.
	Many HCPCS codes contain a unit of service as part of the description. The actual number or amount of the service provided is reported in terms of the designated unit of service.
	To select the correct code, coders must use both the index and tabular list. HCPCS codes consist of a letter followed by four numbers.
	The tabular list is organized into sections according to the letter in the first position of the code. Each section describes a limited number of types of services or supplies. The shortest section has only three HCPCS codes, whereas the larger ones have hundreds of individual codes.
15.2 Identify services described by A-, B-, C-, and E-codes. **Pages 474–478**	A-codes describe transportation services, including emergency and non-emergency transportation; medical and surgical supplies; and certain administrative services.
	B-codes identify products and devices used for enteral and parenteral therapy, including special foods and infusion pumps.
	C-codes describe services reported by hospital outpatient departments. These codes are not used to report professional services or hospital services provided to inpatients.
	E-codes describe durable medical equipment.
15.3 Select codes to report services described by G-, H-, J-, K-, L-, and M-codes. **Pages 478–482**	G-codes describe professional services. These codes may be required by Medicare to report services even if a CPT code describes the same service. These codes are used to report measures for the Physician Quality Reporting Initiative.
	H-codes report alcohol and substance abuse services provided by Medicaid programs.
	J-codes identify drugs provided in physician offices and other outpatient settings. These codes do not describe prescription drugs provided by pharmacies.
	K-codes report wheelchair equipment and other equipment for Medicare.
	L-codes describe orthotic and prosthetic devices.
	M-codes identify certain medical services. There are only six separate M-codes in the entire section.
15.4 Determine codes to report services described by P-, Q-, R-, S-, T-, and V-codes. **Pages 482–485**	P-codes describe pathology and laboratory services.
	Q-codes report certain supplies. These may also include temporary codes for Medicare reporting purposes.
	R-codes describe transporting x-ray and ECG equipment to nursing homes or other facilities to perform tests. There are only three R-codes in this section.
	S-codes are temporary codes used by commercial payers and Medicaid programs. Medicare does not recognize S-codes.
	T-codes report services for State Medicaid programs. These codes may be used by commercial payers but are not recognized by Medicare.
	V-codes describe vision, hearing, and speech-language devices and services.

Learning Outcome	Key Concepts/Examples
15.5 Use HCPCS modifiers. **Pages 485–487**	The HCPCS code set contains modifiers that may be used with both HCPCS codes and CPT codes. There are more HCPCS modifiers than CPT modifiers.

Some modifiers describe anatomical details not contained in CPT or HCPCS codes, such as specific fingers, toes, eyelids, and coronary arteries.

Other modifiers provide greater detail regarding DME, such as whether the equipment is purchased or rented. Modifiers also indicated whether the equipment is purchased new or used.

The HCPCS manual includes four appendices. Appendix 1 (Table of Drugs) is used to locate HCPCS codes that identify specific drugs administered by healthcare providers. These codes are not used to identify prescription medications from pharmacies.

Appendix 2 lists the HCPCS modifiers. Appendix 3 is a list of HCPCS abbreviations and acronyms. Appendix 4 reprints some of the Medicare publications and guidance documents. |

Using Terminology

Match the key terms with their definitions.

_____ **1.** L015.2 Advanced life support (ALS)

_____ **2.** L015.2 Basic life support (BLS)

_____ **3.** L015.2 Durable medical equipment (DME)

_____ **4.** L015.2 Emergency transportation

_____ **5.** L015.2 Enteral and parenteral therapy

_____ **6.** L015.1 Level I HCPCS codes

_____ **7.** L015.1 Level II HCPCS codes

_____ **8.** L015.2 Medical supplies

_____ **9.** L015.2 Non-emergency transportation

_____ **10.** L015.3 Orthotic

_____ **11.** L015.3 Physician Quality Reporting Initiative (PQRI)

_____ **12.** L015.3 Prosthetic

_____ **13.** L015.1 Table of Drugs

_____ **14.** L015.1 Unit of service

A. Transportation used to move a patient who is not in immediate, critical need of medical care

B. The provision of nutrients to prevent or treat malnutrition

C. Codes used by CMS to describe services not covered by CPT codes

D. Supplies used to provide medical care to a patient, classified as either single use or durable

E. A device used to replace or function as a missing part of the body

F. The level of medical care given to patients with life-threatening illnesses or injuries until the patient reaches a hospital

G. Index used to identify specific codes that describe medications provided to patients in physician offices or medical facilities, but not prescription medications provided by a pharmacy

H. Amount of the service provided, used to select the correct HCPCS code

I. CPT codes

J. A higher level of medical care that supports circulation and breathing while the patient is being transported

K. Program used by Medicare to monitor physician quality

L. Items that are used repeatedly over a long period of time

M. Transportation used to bring a critically ill patient to a hospital

N. A device that supports the function of a part of the body

Checking Your Understanding

Select the letter that best completes the statement or answers the question.

1. L015.2 C-codes describe some services, such as drugs, biologicals, radiopharmaceuticals, devices, and supplies, that are provided in the _____ setting.

   a. Inpatient
   b. Office
   c. Outpatient hospital
   d. Nursing home

2. L015.2 Which of the following is/are not an example of a DME?

   a. Canes and crutches
   b. Decubitus care equipment (e.g., a dry pressure mattress)
   c. Oxygen tanks
   d. IV tubing

3. L015.3 CMS creates a G-code that has the same meaning as an existing CPT code. CMS generally requires the use of G-codes to describe services provided to which type of patient?

   a. Patients with commercial insurance
   b. Medicare patients
   c. TRICARE patients
   d. The type of insurance a patient has does not impact the use of this code.

4. L015.3 Which codes are used by state Medicaid agencies that are mandated by state law to have separate codes for identifying mental health services that include alcohol and drug abuse treatment services as well as at-risk prenatal care?

   a. A-codes
   b. C-codes
   c. H-codes
   d. J-codes

5. L015.1 When selecting J-codes to identify drugs administered by injection, infusion, or inhalation, in which part of the HCPCS manual should coders begin?

   a. Alphabetic index
   b. Table of Drugs
   c. Appendix A
   d. Appendix C

6. L015.2 Which two code ranges could be used for DME products?

   a. K and E
   b. J and E
   c. Only E-codes are used.
   d. Q and E

7. L015.3 A device that supports an impaired body part is _____.

   a. A prosthetic device
   b. An orthotic device
   c. Durable medical equipment
   d. Casting

8. L015.4 A portable x-ray machine is transported from a facility to a nursing home. What range of HCPCS codes would be used to report the service?

   a. A-codes
   b. C-codes
   c. R-codes
   d. M-codes

9. L015.4 Which HCPCS codes are temporary codes used by the private sector and some Medicaid agencies, but are not recognized by CMS for Medicare beneficiaries?

   a. S-codes
   b. G-codes
   c. K-codes
   d. T-codes

10. L015.4 T-codes (national codes established for use by state Medicaid agencies) were established when HIPAA eliminated the use of which HCPCS codes?

   a. Level III codes
   b. Level I codes
   c. Level II codes
   d. None of these

11. L015.2 When ambulance services are reported, special modifiers must be used to identify the _____.

   a. Type of service
   b. Pickup point and destination
   c. Pickup point only
   d. Destination only

12. L015.5 A screening mammogram and diagnostic mammogram were performed on the same patient on the same day. The HCPCS II modifier that would be used to report these procedures is _____.

   a. GH
   b. GG
   c. SG
   d. R

13. L015.1 HCPCS codes should generally be used in which of the following circumstances?

   a. There is not a CPT code that describes the item or service provided.
   b. The HCPCS code is more specific than the CPT code.
   c. When instructed to do so by a particular payer.
   d. All of these.

connect™ plus+
Enhance your learning by completing these exercises
and more at mcgrawhillconnect.com!   CHAPTER 15 | INTRODUCTION TO THE HEALTHCARE COMMON PROCEDURE CODING SYSTEM (HCPCS)   491

14. L015.1 HCPCS codes are five-digit alphanumeric codes that begin with a single letter followed by four numerical digits. The first character, which is an alpha character, denotes _____.

   a. Place of service
   b. Type of service
   c. The section of the HCPCS manual in which the code is located
   d. None of these

15. L015.1 When both a CPT code and HCPCS code have essentially identical descriptions and the patient is a Medicare beneficiary, which guideline applies?

   a. The HCPCS code should be used.
   b. The CPT code should be used.
   c. Medicare instructs the use of a HCPCS code
   d. Both codes are always used.

16. L015.5 Which HCPCS code modifier indicates that a resident/teaching physician provided the service?

   a. GC
   b. GE
   c. GF
   d. There is not a modifier for this.

17. L015.3 What HCPCS code describes a bilateral diagnostic mammogram with digital image, all views, for a Medicare patient?

   a. G0204
   b. G0206
   c. G0202
   d. 77051

18. L015.2 A non-emergency patient is transported by wheelchair van. The correct HCPCS code to report is:

   a. A0120
   b. A0130
   c. A0100
   d. A0110

19. L015.3 What is the correct code for documentation of cognitive impairment screening using a standardized tool?

   a. G8435
   b. G8436
   c. G8434
   d. G8430

20. L015.3 What is the difference between HCPCS codes G8560 and G8562?

   a. Whether or not the patient had a history of active drainage within the previous 90 days
   b. Whether or not the patient is eligible for referral for patients with active history of active drainage
   c. Whether or not the patient was referred to a physician for an otologic evaluation
   d. Either code could be used.

Applying Your Skills

Use the HCPCS manual to select the correct HCPCS code, units of service, and modifier as needed for the following services.

1. L015.2 A pair of electrodes for an apnea monitor _____

2. L015.2 Tubing used with a positive airway pressure device _____

3. L015.2 A disposable home glucose monitor, including the test strips _____

4. L015.2 The injection of 20 ml of gadolinium-based magnetic resonance contrast agent _____

5. L015.2 Sixty-four ounces of orally administered food thickener _____

6. L015.2 Eighteen hundred calories of a nutritionally complete enteral formula with intact nutrients, including proteins, fats, carbohydrates, vitamins, and minerals and possibly fiber, that is administered through an enteral feeding tube _____

7. L015.2 An extra-wide mobile commode chair with arms _____

8. L015.2 A water pressure mattress _____

9. L015.2 A moist electric heat pad _____

10. L015.2 A portable paraffin bath and five pounds of paraffin _____

11. L015.2 Purchase of a new intrapulmonary percussive ventilation system and related accessories _____

12. L015.3 The administration of influenza virus vaccine to a Medicare patient _____

13. L015.3 Unilateral diagnostic mammography that produces a direct digital image for a Medicare patient _____

14. L015.3 Intravenous injection of 100 mg of respiratory syncytial virus immune globulin _____

15. L015.3 Injection of 750 mg of human tetanus immune globulin _____

16. L015.2 An emergency helicopter landing at the scene of an accident and transportation of the patient to the nearest hospital heliport _____

17. L015.4 A laser-assisted uvulopalatoplasty (LAUP) _____

18. L015.4 The third visit for sperm procurement and cryopreservation services _____

19. L015.4 The repair or modification of a hearing aid _____

20. L015.4 A telephone amplifier _____

21. L015.2 Technetium Tc-99m apcitide, per study dose, up to 20 millicuries (AcuTect) _____

22. L015.2 Portable parenteral nutrition infusion pump _____

23. L015.3 Heavy-duty wheelchair _____

24. L015.3 Cervical-thoracic-lumbar-sacral orthotic (CTLSO), Milwaukee brace, furnishing initial orthotic _____

25. L015.3 Prefabricated Swedish type knee orthotic _____

26. L015.3 Below-knee prosthesis with molded socket and SACH foot _____

27. L015.4 Low osmolar contrast material, iodine concentration 200–299 mg/ml, per ml _____

28. L015.4 Cast supplies for a plaster shoulder cast for an adult _____

29. L015.4 Transportation of a portable x-ray machine to a nursing home, per patient when more than one patient is seen _____

30. L015.4 AlloSkin skin substitute, per square centimeter _____

Thinking It Through

Use your critical-thinking skills to answer the questions below.

1. Explain when a HCPCS code would be reported if there is a CPT code that describes the same service.

_____

_____

_____

2. Describe the kinds of information provided by HCPCS modifiers.

_____

_____

_____

3. Identify which HCPCS codes Medicare accepts to report services for Medicare beneficiaries and which codes they do not. Identify HCPCS codes that are primarily used to report services for Medicare beneficiaries.

_____

_____

_____

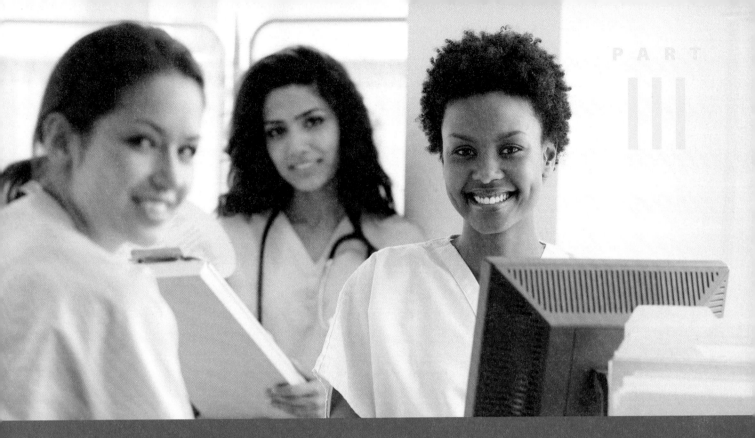

PRACTICUM

16 **Putting It All Together**

16 PUTTING IT ALL TOGETHER

Learning Outcome *After completing this chapter, students should be able to:*

16.1 Code the services and supplies described in short scenarios of healthcare encounters.

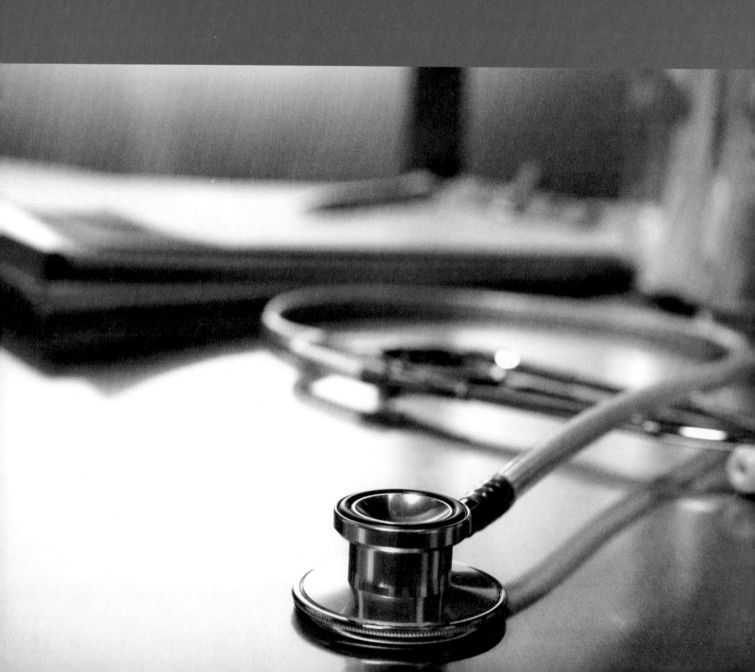

Introduction

Each chapter in this book has addressed a single aspect of coding, concentrating on one type of coding system, such as ICD-9-CM diagnosis codes or CPT procedure codes, or a single section within a particular coding manual. This provided a narrow focus from which to select the codes to answer questions in the exercises.

This chapter will bring you closer to the real experience of being a medical coder. This chapter consists of exercises in which short descriptions of real healthcare situations are provided. Each scenario describes a number of diagnoses, services, and supplies, followed by either multiple choice or fill-in-the-blank questions. Using instructions in the coding manuals and this textbook, determine the codes that most accurately describe the services provided. Each scenario includes sufficient information to identify all codes to best describe the scenario.

Over time, you will likely develop your own methods for coding, but it is usually helpful to take the same approach to all coding situations. For example, you may want to ask yourself the following questions, even if the answers are obvious:

- On what date(s) were the services provided?
- Where were the services provided (outpatient, hospital, other facility, etc.)?
- Has the provider performed evaluation and management services? If so, what codes describe these services? Are any modifiers indicated?
- Has the provider performed any procedures? If so, what codes describe these services? Are any modifiers indicated? How many units should be reported?
- Are other services involved, such as anesthesia, radiology, or pathology? If so, what codes describe those services? Are modifiers indicated? How many units were provided?
- Did the services include any medical supplies, durable medical equipment, orthotics, prosthetics, or other services described by HCPCS codes? What HCPCS codes describe those services? Are modifiers necessary? How many units were provided?
- Why were all these procedures and services provided? What diagnosis codes describe the patient's condition?

So, let's get started and put it all together!

Coding Scenarios

Scenario 1

A 23-year-old obese female presents to her gynecologist's office for her annual exam. The physician performs a Pap smear and pelvic exam. The patient states that she has not had a menstrual cycle in four or five months and complains of bloating and abdominal cramping. The physician performs a problem-focused exam, and the medical decision making is of low complexity. The physician has the patient leave a urine specimen for dipstick analysis and orders a pelvic ultrasound.

a. 99213, 81000, 99395-25, V70.3
b. 99395, 99212-25, 81000, 626.0, V70.0
c. 99394, 99213, 81000, 626.1, V70.2
d. 99213-25, 99395, 81000, 626.2, V70.3

In addition to the above codes, the physician may report the bloating and abdominal cramping with the following codes: _____ and _____.

An imaging center performs the pelvic ultrasound, which is interpreted by an employed radiologist. This is reported with the following code: _____.

(The ICD-10-CM codes that best describe this scenario are _____.)

Scenario 2

The parents of a four-year-old boy present to the emergency room with the child, who had been burned by a campfire. They explain that they were getting their children ready for bed and into their sleeping bags when they noticed the youngest child was not in sight. They then heard a scream and found he had accidentally fallen into the campfire. They rushed him to the emergency room, where the doctor performs a detailed history and exam. He determines that the child sustained a third-degree burn to his left forearm and second-degree burns to his left cheek and forehead. The total body surface area burned is between 5 and 10 percent.

a. 99281-25, 944.35, 941.20, 948.00, E897
b. 99284-25, 944.31, 941.24, 948.00, E896
c. 99205, 944.31, 941.27, 948.10, E896
d. 99284, 944.31, 941.27, 948.00, E897

The child is admitted and taken to the operating room for care of the burns and application of dressings.

CPT code for surgical procedure: _____

CPT code for anesthesia: _____

(The ICD-10-CM codes that best describe this scenario are _____.)

Scenario 3

A patient in labor arrives at the hospital for delivery of the baby. She is taken to the maternity ward and quickly moved to a delivery room. There she delivers twins, only one of which is alive at birth. Her regular physician is not able to get to the hospital in time, and the on-call obstetrician delivers the babies. The pregnancy and delivery are otherwise normal, and her usual obstetrician arrives after the delivery.

a. 59400, 651.02, 656.41, V27.0
b. 59409, 651.01, 656.41, V27.3
c. 59409, 651.01, 656.31, V27.1
d. 59400, 651.03, V27.2

The anesthesiologist provides anesthesia for the delivery. This is reported with the following code: _____.

(The ICD-10-CM codes that best describe this scenario are _____.)

Scenario 4

A patient with chronic back pain is evaluated by a pain specialist and scheduled for a transforaminal epidural steroid injection (TFESI) under fluoroscopic guidance. On the day of the procedure, the patient is taken to the procedure room and placed in the prone position. The patient's back and buttocks are prepped in a sterile fashion. Sterile drapes are applied. Fluoroscopy is used to examine the patient's spine.

The C-arm is positioned oblique to the ipsilateral side of the right L3 pedicle. The skin is infiltrated with 1 percent lidocaine, a 22 gauge spinal needle is advanced until contact is made with the 6 o'clock position of the pedicle. It is then walked off inferiorly to rest within the transforaminal space. The position of the needle is confirmed with fluoroscopy. Aspiration is negative for blood or CSF. A total of 3 cc of 0.125 percent bupivicaine with 20 mg of Kenalog is injected. A similar procedure is repeated for the right L4 pedicle and subsequent transforaminal space.

The needles are flushed and withdrawn. The patient is taken to the recovery room in good condition.

a. 64493, 64494, S0020 X 3, J3301 X 2, 722.52
b. 64483-RT, 64484-RT, S0020 X 3, J3301 X 2, 722.52
c. 64483-RT, 64484-RT, 77003, S0020 X 3, J3301 X 2, 722.52
d. 64493-RT, 64494-RT, J3301 X 3, J3301 X 2, 722.52

(The ICD-10-CM codes that best describe this scenario are _____.)

Scenario 5

A patient in the hospital for other reasons is suddenly found to have an abnormal cardiac rhythm. The nurses call the cardiologist, who evaluates the patient, interprets an ECG rhythm strip, and determines that the patient has paroxysmal supraventricular tachycardia. The evaluation consists of an expanded problem-focused history and physical examination with straightforward medical decision making. The cardiologist performs external cardioversion and successfully converts the heart to a normal sinus rhythm. The cardiologist orders a repeat ECG and interprets it to verify sinus rhythm. The following codes describe the services provided by the cardiologist.

a. 99252, 92961, 93040, 427.1
b. 99232, 92960, 93042, 427.1
c. 99252, 92960, 93042, 93042-76, 427.0
d. 99232, 92960, 93040, 93040-76, 427.0

(The ICD-10-CM codes that best describe this scenario are _____.)

Scenario 6

A patient presents to his physician's office complaining of fatigue, dizziness, and shortness of breath. The physician performs a comprehensive history and exam; medical decision making is of high complexity. The doctor's diagnosis is unstable angina, hypertension, diabetes with hypoglycemia, and a history of myocardial infarction. The patient is sent to the hospital and admitted by the on-call cardiologist for evaluation.

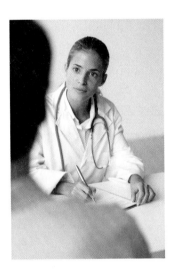

Choose the correct codes to describe the services provided by the patient's physician in his office:

a. 99214, 413.9, 401.9, 250.80, 412
b. 99215, 411.1, 401.9, 250.80, 412
c. 99205, 411.1, 401.1, 250.8, 412
d. 99241, 411.1, 401.9, 250.00, 410.9

The cardiologist who admits the patient performs a comprehensive history and physical examination; medical decision making is of high complexity. The coder reports this service with the following code: _____.

(The ICD-10-CM codes that best describe this scenario are _____.)

Scenario 7

A 42-year-old female presents to her doctor's office with shortness of breath, cough, fever, and tightness in her chest. She has a temperature of 101.5 degrees, and her throat is red in color with white spots. The doctor orders a two-view chest x-ray and a throat culture and sensitivities (disk method) to be completed in his office at the time of visit.

The doctor performs an expanded problem-focused history and exam. The physician determines that the patient has an upper respiratory infection and strep throat.

a. 99213, 71020, 87060, 462
b. 99215, 71010, 87184, 491.9, 034.0
c. 99204, 71020-26, 87060, 462
d. 99213, 71020, 87070, 87184, 465.9, 034.0

(The ICD-10-CM codes that best describe this scenario are _____.)

Scenario 8

A 42-year-old man was experiencing right upper quadrant pain that radiated to the middle of the abdomen. He had tried taking over-the-counter medication to help alleviate the pain. After several hours with no relief, he presents to the emergency room. The ER physician performs an expanded problem-focused history and exam; he also orders a CT exam of the abdomen without contrast for confirmation of his diagnosis. The exam shows multiple small stones in the patient's gallbladder. The medical decision making is of moderate complexity.

a. 99283, 74150-26, 574.41
b. 99284, 74261-26, 574.41
c. 99283, 74240, 574.30
d. 99283, 574.00

The radiologist's services are reported with the following code _____.

(The ICD-10-CM codes that best describe this scenario are _____.)

Scenario 9

A 55-year-old woman presents to her surgeon's office for a follow-up visit to remove her stitches after a bilateral mastectomy. The lower half of each breast is red and warm to the touch. The physician performs a comprehensive history and physical exam. The physician determines that the patient has developed an infection (cellulitis) in her breasts and decides to admit her to the hospital for IV antibiotic therapy. The medical decision making is of moderate complexity.

a. 99214, 99222-25, 174.9, 611.0
b. 99214-25, 99222, 611.1
c. 99222, 174.9, 611.0
d. 99221, 99213-25, 611.1

(The ICD-10-CM codes that best describe this scenario are _____.)

Scenario 10

A patient is airlifted to the hospital by helicopter after a motor vehicle accident on the highway. The transport is 73 miles and takes 55 minutes. The emergency transport is reported as follows:

a. A0431-SH, A0425 X 73
b. A0431-SH, A0436 X 73
c. A0430-HS, A0425 X 73
d. A0431-HS, A0436 X 73

(The ICD-10-CM codes that best describe this scenario are _____.)

Scenario 11

A 15-year-old boy was brought to the emergency department (ED) by ambulance with a 7.8 cm laceration to his head due to blunt force trauma. The boy states he was riding his bike, failed to pay attention, and hit his head on a light pole. The ED physician performs a detailed history and physical examination with decision making of moderate complexity. The ED physician orders a CT scan of the boy's head and cervical spine without contrast material. The CT scan is normal; the physician uses seven staples to close the boy's laceration. The boy is sent home that evening.

a. 99284, 13121, 13122, 873.1, E006.4
b. 99285, 14020, 873.1, E006.4
c. 99283, 13101, 873.0, E006.4
d. 99284, 13121, 13122-51, 873.0, E006.4

The radiologist's services are reported with the following codes: _____ and _____.

(The ICD-10-CM codes that best describe this scenario are _____.)

Scenario 12

An anesthesiologist administers a general anesthetic for a total knee arthroplasty. Following surgery, the orthopedic surgeon requests that the anesthesiologist place a femoral nerve block using an indwelling catheter for a continuous infusion technique. The anesthesiologist places the catheter, performs the requested block, and initiates the infusion. The following codes describe the services provided by the anesthesiologist.

a. 01400, 64447, 715.15
b. 01402, 64448, 715.16
c. 01360, 64447, 715.16
d. 01392, 64448, 715.15

(The ICD-10-CM codes that best describe this scenario are _____.)

Scenario 13

A patient with a personal and family history of breast cancer and previous bilateral mastectomies is admitted to the outpatient hospital to have a scheduled prophylactic laparoscopic oophorectomy due to a positive *BRCA2* test result.

a. 58943, V16.3
b. 58953, V16.40, V84.01
c. 58940, V84.01, V16.3
d. 58956, V16.40

Anesthesia for this procedure is reported with the following code: _____.

(The ICD-10-CM codes that best describe this scenario are _____.)

Scenario 14

A patient presents to his regular doctor's office complaining of pain in both shoulders. He states the pain has been present for the past several days and is getting progressively worse each day. He has tried taking over-the-counter anti-inflammatory medication, but it has not helped at all. The doctor performs a detailed history and exam. He determines that the patient has bursitis and tendonitis of both shoulders. To help alleviate the pain, he injects a steroid preparation into both shoulders. The medical decision making is of moderate complexity.

a. 99214, 20553, 726.0
b. 20552-50, 727.3
c. 99213-25, 20551-RT/LT X 2, 727.3
d. 99214, 20610-50, 726.10

(The ICD-10-CM codes that best describe this scenario are _____.)

Scenario 15

A 15-year-old was playing water polo and sustained an injury to her left hand. Upon her arrival at her regular physician's office, the doctor immediately orders a three-view x-ray of her left hand to be done in his office. After determining that she has a fracture to her left middle metacarpal bone, he refers the patient to an orthopedic surgeon. The doctor performs a detailed history and exam, and the medical decision making is of moderate complexity.

a. 99214, 73120-LT, E002
b. 99204, 73120-LT, E002.2, 815.03
c. 99213, 73130-LT, 815.03, E002.3
d. 99214, 73130-LT, 815.03, E002.2

(The ICD-10-CM codes that best describe this scenario are _____.)

Scenario 16

The patient from Scenario 15 presents to the orthopedic surgeon's office. After performing a comprehensive history and physical exam, including reviewing the x-rays from the other physician's office, the orthopedic surgeon informs the patient that the injury will require open surgery with internal fixation to repair the fracture. The decision making is of moderate complexity. The orthopedic surgeon reports his initial services with the following codes:

a. 99203-57
b. 99241-57
c. 99242-57
d. 99204-57

The surgery is scheduled for the next day as an outpatient procedure in the hospital. Before surgery, an x-ray of the hand is taken to reevaluate the fracture. Select the code that describes the services provided by the orthopedic surgeon:

a. 26615-LT
b. 26608-LT
c. 26608-F2
d. 26615-F2

The radiologist who interprets the x-ray reports her services with code _____.

The anesthesiologist reports his services with code _____.

(The ICD-10-CM codes that best describe this scenario are _____.)

Scenario 17

A female patient visits her urologist's office complaining of pain and chronic urinary incontinence. The urologist performs a detailed problem-focused history and physical exam; the medical decision making is of moderate complexity. The physician determines that the patient requires surgery to relieve the pressure and constant pain. He discusses this with the patient and schedules the patient for an outpatient procedure.

a. 99214-25
b. 99214-57
c. 99213
d. 99204-57

Several days later, the urologist performs a simple Marshall-Marchetti-Krantz type urethropexy at an ambulatory surgery center. Which codes describe this procedure and the patient's diagnosis?

a. 51840, 625.6
b. 58140-50, 788.32
c. 57288, 788.32
d. 58152, 625.6

The anesthesiologist reports the following code: _____.

(The ICD-10-CM codes that best describe this scenario are _____.)

Scenario 18

A patient sees a urologist for the first time because he has problems urinating. He explains that he has difficulty beginning to urinate and has to urinate more often but with less urine each time. The physician performs a detailed history and physical exam and determines that the patient has benign prostatic hypertrophy. The decision making is of moderate complexity. The physician schedules the patient for a transurethral resection of the prostate (TURP). Determine all the correct codes to report these services.

a. 99204-57, 52500, 600.01, 788.64, 788.41
b. 99203-57, 52601, 600.01, 788.64, 788.41
c. 99203-57, 52648, 600.00
d. 99204-57, 53420, 600.00

The anesthesiologist reports the following code: _____.

(The ICD-10-CM codes that best describe this scenario are _____.)

Scenario 19

On Friday afternoon, a 37-year-old patient presents to her doctor's office complaining of pain under her arm in the axilla area. The doctor performs a detailed history and an expanded problem-focused exam. The physician determines that the patient has a small abscess and cellulitis. He prescribes an oral antibiotic. The medical decision making is of moderate complexity.

a. 99214, 788.0
b. 99215, 682.3
c. 99204, 682.2
d. 99213, 682.3

(The ICD-10-CM codes that best describe this scenario are _____.)

Scenario 20

The patient in Scenario 19 has been taking her medication as prescribed, but the pain is getting worse. On Monday morning, she returns to the doctor's office. After an exam, the patient is admitted to the hospital for IV antibiotics. The physician requests a consultation from a general surgeon because the abscess is getting worse. The surgeon performs an inpatient consultation with a problem-focused history and exam and determines that the patient needs surgery for an incision and drainage. The medical decision making is of low complexity. Code for both the consultation and the surgery.

a. 99251-57, 10061, 682.3
b. 99252, 10060, 682.2
c. 99253-57, 10060, 682.3
d. 99251, 10061, 788.0

The anesthetic for this procedure is reported with the following code: _____.

(The ICD-10-CM codes that best describe this scenario are _____.)

Scenario 21

A 28-year-old male was playing baseball. He states that when he went to pitch the ball he heard something snap and his arm was dangling. When he presents to the emergency room, the physician performs a detailed history and an expanded problem-focused physical examination. The medical decision making is of moderate complexity. The ED physician orders AP- and lateral-view x-rays of the patient's upper right arm, which show a closed spiral fracture of the right humerus. He also orders a CT of the humerus without contrast material to ensure there is no pathological reason for the spiral fracture.

An orthopedic surgeon reviews the x-rays and CT scan and schedules surgery for the next day. The surgeon performs a comprehensive history and exam; the medical decision making is of high complexity.

The next day, the surgeon performs an open reduction and internal fixation of the right humerus with plates and screws with the patient under general anesthesia.

Fill in the blanks with all appropriate codes:

ICD-9-CM diagnosis codes
(may be reported by all treating providers):   _____

ED physician: _____

Radiologist: _____

Orthopedic surgeon on day of admission: _____

Orthopedic surgeon on day of surgery: _____

Anesthesiologist: _____

(The ICD-10-CM codes that best describe this scenario are _____.)

Scenario 22

A patient is seen in the emergency department for evaluation of abdominal pain. The ED physician performs an expanded problem-focused history and physical examination. The physician determines that the patient has acute appendicitis and requires surgery right away. This medical decision making is of moderate complexity. The ED physician calls in the on-call surgeon. After examining the patient, the surgeon concurs with the ED physician's original diagnosis of acute appendicitis. He admits the patient after performing a comprehensive history and exam with decision making of moderate complexity. He decides the patient should undergo surgery and performs a laparoscopic surgical appendectomy.

List the codes to report the following:

ICD-9-CM diagnosis codes: _____

ED physician: _____

Surgeon: _____

Anesthesiologist: _____

(The ICD-10-CM codes that best describe this scenario are _____.)

Scenario 23

A physician admits an 83-year-old man with labored breathing to the hospital for chronic obstructive pulmonary disease. The physician performs a comprehensive history and exam. The medical decision making is of high complexity. The patient stays in the hospital for the next four days. On day two, the physician performs an expanded problem-focused history and exam with medical decision making of high complexity. The patient's labored breathing is still present. On day three, the physician examines the patient and there is definite improvement in the patient's condition. The physician performs an expanded problem-focused history and exam and determines that the patient is not ready to be discharged yet. On day four, the physician performs a problem-focused history and exam and determines that there is significant improvement and the patient might be able go home the next day if the improvement continues as expected. On day five, the patient shows significant improvement and the physician discharges the patient home.

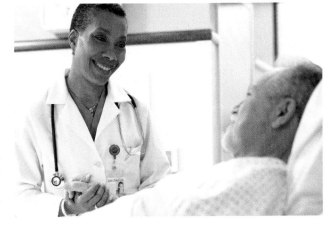

    Describe the physician's services on each hospital day and the diagnosis codes associated with this admission.

Day 1	Day 2	Day 3	Day 4	Day 5	Diagnosis Codes
_____	_____	_____	_____	_____	_____

(The ICD-10-CM codes that best describe this scenario are _____.)

Scenario 24

An 18-month-old child was playing in her yard when she walked behind her brother, who was swinging a baseball bat. She was struck in the head above her right eye and has a 3.0 cm laceration. She is brought to the emergency room for evaluation and treatment of the laceration. The ED physician performs an expanded problem-focused history and exam with medical decision making of high complexity. He orders a CT of the head with and without contrast material to rule out internal injuries. He also closes the laceration with seven stitches.

    The child is seen by her regular pediatrician seven days later to check on the wound and remove the stitches. The pediatrician performs an expanded problem-focused history and a problem-focused physical exam; decision making is of low complexity. The pediatrician proceeds to remove the stitches.

    Report the following:

ICD-9-CM diagnosis codes: _____

ED physician's services: _____

Radiologist's services: _____

Pediatrician's services   _____

(The ICD-10-CM codes that best describe this scenario are _____.)

Scenario 25

A 73-year-old man with known mitral valve insufficiency that is not related to rheumatic heart disease sees his cardiologist because of increasing discomfort and shortness of breath. The cardiologist performs a detailed history and physical exam with decision making of moderate complexity. The cardiologist then refers the patient to a cardiac surgeon. The surgeon performs a comprehensive history and physical exam and decides that the patient should have surgery within the next several weeks. The patient arranges for surgery a week later. Fill in the codes used to describe the following:

ICD-9-CM diagnosis code(s): _____

Cardiologist's services: _____

Cardiac surgeon's services: _____

Anesthesiologist's services: _____

(The ICD-10-CM codes that best describe this scenario are _____.)

The following exercises include information from many chapters. When putting it all together, you may be asked to identify codes from any part of the code sets.

Checking Your Understanding

Select the letter that best completes the statement or answers the question.

1. L016.1 A Medicare patient presents for the trimming of six dystrophic nails. Select the best HCPCS code:
   a. G0127
   b. 11719 X 6
   c. G0127 X 6
   d. 11719

2. L016.1 The HCPCS modifier _____ indicates that an Advance Beneficiary Notice is on file in the doctor's office.
   a. GA
   b. GY
   c. GB
   d. G2

3. L016.1 An established six-year-old patient sees his pediatrician for his annual exam. During the visit, the doctor also performs a venipuncture, a hearing screen, and an eye exam using a Snellen chart. The child's immunizations are up to date and he does not receive any immunizations. This visit would be reported with the following codes:
   a. 99393, 36415, 99173, 92552, V20.2, V70.0, V72.0
   b. 99393, 36415, 92551, 99173, V20.2, V70.0, V72.0
   c. 99393, 36415, V20.0
   d. 99383, 36415, 99251, 99173, V20.2, V70.0, V72.0

4. L016.1 A patient returns to her doctor's office, where she was seen two days ago, for the reading of a PPD (tuberculosis skin test). The nurse documents her reading as negative in the patient's chart. This visit would be reported with code _____.
   a. 99211, 86580
   b. 86580
   c. 99212
   d. 99211

5. L016.1 A patient presents for replacement of a single-chamber pacemaker system with a dual-chamber system including insertion of a new pulse generator and electrodes. The correct code(s) would be:
   a. 33213
   b. 33233, 33214
   c. 33213, 33233
   d. 33214

connect plus+

Enhance your learning by completing these exercises
and more at mcgrawhillconnect.com!

CHAPTER 16 | **PUTTING IT ALL TOGETHER**   507

6. L016.1 A patient with a bronchopleural fistula requires a Schede thoracoplasty for treatment. Code this procedure as _____.

   a. 32900
   b. 32905
   c. 32906
   d. 32999

7. L016.1 A patient suffering from acute maxillary sinusitis undergoes a radical (Caldwell-Luc) procedure with removal of antrochoanal polyps. Codes _____ report this encounter.

   a. 31030, 461.8
   b. 31225, 461.8
   c. 31032, 461.0
   d. 31299, 461.1

8. L016.1 Report the correct procedure code for a deep bone, open biopsy of the femur:

   a. 20220
   b. 20225
   c. 20240
   d. 20245

9. L016.1 A patient with plantar fasciitis undergoes extracorporeal shock wave therapy. Code the procedure:

   a. 28890, 728.71
   b. 0019T, 728.79
   c. 50590, 728.1
   d. 27899, 728.79

10. L016.1 What are the codes for the extensive destruction of seven condyloma acuminatum?

   a. 56515, 078.11
   b. 57061, 078.10
   c. 17000, 17003 X 6, 078.11
   d. 17000, 17003 X 6, 078.19

Thinking It Through

Use your critical-thinking skills to answer the questions below.

1. L016.1 How are multiple laceration repairs reported?

   _____

   _____

   _____

   _____

2. L016.1 Codes in ICD-9-CM category 948 (Burns) are classified according to the extent of the body surface area involved. Explain how this is represented with the codes.

_____

_____

_____

_____

3. L016.1 List the various elements coders should consider when reviewing different scenarios to determine the codes that describe the services provided.

_____

_____

_____

_____

4. L016.1 As a general rule, coders should report all services provided to patients. However, this general rule does not always apply. How would coders know when the general rule does not apply? Name at least one type of procedure to which the general rule does not apply.

_____

_____

_____

_____

5. L016.1 Explain how to code for a large number of lab tests performed at the same time on a single blood sample from a patient.

_____

_____

_____

_____

connect plus+
Enhance your learning by completing these exercises
and more at mcgrawhillconnect.com!   CHAPTER 16 | PUTTING IT ALL TOGETHER   509

Common Medical Abbreviations

Abbreviation	Meaning
a	before
a.c.	before meals
abd	abdomen
ABG	arterial blood gases
ABN	abnormal
ABS	active bowel sounds
AD	right ear
ADD	attention deficit disorder
ADH	antidiuretic hormone
ADHD	attention deficit hyperactivity disorder
ad lib	as desired
AIDS	acquired immunodeficiency syndrome
AK	above the knee
AKA	also known as; above knee amputation
alt. h.	alternate hours
AMA	against medical advice
APTT	activated partial thromboplastin time
aq.	aqueous or water
AS	left ear
ASC	ambulatory surgery center
ASD	atrial septal defect
ASHD	arteriosclerotic heart disease

Abbreviation	Meaning
AU	both ears
B&B	bowel and bladder
b.i.d.	twice a day
b.i.n.	twice a night
BM	bowel movement
BMI	body mass index
BP	blood pressure
BPH	benign prostatic hypertrophy
bpm	beats per minute
BRP	bathroom privileges
BSA	body surface area
BUN	blood urea nitrogen
BV	bacterial vaginosis
Bx	biopsy
C	Celsius
Ca	calcium
CA	cancer
CAD	coronary artery disease
CAO	conscious, alert, and oriented
cap	capsule
CAT	computerized axial tomography
Cath	catheterize

(Continued)

Abbreviation	Meaning
CBC	complete blood count
CBR	complete bed rest
cc	cubic centimeter
CC	chief complaint
CCU	critical care unit
CF	cystic fibrosis
CH	cholesterol
CIS	carcinoma in situ
cm	centimeter
CMS	Centers for Medicare & Medicaid Services
c/o	complains of
CO	cardiac output
Cont.	continue
CP	cerebral palsy
CPK	creatinine phosphokinase
CRF	chronic renal failure
CT	computed tomography
CVL	central venous line
CXR	chest x-ray
D/C	discharge or discontinue
D&C	dilation and curettage
DE	dose equivalent
Def.	deficient or deficiency
D&I	dry and intact
DM	diabetes mellitus
DME	durable medical equipment
DOA	dead on arrival
DOB	date of birth
DOS	date of service
DP	dorsalis pedis
dsg	dressing
DSMT	diabetes self-management training

Abbreviation	Meaning
DT	diphtheria and tetanus toxoids
DTaP	diphtheria, tetanus toxoids, acellular pertussis vaccine
Dx	diagnosis
EBL	estimated blood loss
ECG or EKG	electrocardiogram
ECU	emergency care unit
ED	emergency department
E/M	evaluation and management
Eng.	engorged
EOB	explanation of benefits
EPSDT	Early Periodic Screening, Diagnosis, and Treatment
ER	emergency room
ESRD	end-stage renal disease
ESWL	extracorporeal shock wave lithotripsy
ET	endotracheal
ETOH	ethyl alcohol
F	Fahrenheit
FB	foreign body
FBR	foreign body removal
Fe	iron
FH	family history
FHT	fetal heart tones
fl	fluid
Fluoro	fluoroscopic guidance
FNA	fine needle aspiration
F/U	follow-up
fx	fracture
g	gram
GERD	gastroesophageal reflux disease
gr.	grain
gtts	drops
GU	genitourinary

(Continued)

Abbreviation	Meaning	Abbreviation	Meaning
H.	hypodermically	KO	keep open
h. or hr	hour	KVO	keep vein open
H&H	hematocrit and hemoglobin	L	liter
H&P	history and physical	lb.	pound
HBP	high blood pressure	LLL	left lower lobe
Hct	hematocrit	LLQ	left lower quadrant
Hgb	hemoglobin	LOA	leave of absence
Hib	Hemophilus influenza b vaccine	LUL	left upper lobe
HIV	human immunodeficiency virus	LUQ	left upper quadrant
HLV	herpeslike virus	m	meter
HNV	has not voided	MAP	mean arterial pressure
HPI	history of present illness	mcg	microgram
HPV	human papillomavirus	mEq	milliequivalent
HR	heart rate	mg	milligram
h.s.	hour of sleep	ml	milliliter
HSV	herpes simplex virus	mm	millimeter
Ht	height	MIS	minimally invasive surgery
HTN	hypertension	MNT	medical nutrition therapy
Hx	history	MRI	magnetic resonance imaging
IBW	ideal body weight	NCCI	National Correct Coding Initiative
ICF	intermediate care facility	NEC	not elsewhere classified
ICU	intensive care unit	NKA	no known allergies
ID	intradermal	NKDA	no known drug allergies
I&D	incision and drainage	noc	night
IDDM	insulin-dependent diabetes mellitus	NOS	not otherwise specified
IM	intramuscularly	NPO	nothing by mouth
INF	inferior or infusion	NSAID	nonsteroidal anti-inflammatory drug
INJ	injection	NTG	nitroglycerine
I&O	intake and output	N&V	nausea and vomiting
IPPB	intermittent positive pressure breathing	OD	right eye
IV	intravenous	OM	otitis media
kg	kilogram	OOB	out of bed

(Continued)

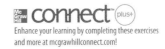

Enhance your learning by completing these exercises
and more at mcgrawhillconnect.com!

APPENDIX | COMMON MEDICAL ABBREVIATIONS   A-3

Abbreviation	Meaning
OP	outpatient
OR	operating room
OS	left eye
OU	both eyes
oz.	ounce
p	after or per (depending on context)
P	pulse
PAM	pulmonary artery mean pressure
PAP or Pap	Papanicolaou smear
PARR	postanesthesia recovery room
Path	pathology
PAWP	pulmonary artery wedge pressure
p.c.	after meals
PCA	patient-controlled analgesia
PCN	penicillin
PCP	primary care physician
PCV	pneumococcal conjugate vaccine
PE	pulmonary embolism
PET	positron emission tomography
PFSH	past, family, and social history
PFT	pulmonary function test
PH	past history
PI	present illness
PICC	peripherally inserted central catheter
PNB	percutaneous needle biopsy
PO	postoperative or by mouth
POS	place of service
Pos.	positive
PPD	purified protein derivative (of tuberculin)
PR	per rectum
p.r.n.	as needed
PTSD	post-traumatic stress disorder

Abbreviation	Meaning
PVR	pulmonary vascular resistance
Px	prognosis
QNS	quantity not sufficient
QS	quantity sufficient
R	respirations
RAP	right arterial pressure
RBC	red blood cell
Rh	Rhesus
Rh neg	Rhesus factor negative
R/O	rule out
ROM	range of motion
RTC	return to clinic
RTO	return to office
RLL	right lower lobe
RLQ	right lower quadrant
ROS	review of systems
RUL	right upper lobe
RUQ	right upper quadrant
RVU	relative value unit
Rx	treatment or prescription
RXN	reaction
SB	spina bifida
SBE	self breast exam
SF	spinal fluid
SH	social history
SNF	skilled nursing facility
SOB	shortness of breath
S/P	status post
SQ, subq, subcu	subcutaneous
Staph	*Staphylococcus*
STAT	immediately
STD	sexually transmitted disease

(Continued)

Abbreviation	Meaning
Strep	*Streptococcus*
supp	suppository
SV	stroke volume
SVR	systemic vascular resistance
T&A	tonsillectomy and adenoidectomy
TB	tuberculosis
Td	tetanus and diphtheria
TKO	to keep open
U/A	urinalysis
U&C	usual and customary
ung	unguent or ointment
US	ultrasound
UTI	urinary tract infection

Abbreviation	Meaning
vd	void
VO	verbal order
VS	vital signs
WBC	white blood count
w/d	warm and dry
WDWN	well developed, well nourished
WNL	within normal limits
Wt	weight
y.o.	years old
#	number, if before a digit; pounds, if after a digit
>	greater than
<	less than

connect plus+

Enhance your learning by completing these exercises
and more at mcgrawhillconnect.com!

APPENDIX | COMMON MEDICAL ABBREVIATIONS   A-5

GLOSSARY

A

abbreviation A shortened form of a commonly used word.

abscess Localized collection of pus found in tissues, organs, or confined spaces. Usually accompanied by inflammation and pain.

acronym A term made up of the beginning letters of a multiword term. An example of an acronym would be *ADH,* which stands for antidiuretic hormone.

add-on code Code that describes services that are in addition to those described by the primary code. Add-on codes cannot be listed alone and require the parent code to be listed. Designated by a plus sign and listed in Appendix D of the CPT.

adjacent tissue transfer Skin repair procedure in which adjacent tissue is transferred or rearranged to cover part of the primary wound.

administration Supplying a substance (e.g., drug, fluid, vaccine, or contrast material) to a patient by one of several routes, such as by injection, by mouth, or through an IV.

admit/discharge code Code that is reported when a patient is admitted and discharged on the same day.

adrenal glands Endocrine glands located just above the kidneys that secrete substances such as epinephrine.

advanced life support (ALS) Type of ground ambulance service that includes equipment and personnel to support circulation and breathing while the patient is being transported.

aftercare Code to describe situations when the initial treatment of a disease or injury has been provided but the patient requires continued care through the recovery or healing process. Aftercare codes are found in categories V51–V59.

allograft Skin graft or organ that is used for a patient and is obtained from another human.

allotransplantation Transplantation of an allograft. Three types are cadaveric donor transplantation, living related donor transplantation, and living unrelated donor transplantation. Also known as *allogenic* or *allogeneic transplantation.*

Alphabetic Index of Diseases (Volume 2) Alphabetical listing of possible diagnosis codes that should always be used first when locating an ICD-9-CM or ICD-10-CM diagnosis code.

ambulance trip Transportation of an individual from the point of pickup to a care facility by ambulance.

American Society of Anesthesiologists Professional network of anesthesiologists that develops and publishes the *Relative Value Guide,* which lists base units for anesthesia services.

analgesia Absence of the sensation of pain.

anatomic pathology Professional services associated with postmortem examinations (autopsies), including gross examination and microscopic examination.

anatomy The physical structure of the body including structures that make up the musculoskeletal system, organs, and glands. The study of anatomy is usually divided into the study of specific systems.

anesthesia Absence of painful sensations. May be provided as general, neuraxial, regional, or local anesthesia.

anesthesia assistant (AA) Non-nurse professional trained to provide anesthesia services under the direction of an anesthesiologist.

anesthesiologist Physician specially trained to administer anesthesia.

aneurysm Weak area of an artery or vein that can suddenly rupture causing extreme blood loss, damage to surrounding anatomical structures, and possible death.

angioplasty Insertion and inflation of a balloon-tipped catheter to clear a circulatory pathway.

antepartum care Care provided to pregnant women prior to delivery.

anterior cranial fossa Anterior subdivision of the floor of the cranial cavity. Supports the frontal lobes and consists of three bones: ethmoid, frontal, and sphenoid.

anterior vertebral structure Vertebral body.

anteroposterior (AP) Direction of a beam that enters at the front of the body (anterior) and exits at the back (posterior).

aphakia Absence of the natural lens in the eye, usually due to surgical excision for cataract or trauma.

appendices Portions of the coding manuals that contain additional information for complete and accurate coding.

appendix Wormlike diverticulum of the cecum.

arterial system Network of arteries that carry blood from the heart to the rest of the body. Part of the cardiovascular system, along with the heart, capillaries, and venous system.

arteriovenous malformation Abnormal communication between an artery and a vein. Also known as *AV malformation.*

arthrodesis Fusion of two bones usually performed with bone grafting and instrumentation.

arthroscopy Examination of the interior of a joint with an arthroscope.

assistant surgeon Additional professional who helps a surgeon perform a procedure.

asymptomatic HIV Condition of patients infected with human immunodeficiency virus (HIV) or "HIV positive" as long as no HIV-related conditions are present.

autograft A graft of tissue derived from another site of the patient's body.

B

backbench work Process to prepare a donor organ for transplantation.

Bartholin's gland One of two glands located just within the opening of the vagina.

base unit Relative value of one anesthetic compared to other anesthetics based on expected or potential difficulties.

basic life support (BLS) Type of ground ambulance service used for a patient with life-threatening illness or injuries until the patient reaches the hospital.

bilateral procedure Same procedure performed bilaterally.

bladder Membranous sac that holds fluid such as urine or bile.

bronchi Large air passage of the lung. Left and right bronchi divide from the trachea.

bronchodilator A drug that opens the breathing tubes in the lungs.

bronchoscopy Examination of the bronchi with a bronchoscope.

C

capillary Tiny blood vessel between the arterial and venous systems. Capillaries form a network in nearly all parts of the body. Their walls allow the transfer of fluids and oxygen between the blood and tissue fluid.

carcinoma in situ A neoplasm in early stages that has not spread beyond the site of origin.

cardiac catheterization Insertion of a catheter from a peripheral vein or artery to the heart and great vessels.

cardiography Technique of graphically recording physical or functional aspects of the heart.

cardiopulmonary bypass Diversion of the flow of blood directly from the venous system to the aorta via a pump oxygenator, avoiding both the heart and lungs.

cardiotomy Opening the heart to explore the interior chambers.

cardiovascular system Network that includes the heart, arterial system, capillaries, and venous system. Sometimes referred to as the circulatory system. The cardiovascular system is responsible for the circulation of blood and delivery of oxygen and other nutrients.

care coordination Organization of a patient's care with multiple healthcare organizations; one of the three contributing components of the determination of the level of E/M services.

carotid body Small neurovascular structure within the carotid arteries. Stimulation by hypoxia, hypercapnia, or elevated hydrogen ion concentration results in an increase in blood pressure, heart rate, and respiratory movements.

cast A rigid dressing, molded while wet and hardening as it dries, to give firm support to allow a fracture to heal.

Category I codes Listing of services that are generally acceptable in the current practice of medicine and are performed by many physicians in multiple clinical locations. Generally considered to be standard medical practice.

Category II codes Performance measures used by Medicare to document the quality of services provided to individual patients and to the patient population under the care of individual providers, groups of providers, or a healthcare system. These codes are four numeric digits followed by the letter *F*.

Category III codes Temporary codes used to designate emerging technologies, services, and procedures. Used to document the extent of use and geographical areas of new procedures. These codes are four digits followed by the letter *T*.

central venous access device A catheter inserted into the heart or the venous trunk through a large vein, as of the arm, leg, neck, or shoulder, for long-term IV use.

certified registered nurse anesthetist (CRNA) Specially trained nurse who provides anesthesia services, often under the direction of a physician.

cervical spine Vertebrae of the neck.

cervix Lower part of the uterus.

cesarean section Incision through the abdominal and uterine walls for delivery of a baby.

chemistry Tests to measure for the presence of substances within blood or other bodily fluids.

chief complaint A brief statement, usually in the patient's own words, that describes the reason the patient is seeing the physician. May be a symptom, condition, problem, diagnosis, or other medical reason for the encounter.

chronic kidney disease A condition in which the kidneys lose their ability to function. Stages of chronic kidney disease are determined by glomerular filtration rate and include stages 1–5 and end-stage renal disease (ESRD).

closed fracture A fracture in which the skin overlaying the fracture site is not compromised and the fracture is not exposed to the external environment.

closed treatment Treatment for a fracture during which the fracture site is not surgically opened.

co-surgeons Two surgeons who perform distinct parts of a single procedure.

code sections Specific grouping of codes.

colonoscopy Endoscopic procedure including the entire colon from the rectum to the cecum and may include a portion of the distal ileum.

colposcopy Examination of the cervix and vagina by means of a colposcope.

combining form A word element created by adding a combining vowel to a root word.

combining vowel A vowel such as "o" or "i" added to a root or base word to facilitate pronunciation.

comminuted fracture Fracture in which the bone is broken into more than two pieces. May be either an open or closed fracture.

complete blood count (CBC) Measures hemoglobin, hematocrit, red blood cells, white blood cells, and platelets.

complete mastectomy Excision of the entire breast.

complex wound repair Repair of a wound that requires more than layered closure.

comprehensive history General multisystem exam or a complete exam of a single body area or organ system.

computed tomography (CT) Imaging technique that uses multiple x-rays to produce cross-sectional images.

concurrent care Two or more physicians provide care to the same patient on the same day.

congenital Present at birth; either inherited or due to an event during gestation up to the moment of birth.

congenital abnormalities Abnormalities that exist at birth.

consultation Type of service provided by a physician when asked for an opinion or advice by another physician.

contrast material Material used to enhance viewing of anatomical structures during radiological procedures.

contributory components Components that contribute to E/M services but are not necessarily provided during every E/M encounter. May include counseling, care coordination, the nature of the presenting problem, and time.

conventions Standards or rules for coding systems.

coronal plane A vertical plane that divides the body into front and back portions. Also known as *frontal plane*.

coronary artery stent A slender tubular device used to hold open one of several arteries branching from the aorta that supply blood to the heart muscle.

counseling Discussions with a patient and/or family regarding aspects of the patient's medical situation, such as diagnostic tests and results; patient prognosis; treatment options, including risks and benefits; patient instructions regarding compliance with treatment; risk factors for disease and reducing those risks; and education of the patient and/or family.

CPT manual Current Procedural Terminology code set created by the AMA to accurately describe services and provide a convenient method of communicating this information.

craniectomy Procedure performed through an opening made in the cranium or upper part of the skull. Removes a portion of the bone either permanently or at least for an extended period of time.

cranioplasty Surgical correction of defects of the skull.

craniotomy Procedure performed through an opening made in the cranium or upper part of the skull. Temporary removal of part of the skull; bone is replaced at the end of the procedure.

critical care Delivery of medical care to a patient who is critically ill or injured.

Current Dental Terminology (CDT) Codes that describe dental procedures. Developed and maintained by the American Dental Association. Updated every two years.

cystocele Hernial protrusion of the urinary bladder, usually through the vaginal wall.

D

debridement Removal of foreign material or contaminated tissue until surrounding healthy tissue is exposed.

decision to perform surgery Physician decision that surgery is necessary.

decubitus Position in which patient is lying with one side down.

deoxygenated blood Blood that has released its oxygen and is returning to the heart through the venous system.

detailed exam An extended exam of the affected body areas or organ systems and other related systems.

diagnosis code Code that designates the reason for a patient's encounter; represents the patient's condition or symptoms obtained through the ICD-9-CM or ICD-10-CM manual.

diagnostic thoracoscopy Examination of the pleural cavity with an endoscope.

digestive system System of tubular structures and attached organs that starts at the mouth and ends at the anus. The major functions of the digestive system are to break down foods into basic elements, absorb nutrients, and eliminate waste.

digital x-ray system Imaging technique that uses computerized data for radiological imaging instead of conventional x-ray film.

distinct procedure Services that are not usually reported with other services, but under certain circumstances may be reported as a separate procedure. Modifier 59 is used to indicate distinct procedures.

drug test Qualitative test to detect the presence of many individual drugs or drug classes from a biological sample.

durable medical equipment (DME) Equipment that is meant to be long lasting, can withstand repeated use, may be used in the home, and is not generally used by those without a medical condition.

E

ectopic pregnancy Pregnancy occurring outside the uterus.

electroencephalogram (EEG) Record of electrical activity of the brain.

embolectomy Surgical removal of an embolus.

emergency transportation Transportation provided by an ambulance service.

emerging technology New technologies and new uses for existing technologies. Listed as temporary codes in Category III of the CPT manual.

encounter Patient's visit for medical treatment or a procedure.

end-stage renal disease (ESRD) Chronic kidney disease requiring regular dialysis.

endocrine system Network of glands that secrete or excrete hormones. Major glands of the system include the hypothalamus, pituitary, pineal, thyroid, parathyroids, thymus, adrenals, pancreas, ovaries, and testes.

endometrium Inner lining of the uterus.

endoscopic retrograde cholangiopancreatography (ERCP) Insertion of a catheter through the ampulla of Vater to inject contrast material for x-ray or other imaging examination of the hepatobiliary system. Includes the pancreatic ducts, hepatic ducts, common bile duct, and gallbladder.

endoscopy Visual inspection of any cavity of the body by means of an endoscope.

enteral and parenteral therapy Provision of nutrients to prevent or treat malnutrition.

enterocele Hernia containing a portion of the intestine.

epididymis Elongated corded structure along the posterior border of the testis. Provides for storage, transit, and maturation of spermatozoa.

epidural Situated upon or outside the dura mater.

epispadius Developmental anomaly consisting of an absence of the upper wall of the urethra. Most common in males in whom the urethral opening is located on the top side of the penis.

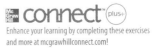

eponym Medical term based on or derived from a person's name. Many identify the person associated with the disease or process.

established patient Patient who has been seen by a particular physician or another physician of the same specialty within the same group practice during the past three years.

ethmoid sinus Air-filled cavity located at the top of the nasal cavities between the eyes.

etiology The causes or origins of a disease or disorder.

evaluation and management services (E/M services) Services commonly associated with "doctor visits" in which a provider takes the patient's history; performs a physical examination; determines the cause of the patient's problem; orders and interprets appropriate tests; decides on necessary treatments; and monitors the patient for changes in his or her health status. These services are divided into many categories based on the setting of services.

evocative/suppression testing Series of tests to determine if a patient responds appropriately to particular agents or chemicals.

excision Full-thickness removal of a lesion and surrounding tissue. Each lesion that is removed is coded separately. The size, location, and whether each lesion was benign or malignant must be known to be coded properly.

Excludes1 An ICD-10-CM notation indicating that the excluded code should not be listed with the code indicated because the two conditions do not occur together.

Excludes2 An ICD-10-CM notation indicating that the excluded condition is not part of the code indicated and an additional code should be assigned.

expanded problem-focused exam Limited exam of the affected body areas or organ systems and other related systems.

external fixation Use of an external mechanism to hold the bones in position to treat bony deformities.

extracorporeal membrane oxygenation (ECMO) Procedure that processes blood externally by taking it from a patient's circulatory system and returning it after processing.

extracranial arteries Arteries located outside the cranium.

F

family history Review of medical history of family members that includes their health status or causes of death. Includes diseases in family members that may relate to a patient's chief complaint or that may put the patient at risk such as hereditary conditions.

fascia Sheet of fibrous connective tissue.

fine needle aspiration Biopsy that uses a needle to collect cells for clinical examination.

first-listed diagnosis Main reason for the visit used in physician's office coding; also referred to as the *primary diagnosis*.

fistula An abnormal passage usually between two body structures or leading from an internal structure to the surface of the body.

fluoroscopy Imaging technique that is used to view real-time images of the body using an x-ray source and a fluoroscope.

frontal bone Large bone of the forehead.

frontal plane A divisional plane that divides the body into front (anterior) and back (posterior) portions.

frontal sinus One of the paired, irregular-shaped paranasal sinuses in the frontal bone. Separated by a bony septum.

G

gastrointestinal Relating to the stomach and intestines. The gastrointestinal tract begins at the lips and continues uninterrupted through irregular tubular structures to the anus.

general anesthesia An anesthesia technique in which the patient is made unconscious.

General Equivalence Mappings (GEMs) System developed to help identify potential ICD-10-CM codes from ICD-9-CM codes.

general guidelines Overall instructions on how to use coding systems.

gestational diabetes Occurs in the second and third trimester in some women who were not diabetic prior to becoming pregnant. Gestational diabetes can cause complications similar to those of preexisting diabetes and increases the mother's risk of becoming diabetic later.

gland Tissue that secretes substances that act elsewhere in the body.

global period Period of time during which some services provided by the physician who performed the original procedure are considered to be related to that procedure.

gonads Testes and ovaries.

guidelines Instructions included in sections of the coding manuals that provide information necessary to correctly report services listed in that section.

H

heart Organ containing cardiac muscle that is divided into four cavities: two atria and two ventricles.

hematoma Localized collection of blood, usually a blood clot, that is commonly caused by a break in the wall of a blood vessel.

hemic system Network of blood-producing tissues and blood cells, including red cells, white cells, and platelets.

hemodialysis An artificial method to remove certain elements from the blood by filtering the blood through a semipermeable membrane. Also known as *dialysis*.

hidradenitis Inflammation of a sweat gland.

history of present illness (HPI) Chronological description of the patient's present illness from onset to the present that includes factors describing the medical reason for the encounter with the physician. Usually includes signs and symptoms associated with the patient's condition.

HIV-positive patient A patient diagnosed with human immunodeficiency virus (HIV) infection.

HIV-related condition A condition related to the presence of human immunodeficiency virus (HIV).

hospital inpatient services Services provided to patients admitted to the hospital.

hospital observation services Provided when it is unclear whether it is medically necessary to admit the patient as an inpatient.

human papillomavirus (HPV) A group of viruses that cause many afflictions such as warts and cervical cancer.

Hypertension Table A table located in Volume 2 of the ICD-9-CM or ICD-10-CM that lists all conditions due to or associated with hypertension.

hypospadius Developmental anomaly where the urethra opens inferior to the usual location. Most common in males in whom the opening is on the underside of the penis.

I

ICD-9-CM Abbreviated title of the *International Classification of Diseases, 9th Revision, Clinical Modification*, the coding system in use in the United States until October 1, 2013. Contains both an alphabetical and a tabular listing of codes associated with medical diagnosis.

ICD-10-CM Abbreviated title of the *International Classification of Diseases, 10th Revision, Clinical Modification*, the system of classification codes that will be implemented in the United States on October 1, 2013. ICD-10-CM is much more detailed than the ICD-9-CM and will allow much more specificity for diagnosis codes.

ICD-10-PCS *International Classification of Diseases, 10th Revision, Procedure Coding System.*

immune globulin Any of the structurally related glycoproteins that function as antibodies. Can be extracted from human blood or produced in a laboratory.

incision and drainage Procedure that punctures the skin or makes an incision but does not close the skin at the end of the procedure, allowing for drainage.

Includes A term indicating that the listed conditions following the term are described by the code.

index Alphabetical listing of main terms in the coding manuals. Should always be used first when selecting and assigning codes to report services, procedures, or devices.

infratentorial Lower part of the brain.

initial treatment Primary treatment for a condition.

integumentary system Largest organ system in the body, which includes skin and accessory organs of the hair, nails, and glands.

intermediate wound repair Multilayer closure of a wound with one or more layers of subcutaneous tissue closure in addition to the skin closure.

internal fixation Treatment in which plates and screws or other devices are attached to fractured bones to allow healing to occur in correct alignment.

intestines Made up of the small and large intestines. The small intestine includes the duodenum, jejunum, ileum, and ileocecal junction. The large intestine includes the ascending colon, transverse colon, descending colon, sigmoid colon, and rectum and ends at the anus.

intracranial arteries Arteries within the cranium.

intrathecal Within the thecal sac of the spinal cord, also known as the subarachnoid space.

K

key components Used to determine the level of E/M services. Includes history, physical examination, and medical decision making.

kidney Organ pair that filters the blood, excretes the end products or waste of body metabolism in the form of urine, and regulates concentrations of hydrogen, sodium, potassium, phosphate, and other ions in the extracellular fluid.

L

laboratory Facility designed to perform tests.

laparoscopy Examination of the interior of the abdomen by means of a laparoscope.

laterality Designation of the right or left side of the body.

left lateral decubitus Patient is lying on the left side of the body.

Level I HCPCS codes Current Procedural Terminology (CPT) codes developed and maintained by the American Medical Association.

Level II HCPCS codes Services, supplies, and equipment that are not identified by CPT codes. Created and maintained by the Centers for Medicare and Medicaid Services (CMS).

local anesthesia Injection of local anesthetic agent into the skin and subcutaneous tissues surrounding the operative area.

lumbar spine Vertebrae located between the thorax and the pelvis.

lymphatic system Network consisting of the lymph vessels, nodes, and spleen that collects excess fluid from the interstitial space and returns it to the heart.

M

magnetic resonance imaging (MRI) Imaging technique that uses a powerful magnetic field to produce an image.

main terms Key terms found in the index of the CPT.

mammography An x-ray of the breast used to screen for breast cancer.

manifestation Symptom or sign of disease.

manipulation Manually applying external forces to align bones or joints to their normal anatomical positions.

maxilla Irregularly shaped bone that is one of two bones that create the upper jaw.

maxillary sinus One of a pair of air cavities in the maxilla (upper jaw) that connect with the nose.

measles, mumps, and rubella (MMR) Combination vaccine for measles, mumps, and rubella.

mediastinum Area between the lungs containing the heart, aorta, venae cavae, esophagus, trachea, and main bronchi.

medical decision making Establishing a diagnosis and/or selecting from among treatment or management options.

medical supplies Supplies provided to patients as part of their treatment. Most of these supplies are single-use disposable items.

meninges Three membranes that envelop the brain and spinal cord: dura mater, pia mater, and arachnoid.

methicillin-resistant *Staphylococcus aureus* (MRSA) A strain of bacteria that is resistant to penicillin.

microscopy Manually looking at a sample under a microscope to determine whether other substances, such as red or white blood cells, are present in the sample. Can be automated or nonautomated.

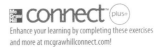
Enhance your learning by completing these exercises and more at mcgrawhillconnect.com!

GLOSSARY   G-5

middle cranial fossa Middle subdivision of the cranial cavity. Supports the temporal lobes and the pituitary gland.

moderate sedation State of depression induced by drugs during which patients respond purposefully to verbal commands.

modified radical mastectomy Breast removal that does not include the removal of the pectoralis major muscle. The pectoralis minor may or may not be removed.

modifier Numbers or letters added to a code to indicate that a procedure was altered by specific circumstances.

modifier 26 Modifier used to report professional services.

modifier 51 exempt Indicates that modifier 51 cannot be added to a code. Designated by the circle-slash symbol ($\oslash$).

modifier TC Modifier reported by an entity that owns or leases the equipment to report the technical component.

modifying terms Listed as indentations under main terms of the CPT index; could have an effect on code selection.

Mohs micrographic surgery Technique for removal of malignant skin lesions and pathological examination of all tissues margins by a single provider acting as both surgeon and pathologist. Also known as *Mohs surgery*.

molar pregnancy A fertilized ovum that develops into a nonviable pregnancy.

monitored anesthesia care (MAC) Anesthesia procedure in which vital signs are monitored and patients sedated to the extent necessary for comfort, but not to the extent that they are unconscious.

multiple procedures More than one procedure performed during single operative session.

myometrium Muscle wall of the uterus.

N

NEC (not elsewhere classifiable) Code that is used when the information supplied indicates a specific condition but listed codes do not identify the specific condition.

necrotizing infection Inflammation that results in the death of tissues.

new patient Patient who has not been seen by a particular physician or another physician of the same specialty within the same group practice during the past three years.

Neoplasm Table A table located in Volume 2 of the ICD-9-CM or ICD-10-CM that lists the different types and locations of neoplasms.

nervous system Composed of the central and peripheral nervous systems, this system contains the brain, spinal cord, cranial nerves, spinal nerves, and peripheral nerves.

newborn services E/M services administered to patients from birth through 28 days of age.

non-emergency transportation Transportation used when patient is not in immediate, critical need of medical care.

NOS (not otherwise specified) Code that is used when there is not sufficient information available for a specific diagnosis.

nuclear medicine Radioactive material is placed within the body and radioactive emissions from those elements are monitored for either diagnostic or therapeutic purposes.

O

oblique Term used when a patient is positioned somewhere between the standard imaging technique positions.

occipital bones Bones of the back of the skull.

open or compound fracture Fracture in which the skin is open and the fracture is exposed to external elements.

open treatment Treatment in which a fracture is surgically exposed as part of the treatment. Usually done through an incision to allow a surgeon to manipulate the bones into proper position.

orchiopexy Surgical fixation in the scrotum of an undescended testis.

organ A part of the body that carries out one or more special functions.

organ/disease panel Predefined cluster of laboratory tests to evaluate a diseased organ, organ system, or disease.

orthotic Device that supports an impaired body part.

osteotomy Surgical cutting of bone.

oxygenated blood Blood that contains oxygen for use by the tissues of the body.

P

pancreas A large, curved gland that lies behind the stomach between the spleen and the duodenum.

parathyroid gland Small endocrine gland situated beside or behind the thyroid.

parent code Primary code for a procedure.

parenthetical note Provides specific information about an individual code or group of codes.

parietal bones Two bones that form the sides and roof of the cranium.

partial mastectomy Surgical procedure in which less than the entire breast is removed.

partial thromboplastin time (PTT) Measurement of the time it takes to form a blood clot to evaluate some coagulation factors in blood plasma.

past, family, and social history (PFSH) Includes information regarding the patient's past, family, and social history as factors in E/M coding.

past medical history History of a patient's previous major illnesses, injuries, operations, hospitalizations, medications, allergies, immunizations, and dietary status.

pathological fracture A broken bone caused by a disease leading to a weakness of the bone, such as a tumor or severe osteoporosis.

penetrating wound A wound that penetrates the skin, such as a stab or gunshot wound.

percutaneous skeletal fixation Treatment in which a fracture is not surgically exposed but pins and other devices are placed through the skin to hold the ends of the fracture in place.

performance measure Supplementary tracking code from Category II of the CPT used to document the quality of care by individual providers and healthcare systems.

performance measurement exclusion modifiers Indicate a provider considered providing a service associated with the performance measure but, because of a medical, patient, or system reason, did not provide the service.

pericardium Sac that surrounds the heart.

peripartum period Six-month period beginning with the last month of pregnancy and lasting five additional months.

physical examination Process by which a physician or other healthcare provider assesses a patient for the presence or extent of an illness or injury.

physical status modifiers Identify the patient's health status before undergoing anesthesia. These are added to CPT codes 00100–01999 by anesthesia providers.

Physician Quality Reporting Initiative (PQRI) Created by CMS for physicians to report their performance of certain services or the reason a particular service was not performed.

physiology The study of how anatomical structures function in a living person.

pineal gland Small, flattened, cone-shaped gland located deep within the brain.

pituitary gland Pea-sized gland at base of the brain.

place of service Location where services were provided.

placeholder Letter "x" inserted into an ICD-10-CM diagnosis code to indicate unused digits.

pleura Membrane covering the lungs and lining the thoracic cavity.

positron emission tomography (PET) Imaging technique that uses positron-emitting radionuclides to capture a clear image of the selected anatomy.

posterior cranial fossa Posterior subdivision of the cranial cavity. Holds the cerebellum, pons, and medulla oblongata.

posterior vertebral structure Bony structures of the back including the spinous process, lamina, and facet joint.

posteroanterior (PA) Imaging technique in which a beam is aimed at the patient's back (posterior) and the film is placed along the front side of the patient.

postpartum care Hospital and office visits following the delivery of a baby.

postpartum period Begins immediately after delivery and ends after six weeks.

prefix A word element added to the beginning of a root word to provide greater specificity.

prenatal visits Encounters that occur during pregnancy before delivery to monitor the mother and fetus.

preventive medicine services Age-appropriate history and physical exam of a patient without specific medical complaint.

primary malignant tumor The original site and type of a tumor.

principal diagnosis Main diagnosis, or main reason for visit, in hospital coding.

problem-focused history Limited exam of the affected body area or organ system.

proctectomy Surgical removal of the rectum.

professional component The portion of a procedure performed by a physician or other professional when the procedure includes both professional and technical components.

prolonged services Services that require more than the usual time for E/M services in the outpatient or inpatient setting.

prone Position in which the patient is lying stomach side down.

prostate Gland in males that surrounds the bladder neck and urethra.

prosthetic Device that replaces a missing body part.

prothombrin time (PT) Test that measures the time needed for clot formation in blood plasma.

puerperium Period from the end of the third stage of labor until the uterus has returned to its normal size.

Q

qualifying circumstances add-on code Code used to report that an anesthetic involved additional anesthesia techniques or the individual patient circumstances made the anesthetic more difficult than usual.

qualitative Result that indicates whether a specific substance is present in the sample but does not show the amount that is in the sample.

quantitative Result that shows the amount of a substance in the sample.

R

radical mastectomy Removal of the entire breast, axillary lymph nodes, and both pectoralis major and pectoralis minor muscles.

radiological supervision and interpretation Term that describes the professional component of radiological services.

rectocele Hernial protrusion of part of the rectum into the vagina.

red blood cell (RBC) A cell that contains hemoglobin that carries oxygen to the body tissues.

refractive state Eye's ability to focus light to form recognizable images.

regional anesthesia Term used when an anesthesia provider performs procedures to interrupt nerve function to make a large portion of the patient's body insensitive to pain while the patient remains awake.

renal calculus Kidney stone.

reproductive system System of organs related to reproduction. Organs of this system vary by gender and include internal and external anatomical structures.

resident physician Individual at a teaching institution who is completing training in the medical field.

respiratory system System whose purpose is to exchange carbon dioxide and waste products for oxygen. Structures included in this system include the nose, pharynx, larynx, trachea, bronchi, bronchioles, and lungs.

review of systems (ROS) Series of questions regarding body and organ systems designed to identify signs and symptoms that a patient is experiencing or has experienced.

right lateral decubitus Patient is lying on the right side of the body.

root word The base of a term that contains the basic meaning of the word.

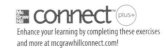
Enhance your learning by completing these exercises and more at mcgrawhillconnect.com!

GLOSSARY   G-7

S

sagittal plane Plane that runs through the body vertically from front to back to divide the body into right and left sides.

secondary diabetes Diabetes that is caused by another primary condition or event.

secondary diagnosis Additional code used to identify other conditions that are present beyond the main reason for the encounter.

secondary malignant tumor A tumor that has metastasized or spread from its original location to another site.

seminal vesicle Sac of the vas deferens that produces seminal fluid.

separate procedure A notation that indicates that the procedure is usually a part of another procedure and not reported separately. These procedures are only reported when performed alone and not part of another procedure.

sepsis Systemic inflammatory response syndrome (SIRS) secondary to infection.

septic shock Circulatory failure associated with severe sepsis.

septicemia Systemic disease caused by the presence of bacteria in the bloodstream.

sequelae Coding term used to identify late effects.

severe sepsis Sepsis associated with acute organ dysfunction.

shunt A tube that temporarily allows blood to bypass the area of the vessel being repaired.

sign Indication of the existence of a disease observed by a medical professional.

simple wound repair Single-layer closure of a skin defect using sutures or a closure device.

sinusotomy Opening a sinus cavity.

social history Review of the patient's nonmedical information, including current employment, occupational history, marital status, education, sexual history, and use of alcohol, tobacco, and drugs.

specimen Sample used for examination or testing.

sphenoid sinus One of two cavities in the sphenoid bone that communicate with the nasal cavities.

spinal instrumentation Metal structures used to hold spinal segments in alignment to allow proper healing.

splint An appliance used to immobilize and protect an injured body part.

staged procedure Procedure that is performed over two or more operative sessions.

standing Upright position during imaging or other procedure.

strapping The use of adhesive strips applied directly to the skin to align bones or immobilize joints.

subcutaneous Beneath the skin.

subsequent encounter Care or treatment following the initial treatment of an injury.

suffix A word element added to the end of a root word to provide greater specificity.

supine Position for imaging technique in which the patient is lying back side down.

supplemental classification Additional information beyond diagnosis codes, including the Factors Influencing Health Status and Contact with Health Services (V-codes) and External Causes of Injury and Poisoning (E-codes).

supratentorial Upper part of the brain.

surgical pathology Examination of tissue samples removed during surgery to determine the cause of underlying disease or whether any disease is present in the tissue.

surgical team Three or more surgeons, often from different specialties.

surgical thoracoscopy Surgical endoscopy done as part of a thoracic procedure.

symbols Identifiers attached to codes to indicate additional information.

symptom Subjective manifestation of disease.

systemic inflammatory response syndrome (SIRS) A systemic response to infection, burns, trauma, or other severe insult. Symptoms may include fever, tachycardia, tachypnea, and leukocytosis.

T

Table of Drugs Identifies specific HCPCS codes that describe medications provided to patients.

Table of Drugs and Chemicals Extensive listing of drugs, industrial solvents, corrosive gases, noxious plants, pesticides, and other toxic agents in Volume 2 of the ICD-9-CM and ICD-10-CM.

Tabular List of Diseases (Volume 1) Listing of disease classification by etiology or site, supplementary classification, and appendixes within the ICD-9-CM or ICD-10-CM manual.

technical component The portion of a procedure that represents the equipment used when the procedure includes both professional and technical components.

temporal Lateral region of the head or one of the lobes of the brain.

testis or testicle Male gonad. Either of the paired egg-shaped glands normally situated in the scrotum.

therapeutic level Presence of a particular medication in sufficient quantity to have a desired effect but not enough to be dangerous.

thoracentesis Removal of fluid from the pleural cavity. Also known as *pleuracentesis*.

thoracic spine Portion of the the spine between the cervical and lumbar spine, generally lying in the region behind the heart and lungs.

thrombectomy Excision of a thrombus from a blood vessel.

thymus Endocrine gland located at the superior mediastinum.

thyroid Endocrine gland in the neck.

time Contributing component of E/M services.

time unit Conversion of minutes into discrete units used to report anesthesia time.

tissue flap Transfer of tissue to a site that is more distant from the donor site than an adjacent tissue transfer (may be a single procedure or completed in stages).

tomogram Two-dimensional image of a plane or slice through the body.

trachea Cartilaginous and membranous tube descending from the larynx and branching into the left and right main bronchi.

traction Application of force to a limb through pins or wires attached to the bones or through strapping applied directly to the skin to align bones to their original length and/or position.

transverse plane Plane that runs through the body horizontally to divide the body into top and bottom portions.

tunica vaginalis Serous membrane covering the front and sides of the testis and epididymis.

turbinate Any of the nasal conchae.

type I diabetes Diabetes characterized by the abrupt onset of symptoms, low insulin production, and the need for insulin administration to properly process glucose.

type II diabetes Diabetes characterized by an inadequate response to normal levels of insulin; may be controlled by diet, although insulin also may be needed to provide sufficient glucose metabolism.

U

ultrasound A procedure using sound waves to record permanent images and measurements of an organ or tissue and as guidance during other procedures.

unit of service Particular amount of a described service.

unlisted procedure No specific code exists that describes the service provided.

ureter Fibromuscular tube that conveys urine from the kidney to the bladder.

urethra Membranous canal that conveys urine from the bladder to the exterior of the body.

urinalysis (UA) Tests on urine samples with dipsticks or reagents to detect a number of chemicals or to determine the specific gravity of a urine sample.

urinary system Anatomical system that removes metabolic waste and maintains fluid and electrolyte balance within the body. System includes the kidneys, ureters, urinary bladder, and urethra.

V

vaccine Attenuated or killed microorganisms administered to prevent infectious diseases.

vagina Genital canal of a female. Extends from the vulva to the cervix uteri.

vaginal delivery Procedure during which a fetus is delivered through the vagina.

vas deferens (spermatic cord) Tube that receives sperm from the epididymis.

VBAC procedure Vaginal birth after cesarean. Attempted vaginal delivery after previous cesarean section.

venous system System of veins that transports deoxygenated blood from the body to the right atrium of the heart.

visit Patient's encounter for medical treatment or a procedure.

vulva Region of the external genital organs of the female.

W

white blood cell (WBC) Cell that helps protect the body from infection and disease.

word elements Parts of a word. These word elements make up medical language.

X

x-ray film X-ray detector upon which the x-ray beam is focused to form an image of the body plane being examined.

xenograft A tissue graft from a nonhuman donor.

connect plus+
Enhance your learning by completing these exercises and more at mcgrawhillconnect.com!

GLOSSARY   G-9

CREDITS

TEXT AND ILLUSTRATION CREDITS

CHAPTER 1

Table 1.4 p. 8: © The Joint Commission, 2011. Reprinted with permission. Figure 1.3, p. 11: *Anatomy & Physiology: The Unity and Form of Function*, (3rd edition), by K. S. Saladin, 2004, Dubuque, IA; The McGraw-Hill Companies, Inc. Reprinted with permission. Figure 1.4, p. 12: *Anatomy & Physiology: The Unity and Form of Function*, (3rd edition), by K. S. Saladin, 2004, Dubuque, IA; The McGraw-Hill Companies, Inc. Reprinted with permission. Figure 1.5, p. 12: *Human Anatomy*, by K. S. Saladin, 2005, Dubuque, IA: The McGraw-Hill Companies, Inc. Reprinted with permission. Figure 1.6, p. 14: *Anatomy & Physiology: The Unity and Form of Function*, (3rd edition), by K. S. Saladin, 2004, Dubuque, IA; The McGraw-Hill Companies, Inc. Reprinted with permission. Figure 1.7, p. 14: *Anatomy & Physiology: The Unity and Form of Function*, (3rd edition), by K. S. Saladin, 2004, Dubuque, IA; The McGraw-Hill Companies, Inc. Reprinted with permission. Figure 1.8, p. 15: *Anatomy & Physiology: The Unity and Form of Function*, (3rd edition), by K. S. Saladin, 2004, Dubuque, IA; The McGraw-Hill Companies, Inc. Reprinted with permission. Figure 1.9, p. 15: *Anatomy & Physiology: The Unity and Form of Function*, (3rd edition), by K. S. Saladin, 2004, Dubuque, IA; The McGraw-Hill Companies, Inc. Reprinted with permission. Figure 1.10, p. 16: *Anatomy & Physiology: The Unity and Form of Function*, (3rd edition), by K. S. Saladin, 2004, Dubuque, IA; The McGraw-Hill Companies, Inc. Reprinted with permission. Figure 1.11, p. 17: *Anatomy & Physiology: The Unity and Form of Function*, (3rd edition), by K. S. Saladin, 2004, Dubuque, IA; The McGraw-Hill Companies, Inc. Reprinted with permission. Figure 1.12, p. 17: *Anatomy & Physiology: The Unity and Form of Function*, (3rd edition), by K. S. Saladin, 2004, Dubuque, IA; The McGraw-Hill Companies, Inc. Reprinted with permission. Figure 1.13, p. 19: *Human Anatomy*, by K. S. Saladin, 2005, Dubuque, IA: The McGraw-Hill Companies, Inc. Reprinted with permission. Figure 1.14, p. 20: Essentials of Medical Language, by D. M. Allan and K. Lockyer, 2009, Dubuque, IA: The McGraw-Hill Companies, Inc. Reprinted with permission. Figure 1.15, p. 21: *Anatomy & Physiology: The Unity and Form of Function*, (3rd edition), by K. S. Saladin, 2004, Dubuque, IA; The McGraw-Hill Companies, Inc. Reprinted with permission. Figure 1.16, p. 21: *Anatomy & Physiology: The Unity and Form of Function*, (3rd edition), by K. S. Saladin, 2004, Dubuque, IA; The McGraw-Hill Companies, Inc. Reprinted with permission. Figure 1.17, p. 21: *Hole's Human Anatomy & Physiology*, (10th edition), by D. Shier, J. Butler, and R. Lewis, 2004, Dubuque, IA: The McGraw-Hill Companies, Inc. Reprinted with permission. Figure 1.18, p. 22: *Anatomy & Physiology: The Unity and Form of Function*, (3rd edition), by K. S. Saladin, 2004, Dubuque, IA; The McGraw-Hill Companies, Inc. Reprinted with permission. Figure 1.19, p. 24: *Anatomy & Physiology: The Unity and Form of Function*, (3rd edition), by K. S. Saladin, 2004, Dubuque, IA; The McGraw-Hill Companies, Inc. Reprinted with permission. Figure 1.20, p. 24: *Anatomy & Physiology: The Unity and Form of Function*, (3rd edition), by K. S. Saladin, 2004, Dubuque, IA; The McGraw-Hill Companies, Inc. Reprinted with permission. Figure 1.21, p. 25: *Hole's Human Anatomy & Physiology*, (10th edition), by D. Shier, J. Butler, and R. Lewis, 2004, Dubuque, IA: The McGraw-Hill Companies, Inc. Reprinted with permission.

CHAPTER 3

Figure 3.8, p. 66: *Anatomy & Physiology: The Unity and Form of Function*, (3rd edition), by K. S. Saladin, 2004, Dubuque, IA; The McGraw-Hill Companies, Inc. Reprinted with permission. Figure 3.9, p. 69: *Anatomy & Physiology*, (7th edition), by R. R. Seeley, T. D. Stephens, and P. Tate, 2006, Dubuque, IA: The McGraw-Hill Companies, Inc. Reprinted with permission.

CHAPTER 4

Figure 4.1, p. 83: *Anatomy & Physiology: The Unity and Form of Function*, (3rd edition), by K. S. Saladin, 2004, Dubuque, IA; The McGraw-Hill Companies, Inc. Reprinted with permission. Figure 4.6, p. 96: *Hole's Human Anatomy & Physiology*, (10th edition), by D. Shier, J. Butler, and R. Lewis, 2004, Dubuque, IA: The McGraw-Hill Companies, Inc. Reprinted with permission.

CHAPTER 10

Figure 10.1, p. 263: *Human Anatomy*, by K. S. Saladin, 2005, Dubuque, IA: The McGraw-Hill Companies, Inc. Reprinted with permission. Figure 10.2, p. 266: *Anatomy & Physiology*, (7th edition), by R. R. Seeley, T. D. Stephens, and P. Tate, 2006, Dubuque, IA: The McGraw-Hill Companies, Inc. Reprinted with permission. Figure 10.3, p. 270: *Human Anatomy*, by K. S. Saladin, 2005, Dubuque, IA: The McGraw-Hill Companies, Inc. Reprinted with permission.

CHAPTER 12

Figure 12.1.1, p. 317: *Hole's Human Anatomy & Physiology*, (10th edition), by D. Shier, J. Butler, and R. Lewis, 2004, Dubuque, IA: The McGraw-Hill Companies, Inc. Reprinted with permission. Figure 12.2.2, p. 330: *Human Anatomy*, by K. S. Saladin, 2005, Dubuque, IA: The McGraw-Hill Companies, Inc. Reprinted with permission. Figure 12.2.3, p. 334: *Hole's Human Anatomy & Physiology*, (10th edition), by D. Shier, J. Butler, and R. Lewis, 2004, Dubuque, IA: The McGraw-Hill Companies, Inc. Reprinted with permission. Figure 12.2.4, p. 334: *Human Anatomy*, by K. S. Saladin, 2005, Dubuque, IA: The McGraw-Hill Companies, Inc. Reprinted with permission. Figure 12.2.5, p. 335: *Human Anatomy*, by K. S. Saladin, 2005, Dubuque, IA: The McGraw-Hill Companies, Inc. Reprinted with permission. Figure 12.6.1, p. 401: *Anatomy & Physiology: The Unity and Form of Function*, (3rd edition), by K. S. Saladin, 2004, Dubuque, IA; The McGraw-Hill Companies, Inc. Reprinted with permission. Figure 12.6.2, p. 402: *Human Anatomy*, by K. S. Saladin, 2005, Dubuque, IA: The McGraw-Hill Companies, Inc. Reprinted with permission. Figure 12.6.3, p. 406: *Human Anatomy*, by M. McKinley and V. D. O'Loughlin, 2006, Dubuque, IA: The McGraw-Hill Companies, Inc. Reprinted with permission. Figure 12.6.4, p. 411: *Human Anatomy*, by M. McKinley and V. D. O'Loughlin, 2006, Dubuque, IA: The McGraw-Hill Companies, Inc. Reprinted with permission. Figure 12.6.5, p. 414: *Anatomy & Physiology: The Unity and Form of Function*, (3rd edition), by K. S. Saladin, 2004, Dubuque, IA; The McGraw-Hill Companies, Inc. Reprinted with permission.

CHAPTER 13

P 13.2, p. 432: *Anatomy & Physiology: The Unity and Form of Function*, (3rd edition), by K. S. Saladin, 2004, Dubuque, IA; The McGraw-Hill Companies, Inc. Reprinted with permission.

PHOTO CREDITS

PART OPENERS

1: © OJO Images/Getty RF; 2: © Janis Christie/Digital Images/Getty RF; 3: © Susan Vogel/UpperCut Images/Getty RF

ICONS

2: © Fuse/Getty RF; 3: © Peter Dazeley/The Image Bank/Getty; 4: © PhotoAlto/Ale Ventura/Getty RF; 5 © Ken Whitmore/Stone/Getty; 6: © Daniel Allan/Photographer's Choice/Getty RF; 7: © Dana Neely/The Image Bank/Getty; 8: © Jose Luis Pelaez Inc/Blend Images/Getty RF; 9: © Chris Ryan/OJO Images/Getty RF; 10: © Fuse/Getty RF; 11: © Fuse/Getty RF; 12.1 © MedicImage/Universal Images Group/Collection Mix: Subjects/Getty; 12.2 © Carol & Mike Werner/Visuals Unlimited; 12.3 © Kurt Drubbel/The Agency Collection/Getty RF; 12.4 © Artpartner-Images/Photographer's Choice/Getty; 12.5 © Stockbyte/Getty RF; 12.6 © CMSP/Custom Medical Stock Photo/Getty; 13: © Justin Gollmer/Brand X Pictures/Getty RF; 14: © Ingram Publishing RF; 15: © Chris Ryan/Getty RF; 16: © Susan Vogel/UpperCut Images/Getty RF

CHAPTER 1

Opener: © Patrick Lane/Blend Images/Getty RF; 1.1: © The McGraw-Hill Companies/JW Ramsey, photographer; 1.2b: © The McGraw-Hill Companies/Joe DeGrandis, photographer; 1.22: © Bill Longcore/Photo Researchers; p. 26: © Corbis RF

CHAPTER 2

Opener: © Fuse/Getty RF; p. 38: © Image Source/Getty RF; p. 42: © Dynamic Graphics Group/IT Stock Free/Alamy RF; p. 45: © Jose Luis Pelaez/Getty RF; p. 47: © Jose Luis Pelaez/Blend Images LLC RF

CHAPTER 3

Opener: © Peter Dazeley/The Image Bank/Getty; 3.1: © Dr. Jack M. Bostrack/Visuals Unlimited; 3.2: © CNRI/SPL/Photo Researchers; 3.3: © Dennis Kunkel Microscopy, Inc./Phototake Inc/Alamy; 3.4 & 3.5: © BioPhoto Associates/Photo Researchers; 3.6: © James Stevenson/Photo Researchers; p. 61: © Image Source/ Veer RF; 3.7: © Meckes/Ottawa/Photo Researchers; p. 66: © Eyewire/Getty RF; p. 68: © McGraw-Hill Companies/Scott Thompson, Photographer; p. 71: © moodboard/Corbis RF; 3.10: © CNRI/SPL/Photo Researchers; 3.11: © Dr. Joseph William/Phototake; 3.12: © SIU Biomedical/Photo Researchers

CHAPTER 4

Opener: © PhotoAlto/Ale Ventura/Getty RF; p. 86: © Jose Luis Pelaez/Blend Images LLC RF; 4.2: © The McGraw-Hill Companies, Inc./Dennis Strete, photographer; 4.3: © Medical-on-line/Alamy; 4.4: © Scott Camazine/Alamy; 4.5a: © Sheila Terry/Photo Researchers; 4.5b: © Dr. P. Marazzi/SPL/Photo Researchers; 4.5c: © John Radcliffe Hospital/Photo Researchers; p. 97: © Ingram Publishing RF; p. 98: © PhotoDisc/Getty RF; p. 99: © Blend Images/Jupiterimages RF; p. 101: © Image Source/Getty RF

CHAPTER 5

Opener: © Ken Whitmore/Stone/Getty; p. 112: © Monashee Frantz/OJO Images/Getty RF; p. 115: © Image Source/Veer RF; p. 119: © Image Source/Getty RF

CHAPTER 6

Opener: © Daniel Allan/Photographer's Choice/Getty RF; p. 132: © Digital Vision RF; p. 135: © Andersen Ross/Blend Images LLC RF; p. 138 & 139: © Ingram Publishing RF; p. 142: © DreamPictures/Pam Ostrow/Blend Images LLC RF

CHAPTER 7

Opener: © Dana Neely/The Image Bank/Getty; p. 155: © Jose Luis Pelaez/Blend Images LLC RF; p. 158: © Andersen Ross/Blend Images LLC RF; p. 162: © Image Source/Getty RF; p. 165: © Rob Melnychuk/Getty RF; p. 169: © Image Source/Getty RF; p. 173: © Erproductions Ltd/Blend Images LLC RF; p. 176: © Ingram Publishing RF

CHAPTER 8

Opener: © Jose Luis Pelaez Inc/Blend Images/Getty RF; p. 189: © Charles Gullung/zefa/Corbis RF; p. 193: © Image Source/Veer RF; p. 196 & 198: © The McGraw-Hill Companies, Inc./Rick Brady, photographer; p. 200: David Fischer/Getty RF

CHAPTER 9

Opener: © Chris Ryan/OJO Images/Getty RF; p. 211: © JGI/Blend Images LLC RF; p. 214: © Erproductions Ltd/Getty RF; p. 217: © Plush Studios/Blend Images LLC RF; p. 219: © Jose Luis Pelaez Inc/Blend Images LLC RF; p. 224: © Ingram Publishing RF; p. 225: © Erproductions Ltd/Blend Images LLC RF; p. 230: © Jose Luis Pelaez Inc/Blend Images LLC RF; p. 233: © Blend Images/Getty RF; p. 234: © Thinkstock Images/Getty RF; p. 236: © Jose Luis Pelaez Inc/Blend Images LLC RF; p. 239: © Ingram Publishing RF

CHAPTER 10

Opener: © Fuse/Getty RF; p. 256: © Ingram Publishing RF; p. 258: © Ingram Publishing RF; p. 274: © Erproductions Ltd/Blend Images/Getty RF

CHAPTER 11

Opener: © Greg Pease/The Image Bank/Getty; p. 286: © Erproductions Ltd/Blend Images LLC RF; 11.1: © SPL/Photo Researchers; 11.2: © ISM/Phototake; 11.3 © Wellcome Trust Images; 11.4: © Zephyr/Photo Researchers; 11.5a: © ALIX/Phanie/Photo Researchers; 11.5b: © TSI/Getty Images

CHAPTER 12

Opener: © Lois Schlowsky/Workbook Stock/Getty

CHAPTER 12.1

Opener 12.1: © MedicImage/Universal Images Group/Collection Mix: Subjects/Getty; p. 311: © Ragnar Schmuck/Getty RF; p. 315: © Andersen Ross/Blend Images LLC RF

CHAPTER 12.2

Opener: © Carol & Mike Werner/Visuals Unlimited; 12.2.1: © SIU/Visuals Unlimited

CHAPTER 12.3

Opener: © Kurt Drubbel/The Agency Collection/Getty RF; 12.3.1: © Phototake; p. 348: © Jim Wehtje/Getty RF; p. 351: © McGraw-Hill Companies, Inc; p. 355: © Creatas/PunchStock RF; p. 359: © McGraw-Hill Companies, Inc

CHAPTER 12.4

Opener: © Artpartner-Images/Photographer's Choice/Getty; p. 371: © McGraw-Hill Companies, Inc; p. 375: © Indeed/Digital Vision/Getty RF

CHAPTER 12.5

Opener: © Stockbyte/Getty RF; p. 385: © McGraw-Hill Companies, Inc; 12.5.1: © McGraw-Hill Companies, Inc; 12.5.2: © Science Photo Library RF/Getty RF; p. 393: © PunchStock/BananaStock RF

CHAPTER 12.6

Opener: © CMSP/Custom Medical Stock Photo/Getty

CHAPTER 13

Opener: © Justin Gollmer/Brand X Pictures/Getty RF; **p. 425:** © Vol. 40/PhotoDisc/Getty RF; **13.1:** © Oliver Meckes/Photo Researchers; **13.2:** © Kathy Park Talaro

CHAPTER 14

Opener: © Ingram Publishing RF; **p. 443:** © Ingram Publishing/SuperStock RF; **p. 445:** © Image Source/Getty RF; **p. 448:** © Science Photo Library RF/Getty RF; **p. 454:** © Don Farrall/Getty RF; **p. 457:** © Jose Luis Pelaez/Blend Images LLC RF; **p. 461:** © Blend Images/Getty RF

CHAPTER 15

Opener: © Chris Ryan/Getty RF; **p. 475:** © Blend Images/Masterfile RF; **p. 476:** © Ingram Publishing RF; **p. 480:** © Image Source/Getty RF; **p. 481:** © Thinkstock/Jupiterimages RF; **p. 485:** © Corbis Images/Getty RF

CHAPTER 16

Opener: © Janis Christie/Digital Vision/Getty Images/RF; **p. 499:** © Photoalto/Odilon Dimier/Getty RF; **p. 505:** © Jon Feingersh/Blend Images LLC RF

connect plus+

Enhance your learning by completing these exercises and more at mcgrawhillconnect.com!

CREDITS   C-3

A

A-codes (HCPCS), 474–476
  for contrast material (imaging agents), 290, 476
  for medical supplies, 476
  for transportation, 474–475
A-V malformations, repair of, 404
Abbreviation(s), 8
  to avoid in medical documentation, 8, 8t
  common medical, A1–A5
  in CPT manual, 140
  in HCPCS, 486, 487t
  in ICD-9-CM, 43
  in ICD-10-CM, 118
Abdomen, CPT coding for, 375–376. *See also specific procedures and disorders*
  anesthesia, 377, 378t
    lower abdomen, 267
    upper abdomen, 266–267
    vascular procedures, 359, 360t
  CT scan with CT of pelvis, 290
Abdominal aortic aneurysm, repair of, 352–353
Abdominal wall tumor, excision of, 333
Abnormality, congenital. *See* Congenital abnormality
Abortion
  CPT coding of, 394
  ICD-9-CM coding of, 86–87
Abscess, 310. *See also* Incision and drainage
Abuse, ICD-9-CM coding of, 102
Accessory sinuses, CPT coding for, 344
Achilles tendon, 8f
Acronyms, 8, 8t. *See also* Abbreviation(s)
Acupuncture, 459
Acute exacerbation, 71
Acute illness, with chronic condition, 120
Acute myocardial infarction (AMI)
  HCPCS coding of, 479
  ICD-9-CM coding of, 69, 70
ADA (American Dental Association), 471, 477
Add-on codes (CPT), 134, 261, 442
  location in manual, 138
  for microsurgery with microscope, 370, 415
  for prolonged E/M services, 193, 195, 201, 223, 224t, 229–231
  qualifying circumstances (anesthesia), 261, 262, 460
Adenoids, 369
Adjacent tissue transfer, 315
Administration, 444. *See also* Drug administration
Admit/discharge codes, 213, 217, 217t, 218
  for newborn, 238
  for observation, 214

Adrenal glands, 401
Adrenalectomy, 401, 416t
Adult, body surface area percentages in, 95, 96f, 273
Advanced life support (ALS), 474
Adverse drug effects, ICD-9-CM coding of, 96
  E-codes, 99–102
  Table of Drugs and Chemicals, 38, 102, 102t–103t
Aftercare, 99
  ICD-9-CM coding of
    fractures, 90, 99
    V-codes, 99
Age conflict edits (ICD-9-CM), 44
Aged person, anesthesia in, 261
Agency for Healthcare Research and Quality (AHRQ), 140
Alcohol and drug abuse treatment services, HCPCS coding of, 479
Allergen immunotherapy, CPT coding of, 455
Allergy tests, CPT coding of, 454–455
Allografts, 316
Allotransplantation, 384
Alphabetic Index (ICD-10-CM), 116, 118, 119, 120
Alphabetic Index of Diseases (Volume 2, ICD-9-CM), 37–39
  Alphabetic Index to External Causes of Injury and Poisoning (E-codes), 38, 101, 102
  Hypertension Table, 38, 67, 68t
  Neoplasm Table, 38, 57–58, 58t, 59
  sample entries, 39f
  sections, 38
  Table of Drugs and Chemicals, 38, 102, 102t–103t
  use of, 38, 39
Alphabetic Index to External Causes of Injury and Poisoning (E-codes) (ICD-9-CM), 38, 101, 102
Alphabetical Clinical Topics Listing (CPT), 137, 139, 141
ALS (advanced life support), 474
AMA. *See* American Medical Association
Ambulance modifiers (HCPCS), 177, 475
Ambulance services
  BLS *vs.* ALS, 474
  HCPCS coding of, 177, 474–475
  interfacility, critical care of infant in, E/M coding of, 239
Ambulance trip, 177
American Dental Association (ADA), 471, 477
American Medical Association (AMA), 131, 139, 471
  and Category II codes (CPT), 140, 141
  and Category III codes (CPT), 143

American Society of Anesthesiologists, 262
Analgesia, 260
Anatomic pathology, 431
  CPT coding of, 431–432
Anatomical modifiers (HCPCS), 167, 176–177, 287, 485
Anatomical planes, 9–10, 10f, 285
  coronal (frontal), 9, 285, 288
  sagittal, 9–10, 285, 288
  transverse, 10, 285, 288
Anatomical positions
  with directional terms, 10f
  for radiology services, 285–288
Anatomy, 2, 9–24
Anemia
  ICD-9-CM coding of, 63, 74
  sickle cell, 63f
Anesthesia, 255
  CPT coding of, 255–275
    by anatomical part, 256, 263–272, 338t
    burn procedures, 273–274
    for cardiovascular system, 359, 360
    for digestive system, 370, 377, 378t
    for esophagus, 377
    for female genital/reproductive system, 395
    for integumentary system, 321
    local anesthesia, 172
    for male genital/reproductive system, 395
    modifiers in, 172, 173, 175, 259–260, 262
    multiple procedures, 257
    for musculoskeletal system, 337–338, 338t
    not-otherwise-specified/-classified procedures, 257, 275
    obstetrical procedures/delivery, 274, 275, 395
    physical status before anesthesia, 175, 259–260
    qualifying circumstances add-on codes, 261, 262, 460
    radiological procedures, 273
    for respiratory system, 359, 360t
    secondary aspects of, 259–261
    surgeon-provided anesthesia, 172
    time calculation and reporting in, 258–259, 262
    units of value in, 257–262
    for urinary system, 395
    for vascular system, 359, 360t
  general, 172, 255
  introduction to, 255
  local, 172, 255
  MAC, 255, 260, 461
  nerve block (*See* Nerve block)
  provider types, 255

Anesthesia—Cont.
  regional, 172, 255
  termination of procedure after
      induction of, 173
  time taken for, 258–259
  types of, 255
Anesthesia assistant, 255
Anesthesia provider(s)
  procedure code modifiers for, 172, 175, 260
  types of, 255
Anesthesia units, 262
  base, 257, 262
  in physical modifiers (P1–P6), 259–260, 262
  in qualifying circumstances add-on codes,
      261, 262
  time, 258–259, 262
  total, calculation of, 262
Anesthesiologist, 172, 255, 260
Aneurysm, 352
  intracranial, 404
  repair of, 352–353, 404
Angiography, 139, 452–453
Angioplasty, 349, 351*f*
  CPT coding of
      cardiovascular vessels, 349
      with coronary artery repair, 349
      with coronary artery stent placement, 450
      with endovascular repairs, 351, 353
      transluminal, 353, 354
Ankle joint, CPT coding for, 270, 336
Annual assessment, of nursing facility patient,
      226, 226*t*
Anoscopy, 374
Antepartum care (prenatal care)
  alcohol and drug abuse assessment as, HCPCS
      coding of, 479
  components of, 392
  CPT coding of, 393, 394
  ICD-9-CM coding of, 84
  prenatal testing, 393
  prenatal visit, 84, 392
Anterior chamber, CPT coding for, 412
Anterior cranial fossa, 403
Anterior sclera, CPT coding for, 412
Anterior segment, CPT coding for, 412
Anterior vertebral structure, CPT coding for,
      331, 332
Anteroposterior (AP) projection, 285, 287
Anticoagulant management, E/M coding of,
      231–232, 236
Antineoplastic therapy. *See also specific types*
  ICD-9-CM coding of, 59, 63
Anus, CPT coding for, 353, 373–374
Aorta, 355. *See also* Great vessels
  catheterization of, 355
  descending thoracic, repair of, 351
  transluminal angioplasty of, 354
Aortic aneurysm, repair of, 352–353
Aortic valve, 348
AP projection, 285, 287
Aphakia, 449
Appendectomy, 372
Appendices
  of CPT manual, 137–140
      A, 138
      B, 138
      C, 138

D, 138, 166, 442
E, 138, 166, 442
F, 138–139, 172
G, 139, 461
H, 139
I, 139, 175
J, 139, 456
K, 139
L, 139, 355
M, 139
N, 140
  of HCPCS manual, 486
  of ICD-9-CM manual, Volume 1, 41
Appendix (body part), 372
Arm, CPT coding for, 271–272, 334
Arrhythmia, induction of, 454
Arterial bypass graft
  coronary (*See* Coronary artery bypass graft)
  extracranial–intracranial, 404
  venous grafts in, 354
Arterial catheterization, CPT coding of, 355–356
  coronary, 356, 452–453
Arterial grafting, CPT coding of
  in aneurysm repair, 353
  in CABG, 349, 350
Arterial studies, 454
Arterial system, 13, 15, 15*f*, 355. *See also*
      Vascular system
  coronary, 67*f*
  location in CPT manual, 139
Arterial-venous grafting, in CABG, 349
Arteriovenous fistula, repair of, 353
Arteriovenous malformations, repair of, 404
Arthrodesis, 332
  CPT coding of, 327
      of spine, 332–333
Arthroscopy, CPT coding of, 336–337
Aspiration, CPT coding of
  joints, 329
  spinal structures, 406–407
Assistant surgeon, 169–170
Assisted living facility care services, CPT coding of
  E/M, 227, 227*t*, 232, 233, 236
  nonphysician services, 461
Asthma, 71
Asymptomatic HIV, 55
Atherectomy
  cardiovascular vessel, 450
  transluminal, 353, 354
Audiologic function tests
  CPT coding for, 449
  HCPCS coding of, 485
Auditory system, CPT coding of, 413–415
  anesthesia, 416*t*
  code subsections/list, 413
  evaluation, 449
  external ear, 414
  inner ear, 415
  middle ear, 414–415
  rehabilitation, 449
  temporal bone, with middle fossa
      approach, 415
Auditory system devices, 449, 485
Autograft, 315
Autonomic nerve block, 409, 410
Autonomic nervous system, CPT coding
  for, 409, 410

Autopsy, 431–432
Avian influenza, 71, 72
Axilla, anesthesia in, 270–271

B

B-codes (HCPCS), 476, 477
Back. *See also* Spine
  soft tissue of, 331
Backbench work, 375
Bacteria
  examples, 56*f*
  laboratory tests for, 430–431
Bariatric surgery, 371
Bartholin's gland, 390
Base units (anesthesia), 257, 262
Basic life support (BLS), 474
BCBSA. *See* Blue Cross and Blue Shield
      Association
Behavior change assessment/intervention
  by nonphysicians, 456
  by physicians, 235
Benign neoplasms (tumors/lesions)
  CPT coding of, skin and subcutaneous, 311,
      317–318
  ICD-9-CM coding of, 57, 58
Bilateral procedure, 164
  CPT modifier 50 for, 164–165, 287
Biliary tract, 375
Biofeedback training, 447
Biologic agents, administration of, 458
Biopsy, CPT coding of
  breast, 319
  fine needle aspiration, 309
  percutaneous needle, 309
  skin lesions, 310
Birthing room attendance. *See* Delivery room
      attendance
Biventricular pacing, 348
Bladder, 384
  CPT coding for, 385–387
Blood. *See also* Hemic system
  components of, 24
  deoxygenated, 15
  ICD-9-CM coding for, 63
  medical terms related to, 24*t*
  oxygenated, 15
Blood cell count, 429
Blood cells
  red, 24, 24*f*, 429
  white, 24, 429
Blood clot, 430*f*
Blood clot removal. *See* Thrombectomy
Blood coagulation tests, 429
Blood component tests, 429
Blood count, complete (CBC), 429
Blood-forming organs. *See* Hemic system
Blood transfusion services, 430, 482
Blood vessels. *See* Arterial system; Vascular
      system; Venous system; *specific vessels*
BLS (basic life support), 474
Blue background (ICD-9-CM), 44
Blue Cross and Blue Shield Association (BCBSA),
      471, 483
Body surface area (BSA), 95
  total (TBSA), 273, 274, 316

Bone graft, 329
    in spine, 332–333
Bone marrow, preparation of, 358
Bone studies, 292
Brachial plexus, 406*f*
Brachytherapy, 287, 293, 450
Brackets
    in ICD-9-CM, 43
    in ICD-10-CM, 118
Brain, 21, 21*f*
    CPT coding for, 402–405, 416*t*
Brain tumors. *See* Intracranial lesions
Breast, CPT coding for, 319–320
Bronchi, CPT coding for, 345–346
Bronchitis, 71
Bronchodilator, 454
Bronchoscopy, 345
Bundling rules, 442
Burns
    calculation of body surface involvement,
        273–274
        Rule of Nines for, 95, 96*f*, 316, 317*f*
    classification of, 95, 95*f*
    CPT coding of, 273–274, 316
    ICD-9-CM coding of, 95–96, 96*f*
    late effects of, 96
Burr hole, 403
Bypass graft, CPT coding of
    coronary artery (*See* Coronary artery
        bypass graft)
    extracranial–intracranial, 404
    venous grafts in, 354

C

C-codes (HCPCS), 477
CABG. *See* Coronary artery bypass graft
Callus, 310
Cancer. *See* Neoplasms
Capillaries, 13
Carcinoma in situ, 58
Cardiac anomaly, congenital
    catheterization for, 453
    repair of, 350–351
Cardiac assist procedures, 351
Cardiac catheterization, CPT coding of, 356,
    452–453, 454
Cardiac device. *See also* Cardioverter-defibrillator;
    Pacemaker
    evaluation and programming of, 451–452
    insertion/replacement of, 347–348
Cardiac mapping, 454
Cardiac recording device, CPT coding of
    evaluation and programming, 451, 452
    insertion/removal of, 348
Cardiac rhythm assessment, 451
Cardiac tumor, excision of, 347
Cardiac valve(s), 348
    artificial, 359*t*
    repair/replacement of, 348, 359
Cardiography, 451
Cardiopulmonary bypass, 348, 360
Cardiotomy, 348
Cardiovascular monitoring services, 451
Cardiovascular system, 13–15
    components of, 13, 344

CPT coding for, 344, 347–351, 450–454
    anesthesia, 359, 360
    anomaly repair for heart or great vessels,
        350–351
    CABG, 349–350, 360, 453
    cardiac assist, 351
    cardiac catheterization, 356, 452–453, 454
    cardiac device, 347–348, 451–452
    cardiac recording device, 348, 451, 452
    cardiac valve repair/replacement, 348, 359
    cardiography, 451
    coronary artery repair, 349
    coronary artery stent placement, 450, 451
    echocardiography, 452
    electrophysiologic operative procedures, 348
    electrophysiological studies, 454
    heart and heart-lung transplant, 351
    infant anesthesia, 359, 360
    monitoring, 451
    noninvasive physiologic, 454
    nonsurgical procedures/medical services,
        450–454
    pacemaker, 347–348, 451
    pericardiocentesis, 347
    therapeutic, 450
    transmyocardial revascularization, 347
    tumor excision, 347
    vascular procedures, 450, 451
    wound repair for heart or great vessels, 348
ICD-9-CM coding for, 67–70
medical terms related to, 14*t*
Cardioverter-defibrillator
    evaluation and programming of, 451
    insertion/removal of, 347, 348, 359
Care coordination, E/M coding of, 195, 201
Care plan oversight services, E/M coding of,
    232–233, 236
Caridiotomy, 348
Carotid body, CPT coding for, 401
Case management services, E/M coding of,
    231–232
    anticoagulant management, 231–232, 236
    medical team conference, 232
Cast, 336
    application of, 336, 337
    supplies, 483
Category I codes (CPT), 131
    and Category III codes, 143
    code sections, 132–133
    format of, 473
    update of, 132
Category II codes (CPT), 131, 132,
    140–142, 473
Category III codes (CPT), 131, 132, 143, 473
Catheterization
    cardiac, 356, 452–453, 454
    spinal, 407
    vascular, 354–356
CBC (complete blood count), 429
CCI (Correct Coding Initiative), 166, 167
CCI tables, 167–168, 167*t*
CDT (Current Dental Terminology) codes,
    471, 477
Centers for Disease Control and Prevention
    (CDC), and ICD-10-CM, 112, 113
Centers for Medicaid and Medicare
    Services (CMS)

    and CDT codes, 471, 477
    and CPT codes, 140, 155
    and HCPCS codes, 471, 478–479, 480, 481
    and ICD-9-CM, 37
    and ICD-10-CM, 112, 113
Central nervous system, 21
Central venous access, CPT coding of,
    354–355, 356
Central venous access device, 354
Cerebral infarction, ICD-9-CM coding of, 69
Cerebrospinal fluid leak repairs, 408
Cerebrospinal fluid shunt, 405, 408
Cerebrovascular accident (CVA), 69
Cerebrovascular disease, 69
Certified registered nurse anesthetists (CRNAs),
    172, 255, 260
Cervical spine, 331
Cervix (cervix uteri), 391
Cesarean section/delivery, 393
    CPT coding of, 274, 394
    ICD-9-CM coding of, 85
    repeat, 394
    vaginal delivery after (VBAC), 394
Chemistry and Toxicology Tests (HCPCS),
    482, 483
Chemistry test, CPT coding of, 429
Chemotherapy
    CPT coding of, 458
    HCPCS coding of, 480, 483
    ICD-9-CM coding of, 59
Chest wall anesthesia, 264–265
Chief complaint, 191
Child. *See also* Infant; Newborn
    body surface area percentages in, 95
    critical care of, 224, 239–240
    E/M coding for, 238–240
    immunization in, 444–445
    skin replacement surgery in, 315, 316
Child abuse, 102
Childbirth, stages of, 83*f. See also* Delivery
Chiropractic manipulation, 460
Chronic illness, 63, 71, 120
Chronic kidney disease (CKD), 74
    ICD-9-CM coding of, 74
        with anemia, 63, 74
        hypertensive, 67, 68
        with hypertensive heart disease, 67, 69
        staging, 74
Chronic obstructive pulmonary disease
    (COPD), 71
Circulatory assistance, 351
Circulatory system. *See also* Cardiovascular
    system; Vascular system
    arterial, 13, 15, 15*f*, 355
    coronary arterial, 67*f*
    ICD-9-CM coding of, 67–70
    venous, 13, 15, 15*f*
Cirrhosis of liver, 73*f*
CKD. *See* Chronic kidney disease
Cleft lip and palate, 91*f*
    repair of, 367, 368
Clinical brachytherapy, 287, 293
Clinical immunology services, 454–455
Clinical pathology consultation, 428
Clinical topics listing (CPT), 137, 139, 141
Clinical treatment planning (radiation
    oncology), 292

Enhance your learning by completing these exercises
and more at mcgrawhillconnect.com!

INDEX   I-3

Closed fracture, 328, 329
Closed treatment, 327
CMS. *See* Centers for Medicaid and Medicare Services
Co-surgeon, 170
  in spinal procedures, 332, 407–408
Coagulation tests, 429
Code(s)
  add-on (CPT), 134, 138, 261, 442
  default, 119
  diagnosis, 25
  medical, purposes of, 2
  parent, 134
"Code first underlying disease" instruction (ICD-9-CM), 43
Code sections (CPT), 132–133
Coding systems, 37. *See also* CPT; HCPCS; ICD-9-CM; ICD-10-CM
  purposes of, 2
Cognitive function tests, 456
Colonoscopy, 372, 373, 479
Colons
  in ICD-9-CM, 43
  in ICD-10-CM, 118
Color designations (ICD-9-CM), 44
Colposcopy, 391
Column 1 codes (CCI), 167
Column 2 codes (CCI), 167
Combination code(s), 45
  ICD-9-CM, 45
  ICD-10-CM, 120
Combination coding (CPT), 286
  for psychotherapy and E/M services, 446, 447
  for radiology services
    abdominal and pelvic CT, 290
    with non-radiology services, 286, 309
    nuclear medicine therapy, 294
    radiologic guidance, 292, 309, 351
Combining form, 2
Combining vowel, 2, 5
Comminuted fracture, 328, 329
Communicable diseases. *See* Infectious diseases
Complete mastectomy, 319
Complete blood count (CBC), 429
Complex wound repair, 313, 314
Complications of care
  CPT modifier for second procedure related to, 159–160
  ICD-9-CM coding of, 97
Component coding. *See* Combination coding
Compound fracture. *See* Open fracture
Comprehensive history, 196, 196t
Comprehensive physical examination, 198
Comprehensive service, 233
Computed tomography (CT), 285. *See also* Radiology services
  CPT coding of
    abdominal-pelvic scans, 290
    diagnostic, 289
    as radiologic guidance, 291
    unlisted procedures, 287
  and tomogram, 285, 288
Concurrent care, 191
Congenital, definition of, 452
Congenital abnormality
  cardiac (*See* Cardiac anomaly, congenital)
  diagnosis coding for

ICD-9-CM, 91, 92
ICD-10-CM, 116
  repair of, CPT coding of
    in heart or great vessels, 350–351
    in penis, 388
Conjunctiva, CPT coding of, 413
Connective tissue diseases, 89–90
Conscious sedation. *See* Moderate sedation
Consultation, 190, 219
  E/M
    inpatient, 215, 220–221, 221t
    office/outpatient, 219–220, 220t
    and transfer of care, 191, 219
  medical
    clinical pathology, 428
    surgical pathology, 433
Contact lenses, 449, 485
Contrast material (imaging agents), 289
  CPT coding of, 286, 289, 290
  HCPCS coding of, 290, 476, 483
Contributory components (E/M codes), 195
Corn, 310
Cornea, CPT coding of, 412
Corneal transplant (keratoplasty), 412
Coronal (frontal) plane, 9, 285, 288
Coronary arterial circulation, 67f
Coronary artery anomaly, repair of, 349
Coronary artery bypass graft (CABG), CPT coding of, 349–350
  anesthesia, 359, 360
  Doppler probe placement, 453
Coronary artery catheterization, 356, 452–453
Coronary artery stent, placement of, 450, 451
Coronary vessels, CPT coding of, 450, 451
Corpus uteri, CPT coding of, 391
Correct Coding Initiative (CCI), 166, 167–168, 167t
Corticotropin-releasing hormone (CRH) stimulation panel, 427
Counseling, 191–192. *See also* Psychotherapy
  E/M coding of, 191–192, 201, 233, 235
  genetic, CPT coding of, 456
CPT (Current Procedural Terminology), 131–143
CPT code(s), 37, 131–143
  Category I, 131, 132–133, 473
  Category II, 131, 132, 139, 140–142
  Category III, 131, 132, 143
  code sections/categories, 132–133
  code series format, 133
  conventions of, 133–136
  deleted, 138, 139, 143
  and HCPCS codes, 471, 472, 478–479
  and HCPCS modifiers, 176–178, 260
  maintenance and update of, 131, 132, 138
  new, 138
  out-of-sequence, 140, 143
  renumbered, 139
  revised, 138
  "separate procedure" designation in, 135–136, 307, 442, 443
CPT code modifiers. *See* CPT modifiers
CPT Editorial Panel, 131, 132
CPT manual, 131–143
  appendices, 137–140
  conventions, 133–136
  index, 136–137, 143

inside front and back covers, 140
introductory pages, 140
maintenance and update of, 131, 132, 138
parenthetical notes, 134–135, 309
CPT modifiers, 135, 152–178
  for additional providers, 169–170
  for anesthesia services, 259–260, 262
    physical status (P1–P6), 175, 259–260, 262
    by surgeon (modifier 47), 172
  for assistant surgeon (modifiers 80–82), 169
  Category II, 141–142
  and CCI tables, 167–168, 167t
  for co-surgeons (modifier 62), 170, 332, 407–408
  for components of procedure by different providers, 161–164
    professional components (modifier 26), 162, 163, 286, 287, 289
    surgical procedure components (modifiers 54–56), 163, 164
    technical components (modifier TC), 162, 163, 287
  for decision to perform surgery (modifier 57), 157–158
  for E/M services, 155–158
  function of, 152–154
  for genetic tests, 139, 175–176
  for global period services, 154–161, 163, 164
  HCPCS modifiers as (*See* HCPCS modifiers)
  informational, 152
  for laboratory test, repeated (modifier 91), 159, 168, 431
  list of, 153t–154t
  location in CPT manual, 138, 139, 140
  for mandatory services (modifier 32), 174
  for multiple procedures on same day, 164–168
    bilateral (modifier 50), 164–165, 287
    distinct/"separate" (modifier 59), 166–168, 286, 288, 307
    multiple (modifier 51), 165–166
    repeated laboratory tests (modifier 91), 159, 168, 431
  payment, 152, 154
  performance measurement exclusion, 141–142
  physical status (P1–P6), 175, 259–260
  for postoperative E/M (modifier 24), 155–156
  for procedure terminated after induction of anesthesia (modifier 53), 173–174
  for procedures involving more/less work than is typical, 171–174
    less than typical (modifier 52), 173
    more than typical (modifier 22), 171–172
  professional components (modifier 26), 162, 163, 286, 287, 289
  for radiology services, 162, 163, 287–288
  for repeated procedure
    by different provider (modifier 77), 158–159
    laboratory test (modifier 91), 159, 168, 431
    by same provider (modifier 76), 158–159, 288
  for separate procedures/services
    distinct/"separate" (modifier 59), 166–168, 286, 288, 307
    E/M (modifier 25), 156–157, 195, 233
  for staged procedures (modifier 58), 158

for surgery on infant less than 4kg (modifier 63), 138–139, 172
for surgical procedure components (modifiers 54–56), 163, 164
for surgical team (modifier 66), 170
technical components (modifier TC), 162, 163, 287
for unplanned second procedure (modifier 78), 159–160
for unrelated procedure by same surgeon (modifier 79), 160–161
use of, 152–154
Cranial fossa, 403
Craniectomy, 403
Cranioplasty, 403
Craniotomy, 403
CRH stimulation panel, 427
Critical care services, 190
    E/M coding of, 223–224
        in emergency department, 222
        for infant, 224, 239–240
        time codes, 223, 224, 224t
Critical care transport. See also Emergency transportation
    of infant, E/M coding of, 239
Critical care units, 223
Critical illness/injury, 223
CRNA. See Certified registered nurse anesthetists
CT. See Computed tomography
Current Dental Terminology (CDT) codes, 471, 477
Current Procedural Terminology (CPT), Fourth Edition, code set. See CPT manual
Custodial care services. See Domiciliary care services
Cutting, of skin lesions, 310
CVA (cerebrovascular accident), 69
Cystocele, 391
Cystoscopy, 386
Cystourethroscopy, 386–387
Cytogenetic studies, 432
Cytopathologic tests, 432

D

D-codes (HCPCS), 477
Debridement, 310
    CPT coding of
        burn tissue, 273–274, 316
        skin, 310
Decision to perform surgery, 157–158
Decubitus position, 285, 286
    left lateral, 285, 288
    right lateral, 285, 287
Decubitus ulcer. See Pressure (decubitus) ulcer
Default code, 119
Deleted codes (CPT), 138, 139, 143
Delivery
    by cesarean section, 85, 274, 393, 394
    CPT coding of, 393–394
        anesthesia, 274, 275, 395
        cesarean section, 274, 394
        newborn E/M services, 238, 239
        vaginal/normal, 393, 394
        VBAC, 394
    ICD-9-CM coding of

after attempted abortion, 87
    cesarean section, 85
    complication after, 86
    HIV infection in, 85
    newborn condition resulting from, 92
    V-codes, 84, 85, 99
    vaginal/normal, 86
outside hospital, visit after, 86
service components, 393
stages of, 83f
vaginal/normal, 86, 393, 394
VBAC, 394
Delivery room attendance, for newborn E/M, 238, 239
Delivery room resuscitation, of newborn, 238, 239
Dental procedures, 368, 471, 477
Dentoalveolar procedures, 368
Deoxygenated blood, 15
Dermatological procedures, 459
Descending thoracic aorta, repair of, 351
Detailed history, 196, 196t
Detailed physical examination, 198
Diabetes mellitus
    complications of, 60–61
    gestational, 85
    ICD-9-CM coding of, 60–62
        in CKD, 74
        in pregnancy, 85, 86
        secondary, 61–62
        type I, 60, 61
        type II, 60, 61
Diagnosis
    first-listed, 39, 46–47
    principal, 39
    secondary, 39
Diagnosis codes and coding, 25
    combination, 45
    ICD-9-CM (See ICD-9-CM)
    ICD-10-CM (See ICD-10-CM)
    purposes of, 37
"Diagnosis to procedure code" relationships, 37
Diagnostic and Statistical Manual of Mental Disorders, Fourth Edition (DSM-IV), 64
Diagnostic evaluation services. See Evaluation and management (E/M) services
Diagnostic interview, psychiatric, 446
Diagnostic radiology, 285. See also Radiology services
    CPT coding of, 289–290
    HCPCS coding of, 483
    imaging techniques in, 285
    professional component of, 162, 163, 286, 287, 289
    technical component of, 162, 163, 287
Diagnostic thoracoscopy, 346
Diagnostic ultrasound, 290–291
Dialysis. See also Hemodialysis
    CPT coding of, 447–448
Diapers, 484
Digestive system, 18, 18f
    CPT coding of, 367–377
        anesthesia, 377, 378t
        code list, 367
        gastrointestinal tract, 369–374
        mouth and throat, 367–369
        organs, 374–376

ICD-9-CM coding of, 72–73
    medical terms related to, 19t
Digital x-ray system, 285
Directional terms, 10f, 10t
Disability examination, 237
Discharge services, E/M coding of
    for hospital inpatients, 218
        newborn, 238
        in observation, 214, 218
        on same day as admission, 213, 217, 217t, 218, 238
    for nursing facilities, 226
Disease-oriented panels. See Organ/disease-oriented panels
Distinct procedure(s), 166
    and CPT modifier 59, 166–168, 286, 288, 307
DME. See Durable medical equipment
Domiciliary care services, CPT coding of
    E/M, 227, 227t, 232, 233, 236
    nonphysician services, 461
Doppler probe placement, coronary, 453
Dosimetry, 293
Drainage. See Incision and drainage
Drug(s)
    CPT coding of
        immune globulins, 444
        vaccines/toxoids, 444–445
    HCPCS coding of
        non-oral (J-codes), 480
        oral (Q-codes), 483
        temporary national (S-codes), 483
    in Table of Drugs (HCPCS), 472, 480, 486
    in Table of Drugs and Chemicals (ICD-9-CM), 38, 39, 102, 102t–103t
Drug abuse treatment services, HCPCS coding of, 479
Drug administration, 444
    CPT coding of, 457, 458
        chemotherapy and biologic agents, 458
        immune globulins, 444
        vaccines/toxoids, 444–445
    HCPCS coding of
        non-oral (J-codes), 480
        oral (Q-codes), 483
Drug poisoning. See also Adverse drug effects
    ICD-9-CM coding of, 96
Drug test, 426
    CPT coding of, 426, 427
    qualitative vs. quantitative, 426
DSM-IV, 64
Durable medical equipment (DME), 476
    HCPCS coding of
        E-codes, 476, 477–478
        K-codes, 480
        modifiers, 178, 486
Dysrhythmias, supraventricular, excision procedures for, 348

E

E-codes (HCPCS), 476, 477–478
E-codes (ICD-9-CM), 38, 40, 100–102
    categories of, 101
    hierarchy of, 101–102
    and ICD-10-CM, 116
    for toxic effects, 96

E/M codes. *See* Evaluation and management codes

Ear, 414*f*. *See also* Auditory system

Eardrum, 414–415

ECG (electrocardiogram), 451, 454

ECG monitors, external, 451

Echocardiography, 452

ECMO. *See* Extracorporeal membrane oxygenation

Ectopic pregnancy, 83
  CPT coding for, 393

EEG (electroencephalogram), 455

Elbow, CPT coding for, 271–272, 334

Electrocardiogram (ECG), 451, 454

Electrode implants. *See* Neurostimulators

Electroencephalogram (EEG), 455

Electrophysiologic procedures, cardiac
  intracardiac studies, 454
  operative, 348

Embolectomy, 352

Emergency department services, E/M coding of, 222–223
  code requirements, 222*t*
  critical care, 222, 240
  observation, 222
  remote medical direction, 222–223, 239

Emergency medical services. *See also* Emergency transportation
  remote direction of, 222–223, 239

Emergency surgery, anesthesia in, 261

Emergency transportation, 474
  E/M coding of, critical care of infant in, 239
  HCPCS coding of
    A-codes, 474–475
    ambulance modifiers, 177, 475

Emerging services/procedures, CPT coding for, 131, 143

Emerging technology, CPT coding for, 131, 143

Encounter, 46
  subsequent, 115

End-stage renal disease (ESRD), 74
  hemodialysis in (*See* Hemodialysis)
  ICD-9-CM coding of, 68, 69, 74

Endocrine system, 23, 401
  CPT coding of, 401, 402, 455
  ICD-9-CM coding of, 57–59
  major glands, 23*f*, 401
  medical terms related to, 23*t*

Endometrium, CPT coding for, 391

Endoscopic retrograde cholangiopancreatography (ERCP), 370, 375

Endoscopy, 344, 367
  bilateral, 346
  CPT coding of, 357
    of anus, 374
    of biliary tract, 370, 375
    of bladder, 386
    of bronchi, 345
    for cardiac tissue excision, 348
    of cervix (cervix uteri), 391
    of esophagus, 370
    of intracranial, 405
    of joint, 336–337
    of kidney, 385
    of large intestine, 373
    of larynx, 345
    of lungs and pleura, 346
    of sinus, 344–345

    of small intestine, 372
    stomal, 372
    of upper gastrointestinal tract, 370
  diagnostic included in surgical, 344–345, 346

Endovascular procedures, CPT coding of
  intracranial and extracranial, 404
  repairs
    aortic aneurysm, 352–353
    descending thoracic aorta, 351
    iliac aneurysm, 353
  revascularization, 357

Enteral and parenteral therapy, 476
  supplies for, HCPCS coding of, 476, 477

Enterocele, 391

Enterolysis, 371

Enterostomy, 372

Enucleation of eyeball, 411

Epididymus, 389

Epidural, definition of, 407

Epidural adhesions, CPT coding for, 406

Epidural catheterization, CPT coding of, 407

Epidural injections, CPT coding of, 406, 409

Epispadius, 388

Eponyms, 7–8

Equipment, medical
  durable (*See* Durable medical equipment)
  single-use (*See* Medical supplies)

Equipment modifiers (HCPCS), 178, 486

ERCP (endoscopic retrograde cholangiopancreatography), 370, 375

Escharotomy, 316
  CPT coding of, 316

Esophagus, CPT coding for, 369–370, 377

ESRD. *See* End-stage renal disease

Established patient, 191
  E/M coding for, 191, 200
    domiciliary care services, 227, 227*t*
    home services, 228, 229*t*
    outpatient services, 212–213, 212*t*
    preventive medicine services, 234, 235*t*

Ethmoid sinus, 346

Etiology, 40
  ICD-10-CM coding of, 119

Evaluation and management (E/M) codes (CPT), 189
  categories of, 189
  and Category II codes, 140
  components of, 195–199
  format of, 190
  key components of, 195–199, 201*t*, 211*t*
  location in CPT manual, 132
  time components of, 193–194, 195
  for unlisted services, 194, 211

Evaluation and management (E/M) services
  categories and subcategories, 189–190, 195
  CPT coding of, 189–201, 211–240
    (*See also specific services and categories of service*)
    consultation services, 219–221
    critical care services, 223–224
    domiciliary care services, 227
    emergency department services, 222–223, 239
    guidance in CPT manual, 138
    home services, 228
    hospital services, 190, 213–218

    introduction to, 189, 211
    key components in, 195–199, 201*t*, 211*t*
    key terms and concepts, 191–194
    level-of-service selection, 195, 200–201
    medical decision making in, 193, 195, 198–199, 199*t*, 201*t*, 211*t*
    modifiers in, global period, 155–158
    with neurological tests, 455
    nursing facility services, 220–221, 225–226, 232, 233
    outpatient services, 190, 211–213
    overview, 189–201
    patient histories, 192–193, 196–197, 196*t*, 201*t*, 211*t*
    physical examinations, 193, 195, 197–198, 201*t*, 211*t*
    and place of service, 189–190, 195
    with psychotherapy services, 446, 447
    special reports in, 194
    special services, 236–237
    time component in, 193–194, 195, 201
    unlisted services, 194, 211
  definition of, 189
  level of, 195, 200–201
  place of, 189–190, 195
  special reports in, 194
  time components of, 193–194, 195
  unlisted, 194, 211

Evisceration of eyeball, 411

Evocative/suppression testing, CPT coding of, 427

Excision(s), 311. *See also* Tumor/lesion excision; *specific anatomic parts and procedures*
  in breast, 319
  of cardiac tissue, 348
  in endocrine system, 401
  in female genital/reproductive system, 390, 391
  in gastrointestinal tract, 371, 373, 374
  in musculoskeletal system, 327, 328, 330, 331, 333, 334, 335
  of nerves, 410
  in respiratory system, 344, 345, 346
  in skin and subcutaneous tissue, 311, 312, 315, 319
  for vascular grafts, 354

"Excludes" instruction (ICD-9-CM), 43, 60

"Excludes1" instruction (ICD-10-CM), 119

"Excludes2" instruction (ICD-10-CM), 119

Expanded problem-focused history, 196, 196*t*

Expanded problem-focused physical examination, 198

External ear, 414, 414*f*

External fixation, 328

Extracorporeal circulation
  CPT coding of, 351, 357
  ICD-10-PCS coding of, 121

Extracorporeal membrane oxygenation (ECMO), 357

Extracranial arteries, 404

Extracranial nerves, CPT coding of, 409–410

Extracranial–intracranial arterial bypass, 404

Eye procedures. *See* Ocular structure procedures

Eyeball
  anatomy of, 411*f*
  CPT coding for, 411–412
  removal, 411

F

Facial bones, 330, 330*f*
Fallopian tubes. *See* Oviducts
Family history, 192, 197
Fascia, 328, 329
FDA approval, products yet to receive, 139, 445
Female genital/reproductive system
   CPT coding for, 390–392, 395
   medical terms related to, 21*t*
Female urinary system, 384
Femoral artery, revascularization of, 357
Femoral fracture, 26
Femur, CPT coding for, 336
Fertilization, in vitro, 391*f*, 392, 433
Fetal conditions, affecting mother, 85
Fetal invasive services, 393
Fibula, 336
Fine needle aspiration, 309
Fingers, 334
First-listed diagnosis/condition, 39
   in ICD-9-CM, 39, 46–47
   in ICD-10-CM, 119
First-order vessels, 355
Fistula, 372
Fistula repair, CPT coding of
   anus, 373–374
   arteriovenous, 353
   intestinal-bladder, 386
   intestine, 372
   rectum, 373
   vagina, 391
Fixation, types of, 327, 328
Flags (in GEM sets), 112–113
Flank, CPT coding of, 331
Flaps, tissue, 316
Floor of mouth, 368
Fluid therapy, 457, 458
Fluoroscopy, 285, 286
   diagnostic, 289
   as guidance, 291–292, 309
      in endovascular repairs, 351, 353
      in nerve block, 309, 409
      in spinal injection, drainage, and aspiration, 406
   sample, 289*f*
   unlisted procedures, 287
Follow-up care, CPT coding of, 306
   modifiers in, 154–161
Foot, CPT coding of, 270, 336
Forearm, CPT coding of, 272, 334
Forms, combining, 2
Fracture
   comminuted, 328, 329
   ICD-9-CM coding of
      aftercare, 90, 95, 99
      E-codes, 101
      femoral, 26
      pathological, 89–90
      traumatic, 95
   ICD-10-CM coding of, 26
   open, 328, 329
   terminology, 327–328
   traumatic, 95
   types of, 327–328

Fracture treatments, 327–328
   closed, 327
   CPT coding of, 327, 334
      arm and hand, 334
      cast/splint application, 336, 337
      debridement, 310
      head, 330
      pelvis and hip joint, 335, 336
      strapping, 336
      thorax, 331
   open, 327
   terminology, 327–328
   types of, 327–328
Frontal bone, 403
Frontal (coronal) plane, 9, 285, 288
Frontal sinus, 344

G

G-codes (HCPCS), 292, 478–479
Gastric intubation, 371
Gastroenterology study measurement techniques, 448–449
Gastrointestinal endoscopy, 370
Gastrointestinal system, 367
Gastrointestinal tract, 367
   CPT coding of, 369–374
      anesthesia, 370, 377, 378*t*
      anus, 373–374
      appendix, 372, 373
      esophagus, 369–370, 377
      intestines, 371–372, 386
      Meckel's diverticulum, 372
      mesentery, 372
      rectum, 373
      stomach, 371
GEMs (General Equivalence Mappings), 112–113
General anesthesia, 172, 255
General Equivalence Mappings (GEMs), 112–113
General guidelines, for ICD-10-CM, 118, 119–120
Genetic counseling, 456
Genetic modifiers (CPT), 139, 175–176
Genetic tests, CPT coding of, 432
   modifiers in, 139, 175–176
Genitourinary system. *See also* Female genital/reproductive system; Male genital/reproductive system; Urinary system
   ICD-9-CM coding for, 74
Gestational diabetes, 85
GFR (glomerular filtration rate), 74
Gland(s), 9
Glasses, 449, 485
Global codes, 287, 290
Global period, 154, 155, 157, 160
Global period modifiers, 154–161, 163
   for decision to perform surgery (modifier 57), 157–158
   for E/M services, 155–158
   for postoperative E/M services (modifier 24), 155–156
   for repeated procedure
      by different provider (modifier 77), 158–159

      by same provider (modifier 76), 158–159, 288
   for second unplanned procedure (modifier 78), 159–160
   for separate E/M services on same day (modifier 25), 156–157, 195, 233
   for staged procedures (modifier 58), 158
   for surgical procedure components (modifiers 54–56), 163, 164
   for unrelated procedure by same surgeon (modifier 79), 160–161
Glomerular filtration rate (GFR), 74
Glucose monitoring, 455
Gonads, 401
Graft harvesting procedures, CPT coding of, 329
   in CABG, 349, 350
   of veins, 349, 350, 354
Great vessels. *See also* Aorta; Pulmonary artery; Vena cava
   CPT coding of, 347
      anomaly repair, 350–351
      wound repair, 348
Group counseling, 235
Guidelines, for CPT Category I code sections, 132–133
Gums, CPT coding for, 368

H

H-codes (HCPCS), 479
HAC indicator, 44–45
Hand, CPT coding for, 272, 334
HCPCS (Healthcare Common Procedure Coding System), 37, 471–486
HCPCS codes, Level I, 471
HCPCS codes, Level II, 471
   availability of, 471
   categories of, 473, 473*t*
      A-codes, 290, 474–476
      B-codes, 476, 477
      C-codes, 477
      D-codes, 477
      E-codes, 477–478
      G-codes, 292, 478–479
      H-codes, 479
      J-codes, 480
      K-codes, 480, 481
      L-codes, 481
      M-codes, 482
      P-codes, 482, 483
      Q-codes, 483
      R-codes, 483
      S-codes, 483–484
      T-codes, 484
      V-codes, 485
   and CPT coding, 471, 472, 478–479
   definition of, 471
   format of, 473
   functions of, 471
   modifiers (*See* HCPCS modifiers)
   for radiology services, 287, 290, 292, 486
   units of service in, 472
   update and maintenance of, 471
   uses of, 472
HCPCS codes, Level III ("local codes"), 484

Enhance your learning by completing these exercises and more at mcgrawhillconnect.com!

INDEX   I-7

HCPCS manual
  abbreviations used in, 486, 487t
  appendices, 486
  and dental procedures, 471, 477
  index, 472
  instructions and guidance in, 473
  modifier list (Appendix 2), 486
  Table of Drugs (Appendix 1), 472, 480, 486
  tabular list of services, 472
HCPCS modifiers, 152, 176–178, 471, 485–486
  ambulance, 177, 475
  anatomical, 167, 176–177, 287, 485
  anesthesia provider, 260
  equipment/DME, 178, 486
  location in manual, 486
  in MAC, 260
  pick-up/destination, 475
  place of service, 486
  radiology, 486
  in radiology services, 287, 486
Head. See also Brain; Skull
  CPT coding for, 263–264, 330, 404
Health Insurance Association of American (HIAA), 471, 483
Health screening, 99
Hearing devices, 449, 485
Hearing services, 485
Hearing tests, 449, 485
Heart, 13, 14f. See also Cardiovascular system; Coronary artery
  CPT coding of, 347–351, 450–454
    anesthesia, 359, 360
    anomaly repair, 350–351
    cardiac assist, 351
    cardiac device evaluation and programming, 451–452
    cardiac device insertion/replacement, 347–348
    cardiography, 451
    catheterization, 356, 452–453, 454
    electrophysiologic operative, 348
    intracardiac electrophysiological studies, 454
    monitoring, 451
    noninvasive physiologic, 454
    recording device, 348, 451, 452
    therapeutic, 450
    transmyocardial revascularization, 347
    transplant, 351
    tumor excision, 347
    valve repair/replacement, 348, 359
    wound repair, 348
Heart anomaly
  catheterization for, 453
  repair of, 350–351
Heart disease, ICD-9-CM coding of, 67–70
Heart failure, ICD-9-CM coding of, 68
Heart-lung transplant, 351
Heart transplant, 351
Heart tumor, excision of, 347
Heart wound, repair of, 348
Hematologic tests, 429
Hematoma, 310
Hemic system, 24
  components of, 24, 344
  CPT coding of, 358, 429

ICD-9-CM coding of, 63
  medical terms related to, 24t
Hemodialysis, CPT coding of, 357, 447–448
Hemorrhoids, 373, 374
Hepatobiliary system, 370, 374–375
Hernia repairs, CPT coding of, 376
  vaginal, 391
HIAA. See Health Insurance Association of American
Hidradenitis, 311
Hip joint surgery, 334–335
History of disease, 99, 100
History of present illness (HPI), 192, 196
HIV (human immunodeficiency virus) infections, ICD-9-CM coding of, 55, 85
HIV-positive patient, 55
HIV-related condition, 55
Hodgkin's disease, staging laparotomy for, 375–376
Holter monitors, 451
Home health agency patient, 232, 236
Home services
  E/M coding of, 228
    care plan oversight, 232, 233, 236
    established patient, 228, 229t
    new patient, 228, 228t
    by nonphysician, 461
  HCPCS coding of, 483, 484
  by nonphysicians, 461
Hospice
  care plan services, 232–233, 236
  pre-election evaluation, 479
Hospital(s), and ICD-9-CM for procedure coding, 41–42
Hospital-acquired condition (HAC) indicator, 44–45
Hospital discharge, E/M coding of, 213, 218
  for newborn, 238
  from observation, 214, 218
  on same day as admission, 213, 217, 217t, 218, 238
Hospital inpatient services, 215
  E/M coding of, 215–217
    admission/discharge on same day, 213, 217, 217t, 218, 238
    consultation, 215, 220–221, 221t
    discharge (See Hospital discharge)
    initial care, 215–216, 216t
    for newborn, infant, and young child, 238–240
    prolonged services, 229–230, 231
    subsequent care, 216–217, 216t
Hospital observation services, 213
  E/M coding of, 213–215
    admission/discharge on same day, 213, 217, 217t
    discharge, 214, 218
    in emergency department, 222
    initial care, 214, 214t
    subsequent care, 214–215, 215t
  ICD-9-CM coding of, 47
Hospital outpatient services, HCPCS coding of, 477
Hospital outpatient supplies, HCPCS coding of, 477
Hospital services. See also specific types
  E/M coding of, 213–218

consultation, 215, 220–221, 221t
  time components in, 194
  HCPCS coding for, outpatient, 477
HPI. See History of present illness
Human immunodeficiency virus (HIV) infections. See HIV infections
Human papillomavirus (HPV), 445
Humerus, CPT coding of, 334
Hydration, intravenous, 457, 458
Hyperkeratotic lesions, paring/cutting of, 310
Hypertension
  ICD-9-CM coding of, 67–69
  portal, 357
  secondary, 67, 69
Hypertension table, 39
Hypertension Table (ICD-9-CM), 38, 67, 68t
Hyperthermia (therapeutic), 293
Hypospadius, 388
Hypotension, 261
Hypothermia, total body, 261
Hysterectomy, 391, 394
Hysteroscopy, 391

I

ICD-9-CM, 25, 37–47
  conventions, 42–45
  diagnosis code categories/chapters, 40t
  diagnosis code structure, 40, 44, 47, 114
  diagnosis coding with, 37, 38–47 (See also specific diseases and disease categories)
  ICD-10-CM compared to, 25–26, 112, 114, 116
  ICD-10-PCS compared to, 121
  introduction to, 37–47
  maintenance and updates of, 37
  medical terminology in, 9
  procedure coding with, 37, 38, 41–42, 121
  shortcomings of, 112
  structure of manual, 37–38
  Volume 1: Tabular List of Diseases, 37–41, 40t
  Volume 2: Alphabetic Index of Diseases, 37–39
    Alphabetic Index to External Causes of Injury and Poisoning (E-codes), 38, 101, 102
    Hypertension Table, 38, 67, 68t
    Neoplasm Table, 38, 57–58, 58t, 59
    sample entries, 39f
    Table of Drugs and Chemicals, 38, 102, 102t–103t
  Volume 3: Tabular List and Alphabetic List for Procedure Codes, 37, 38, 41–42
ICD-9-CM Maintenance Committee, 37
ICD-10, 112
ICD-10-CM, 25, 112–120
  Alphabetic Index, 116, 118, 119, 120
  benefits of, 112, 114, 120
  code structure, 114–116
  coding guidelines, 118, 119–120
  conventions, 118–119
  expandability/capacity of, 112
  ICD-9-CM compared to, 25–26, 112, 114, 116
  medical terminology in, 9, 25–26

structure of, 116, 117t
Tabular List of Codes, 116, 118, 119
transition to, 25, 37, 112–113
ICD-10-PCS, 120
code structure, 120–121
introduction to, 120–121
sections, 120–121
transition to, 37, 112
ICS-9. *See* ICD-9-CM
Iliac aneurysm, repair of, 353
Iliac artery, revascularization of, 357
Ill-defined conditions, ICD-9-CM coding of, 93
Imaging agents. *See* Contrast material
Imaging techniques, 285. *See also* Diagnostic radiology
Immune globulins, 444
Immunization administration. *See* Vaccination
Immunologic tests, 430, 454–455
Immunotherapy, 59, 455
"In diseases classified elsewhere" designation, 119
In vitro fertilization, 391f
CPT coding of, 392, 433
In vivo laboratory procedures, 433
Incision(s). *See also specific anatomic parts and procedures*
in breast, 319
in digestive system, 374, 375
in gastrointestinal tract, 369, 371, 373–374
in male genital/reproductive system, 388
in musculoskeletal system, 327, 329, 333, 334, 335
in respiratory system, 344, 346
in urinary system, 384, 385
Incision and drainage, 310
CPT coding of
of appendix, 372
of rectum, 373
of skin and subcutaneous tissue, 310
of spinal structures, 406–407
of subfascial soft tissue, 329
"Includes" instruction, 119
in ICD-9-CM, 43
in ICD-10-CM, 119
Index
of CPT manual, 136–137, 143
of HCPCS manual, 472
Index to External Causes. *See* Alphabetic Index to External Causes of Injury and Poisoning
Infant. *See also* Child; Newborn
anal repair in, 374
anesthesia in, 261, 359, 360
body surface area percentages in, 95
critical care of, 224, 239–240
E/M coding for, 224, 239–240
heart/great vessel anomaly repair in, 350
less than 4 kg, surgery in, 138–139, 172
Infectious diseases
CPT coding of, laboratory tests, 430–431
exposure to, 99
ICD-9-CM coding of, 55–56, 99
Influenza, 71, 72
Informational modifiers (CPT), 152
Infratentorial, definition of, 404
Infusion drugs, 480

Infusions
CPT coding of, 457–458, 461
enteral and parenteral, 476, 477
HCPCS coding for, 476, 477
Inhalation drugs, 480
Initial nursing facility care, 225, 226t
Initial treatment, 115
Injections
CPT coding of
in cardiac catheterization, 453
of chemotherapy and biologic agents, 458
of drugs, 457, 458
general, 329
for nerve block, 409–410
for nerve destruction, 410
in spinal structures, 406–407, 409, 410
trigger point, 329, 409
HCPCS coding of, of drugs, 480
vascular, 354–356
Injuries. *See also* Burns
ICD-9-CM coding of, 94–95, 100–102
Inner ear, 414f, 415
Inpatient services. *See* Hospital inpatient services
Instructional notations, in ICD-9-CM, 43
Insulin therapy, 61, 62
Integumentary system, 11. *See also* Burns; Skin and subcutaneous lesions
CPT coding for, 309–321
anesthesia, 321
biopsies, 310
breast procedures, 319–320
debridement, 310
excision of lesions, 311, 312
incision and drainage, 310
lesion destruction, 317–318
nail procedures, 311–312
paring or cutting, 310
pilonidal cyst excision, 312
shaving of lesions, 311
skin repair, 315–316
skin tag removal, 310–311
superficial procedures, 309–312
wound repair (closure), 313–314
ICD-9-CM coding for, 88, 89
medical terms related to, 11t
Intensive care, for newborn, 240
Interfacility transport, critical care of infant in, 239
Intermediate care facility services. *See* Nursing facility services
Intermediate wound repair, 313, 314
Internal fixation, 327, 328f
Internal mammary artery, 349
International Classification of Diseases, 9th Revision, Clinical Modification. *See* ICD-9-CM
Intersex surgery, 389
Interventional radiology, 285
Intestinal fistula
creation, 372
repair, 372, 386
Intestinal graft, 370
Intestinal perforation, repair of, 372
Intestines, 371–372
Intracardiac electrophysiological studies, 454
Intracranial aneurysm, repair of, 404

Intracranial arteries, 404
Intracranial lesions, 404–405
Intracranial neurostimulator implant, 405
Intracranial procedures, CPT coding of, 402–405, 416t
Intracranial–extracranial arterial bypass, 404
Intraservice time (E/M), 194
Intrathecal, definition of, 407
Intrathecal catheterization, 407
Intravascular ultrasound, 357
Italic brackets (ICD-9-CM), 43

J

J-codes (HCPCS), 480
Joint Commission, The (TJC), 8, 140
Joint studies, 292

K

K-codes (HCPCS), 480, 481
Keratoplasty, 412
Key components (E/M codes), 195–199, 201t, 211t
Kidney, CPT coding for, 384–385
Kidney disease. *See* Chronic kidney disease; End-stage renal disease
Kidney transplant
CPT coding of, 384, 401
ICD-9-CM coding of CKD after, 74, 97
Knee joint, 270f
CPT coding of, 269, 336

L

L-codes (HCPCS), 481
Labor anesthesia, 274, 275, 395
Laboratory, 423
Laboratory panels, 423–426, 424t–425t
Laboratory services. *See also* Pathology services
for reproductive procedures, 433
Laboratory tests
CPT coding of, 423–433
chemistry tests, 429
clinical pathology consultation, 428
coagulation tests, 429
code list/sections, 423
cytopathologic, 432
drug testing, 426, 427
evocative/suppression testing, 427
hematologic tests, 429
immunologic tests, 429
in vivo, 433
microbiological tests, 430–431
organ/disease-oriented panels, 423–426, 424t–425t
repeated, and modifier 91, 159, 168, 431
therapeutic drug assay, 427
transfusion services, 429
urinalysis, 428
HCPCS coding of, 482, 483
Laceration repair. *See also* Wound repair (closure)
of eyeball, 412
Laminectomy, 332, 408

Laparoscopy, 367
    CPT coding of
        of abdomen, 376
        bladder, 386
        of esophagus, 370
        of intestine, 372
        of kidney, 385
        of liver, 375
        of rectum, 373
        of stomach, 370, 371
        uterus (corpus uteri), 391
Laparotomy, 375–376
Large intestine, 371
Laryngoscopy, 345
Larynx, 345f
    CPT coding for, 345, 359
Laterality, in ICD-10-CM coding, 114–115
Left lateral decubitus position, 285, 288
Leg, CPT coding for, 269, 270, 335
Lens, 412
Lesions. See Neoplasms; Skin and subcutaneous
    lesions; Tumor/lesion destruction; Tumor/
    lesion excision
Level I HCPCS codes, 471
Level II HCPCS codes. See HCPCS codes,
    Level II
Level III HCPCS codes ("local codes"), 484
Life insurance examination, 237
Ligation, 357
Lip, 367
    cleft, 91f, 368
Liver, 374–375
    cirrhosis of, 73f
Liver transplant, 374
Local anesthesia, 172, 255
Local codes (HCPCS), 484
Long-term care facility services. See Nursing
    facility services
Loop recorder, 451, 452. See also Cardiac record-
    ing device
Lower extremities. See also Ankle joint; Foot; Leg
    CPT coding for, 270, 335, 357
Lumbar spine, 331
Lung, CPT coding for, 346, 359
Lung transplant, 346
Lymphadenectomy, 358, 390
Lymphatic system, 16, 16f, 16t, 344, 358

M

M-codes (HCPCS), 482
MAC. See Monitored anesthesia care
Magnetic resonance imaging (MRI), 285. See also
    Radiology services
    composite projection in, 285
    CPT coding of
        diagnostic, 289
        as radiologic guidance, 291
        unlisted procedures, 287
    sample, 289f
Main terms, 136
Male genital/reproductive system, 20f
    CPT coding of, 387–389, 395
    medical terms related to, 21t
Male urinary system, 384
Malignant neoplasms (tumors/lesions)

CPT coding of
    musculoskeletal, 328
    skin and subcutaneous, 311, 318, 458
examples, 59f
ICD-9-CM coding of, 57–58, 59
in Neoplasm Table (ICD-9-CM), excerpt, 58t
primary, 57, 59
secondary, 57, 59
types of, 57–58
Mammography, 292, 292f
    CPT coding of, 292
        HCPCS modifiers in, 292, 486
Mandatory services, and CPT modifier
    32, 174
Manifestation(s), 119
Manipulation, 328, 460
Mapping, cardiac, 454
Mastectomy, 319–320
Mastoidectomy, 414
Maternal care and delivery, 392–394. See also
    Antepartum care; Delivery; Pregnancy
    CPT coding for
        anesthesia, 395
        code sections/list, 393
        service components, 392, 393
Maxillary sinus, 346
Measles, mumps, and rubella (MMR), 445
Meatus, 387
Meckel's diverticulum, 372
Mediastinum, 344
Medicaid, 131, 471, 475, 483, 484
Medical decision making, 193, 195
    complexity level of, 193, 198–199,
        199t, 201t
    types of, 198, 199t
Medical direction, remote, 222–223, 239
Medical equipment and supplies. See also
    Drug(s)
    CPT coding of, physician-provided, 443
    HCPCS coding of, 471
        casts and splints (Q-codes), 483
        contrast material (imaging agents), 290,
            476, 483
        durable medical equipment (DME), 178,
            476, 477–478, 480, 486
        enteral and parental therapy (B-codes),
            476, 477
        miscellaneous (Q-codes), 483
        orthotics and prosthetics (L-codes), 481
        outpatient hospital (C-codes), 477
        single-use (A-codes), 476
        temporary national (S-codes), 483
        vision and hearing (V-codes), 485
        wheelchairs (K-codes), 480, 481
Medical nutrition management, 459
Medical services
    CPT coding of, 441–462
        acupuncture, 459
        add-on codes in, 442
        allergy and clinical immunologic, 454–455
        cardiovascular, 450–454
        central nervous system assessments/
            tests, 456
        chiropractic manipulation, 460
        code sections/list, 441
        dermatological procedures, special, 459
        endocrinologic, 455

        gastroenterologic, 448
        general guidelines for, 442–443
        genetic counseling, 456
        health and behavior assessment/
            intervention, 456
        hemodialysis, 357, 447–448
        home health procedures/services, 461
        immune globulins, 444
        immunization administration, 444–445
        injections and infusions, 457–458
        medication therapy management, 461
        moderate sedation, 460–461
        for multiple procedures/services, 442
        neurologic and neuromuscular, 455–456
        non-face-to-face nonphysician
            services, 460
        nutrition management, 459
        ophthalmologic, 448–449
        osteopathic manipulation, 460
        otorhinolaryngologic, 449
        patient self-management education and
            training, 460
        photodynamic therapy, 458
        physical medicine and rehabilitation, 459
        psychiatric, 446–447
        pulmonary, 454
        qualifying circumstances for
            anesthesia, 460
        for "separate" procedures/services,
            442, 443
        special services, procedures, and
            reports, 460
        supplies provided by physician, 443
        unlisted services/procedures, 443
        vaccines/toxoids, 132, 139, 445
        vascular studies, noninvasive, 454
    E/M (See Evaluation and management (E/M)
        services)
    HCPCS coding of
        alcohol and drug abuse treatment
            (H-codes), 479
        miscellaneous services, 478–479, 482, 483
        outpatient hospital (C-codes), 477
        pathology and laboratory (P-codes),
            482, 483
        physician performance (G-codes), 479
        temporary national codes (S-codes),
            483–484
        transportation (A-codes), 474–475
        vision, hearing, speech-language
            (V-codes), 485
Medical supplies (single-use). See also Medical
    equipment and supplies
    HCPCS coding of, 178, 476, 484, 486
Medical team conference, 232
Medical terminology, 2–24
    abbreviations and acronyms, 8, 8t
    anatomical, 9–24
    eponyms, 7–8
    in ICD-10-CM, 9, 25–26
    in ICD-10-PCS, 9
    physiological, 9–24
    word elements, 2–6, 7
Medicare
    anesthesia coding for, 255, 258, 259,
        260, 262
    and assistant surgeons, 169

and Category I codes (CPT), 131
and Category II codes (CPT), 131, 140
and consultation coding, 221
and CPT modifier 57, 157
and HCPCS codes, 471, 472
  B-codes, 476
  C-codes, 477
  G-codes, 478–479
  K-codes, 480, 481
  M-codes, 482
  P-codes, 483
  S-codes, 483, 484
  T-codes, 484
and intraoperative and postoperative care by
    different physicians, 164
and multiple procedures, 164, 422
and radiology services, 290, 292
Medicare Physician Fee Schedule, 155, 163, 165,
    166, 169
Medication therapy management, 461
Medicine services. *See* Medical services
Meninges, 402
Meningocele, 408
Mental disorders. *See also* Psychiatric services
  HCPCS coding of, 479
  ICD-9-CM coding of, 64
Metabolic diseases, 57–59
Methicillin-resistant *Staphylococcus aureus*
    (MRSA), 56
Microbiological tests, 430–431
Microbiology, 430
Microscopy, 428, 432, 433, 482
Microsurgical techniques add-on code,
    370, 415
Middle cranial fossa, 403, 415
Middle ear, 414–415, 414f
Mitral valve, 348
MMR (measles, mumps, and rubella), 445
Moderate sedation, CPT coding of, 139, 172,
    370, 460–461
Modified radical mastectomy, 319
Modifier(s), 135
  CPT (*See* CPT modifiers)
  HCPCS (*See* HCPCS modifiers)
  ICD-10-CM, 118
Modifier 22, 171–172
Modifier 24, 155–156
Modifier 25, 156–157, 195
Modifier 26, 162, 163, 286, 287, 289
Modifier 32, 174
Modifier 47, 172
Modifier 50, 164–165, 287
Modifier 51, 165–166
Modifier 51 exempt codes, 134, 166, 442
Modifier 52, 173
Modifier 53, 173–174
Modifier 54–56, 163–164
Modifier 57, 157–158
Modifier 58, 158
Modifier 59, 166–168, 286, 288, 307
Modifier 62, 170, 332, 407–408
Modifier 63, 172, 388
Modifier 63 exempt codes, 138–139, 172, 388
Modifier 66, 170
Modifier 76, 158–159, 288
Modifier 77, 158–159, 288
Modifier 78, 159–160

Modifier 79, 160–161
Modifier 80, 169–170
Modifier 81, 169–170
Modifier 82, 169–170
Modifier 91, 159, 168, 431
Modifier E1–E4, 176f
Modifier TC, 162, 163, 287, 289
Modifying terms, 136
Mohs micrographic surgery, 318
Molar pregnancy, 83
Molecular Pathology, 429
Monitored anesthesia care (MAC), 255, 260, 461
Mouth, 367–368
MRI. *See* Magnetic resonance imaging
MRSA (methicillin-resistant *Staphylococcus
    aureus*), 56
Multiple Procedure Reduction rules, 138
Multiple procedures modifier (CPT modifier 51),
    165–166
Multiple procedures/services. *See also* Repeated
    procedures
  CPT coding of, 164–165, 306–307
    anesthesia, 257
    bilateral procedures, 164–165, 287
    distinct/"separate" procedures, 166–168,
      286, 288, 307
    medical services, 442
    modifiers for, 164–168
    and payment, 164, 422
    and "separate procedure" designation,
      135–136, 286, 307, 442, 443
Muscle, 12f
Musculoskeletal system, 12
  CPT coding for, 327–338
    by anatomical part, 327, 330–336
    anesthesia, 337–338, 338t
    general procedures, 329
    by procedure type, 327, 336–337
  ICD-9-CM coding for, 89–90
  medical terms related to, 13t
  procedure types and terminology, 327–328
Myelomeningocele, 408
Myocardial infarction, acute
  HCPCS coding of, 479
  ICD-9-CM coding of, 69, 70
Myometrium, 391
Myringotomy, 414

N

Nails, CPT coding for, 311–312
National Center for Health Statistics, 37
NEC (not elsewhere classifiable), 43, 45, 118
Neck, CPT coding of
  anesthesia, 264
  endovascular procedures, 404
  soft tissue, 330–331
Neck bones. *See* Cervical spine
Necrotizing infections, 310
Neonate. *See* Newborn
Neoplasm Table (ICD-9-CM), 38, 39, 57–58, 59
  excerpt, 58t
Neoplasms. *See also* Benign neoplasms; Malig-
    nant neoplasms; *specific sites and types*
  ICD-9-CM coding of, 57–59, 63, 65, 66
Nephrectomy, 384, 385
Nerve block, 309, 409–410

Nerve conduction studies, 139, 456
Nerve stimulators. *See* Neurostimulators
Nervous system, 21–22
  brain, 21, 21f
  central, 21
  CPT coding of, 139, 402–410, 455–456
    anesthesia, 416t
    autonomic nervous system, 409, 410
    cognitive function tests, 456
    extracranial nerves, 409
    intracranial, 402–405
    neurological tests, 455–456
    peripheral nerves, 409–410
    spine and spinal cord, 405–408
  ICD-9-CM coding of
    diseases, 65–66
    injuries, 94–95
  medical terms related to, 22t
  peripheral, 21, 409–410
  spinal cord, 21, 22f, 65f, 406f
Neuroendoscopy, 405
Neurological tests, 455–456
Neurolytic agent use, 410
Neuromuscular tests, 455–456
Neurophysiology services, intraoperative, 456
Neuroplasty, 2, 410
Neurostimulators, CPT coding of
  intracranial, 405
  peripheral nerve, 410
  spinal, 408
New patient, 191
  E/M coding for, 200
    domiciliary care services, 227, 227t
    home services, 228, 228t
    outpatient services, 211–212, 212t
    preventive medicine services, 234, 234t
Newborn
  CPT coding for
    critical care, 224, 238, 239–240
    delivery room attendance, 238, 239
    delivery room resuscitation, 238, 239
    E/M services, 238–240
    heart or great vessel anomaly repair, 350
    intensive care, 238, 240
    normal services, 238
    penile incisions, 388
  ICD-9-CM coding for, 92, 99–100
  less than 4kg, CPT modifier 63 for,
    138–139, 172
Newborn sepsis, 92
Newborn services, 238–239
Non-emergency transportation, HCPCS coding
    of, 474, 475
Non-surgeon services, 441
Nonessential modifiers (ICD-10-CM), 118
Nonphysician services
  CPT coding of, 441, 460, 461
  HCPCS coding of, 471, 477
Nonprofessional services, 477
Nonsegmental instrumentation, 333
Non–ST elevation myocardial infarction
    (NSTEMI), 69, 70
NOS (not otherwise specified), 43, 118
Nose, CPT coding for, 344, 359, 360t
Nuclear medicine, 285, 293
  CPT coding of, 287, 293–294
Nursing facility discharge services, 225, 226

Enhance your learning by completing these exercises
and more at mcgrawhillconnect.com!

INDEX   I-11

Nursing facility services
  CPT coding of, nonphysician, 461
  E/M coding of, 225–226
    annual assessment, 226, 226t
    care plan oversight, 232, 233, 236
    consultation, 220–221, 221t
    discharge, 226
    initial care, 225, 226t
    "other," 226, 226t
    subsequent care, 225, 226t
  HCPCS coding of, 483
Nursing services, 484
Nutrition management, 459
Nutritional diseases, 57–59

O

Oblique positions, 285, 287
Observation services. See Hospital observation
    services
Obstetric care. See Antepartum care; Delivery;
    Postpartum care; Pregnancy
Occipital bone, 403
Ocular adnexa, 413
Ocular devices, 449, 485
Ocular implant, 411, 412
Ocular prosthetic, 485
Ocular structure procedures, CPT coding of,
    411–413, 416t
Office of the Inspector General (OIG), 481
Office patient services. See Outpatient services
Omentum, 375, 376
Online medical evaluation, 236–237, 460
Open fracture, 328, 329
Open treatment, 327
Operating microscope, 370, 415
Ophthalmology procedures. See Ocular structure
    procedures
Ophthalmology services, 448–449
OPPS (outpatient prospective payment
    system), 477
Orbit, CPT coding of, 413
Orchiectomy, 388, 398
Orchiopexy, 389
Organ(s), 9
Organ/disease-oriented panels, 423–426,
    424t–425t
Organ harvesting. See also under specific organ
    anesthesia, 175, 259–260, 275
Organ system(s), 10, 11–24
    in physical examination, 198
Organ transplant. See also under specific organ
    backbench work for, 375
    CPT coding of, 351
    ICD-9-CM coding of, complications and
        rejections, 97
Orthotic(s), 481
Osteopathic manipulation, 460
Osteotomy, 332
"Other" code (ICD-9-CM), 45
Otorhinolaryngologic services, 449
Outpatient coding, ICD-9-CM, 39, 46–47
Outpatient equipment and supplies,
    hospital, 477
Outpatient prospective payment system
    (OPPS), 477

Outpatient services
  E/M coding of, 190, 211–213
    consultations, 219–220, 220t
    emergency department, 222–223, 222t, 239
    for established patient, 212–213, 212t
    for new patient, 211–212, 212t
    prolonged services, 229–230, 231
  HCPCS coding of, 477
  ICD-9-CM coding of, 39, 46–47
Ovary, 401
  CPT coding for, 391, 392
Oviducts, 391
Oxygenated blood, 15

P

P-codes (HCPCS), 482, 483
P modifiers (CPT), 175, 259–260
PA projection, 285, 287
Pacemaker, 347, 348f
  evaluation and programming, 451
  insertion/replacement, 347–348, 359
Pain, 65–66
Pain control, 65, 66
Palate
  cleft, 91f, 368
  CPT coding for, 368
Pancreas, 375, 401
Pancreatic transplant, 375
Pap smears, 432, 482, 483
Parasitic diseases, 55–56
Parathyroid glands, 401
Paravertebral facet, nerve procedures in,
    409, 410
Parent code, 134
Parenteral therapy. See Enteral and
    parenteral therapy
Parentheses
  in ICD-9-CM, 43, 44
  in ICD-10-CM, 118
Parenthetical notes, in CPT codes,
    134–135, 309
Parietal bone, 403
Paring, of skin lesions, 310
Parotid gland, 368
Partial mastectomy, 319
Partial thromboplastin time (PTT), 429
Past, family, and social history (PFSH), 197
Past medical history, 192, 197
Pathological fracture, ICD-9-CM coding of,
    89–90
Pathology services, 423. See also
    Laboratory tests
  CPT coding of, 423, 431–433
    anatomic pathology (autopsy), 431–432
    clinical pathology consultation, 428
    code list/sections, 423
    cytogenetic studies, 432
    cytopathologic tests, 432
    in vivo procedures, 433
    in Mohs micrographic surgery, 318
    reproductive medicine procedures, 433
    surgical pathology, 432–433
  HCPCS coding of, 482, 483
Patient-activated event recorder, 348. See also
    Cardiac recording device

Patient history, 195, 196–197
    elements of, 192–193, 196–197, 196t
    types of, 196, 196t, 201t
Patient self-management, education and
    training for, 460
Payers. See also Medicaid; Medicare
    and CPT, 131, 140, 472
    and global period, 155
    and HCPCS, 472
    and ICD-10-CM, 120
Payment
    and add-on codes, 138
    and anesthesia units, 257–262
    CPT modifiers affecting, 152, 154
    and "diagnosis to procedure code"
        relationships, 37
    for MAC, 255, 260
    and modifier 51 exempt codes (CPT), 138
    for multiple procedures/services on same day,
        164, 442
Payment modifiers (CPT), 152, 154
PCPI (Physician Consortium for Performance
    Improvement), 140
Pediatric patients. See Child; Infant; Newborn
Pelvic exenteration, 385
Pelvic floor defect, repair of, 391
Pelvis. See also Female genital/reproductive
        system; Male genital/reproductive system;
        Urinary system
    bony, anatomy of, 335f
    CPT coding for, 268, 290, 334–335, 385
Penetrating wound, 329
Penile revascularization, 357
Penis, 357, 388f
Peptic ulcer, 73f
Percutaneous needle biopsy, 309
Percutaneous skeletal fixation, 327
Performance measure percentage
        calculation, 141
Performance measurement exclusion modifiers
        (CPT Category II), 141–142
Performance measures, 140. See also
        Category II codes
Performance Measures Advisory Group
        (PMAG), 140
Pericardiocentesis, 347
Pericardium, 347
Perinatal period, 92. See also Newborn
    diagnosis coding for
        ICD-9-CM, 92
        ICD-10-CM, 116
Perineum, CPT coding for, 267–268, 390
Peripartum period, 86
Peripheral nerve block, 409
Peripheral nerve stimulators, 410
Peripheral nervous system, 21
    CPT coding for, 409–410
Peritoneum, 375
Peroneal artery, revascularization of, 357
PET. See Positron emission tomography
PFSH (past, family, and social history), 197
Pharynx, 369
Photodynamic therapy, 458
Physical examination, 193
    E/M coding of, 193, 195, 197–198
    types of, 198, 201t
Physical medicine and rehabilitation, 459

Physical status modifiers (CPT codes P1-P6), 175, 259–260, 262
Physician Consortium for Performance Improvement (PCPI), 140
Physician performance, HCPCS coding of, 479
Physician-provided supplies, CPT coding of, 443
Physician Quality Reporting Initiative (PQRI), 479
Physician standby services, 231
Physiology, 2, 9–24
Pick-up/destination modifiers (HCPCS), 475
Pilonidal cyst, 312
Pineal gland, 401
Pituitary gland, 401
Place of occurrence, E-codes (ICD-9-CM) for, 102
Place of service, 140
  CPT coding of, 140
  E/M coding of, 189–190, 195, 212
  HCPCS coding of, 486
Placeholder, 115, 118
Planes, anatomical. See Anatomical planes
Pleura, 346
PMAG (Performance Measures Advisory Group), 140
Pneumococcal vaccine, 479
Pneumonia, 56, 72, 97
Poisoning, ICD-9-CM coding of, 96
  E-codes, 100–102
  Table of Drugs and Chemicals in, 38, 102, 102t–103t
Popliteal artery, revascularization of, 357
Popliteal region, anesthesia in, 269
Portal decompression, 357
Portal hypertension, 357
Positions
  with directional terms, 10f
  for radiology services, 285–288
Positron emission tomography (PET), 285, 289, 289f
Posterior cranial fossa, 403
Posterior segment, 412
Posterior vertebral structure, 331
Posteroanterior (PA) projection, 285, 287
Postmortem examination, 431–432
Postoperative period. See Global period
Postoperative services/procedures
  CPT modifiers for, 154–161
  by different physician, 163, 164
  E/M, 155–156
  repeated
    by different provider, 158–159, 288
    by same provider, 158–159
  unplanned second, 159–160
  unrelated, by same surgeon, 160–161
Postpartum care, 392, 393
  CPT coding of, 393, 394
  ICD-9-CM coding of, 86, 99
Postpartum complications, 86
Postpartum period, 83, 85, 86
Postservice time, 194
PQRI (Physician Quality Reporting Initiative), 479
Prefixes, 5, 5t
Pregnancy
  care during (See Antepartum care)
  CPT coding in, 392–394

diabetes mellitus in, 85, 86
diagnosis coding in
  ICD-9-CM, 83–87, 99
  ICD-10-CM, 115, 116
ectopic, 83, 393
high-risk, 84
HIV infection in, 85
molar, 83
trimester specification in, 115
Premalignant lesions, skin and subcutaneous, 317
Prenatal care. See Antepartum care
Prenatal testing, 393
Prenatal visits, 84, 392
Preoperative services, by different physician, 163
Presenting problem, 192, 195
Preservice time, 194
Pressure (decubitus) ulcer, 88f
  CPT coding of, 316
  ICD-9-CM coding of, 88
  stages, 88
Preventive medicine services, 233
  comprehensive, 233
  E/M coding of, 233–235
    behavior change interventions, 235
    counseling, 233, 235
    established patient, 234, 235t
    new patient, 234, 234t
    unlisted services, 194
Primary malignant tumor, 57, 59
Principal diagnosis, 39
Problem-focused history, 196, 196t
Problem-focused physical examination, 198
Procedure(s)
  distinct/"separate," 166–168, 286, 288, 307
  global period for, 154, 155, 157, 160
  professional component of, 162
  repeated, 158–159, 288
  "separate," designation of, 135–136, 307, 442, 443
  staged, 158
  technical component of, 162
  unlisted, 132
  unplanned second, 159–160
Procedure codes and coding
  CPT (See CPT)
  HCPCS (See HCPCS)
  ICD-9-CM, Volume 3, 37, 41–42, 112, 121
  ICD-10-PCS, 112, 120–121
Procedure Coding System. See ICD-10-PCS
Proctectomy, 373
Proctosigmoidoscopy, 373
Professional component, 162
Professional component modifier. See Modifier 26
Projections (x-ray), 285, 287
Prolonged services, E/M coding of, 229–231
  add-on codes, 193, 195, 201, 223, 224t, 229–231
  critical care, 223, 224t
  face-to-face services, 229–230
  non-face-to-face services, 230, 231
  physician standby services, 231
Prone position, 285, 286
Prostate gland, 389f

Prostate procedures, 387, 389
Prosthetic(s)
  CPT coding of
    head, 330
    pelvis/hip joint, 335
  HCPCS coding of, 481
Prothrombin time (PT), 429
Proton beam treatment delivery, 293
Psychiatric services
  CPT coding of, 446–447
  HCPCS coding of, 479
Psychotherapy, 446, 447
PT. See Prothrombin time
PTT. See Partial thromboplastin time
Puerperium, 83. See also Postpartum period
  HIV infection in, 85
Pulmonary artery. See also Great vessels
  catheterization of, 356
Pulmonary medicine, 454
Pulmonary valve, 348
Pulmonary vein. See Great vessels
Pump oxygenator, 359
Punctuation
  in ICD-9-CM, 43
  in ICD-10-CM, 118

Q

Q-codes (HCPCS), 290, 483
Qualifying circumstances add-on codes, 261, 262, 460
Qualitative test, 426, 427
Quality measures. See Performance measures
Quantitative test, 426, 427

R

R-codes (HCPCS), 483
Radiation oncology, 285
  CPT coding of, 292–293
    for intracranial lesion/tumor, 404–405
    for spinal/spinal cord lesion, 408
    stereotactic radiosurgery, 404–405, 408
  ICD-9-CM coding of, 59
  stages of therapy, 292–293
Radiation therapy. See Radiation oncology
Radiation treatment delivery, 293
Radiation treatment management, 293
Radical mastectomy, 319–320
Radical resection, of tumor/lesion, 328, 331, 333
Radiologic guidance, CPT coding of, 291–292
  in endovascular repairs, 351, 353
  in nerve block, 309, 409
  in percutaneous needle biopsies, 309
  in spinal injection, drainage, and aspiration, 406
  in ultrasound, 291
Radiologic imaging agents. See Contrast material
"Radiological supervision and interpretation," 286, 288
Radiology, 285
Radiology codes (CPT)
  sections/general categories, 288
  unlisted, 287
Radiology modifiers (HCPCS), 486

Radiology services, 285. *See also specific types*
 anatomical planes, 9–10, 10*f*, 285, 288
 CPT coding of, 286–294
  anesthesia, 273
  bilateral procedures, 287
  bone and joint studies, 292
  in combination with other procedures, 286, 290, 309
  with contrast material, 286, 289, 290
  mammography, 292, 486
  modifiers in, 162, 163, 287–288
  professional components, 162, 163, 286, 287, 289
  repeated procedures, 288
  sections/general categories, 288
  "separate procedures," 286, 288
  technical components, 162, 163, 287
  unlisted procedures/codes, 287
 HCPCS coding of, 287, 290, 292, 483, 486
 modifiers used with
  CPT, 287–288
  HCPCS, 287, 486
 non-CPT coding of, 292
 positions, 285–288
 projections, 285, 287
Radiopharmaceuticals, 293, 294, 476, 477
RBCs. *See* Red blood cells
Rectocele, 391
Rectum, 371
Red background (ICD-9-CM), 44
Red blood cells (RBCs), 24, 24*f*, 429
Red brackets (ICD-9-CM), 43
Red code (ICD-9-CM), 44
Red parentheses (ICD-9-CM), 44
Refractive state, 448, 449
Regional anesthesia, 172, 255
Rehabilitation services, 459
Relative Value Guide (American Society of Anesthesiologists), 262
Remote medical direction, 222–223, 239
Renal calculus, 384
Repeated procedures, CPT coding of
 different provider (modifier 77), 158–159
 laboratory test (modifier 91), 159, 168, 431
 same provider (modifier 76), 158–159, 288
Reporting modifier, 141, 142
Reproductive system, 20, 20*f*. *See also* Female genital/reproductive system; Male genital/reproductive system
 CPT coding for
  in vitro fertilization, 392, 433
  laboratory services, 433
  non-sex-specific procedures, 389
 medical terms related to, 21*t*
Resident physicians, 169, 260
Respiratory failure, acute, ICD-9-CM coding of, 71
Respiratory system, 17, 17*f*
 components of, 344
 CPT coding for, 344–346, 359, 360*t*
 ICD-9-CM coding for, 70–72
 medical terms related to, 18*t*
Respiratory tract, lower, 17*f*
Rest home care services. *See* Domiciliary care services
Resuscitation, of newborn, 238, 239
Retina, 412, 449

Revascularization, 347, 357
Review of systems (ROS), 193, 197
Revised codes (CPT), 138
Right lateral decubitus position, 285, 287
Risk factor reduction counseling, 233, 235
Root word(s), 2, 3*t*–4*t*
ROS (review of systems), 193
Rotator cuff muscles, 334*f*
Rule of Nines, 95, 96*f*, 316, 317*f*

S

S-codes (HCPCS), 483–484
Sagittal plane, 9–10, 285, 288
Salivary glands and ducts, 368
Salpingectomy, 391
Salpingo-oophorectomy, 391
Saphenous vein harvesting, 349, 353
Screening V-codes (ICD-9-CM), 99
Second-order vessels, 355
Secondary diabetes mellitus, 61–62
Secondary diagnosis, 39
Secondary malignant tumor, 57, 59
Sedation, moderate. *See* Moderate sedation
"See also" instruction (ICD-9-CM), 45
"See" instruction (ICD-9-CM), 45
Segmental instrumentation, 333
Self-management, by patient, 460
Semicolon, 133, 134
Seminal vesicle, 389
Sense organ diseases, 65–66
Separate procedure(s), 135
 code designation as, 135–136, 286, 307, 442, 443
 and CPT modifier 59, 166–168, 286, 288, 307
Sepsis, ICD-9-CM coding of, 56, 92, 96
Septic shock, 56
Septicemia, 56
Sequelae, 115
Seton placement, 373–374
Severe sepsis, ICD-9-CM coding of, 56, 92, 96
Sex conflict edits (ICD-9-CM), 44
Shaving, of skin lesions, 311
Shoulder, 333, 334*f*
 CPT coding of, 270–271, 333–334
Shoulder girdle, anesthesia in, 264–265
Shunt, 348
Shunt insertion/placement, CPT coding of
 CSF shunt, 405, 408
 for extracorporeal circulation, 348
Sickle cell anemia, 63*f*
Sigmoidoscopy, 373
Signs, 45
 ICD-9-CM coding of, 45, 46, 93
 ICD-10-CM coding of, 119, 120
Simple wound repair, CPT coding of, 313, 314
Sinuses, CPT coding of, 344–345, 359, 360*t*
SIRS. *See* Systemic inflammatory response syndrome
Skeletal muscle, 12*f*
Skeletal system, 12*f*. *See also* Musculoskeletal system
Skilled nursing facility services. *See* Nursing facility services
Skin. *See also* Integumentary system

structure of, 11*f*, 88*f*
Skin and subcutaneous lesions
 benign, 317–318
 calculation of total diameter, 312
 CPT coding for, 311
  biopsy, 310
  destruction, 317–318
  excision, 311, 312, 318
  Mohs micrographic surgery, 318
  photodynamic therapy, 458
  shaving, 311
 malignant, 311, 318, 458
 premalignant, 317
Skin graft, 315–316
Skin repair, CPT coding of, 315–316
 in burns, 273–274, 316, 317*f*
Skin replacement surgery, 315–316
Skin substitutes, 315–316
Skin tag removal, 310
Skull
 bones of, 263*f*, 402*f*, 403
 CPT coding of, 330, 402–405, 416*t*
Skull base, CPT coding for, 403–404
Small intestine, 371
Social history, 193, 197
Soft tissue tumors. *See also* Skin and subcutaneous lesions
 excision of, 328
Somatic nerves, 409, 410
Special report, 194
Specimen, 429, 433
Speech-language pathology services
 CPT coding of, 449
 HCPCS coding of, 485
Spermatic cord, 389
Sphenoid sinus, 346
Spinal cord, 21. *See also* Spine
 cross section, 65*f*
 nerves, 406*f*
 regions, 22*f*
Spinal deformity, correction of, 332
Spinal instrumentation, CPT coding of, 332–333
Spinal lesions, 408
Spinal nerves, 406*f*
 paravertebral, CPT coding for, 409, 410
Spinal neurostimulator implant, 408
Spinal puncture, 406
Spine. *See also* Spinal cord
 CPT coding for, 405–408
  anesthesia, 266, 416*t*
  and approach, 407
  arthrodesis, 332
  aspiration, 406
  catheter implantation, 407
  code subsections/list, 405–406
  CSF shunt, 405, 408
  drainage, 406
  excisions, vertebral, 331
  injections, 406–407, 409, 410
  and level of spine, 407
  multiple surgeons, modifiers for, 332–333, 407–408
  nerve block, 409
  nerve destruction, 410
  neurostimulator implant, 408
  osteotomy, 332

repair, 408
spinal instrumentation, 332–333
stereotaxis and stereotactic
radiosurgery, 408
vertebral column, 331–333
nerves of, 406f
vertebral column of, 266f
Spleen, 358
Splint, 336
application of, 336
supplies for, 483
ST-elevation myocardial infarction (STEMI),
69, 70
Staged procedures, 158
Standing position, 285, 286
Status asthmaticus, 71
Status codes (V-codes) (ICD-9-CM), 99
Stem cells, preparation of, 358
Stereotactic assistance, in intracranial
procedures, 404
Stereotactic radiosurgery, CPT coding of
for intracranial lesions, 404–405
for spinal and spinal cord lesions, 408
Stereotaxis procedures, CPT coding of
intracranial, 404
spinal and spinal cord, 408
Stomach, CPT coding for, 371
Stomach ulcer, bleeding, 371f
Strapping, 336
Stroke, 69
Subcutaneous, definition of, 328
Subcutaneous tissue, 11f. See also Integumentary
system
Subcutaneous tumors, 328. See also Skin and
subcutaneous lesions
Subfascial tumors, 328
Subsequent encounter, 115
Subsequent nursing facility care, 225, 226t
Suffixes, 6, 6t
Supine position, 285, 286
Supplemental classifications (ICD-9-CM),
40, 47
Supplementary Classification of External Causes
of Injury and Poisoning (E-codes). See
E-codes (ICD-9-CM)
Supplementary Classification of Factors Influ-
encing Health Status and Contact with
Health Services (V-codes). See V-codes
(ICD-9-CM)
Supratentorial, definition of, 404
Supraventricular dysrhythmias, excision proce-
dures for, 348
Surgical codes (CPT), 306, 307
listed by section, 132, 307t
Surgical implant, pain from, 66
Surgical pathology, 432–433
Surgical pathology consultation, 433
Surgical procedure(s), 306
with additional providers, 169–170
anesthesia (See Anesthesia)
bilateral, 164–165
components of, 163
CPT coding of, 132–133, 306–307, 307t (See
also specific anatomic parts and
procedures)
CPT modifiers for (See CPT modifiers)
decision to perform, 157–158

distinct/"separate," 166–168, 307
emergency, anesthesia for, 261
follow-up care, 154–161, 306
global period for, 154, 157
HCPCS anatomical modifiers for, 167,
176–177, 485
involving more or less work than is typical,
171–174
multiple, 164–168, 306–307
on newborn/infant less than 4kg, 138–139,
172, 388
by non-surgeon, 441
non-surgical services covered by, 306
repeated, 158–159
and "separate procedure" designation,
135–136, 307, 442, 443
staged, 158
terminated after induction of anesthesia,
173–174
unplanned second, 159–160
Surgical team, 170
Surgical thoracoscopy, 346
Surgical wounds, 94
Suture repairs, of great vessels, 348
Swine flu, 71–72
Symbols
to avoid in medical documentation, 8t
in CPT manual, 134, 140
in ICD-9-CM, 44
Symptoms, 45
ICD-9-CM coding of, 45, 46, 93
ICD-10-CM coding of, 119, 120
Syndromes, 119
System(s), 10, 11–24. See also specific
systems
in physical examination, 198
Systemic inflammatory response syndrome
(SIRS), ICD-9-CM coding of,
56, 96–97

T

T-codes (HCPCS), 484
Table of Drugs (HCPCS), 472, 480, 486
Table of drugs and chemicals, 39
Table of Drugs and Chemicals (ICD-9-CM), 38,
102
excerpt, 102t–103t
Tabular List and Alphabetic List for Procedure
Codes (Volume 3, ICD-9-CM), 37, 38,
41–42
conversion to ICD-9-PCS, 112, 121
Tabular List of Codes (ICD-10-CM), 116,
118, 119
Tabular List of Diseases (Volume 1, ICD-9-CM),
37, 38, 40–41, 45
in E-code selection, 101
organization of, 40–41, 40t
sample entries, 41f
Tabular list of services (HCPCS), 472
Technical component modifier (modifier TC),
162, 163, 287
Technology, emerging, 143
Telephone services, 236–237, 460
Temporal bone, 403, 415
Temporary codes

Category III (CPT), 131, 132, 143, 473
G-codes (HCPCS), 478–479
K-codes (HCPCS), 480
Q-codes (HCPCS), 483
S-codes (HCPCS), 483–484
Temporary national codes (HCPCS S-codes),
483–484
Temporomandibular joint, 330
Tenotomy, 335
Terminology, medical. See Medical
terminology
Terrorism, 102
Testis (testicle), 388–389, 401
Therapeutic drug assay, 427
Therapeutic level, 427
Third-order vessels, 355
Thoracic aorta, descending, repair of, 351
Thoracic spine, 331
Thoracoscopy, 346
Thorax. See also Cardiovascular system;
Respiratory system
CPT coding for
anesthesia, 264–265, 359, 360t, 377
diaphragm, 358
mediastinum, 358
musculoskeletal procedures, 330–331
Throat, 369
Thrombectomy, CPT coding of, 352
from heart, 348
percutaneous transluminal coronary, 450
Thromboendarterectomy, 353
Thymus, 401
Thyroid, 401, 401f
CPT coding for, 401, 402, 416t
Thyroidectomy, 401, 402
Tibia, 336
Tibial artery, revascularization of, 357
Time, in CPT coding
of anesthesia, 258–259, 262
of physician standby services, 231
of prolonged services, 193, 195, 201, 223,
224t, 229–231
Time units (anesthesia), 258–259, 262
Tissue flap, 316
Tissue graft. See also Bone graft;
Vascular graft
CPT coding of
in larynx, 345
in nerves, 410
non-anatomically specific, 329
skin, 315–316
Tissue specimen examination, 432–433
Toe, 336
Tomogram, 285, 288
Tomography, computed. See Computed
tomography
Tongue, 368
Tonsils, 369
Total body surface area (TBSA), 273,
274, 316
Toxic effects, 96
Toxoid administration. See Vaccination
Toxoids, 445
Trachea, 17f, 345
CPT coding for, 345–346, 359
Traction, 328
Transcatheter procedures, 357

connect plus+
Enhance your learning by completing these exercises
and more at mcgrawhillconnect.com!
INDEX   I-15

Transfer of care, 191, 219, 239
Transforaminal epidural injections, 409
Transfusion services, 430
Transluminal angioplasty, 353, 354
Transluminal atherectomy, 353, 354
Transmyocardial revascularization, 347
Transportation
    emergency, 474–475
    interfacility, critical care of infant in, 239
    non-emergency, 474, 475
Transportation codes (HCPCS),
        474–475
Transurethral resection of the prostate
        (TURP), 387
Transverse plane, 10, 285, 288
Traumatic fracture, 95
Treatment
    initial, 115
    open, 327
Treatment complications. *See* Complications
        of care
Treatment simulation, 292
Tricuspid valve, 348
Trigger point injections, 329, 409
Trimester specification, 115
Tubal ligation, 391
Tubuloalveolar glands, 389*f*
Tumor/lesion destruction, CPT coding of
    in abdomen, 375, 376
    in anus, 374
    intracranial, 404–405
    in penis, 388
    in rectum, 373
    in skin and subcutaneous tissue,
        317–318
    in spine and spinal cord, 408
    stereotactic radiosurgery for, 404–405, 408
Tumor/lesion excision
    CPT coding of, 328
        in abdomen, 333, 375, 376
        in back and flank (soft tissue), 331
        in bladder, 385
        in breast, 319–320
        in face and scalp, 330
        in heart, 347
        in neck (soft tissue) and thorax, 330–331
        in shoulder, 333
        skin and subcutaneous, 311, 312
        subfascial *vs.* subcutaneous, 328
    ICD-9-CM coding of, 59
Tumors. *See* Neoplasms; *specific sites and types*
Tunica vaginalis, 389
Turbinate, 344
TURP. *See* Transurethral resection of the prostate
Tympanoplasty, 414–415
Tympanostomy, 414
Type I diabetes mellitus, 60, 61
Type II diabetes mellitus, 60, 61

U

UB-04 claim form, 477
Ulcer
    bleeding, 73*f*, 371*f*
    pressure (decubitus) (*See*
        Pressure ulcer)

Ultrasound, 285
    CPT coding of
        cardiac, 452
        diagnostic, 289, 290–291
        intravascular, 357
        unlisted procedures, 287
Ultrasound guidance, 291
Unit of service (HCPCS), 472
Unlisted procedure/service (CPT), 132
    E/M, 194, 211
    medical, 443
    preventive medicine, 194
    radiology, 287
"Unspecified" code (ICD-9-CM), 45
Update notations (ICD-9-CM), 44
Ureter, CPT coding for, 384–387
Ureteral stent, CPT coding of
    placement, 384–385, 386–387
    removal, 384
Urethra, 384
Urinalysis, 428, 482
Urinary system, 19, 19*f*
    components of, 384
    CPT coding for, 384–387
        anesthesia, 395
        bladder, 385–387
        kidneys, 384–385
        ureter, 384–385, 386–387
        urethra, 387
    ICD-9-CM coding of, 74
    male *vs.* female, 384
    medical terms related to, 20*t*
Urodynamic measurement procedures,
        385, 386
"Use additional code" instruction
        (ICD-9-CM), 43
Uterus, 391
Uvula, 368

V

V-codes (HCPCS), 485
V-codes (ICD-9-CM), 40, 47, 98–100
    groupings, 98–99
    for obstetric care, 84, 85, 99
    uses of, 98, 99–100
Vaccination
    CPT coding of, 444–445
    HCPCS coding of, 479
    ICD-9-CM coding of, 99
Vaccine(s), CPT codes for, 445
    not-yet-approved vaccines, 139, 445
    update of, 132
Vagina, 391
Vaginal delivery, 393, 394
Vaginal delivery after cesarean section
        (VBAC), 394
Vaginal specimen tests, 432, 482. *See also*
        Pap smears
Vas deferens, 389
Vascular graft, CPT coding of, 349, 350,
        352–353, 354
Vascular injections (catheterization), 354–356
Vascular injuries, 94–95
Vascular lesions, destruction of, 317–318
Vascular studies, noninvasive, 454

Vascular system. *See also* Venous system; *specific*
        arteries and veins
    anatomy of, 355
    arterial, 13, 15, 15*f*, 67*f*, 355
    CPT coding for, 352–357
        anesthesia, 359, 360*t*
        aneurysm repair, 352–353, 404
        bypass graft, 349, 350, 354
        catheterization, 354–356
        on coronary vessels, 450, 451
        embolectomy, 352
        endovascular repairs, 351, 352–353
        endovascular revascularization, 357
        exploration, repair, revision, or
            excision, 354
        extracorporeal circulation, 357
        fistula repair, 353
        graft repair, revision, or excision, 354
        hemodialysis, 357
        intracranial and extracranial
            arteries, 404
        intravascular ultrasound, 357
        ligation, 357
        location in manual, 139
        portal decompression, 357
        studies, 454
        thrombectomy, 348, 352, 450
        thromboendarterectomy, 353
        transcatheter, 357
        transluminal angioplasty, 353, 354
        transluminal atherectomy, 353, 354
        vein harvesting, 349, 350, 354
        venous reconstruction, 352
    ICD-9-CM coding of, 94–95
VBAC procedures, 394
Veins. *See* Venous system; *specific veins*
Vena cava. *See also* Great vessels
    catheterization of, 355, 356
Venous catheterization, 356
Venous graft, 349, 350, 354
Venous reconstruction, 352
Venous system, 13, 15, 15*f*, 355. *See also*
        Vascular system
    CPT coding for, 352
        catheterization, 356
        location in manual, 139
        reconstruction, 352
        thrombectomy, 352
        venous graft, 349, 350, 354
Ventilator-associated pneumonia, 97
Ventilator management, 454
Vertebral column, 266*f*
    CPT coding for, 331–333
Vessels, great. *See* Great vessels
Vestibule of mouth, 367–368
Vision services and devices, HCPCS
        coding of, 485
Visit, 46
Vowel, combining, 2, 5
Vulva, 390

W

Well visits. *See* Preventive medicine services
Wheelchairs, 480, 481
White blood cells (WBCs), 24, 429

Word(s), root, 2, 3*t*–4*t*
Word elements, 2–6, 7
World Health Organization (WHO)
   and ICD-9, 37
   and ICD-10, 112
Wound. *See also* Injuries
   penetrating, 329
   surgical, 94
Wound exploration, 329
Wound repair (closure), 313

   CPT coding of, 313–314
      in adjacent tissue transfer, 315
      heart and great vessels, 348
      ocular (eyeball), 412
      skin and subcutaneous tissue
         excisions, 311
   levels of, 313
   and wound length, 313, 314
Wrist, 272, 334

X

X-ray film, 285, 289*f*
X-ray system
   digital, 285
   HCPCS coding of, 483
X-rays, 285, 289. *See also* Radiology services
Xenografts, 316

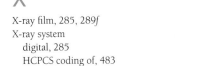

Enhance your learning by completing these exercises
and more at mcgrawhillconnect.com!

INDEX   I-17